Imaging of PAIN

Imaging of PAIN

STEVEN D. WALDMAN, MD, JD
Clinical Professor of Anesthesiology
University of Missouri-Kansas City School of Medicine
Kansas City, Missouri, United States

ROBERT S. D. CAMPBELL, FRCR
Consultant Musculoskeletal Radiologist
Department of Radiology
Royal Liverpool University Hospital
Liverpool, United Kingdom

SAUNDERS
ELSEVIER

SAUNDERS
ELSEVIER

1600 John F. Kennedy Blvd.
Ste 1800
Philadelphia, PA 19103-2899

IMAGING OF PAIN
ISBN: 978-1-4377-0906-3

Library of Congress Cataloging-in-Publication Data

Waldman, Steven D.
Imaging of pain / Steven D. Waldman, Robert S.D. Campbell. – 1st ed.
p. ; cm.
ISBN 978-1-4377-0906-3
1. Pain–Imaging. I. Campbell, Robert S. D., 1961- II. Title.
[DNLM: 1. Pain–diagnosis. 2. Diagnostic Imaging–methods. WL 704 W164i 2010]
RB127.W3483 2010
616'.0472–dc22

2010012846

Acquisitions Editor: Pamela Hetherington
Developmental Editor: Julia Bartz
Project Manager: Vijay Antony Raj Vincent / David Saltzberg
Design Direction: Ellen Zanolle
Publishing Services Manager: Radhika Pallamparthy

Printed in China

Last digit is the print number: 9 8 7 6 5 4 3 2 1

For my wife, Maggie, and my children,
Alex and Sarah. I thank them for all their
generous support and tolerance.

RC

In loving memory of David Waldman
1909-2009

SDW

CONTRIBUTORS

Assistant Editor

Andrew Dunn, FRCR
Consultant Musculoskeletal Radiologist
Royal Liverpool University Hospital
Liverpool, United Kingdom

Contributing Authors

Hifz-ur-Rahman Aniq, MBBS, FRCR
Consultant Radiologist
Royal Liverpool University Hospital
Prescott Street
Liverpool, United Kingdom

Kumar S. V. Das, MRCP, DMRD, FRCR
Consultant Neuroradiologist
Neuroradiology Department
The Walton Centre
Lower Lane
Fazakerley, United Kingdom

Andrew J. Grainger, MRCP, FRCR
Consultant Musculoskeletal Radiologist
Leeds Teaching Hospitals
Chapel Allerton Orthopaedic Centre
Leeds, United Kingdom

Theodore T. Miller, MD, FACR
Attending Radiologist
Hospital for Special Surgery
Professor of Radiology
Weill Medical College of Cornell University
New York, New York

James J. Rankine, MD
Consultant Radiologist
Leeds Teaching Hospitals
Leeds, United Kingdom

PREFACE

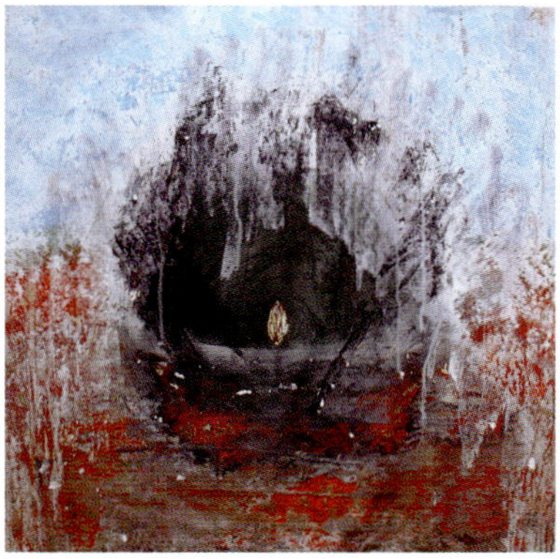

Figure P1 Pool of darkness. Copyright Julie Meese.

It is really hard to know who wants a picture of pain more ... the patient in pain or the physician treating the patient's pain. Efforts to measure, quantify, or take a picture of pain are nothing new. For a brief time in 1895, it seemed that Wilhelm Roentgen had in fact discovered a way to take a picture of pain. But it did not take long for physicians to figure out that it was only a picture of a hand!

Fast forward 100 years, and where are we? Articles in both the lay press and scientific literature suggest that functional MRI and diffusion tensor imaging can now show the physician and patient alike a picture of pain. But are these highly sophisticated imaging modalities, in fact, showing us a picture of pain any more than the x-ray of Roentgen's hand did? Well, at one level the answer must be a loud and emphatic yes, but at another level, the answer unfortunately remains an embarrassed and barely audible no.

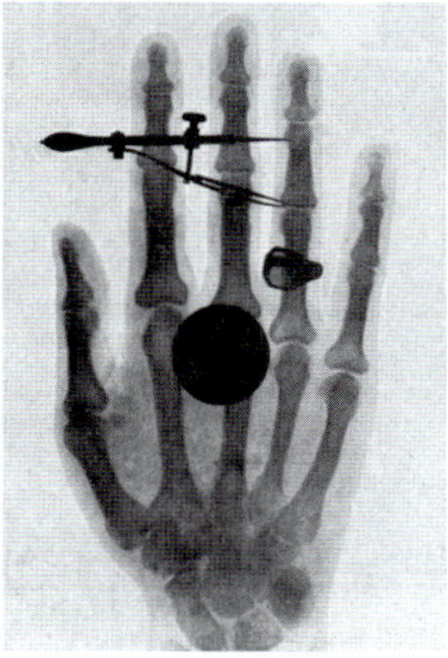

Figure P2 Wilhelm Roentgen's X-ray photograph of his wife's hand.

At this point in our discussion, it is probably time to ask the obvious. If you can't take a picture of pain, why bother to write a book about taking a picture of pain? This is a very good question that I will try to briefly answer. The short answer is: See the first sentence of this Preface. The slightly longer answer is that like every other physician who treats patients in pain, I want to see a picture of my patient's pain with an eye (pardon the pun) to treating it. Like those physicians who came before me, I want something tangible to exterminate or extirpate. When I see a patient in pain, I immediately want to search out the pain and get rid of it. The harder it is for me to "find" the patient's pain, the harder I want to look for it. Hence, the desire to image the patient's pain and to write a book to aid others on a similar quest.

Throughout this text, Rob Campbell and I have tried to put together pictures of what we believe a number of common and sometimes not so common pain syndromes look like. We have endeavored to guide the reader in choosing the best and, whenever possible, least invasive imaging modalities to aid in diagnosing the condition causing the patient's pain. Since, in a clinical situation many painful conditions can mimic one another, we have provided the reader with a comprehensive differential diagnosis, with an emphasis on how appropriate imaging can often help the clinician avoid going down the wrong diagnostic path. We have purposefully avoided discussing the cost of "taking a picture of pain," because both of Rob and I are thoroughly convinced that the cost of undiagnosed or improperly diagnosed pain (in terms of both patient suffering and cost to society) far exceed the cost of an x-ray, CT, or MRI. Rob has worked tirelessly to accumulate the excellent images in this book that are illustrative of the painful conditions presented. Our editors at Elsevier have designed an easily readable text with the images laid out for ready reference by the reader. We both hope this text helps you in your efforts to treat pain and expands your differential diagnosis of some of the less commonly encountered painful conditions we have presented.

Steven D. Waldman M.D.

CONTENTS

PART 1 • IMAGING MODALITIES USED IN THE DIAGNOSIS OF PAIN

PART 2 • SPINE

THE CERVICAL SPINE

THE THORACIC SPINE

THE LUMBAR SPINE

PELVIC, HIP, AND LOWER EXTREMITY PAIN SYNDROMES

THE KNEE

THE ANKLE AND FOOT

PART 1 • IMAGING MODALITIES USED IN THE DIAGNOSIS OF PAIN

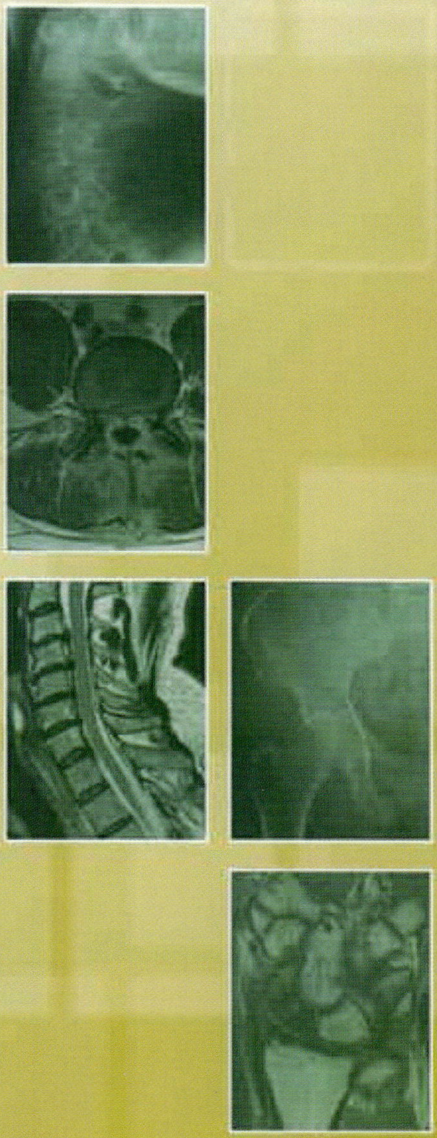

CHAPTER 1

Radiography

CONCEPT

- Radiography uses ionizing radiation of the x-ray variety, which is directed in a beam from an x-ray source over the anatomic area of interest.
- The x-ray beam is detected on a film or screen cassette (conventional radiography) or a bank of thermoluminescent detectors (digital radiography).
- The resulting image is called a *radiograph*.
- Either technique results in a gray-scale image. The density of a tissue is proportional to the degree to which that tissue attenuates the x-ray beam, and thus, to how bright that tissue appears on the resulting "x-ray" image.
- Typical densities (from low to high) that can be visualized on a radiograph are:
  - Air.
  - Fat.
  - Water/soft tissue.
  - Calcium and bone.
  - Metal.

CLINICAL PRACTICE

- Radiography produces high-resolution two-dimensional images and provides a rapid and low-cost means of assessing bone and joint disease and soft tissue calcification.
- Radiography remains the first-line investigation for suspected bone pathology, before other imaging modalities such as MRI or CT.
- Radiography is also a relatively accurate means of evaluating orthopaedic hardware and its relationship to bone.
- Radiography is also of use in areas of high contrast between soft tissue and low density gas, such as the lungs and the gas-filled bowel. However, the intrinsic soft tissue contrast of radiography is very limited.

LIMITATIONS

- The poor soft tissue contrast of radiography limits its use in assessment of soft tissue pathology.
- This modality is unable to demonstrate cartilaginous structures unless they have become calcified.
- Radiography has a limited role in lumbar spine pathology and delivers a significant radiation exposure.

COMMON MUSCULOSKELETAL INDICATIONS

- Acute skeletal trauma.
- Bone pain.
- Follow-up of fracture fixation (including spinal fixation).
- Assessment of arthritis.
- Follow-up of arthroplasty.
- Suspected bone and joint infection.
- Diagnosis of bone tumors.
- Soft tissue calcification.

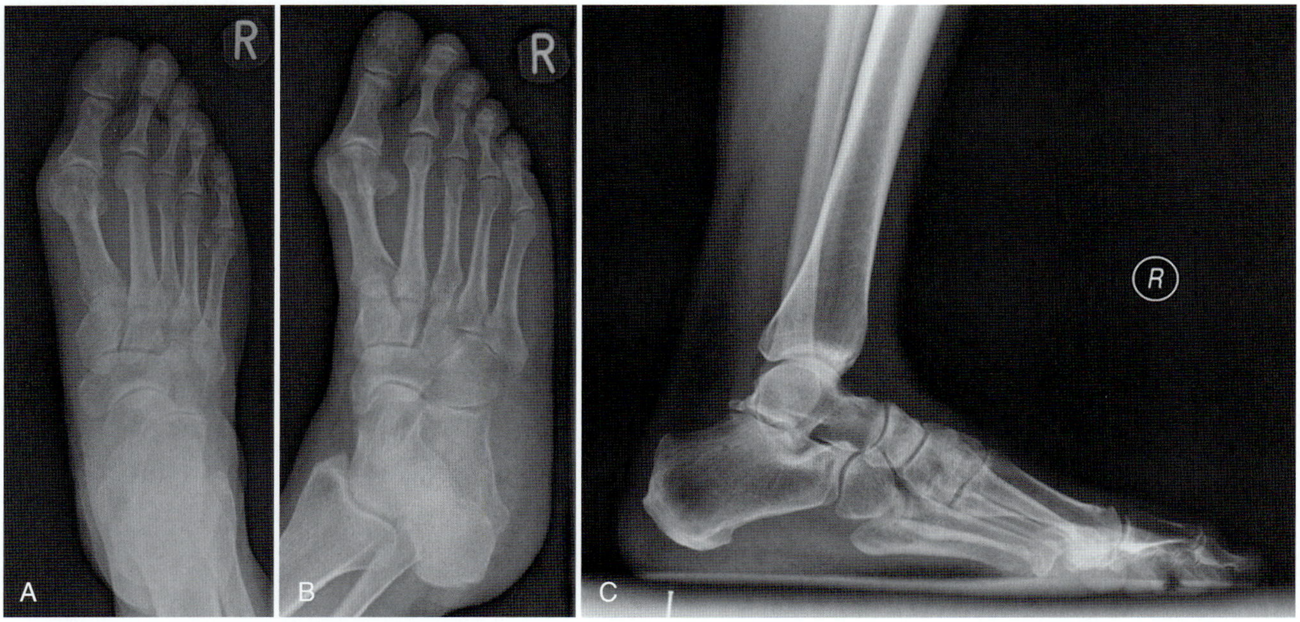

Figure 1.1 AP (**A**), oblique (**B**), and lateral (**C**) radiographs of the foot. It is important to obtain at least two views in all radiographic examinations of the extremities, and these should be performed according to clinical indications. For example, the AP and oblique views are useful to demonstrate joint pathology, and the midfoot joints are fully visualized only through evaluation of both AP and oblique views. The lateral view is useful in orthopaedics for evaluating the plantar arch and foot deformities.

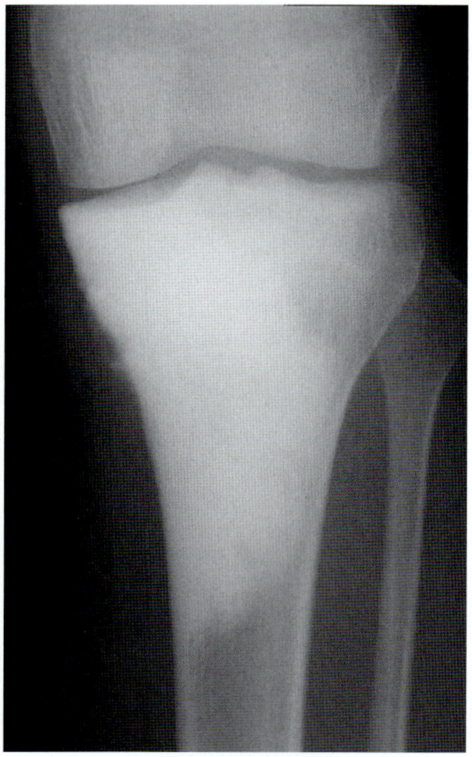

Figure 1.2 Radiograph of a young man with lower leg pain. There is a densely sclerotic lesion in the proximal tibia, which is typical of a conventional osteosarcoma. Radiography remains the primary investigation for most cases of unexplained bone pain.

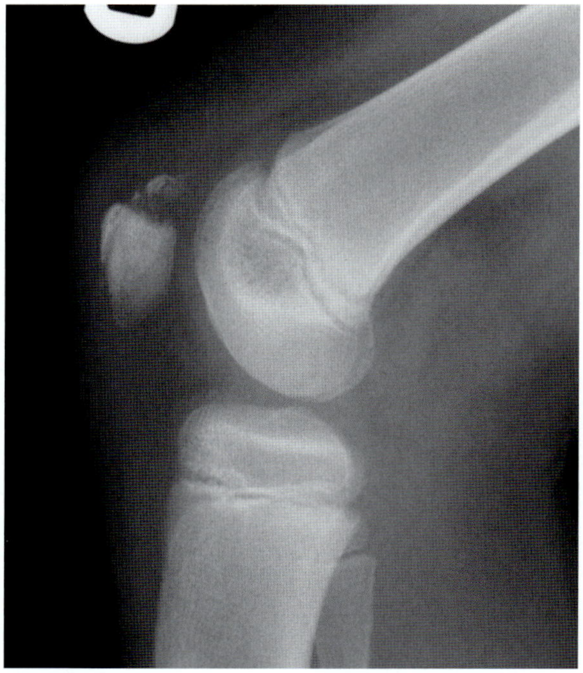

Figure 1.3 Radiograph of a young man with insertional tendinopathy of the quadriceps insertion on the patella. There is marked bony fragmentation. Radiographs are very useful for identifying early new bone formation at entheses.

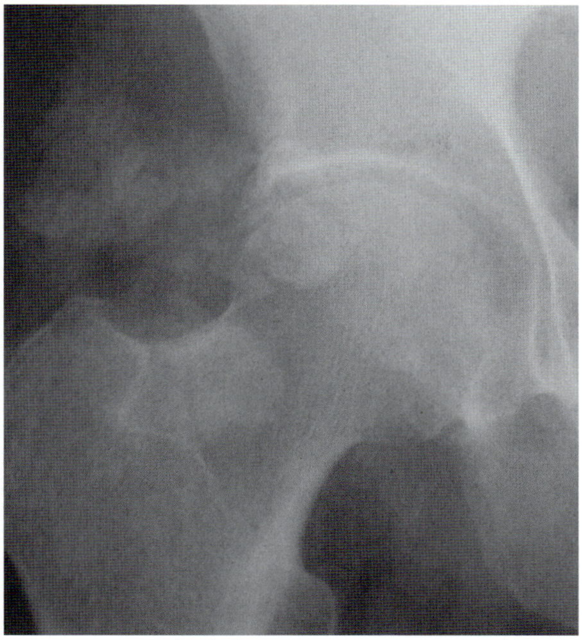

Figure 1.4 Periarticular tumoral calcinosis in the soft tissues around the hip joint in a patient with renal osteodystrophy. Radiographs can be very helpful in characterizing soft tissue calcifications. Early calcification can easily be missed on MRI.

CHAPTER 2

Fluoroscopy

CONCEPT

- Fluoroscopy uses a mobile x-ray source that produces x-rays continuously or in short pulses.
- The x-ray beam is focused on the patient in a relatively small field of view and is detected by a device called an *image intensifier*, which projects the resulting image on a monitor as a real-time image.
- The x-ray source is usually positioned over a patient table and may be fitted to a multiplanar mobile device, called a *C-arm*, or to a unit that is mobile in two directions, called an *over-couch unit*.
- Conventional x-ray exposures can be taken at any point during fluoroscopy to give a "snapshot" of the examination.
- Radiopaque contrast agents are often administered during fluoroscopy to acquire anatomic and functional information. Examples are angiography using an intra-arterial contrast agent and arthrography using an intra-articular contrast agent.
- During angiography, the structures in the background of the image, such as bones, may obscure visualization of vessels; these structures can be removed from the image in a process known as *digital subtraction*.
- Modern fluoroscopy units can acquire and store real-time video clips of fluoroscopic examinations that can be stored and reviewed on a *picture archive and communication system* (PACS).

CLINICAL PRACTICE

- A common clinical indication for fluoroscopy is angiography, which may be diagnostic or therapeutic as in the case of angioplasty.
- Interventional urologic procedures, such as nephrostomy and ureteric stenting, are another common application of fluoroscopy.
- Musculoskeletal (MSK) fluoroscopic procedures include image-guided spine and image-guided joint injections (such as of the hip and subtalar joints) as well as arthrography.

LIMITATIONS

- There are very few limitations to fluoroscopy.
- The patient must be able to lie flat, either prone or supine depending on the procedure.
- Obesity results in decreased image quality and may impair visualization of needles, contrast agent, etc.

COMMON MUSCULOSKELETAL INDICATIONS

- Arthrography (usually combined with CT/MRI).
- Selective lumbar and cervical nerve root blocks.
- Image-guided facet joint injection and medial branch block.
- Lumbar puncture and epidural injections in which non-guided needle location is difficult.
- Image-guided diagnostic and therapeutic joint injection (e.g., hip, subtalar joints).
- Vertebroplasty.

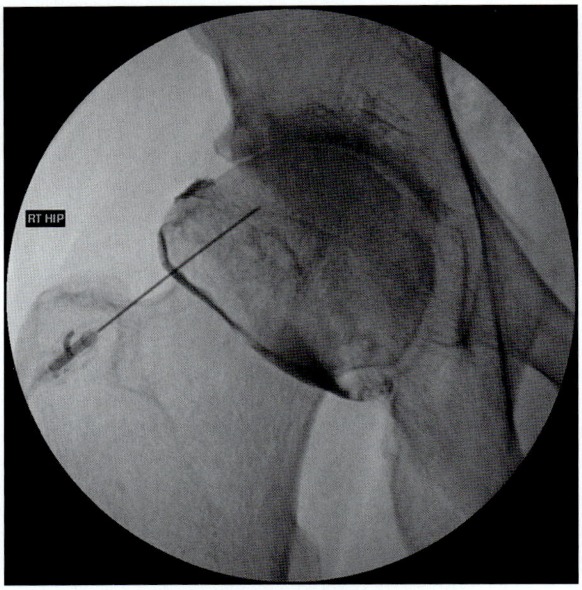

Figure 2.1 Fluoroscopic image acquired during a therapeutic injection of steroid and anesthetic into the hip of a patient with severe osteoarthritis secondary to juvenile chronic arthritis. Contrast agent confirms the intra-articular location of the needle.

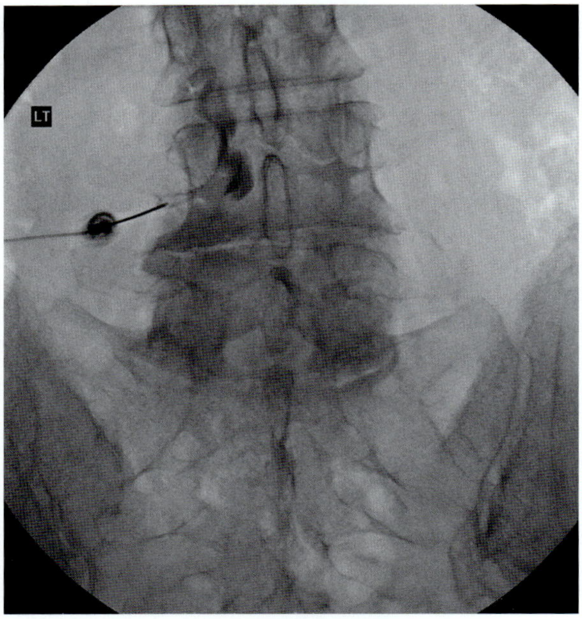

Figure 2.2 Fluoroscopic image of a L4 nerve root block in a patient with exit canal stenosis at the L4-L5 level. There are established spondylotic changes with osteophyte formation. Injection of contrast agent prior to infiltration of a steroid and anesthetic outlines the nerve root and helps prevent intravascular injection.

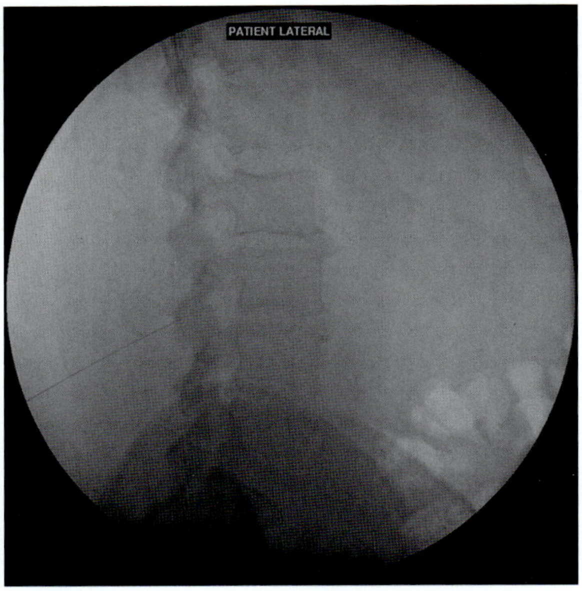

Figure 2.3 Fluoroscopic image acquired during lumbar puncture (LP) in an obese patient in whom a previous non-guided LP attempt failed. The image quality is poor but is sufficient to visualize the 15-cm needle required to reach the cerebrospinal fluid space at the L3/-L4 level.

CHAPTER 3

Ultrasonography

CONCEPT

- Ultrasound imaging, or ultrasonography (US), uses high-frequency sound pulses that are emitted from a hand-held ultrasound transducer, or probe.
- The transducer is applied to the patient's skin via a coupling gel, and the sound pulses are reflected back to the transducer from structures within the patient.
- The magnitude of the reflected sound, or "echo," is converted into a gray-scale image.
- Tissues that are highly reflective of the sound, or "echogenic," such as bone, appear bright. Tissues that allow transmission of the sound pulses, or are poorly echogenic, such as fluid, appear dark or black.
- Substances that are moving, such as flowing blood, can be evaluated using a technique known as *Doppler imaging*, which demonstrates the direction and velocity of movement.
- Images are acquired and viewed in real time and are therefore amenable to image-guided procedures such as biopsy, injection, and aspiration.
- US does not use ionizing radiation and is therefore safe to use during pregnancy and in the pediatric population.

CLINICAL PRACTICE

- The most common clinical application of US is in the assessment of abdominal and pelvic pathology.
- US of the musculoskeletal system, now a well-developed and widely available modality, is often the imaging modality of choice for evaluating superficial soft tissues such as rotator cuff tendons as well as tendons in the hand, wrist, ankle, and foot.
- The application of Doppler imaging allows accurate assessment of superficial vessels, such as the carotid vessels in the neck. Highly sensitive Doppler imaging, known as "power Doppler," can detect flow in very small vessels and inflammatory tissue and is now well established as a diagnostic tool for the early assessment of inflammatory arthritis.

LIMITATIONS

- Ultrasound is transmitted poorly through gas, so structures such as the bowel may impair visualization of deeper structures.
- Ultrasound does not penetrate bone or metal, so US is unable to evaluate the bone marrow or the stability of orthopaedic hardware. However, the relationship of hardware to adjacent soft tissue structures is possible.

COMMON MUSCULOSKELETAL INDICATIONS

- Assessment of acute tendon and muscle injury.
- Assessment of superficial tendinopathy.
- Assessment of superficial soft tissue masses.
- Assessment of synovitis and bursal disease.
- Diagnosis and aspiration of joint effusion.
- Image-guided joint and soft tissue injection and nerve blocks.

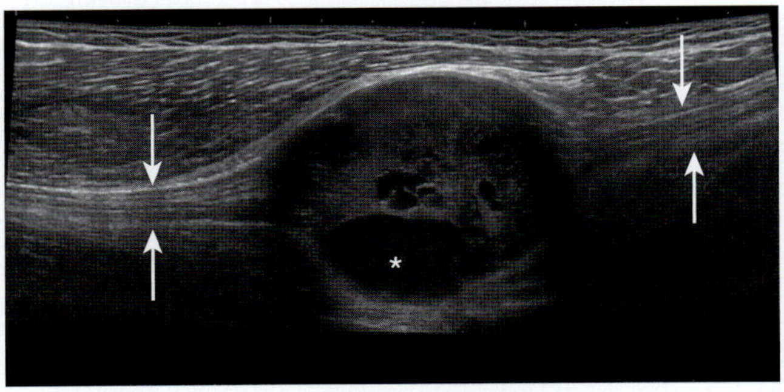

Figure 3.1 US image of a patient with a mass in the posterior thigh. There is a large mass arising from the sciatic nerve (*white arrows*). The mass contains some areas of central cystic degeneration (*asterisk*). These appearances are typical of a schwannoma.

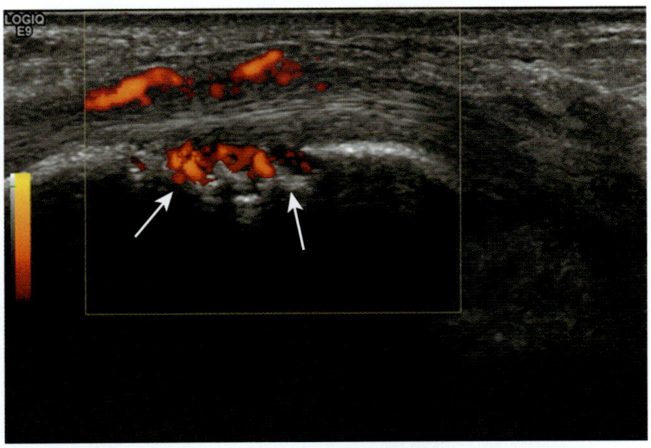

Figure 3.2 Doppler US image of the posterior tibial nerve in a patient with rheumatoid arthritis. There is increased vascularity in the tendon sheath, and an erosion can be seen on the underlying medial malleolus (*white arrows*).

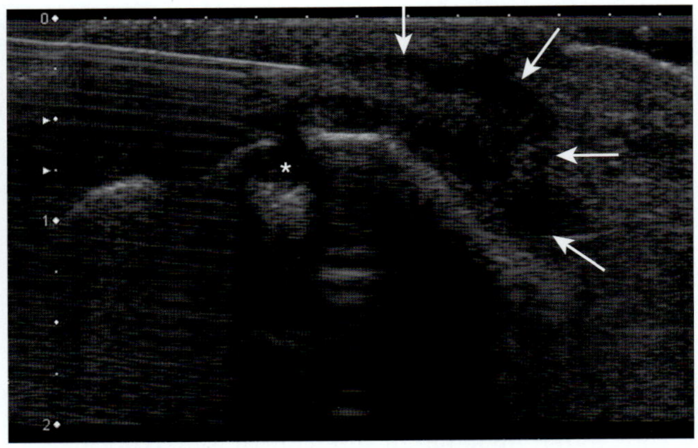

Figure 3.3 US image acquired during image-guided injection of the metatarsophalangeal joint in a patient with rheumatoid arthritis. The needle is clearly visible entering the area of hypoechoic synovitis (*white arrows*), and an erosion of the metatarsal head can also be seen (*asterisk*).

CHAPTER 4

Nuclear Medicine and Positron Emission Tomography

CONCEPT

Nuclear Medicine

- Nuclear medicine (NM) involves the administration of a radioactive isotope to a patient.
- The radioisotope is usually bound to a biologically active agent, or *radiopharmaceutical*.
- The radioisotopes emit radiation that is detected by a device called a *gamma camera*. The intensity and location of the radiation emission are then converted into an image.
- The type of radiopharmaceutical used is determined by the type of tissue being studied. For example, a bone scan uses a commonly used radioisotope called technetium Tc 99m (^{99m}Tc), which is bound to an agent called methylenediphosphonate (MDP). MDP is taken up by active osteoblasts and thus emits the most radiation at sites of bone production and resorption.
- Radiopharmaceuticals may be administered by intravenous injection, ingestion, or inhalation. After certain NM examinations, the patient may emit radiation for some time, and contact with radiosensitive individuals such as pregnant women and babies must be avoided.

Positron Emission Tomography

- Positron emission tomography (PET) uses radioisotopes that emit high-energy positrons that are of a consistent energy in multiple directions.
- The most commonly used isotope is fluorine F 18, which is bound to deoxyglucose to make a radiopharmaceutical called FDG (fluorodeoxyglucose). FDG is metabolized by the body in the same way as glucose.
- FDG is preferentially taken up by hypermetabolic cells, such as malignant tumor cells, myocardium, and some inflammatory tissues.
- In a PET-CT scanner, the detectors of the high-energy positrons are combined with the x-ray detectors of a CT scanner so that a simultaneous, fused CT and PET scan can be generated.
- Functional images of the FDG uptake can be superimposed on the anatomic image of the CT scan to enhance the specificity of the examination.

CLINICAL PRACTICE

- In the musculoskeletal system, the ^{99m}Tc MDP bone scan is a useful "screening" examination of the whole body for the detection of osteoblastic or osteolytic metastasis.
- Uptake is also seen in disease processes such as degenerative and inflammatory joint diseases, which must be considered during interpretation of the images. Correlation with other imaging modalities, such as radiography and MRI, is often necessary.
- Radioisotopes may be tagged to white blood cells (WBCs), for an indium In 111 (^{111}In) WBC scan. The radiolabeled WBCs migrate to sites of active infection. This type of scan is often combined with a ^{99m}Tc MDP bone scan to investigate sites of suspected osteomyelitis.

LIMITATIONS

- Nuclear medicine examinations are highly sensitive but have a significant number of false-positive results and lower specificity. For example, uptake related to degenerative disc disease can mimic uptake due to spinal metastases on a ^{99m}TC MDP bone scan.
- The resolution of NM and PET imaging is limited to around 1 cm, so it is often necessary to correlate the images with modalities such as radiography, CT, and MRI, which have far superior image resolution.
- The radiation dose to the patient must also be considered. Certain NM studies involve very high doses; for example a thallous chloride Tl 201 cardiac stress study delivers an effective dose of 20 mSv, which is equivalent to 1000 chest x-rays or 10 CT scans of the head.

COMMON MUSCULOSKELETAL INDICATIONS

- ^{99m}Tc MDP bone scanning is often used as a whole-body scan for skeletal metastasis, occult fractures, or Paget disease.
- Combined ^{111}In WBC and ^{99m}Tc MDP bone scans for investigation of suspected osteomyelitis.

- FDG PET-CT is frequently used as a whole-body scan for metastases in lung, breast, lymphoma, and head and neck cancers.
- MIBG (meta-iodobenzyl guanidine I 123) scan for hypersecretory neuroendocrine tumors.
- Iodine I 131 is used diagnostically and therapeutically for hyperthyroidism.

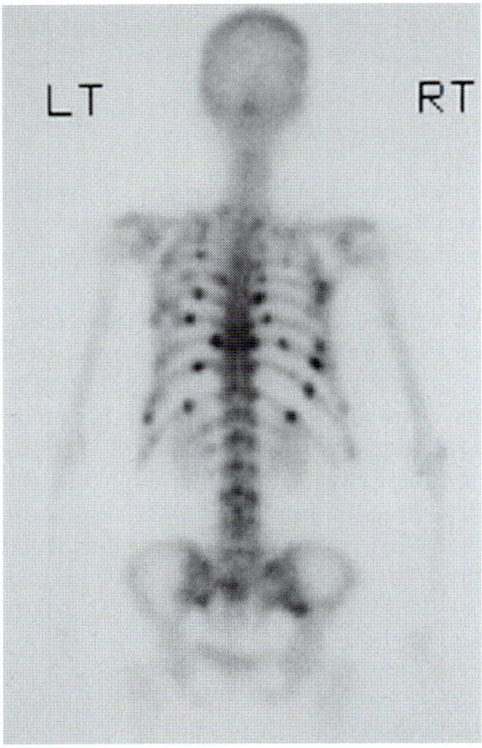

Figure 4.1 ^{99m}Tc MDP bone scan demonstrating widespread osteoblastic metastases within the ribs as areas of "hot spots."

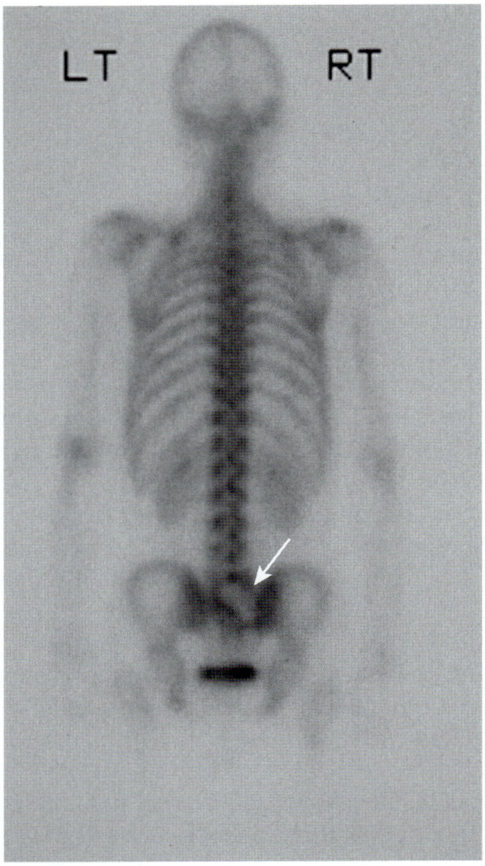

Figure 4.2 ^{99m}Tc MDP bone scan showing a photopenic lesion in the sacrum (*white arrow*), which is due to an osteoclastic or purely lytic metastasis from a primary hepatoma. Photopenic lesions are often more difficult to visualize than lesions with increased uptake.

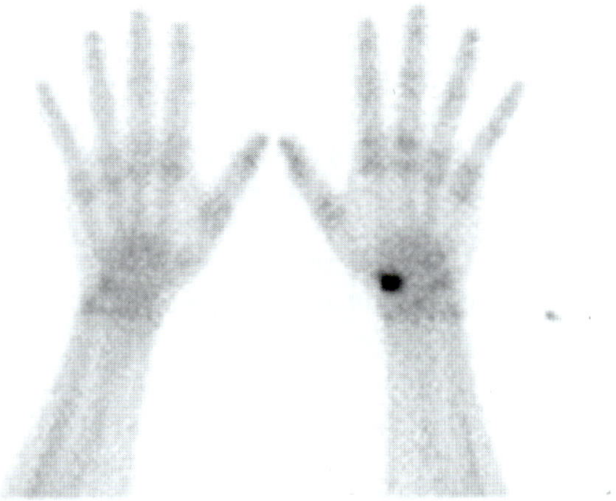

Figure 4.3 ^{99m}Tc MDP bone scan demonstrating increased uptake in an occult scaphoid fracture of the wrist.

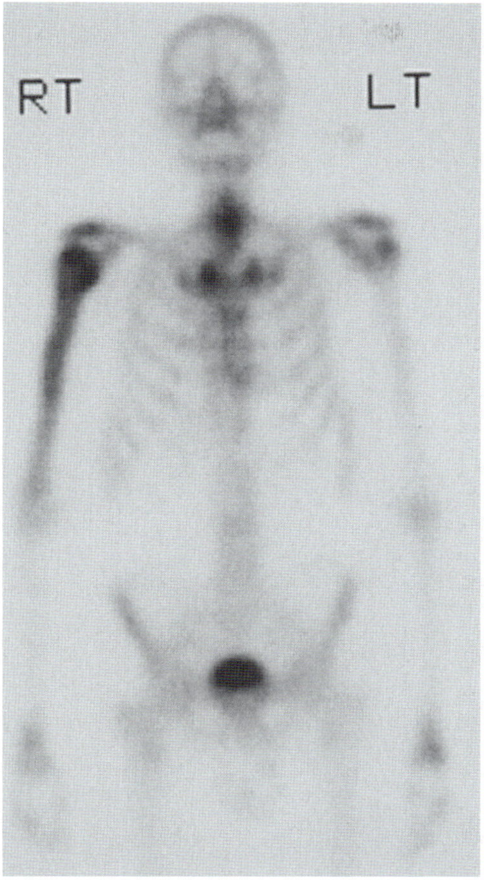

Figure 4.4 ^{99m}Tc MDP bone scan of a patient with upper limb pain and increased uptake involving the proximal and mid humerus. This pattern of uptake is typical of Paget disease.

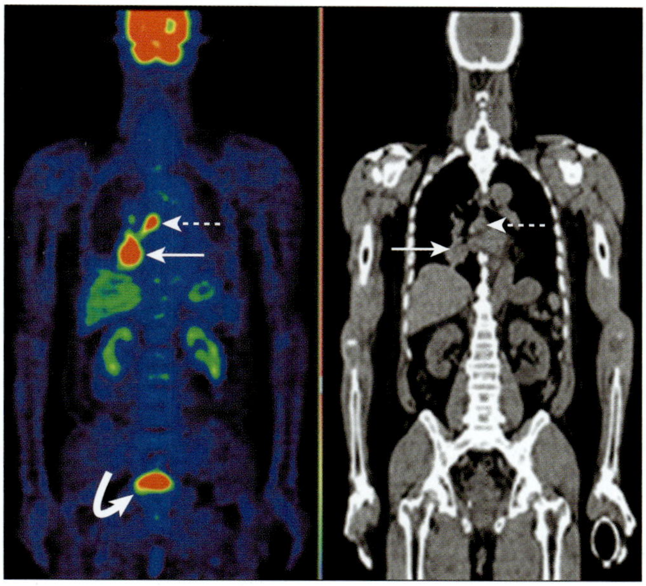

Figure 4.5 FDG PET-CT examination of a patient with carcinoma of the lung. The primary tumor is seen on both the PET image and CT scan (*white arrows*), and there is a metastatic lymph node in the mediastinum (*broken white arrows*). There is also increased uptake on the PET image in the liver, kidneys, and stomach, with very high uptake in the bladder (*curved white arrow*) due to urinary excretion of isotope.

CHAPTER 5

Computed Tomography

CONCEPT

- Computed tomography (CT) uses ionizing x-radiation to generate images by emitting x-rays from a fan-beam source that rotates around the patient.
- After passing through the patient, the beam is incident on a ring of x-ray detectors, which register a value for the degree of attenuation of the x-ray beam known as a *Hounsfield unit*.
- These values reflect the density of the tissue in tiny volumes of space within the patient known as a *voxels,* which are then demonstrated in the resulting image (scan).
- Computational models are applied to assign a gray scale to the individual voxels to make up a two-dimensional (2D), cross-sectional image.
- Voxels contain three-dimensional (3D) information and can be reconstructed into an image in any desired orthogonal plane (multiplanar reformats [MPRs]).
- The CT data set may also be reconstructed into a 3D computer-generated model, in which colors can be applied to represent tissues of different density.
- The contrast of soft tissue structures can be increased with the use of contrast agents, which may be injected into the cardiovascular system, such as iodine-based intravenous contrast agents, or administered into the gastrointestinal system, such as diatrizoic acid (Gastrografin) and barium-based oral contrast agents.
- Lower-density media, such as air and water, may be used to enhance bowel soft tissue contrast.

CLINICAL PRACTICE

- CT produces high-resolution 2D and 3D images and provides rapid evaluation of bone and soft tissue structures.
- It is the imaging modality of choice for the majority of abdominal and thoracic disorders as well as for the brain in the setting of head trauma or acute stroke.
- CT provides an excellent 3D assessment of bone in the setting of trauma and can be utilized to assess fractures with metallic fixation hardware in situ.
- As an alternative to MRI, CT can be combined with arthrography to assess intra-articular derangement of joints.

LIMITATIONS

- CT may be limited by patient motion artifact, so it is important, during consideration of a referral for certain CT examinations, that the patient is able to lie still and to hold his or her breath.
- The soft tissue contrast of CT is inferior to that of MRI and US, so CT is of limited value for assessment of soft tissue disease and bone marrow imaging.

COMMON MUSCULOSKELETAL INDICATIONS

Conventional CT

- Complex fractures.
- Spinal trauma.
- Fracture complications such as non-union and infection.
- Assessment of complex bony anatomy for surgical planning.
- Intra-articular loose bodies.
- Characterization of bone lesions.
- Image-guided spinal injections.

CT Arthrography

- Chondral and osteochondral defects.
- Fibrocartilage tears (especially in the shoulder, wrist, hip, and knee).

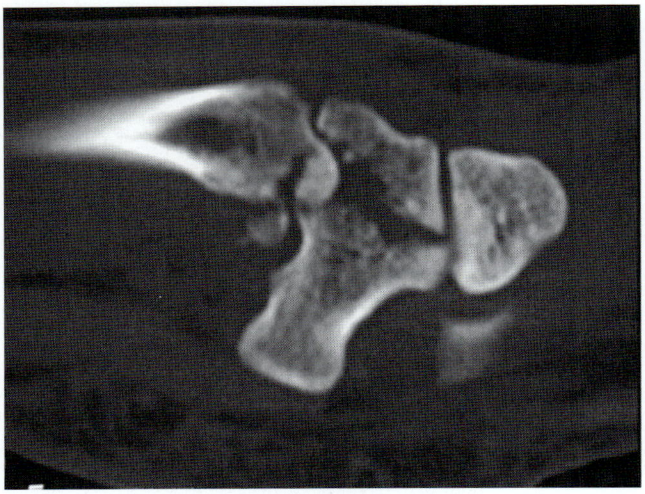

Figure 5.1 Sagittal CT reconstruction of a hamate fracture with proximal dislocation of the base of the fourth metacarpal into the hamate fracture line, which requires reduction to achieve bony healing.

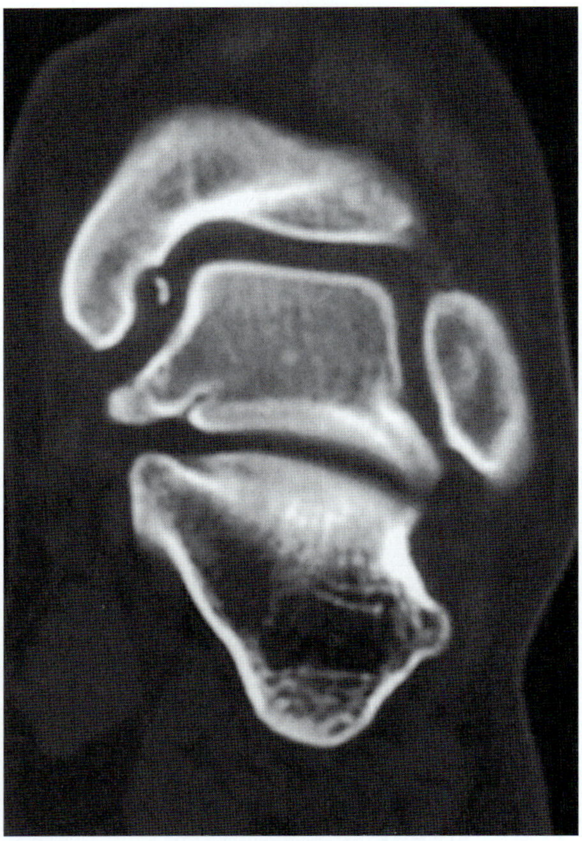

Figure 5.2 Coronal CT reconstruction of the ankle showing an obvious loose body that was not seen on radiographs

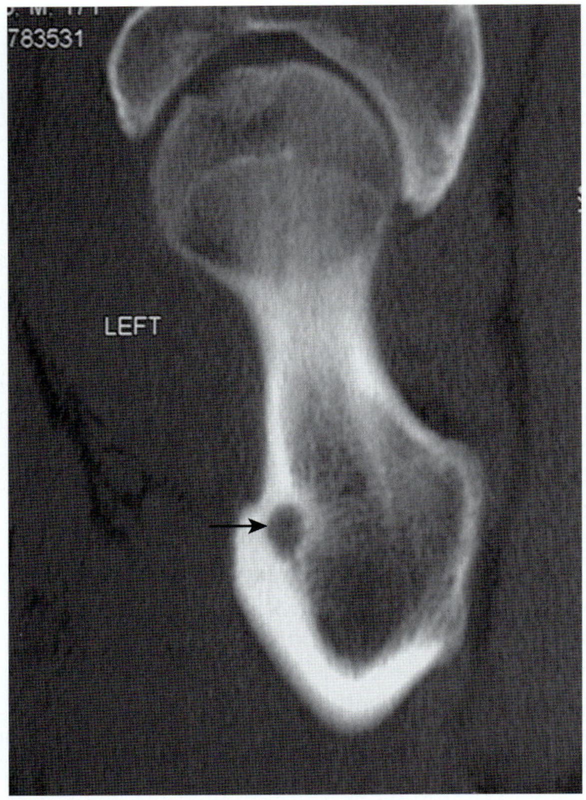

Figure 5.3 Sagittal CT reconstruction of the hip in a patient with a radiolucent osteoid osteoma nidus (*black arrow*) lying on the endosteal surface of the proximal femur. The nidus was not visible on radiographs.

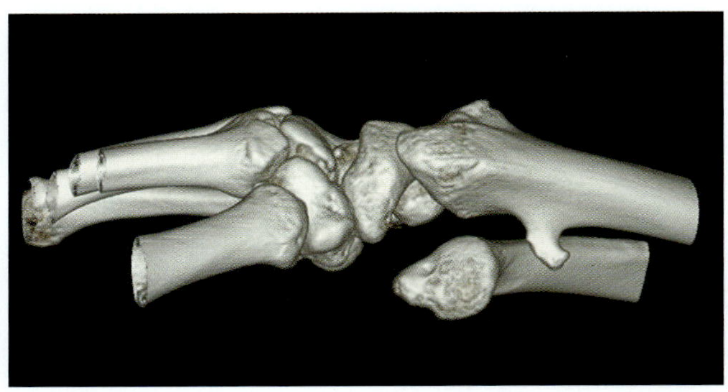

Figure 5.4 3D CT reconstruction of the wrist, viewed from the radial aspect, of a patient with Madelung deformity secondary to diaphyseal aclasia (multiple osteochondromas). The subluxation of the ulna with respect to the distal radius is clearly evident, and there is a bony exostosis (osteochondroma) arising from the distal radius.

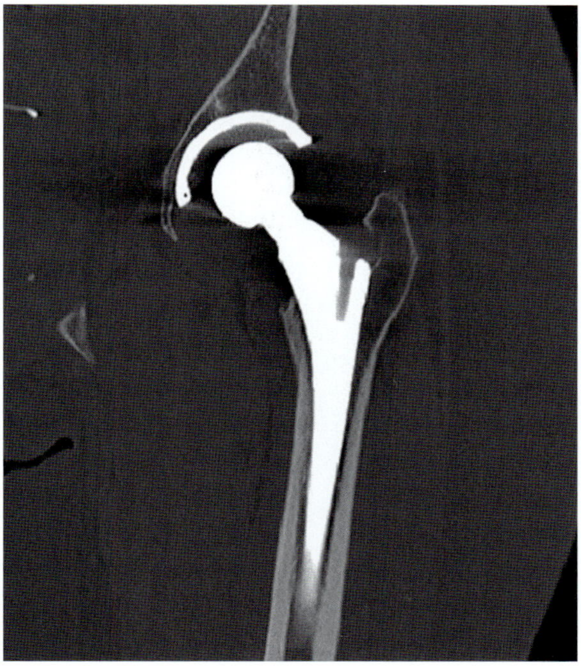

Figure 5.5 Coronal CT reconstruction of a normal hip prosthesis. There is minimal artifact from the prosthesis, and the CT scan provides excellent bony detail.

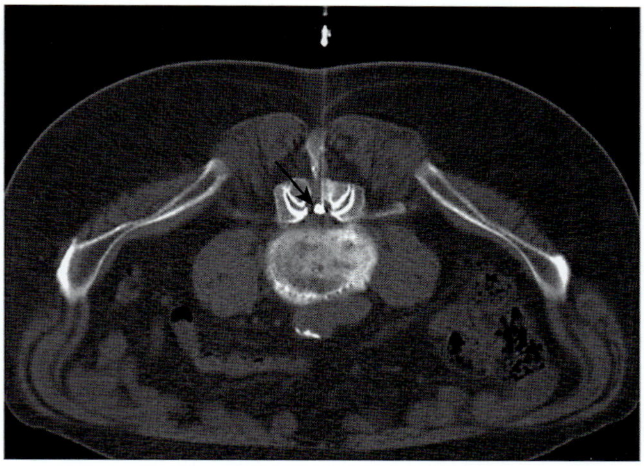

Figure 5.6 Axial scan acquired during a CT-guided epidural injection for pain relief. The spinal needle is clearly visible, and a small injection of contrast material (*black arrow*) confirms the location of the needle within the epidural space prior to injection of the anesthetic and steroid. The procedure is very safe and can be performed in 10 to 15 minutes.

CHAPTER 6

Magnetic Resonance Imaging

CONCEPT

- Magnetic resonance imaging (MRI) uses the movement of protons within a magnetic field to generate an image.
- Within the constant magnetic field of an MRI scanner, tissues that contain free hydrogen nuclei (protons) generate varying signals when pulses of radiofrequency (RF) energy are applied to them.
- These signals, which depend on the type of tissue and the speed at which the tissue "relaxes" or gives up its movement, are then mathematically converted into an image.
- The contrast of the image thus depends on the signal intensity (SI) of different tissues. Certain tissues that are rich in free protons, such as water and fat, are very responsive to the RF pulses. Other tissues with fewer free protons, such as cortical bone and air, are less responsive and generate much less signal.
- Different tissue contrasts can be determined, depending on the strength and timing of the RF pulse; this parameter is known as an *MR sequence*. The most basic forms of MR sequences include:
  - T1-weighted (T1W) imaging, on which fluid appears dark and fat appears bright.
  - T2-weighted (T2W) imaging, on which both fluid and fat appear bright.
  - Proton density (PD) imaging, on which fluid appears intermediate-SI and fat appears bright.
- Manipulating the MR sequences allows the demonstration of different tissue characteristics. For instance, the signal from fat can be cancelled out (made dark) using a technique known as *fat suppression*. Fat suppression with T2 weighting is very useful in musculoskeletal imaging to increase contrast between bright pathologic tissue and fat. Common fat suppression techniques include:
  - Short TI inversion recovery (STIR) imaging.
  - Fat suppression with T2 weighting (FST2W imaging).
- Intravenous contrast agents such as gadolinium can be administered to enhance the visualization of vessels and inflammatory tissue. T1W with fat suppression (FST1W) images are often used to improve contrast between enhanced tissue and adjacent fat structures.
- Intra-articular contrast agents may also be administered, producing an MR arthrogram effect to enhance the evaluation of intra-articular structures such as articular cartilage, fibrocartilage, and ligaments. This method is often employed in shoulder, wrist, elbow, and hip imaging.
- Certain metals, such as stainless steel and cobalt-chrome, distort the magnetic field and thus produce *image artifact*. Other metals, such as titanium, produce much less image distortion. Such distortion may degrade the image quality and is an important consideration in referring patients with metal devices such as orthopaedic hardware for evaluation by MRI.
- Implantable electronic devices, such as cardiac pacemakers and neural stimulators, are affected by the magnetic field and are also incompatible with MRI evaluation.

CLINICAL PRACTICE

- MRI is the investigation of choice for most brain and spine pathology.
- This modality provides excellent contrast between soft tissues, such as articular cartilage, bone marrow, muscle, and ligaments. It is the primary imaging modality for most joint and extremity pathology.
- It is also useful in evaluation of the pelvic soft tissues and can be utilized to investigate abdominal structures, although the evaluation can be limited by movement of the bowels and by respiratory motion.
- MRI is used extensively in pediatrics because it does not use potentially harmful ionizing radiation.

LIMITATIONS

- MRI is particularly limited by patient motion, which produces image artifacts.
- Also, the image acquisition time can be quite long, so MRI is of limited use in the setting of acute trauma.
- Conventional MRI scanners are very confining and may be unsuitable for claustrophobic patients. "Open" MRI scanners are widely available for

such patients, although image quality may be compromised.

- MRI-incompatible hardware, such as stainless steel plates and cobalt-chrome prostheses, produce artifacts; these components may be better imaged with CT.
- Imaging of the thorax is subject to respiratory motion and demonstrates poor MR image contrast properties, making CT a better alternative for investigating lung pathology; however, advances in MR sequences have made cardiac MRI a valuable diagnostic tool.

COMMON MUSCULOSKELETAL INDICATIONS

- Spinal pathology.
- Suspected internal derangement of joints.
- Investigation of skeletal metastasis and other bone lesions.
- Bone and soft tissue infections.
- Soft tissue tumors and masses.
- Compressive neuropathy.

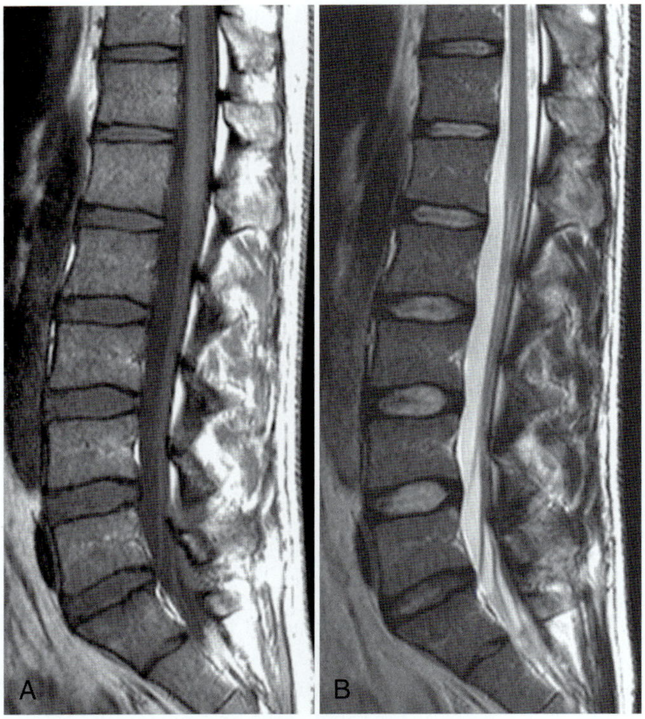

Figure 6.1 Sagittal MR images of the lumbar spine. **(A)**, The T1W MR image demonstrates the cerebrospinal fluid (CSF) as low-SI, with high SI in the marrow and subcutaneous fat. The intervertebral discs are intermediate-SI. **(B)**, By comparison, the CSF and the intervertebral discs on the T2W MR image are bright, or high-SI. Fatty tissues are also bright on T2W MR images.

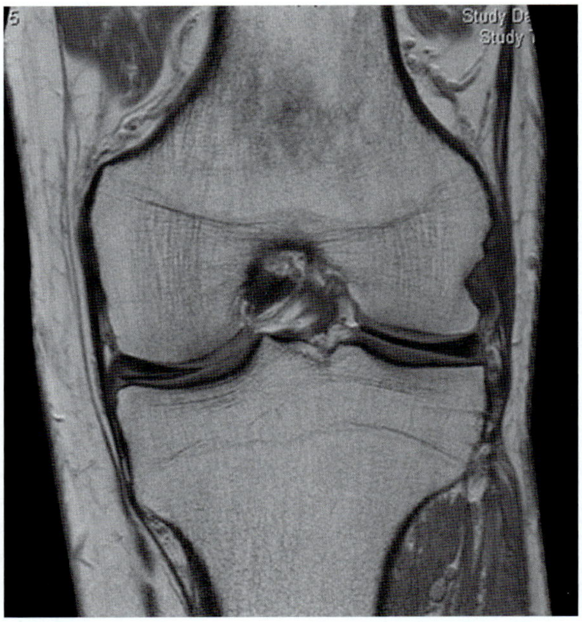

Figure 6.2 Coronal PD image of the knee. There are excellent image resolution and contrast, with clear detail of the ligaments, subchondral bone, articular cartilage, and fibrocartilage. The image is similar to T1W MR images, but fluid is intermediate-SI, depending on pulse sequence parameters.

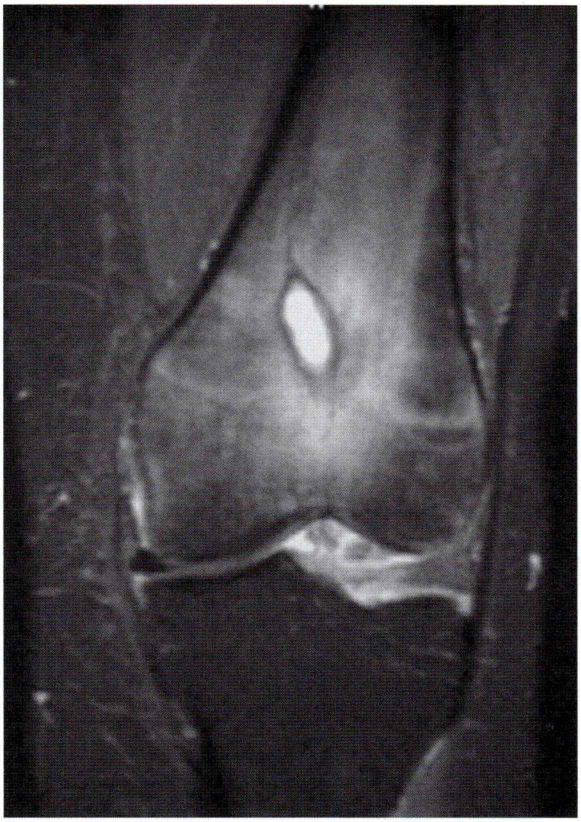

Figure 6.3 Coronal STIR image of the knee in a patient with Brodie abscess. The fluid in the abscess cavity is high-SI, and there is surrounding marrow edema. The marrow edema is particularly well shown because fat suppression improves the contrast between pathologically edematous tissue and the normally high-SI fatty marrow. This image is very similar to FST2W MR images.

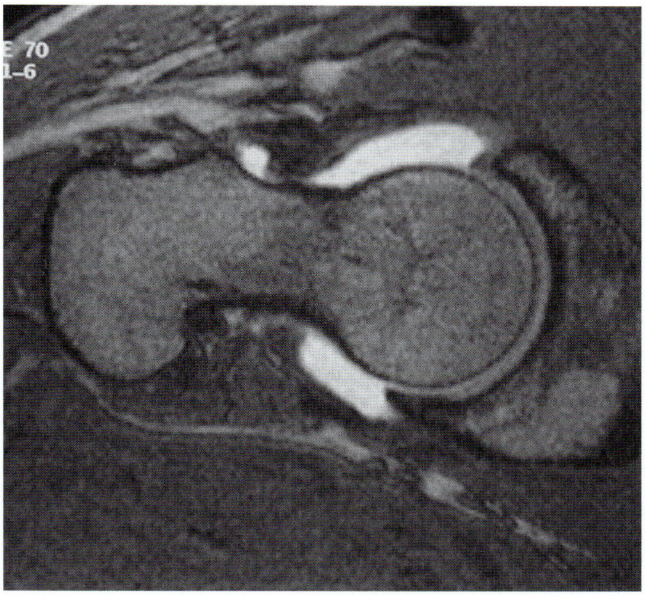

Figure 6.4 T1W gradient echo image from an MR arthrogram of the hip. The high SI of the intra-articular contrast agent provides excellent delineation and contrast for the labroligamentous structures, which are normally closely applied to the bony structures. Gradient echo images maybe useful when thin slices are required for demonstration of fine anatomic detail.

PART 2 • SPINE

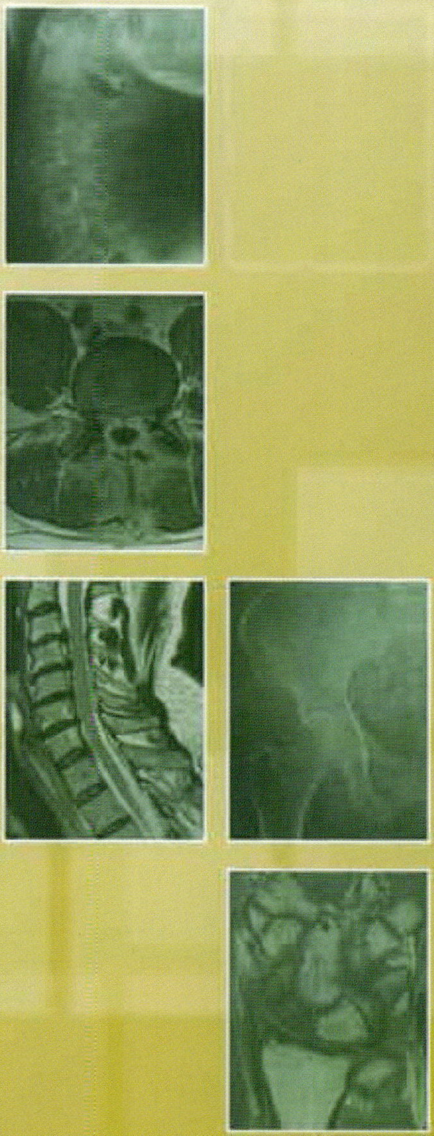

CHAPTER 7

Anatomy: Special Imaging Considerations of the Cervical Spine

OSSEOUS STRUCTURES

Atlas (C1). The first cervical vertebra is a bony ring with a thin anterior arch and posterior laminae, which are joined by lateral masses having articular facets that articulate with the occipital condyles superiorly and the lateral masses of C2 inferiorly.

Axis (C2). The second cervical vertebra has a vertebral body with a superiorly projecting odontoid process that articulates with a concave facet on the anterior arch of C1 to form the atlantoaxial articulation. The axis possesses lateral masses that articulate with those of C1 and a short, bifid spinous process posteriorly.

Cervical Vertebrae (C2-C7). The cervical vertebral bodies are rounded and triangular in cross section, with superior end plates that are slightly anteriorly downsloping. The transverse processes are short and bifid and contain the foramen transversarium for the sympathetic plexus vertebral arteries and veins. Each vertebra has two laminae posteriorly that fuse to form small bifid spinous processes, with the exception of C7, which has a long prominent spinous process. The inferior and superior articular processes arise at the junction of the transverse process and the laminae. The superior process or facet projects posteroinferiorly, and the inferior process projects anteroinferiorly. The intervertebral foramina lie anterior to the inferior articular processes.

Cervical Facet (Zygapophyseal) Joints. Synovial articulations formed between the inferior articular process of the vertebra for which the joint is named, and the superior articular process of the vertebra below. The articular surfaces are coronally oriented, thus preventing forward intervertebral translation. The facet joint capsules are loose, facilitating anterior sliding movement during neck flexion. The facet capsules are innervated by the medial branches of the dorsal rami of the spinal nerves.

LIGAMENTS

Discs and Ligaments. Composed of a tough outer annulus fibrosis that is deficient posteriorly, where each disc is contained by the posterior longitudinal ligament. The central nucleus pulposus is a semifluid material composed of proteoglycans.

Longitudinal Ligaments. The anterior (ALL) and posterior (PLL) longitudinal ligaments are bands of type 1 collagen fibers that attach to the anterior and posterior periosteal surfaces of the vertebral bodies and intervertebral discs. They resist tension and separation of the vertebral bodies during flexion and extension.

Atlantoaxial Ligaments. Anterior atlantoaxial stability is maintained by the apical and alar ligaments, which attach to the skull base and odontoid process. The transverse ligament extends from the posterior surfaces of the C1 anterior arch and over the posterior aspect of the odontoid process, restricting forward translation of C1 on C2.

Posterior Ligaments. The posterior elements are stabilized by a group of three ligaments. The ligamenta flava are composed of elastic collagen fibers that run the whole length of the spine, attaching to the internal surface of the laminae. The spinous processes are stabilized by the interspinous and supraspinous ligaments.

MUSCLES

The cervical spinal musculature is multilayered and can be divided into three groups:

Anterior Muscles. The anterior muscles consist of the paired longus colli, longus capitis, and anterior and lateral rectus capitis muscles. The anterior muscles flex the neck, resist neck hyperextension, and act independently to turn the head.

Lateral Muscles. The lateral group consists of the anterior, middle, and posterior scalene muscles, and the sternocleidomastoid. The scalene muscles act to laterally flex the neck and assist inspiration by elevating the first and second ribs.

Deep Posterior Muscles. The deep posterior cervical muscles consist of the splenius colli, semispinalis, and splenius capitis. They act along with the trapezius muscle to extend the neck and resist hyperflexion.

NEURAL STRUCTURES

The Spinal Nerves. These are made up of a confluence of dorsal and ventral roots, each root being composed of smaller rootlets. The dorsal root contains a spinal ganglion located just proximal to the junction with the ventral root. Each spinal nerve emerges through the intervertebral foramen of the vertebra below its ascribed level; for example, the C6 nerve passes through the C5 neural foramen.

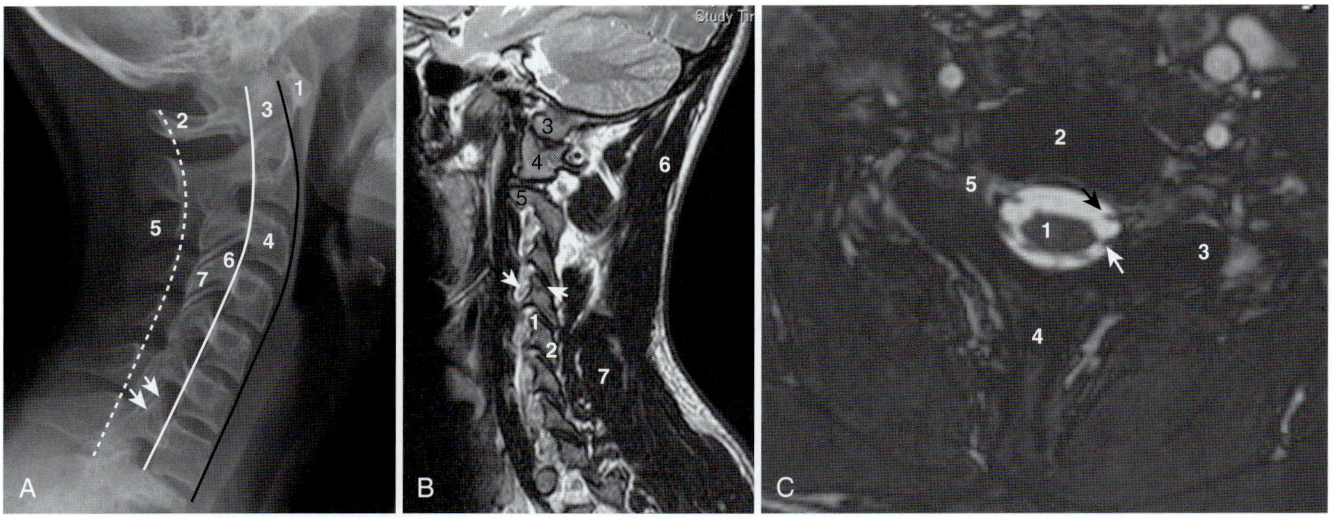

Figure 7.1 (A), Lateral radiograph of the cervical spine: 1, anterior arch of C1; 2, posterior arch of C1; 3, odontoid process of C2; 4, vertebral body of C3; 5, spinous process of C3; 6, superior articular process of C4; 7, inferior articular process of C4; *black line,* anterior spinal line; *white line,* posterior spinal line; *dashed line,* spinal laminar line; *black arrows,* facet (zygapophyseal) joint of C6-C7. (B), Sagittal T2-weighted (T2W) MR image of the cervical spine: 1, superior articular process; 2, inferior articular process; 3, occipital condyle; 4, lateral mass of C1; 5, lateral mass of C2; 6, splenius capitis muscle; 7, splenius colli muscle; *open white arrow,* C3-C4 facet joint (posterior margin); *white arrow,* spinal nerve in neural foramen. (C), Axial three-dimensional T2W MR image of the cervical spine: 1, cervical cord; 2, vertebral body; 3, transverse process; 4, spinous process; 5, neural exit foramen; *open black arrow,* ventral root; *white arrow,* dorsal root.

CHAPTER 8

Arnold-Chiari Malformation Type I

DEFINITION

- Elongation of the cerebellar tonsils extending below the foramen magnum into the cervical spinal canal that is often associated with syrinx of the cervical spinal cord.

SIGNS AND SYMPTOMS

- Suboccipital headache.
- Ocular disturbances.
- Compression of the cervical spinal cord with motor and sensory deficits.
- Gait abnormalities.
- Trauma is often the precipitating event for onset of symptoms.
- Syrinx of brainstem and cervical spinal cord is often present.

DEMOGRAPHICS

- Female preponderance.
- Incidence of approximately 0.3% to 0.4% in all age groups.
- Symptoms may occur from infancy to old age.
- Extent of cerebellar tonsillar herniation correlates with severity of symptoms, with greater than 12 mm of herniation almost always symptomatic.

IMAGING RECOMMENDATIONS

- MRI of the cervical spine:
  - Include axial imaging of the craniocervical junction.

IMAGING FINDINGS

- Tonsils protrude more than 5 mm below the foramen magnum on sagittal T2-weighted (T2W) MR images.
- Normal brainstem location.
- Normal position of fourth ventricle.
- Syringomyelia present in 20% to 73% of cases.
- Occasional association with:
  - Klippel-Feil syndrome.
  - Short clivus.
  - C1 and odontoid process abnormalities.

OTHER RECOMMENDED TESTING

- Evoked potential testing should be performed if myelopathy is considered.

DIFFERENTIAL DIAGNOSIS

- Syringomyelia.
- Hydrocephalus.
- Pseudotumor cerebri.
- Brainstem tumors affecting the lower cranial nerves.
- Acquired tonsillar herniation from Paget disease, osteogenesis imperfecta, rickets, or intracranial hypotension.

TREATMENT

- The patient with Arnold-Chiari malformation I who is asymptomatic without syrinx is treated conservatively.
- The patient who is symptomatic with syrinx may require surgery.
- The patient who is symptomatic, with or without syrinx, is usually treated surgically with the goal of restoring normal flow of cerebrospinal fluid at the foramen magnum.
- Surgical options include posterior fossa decompression and decompression of the posterior arch of C1.

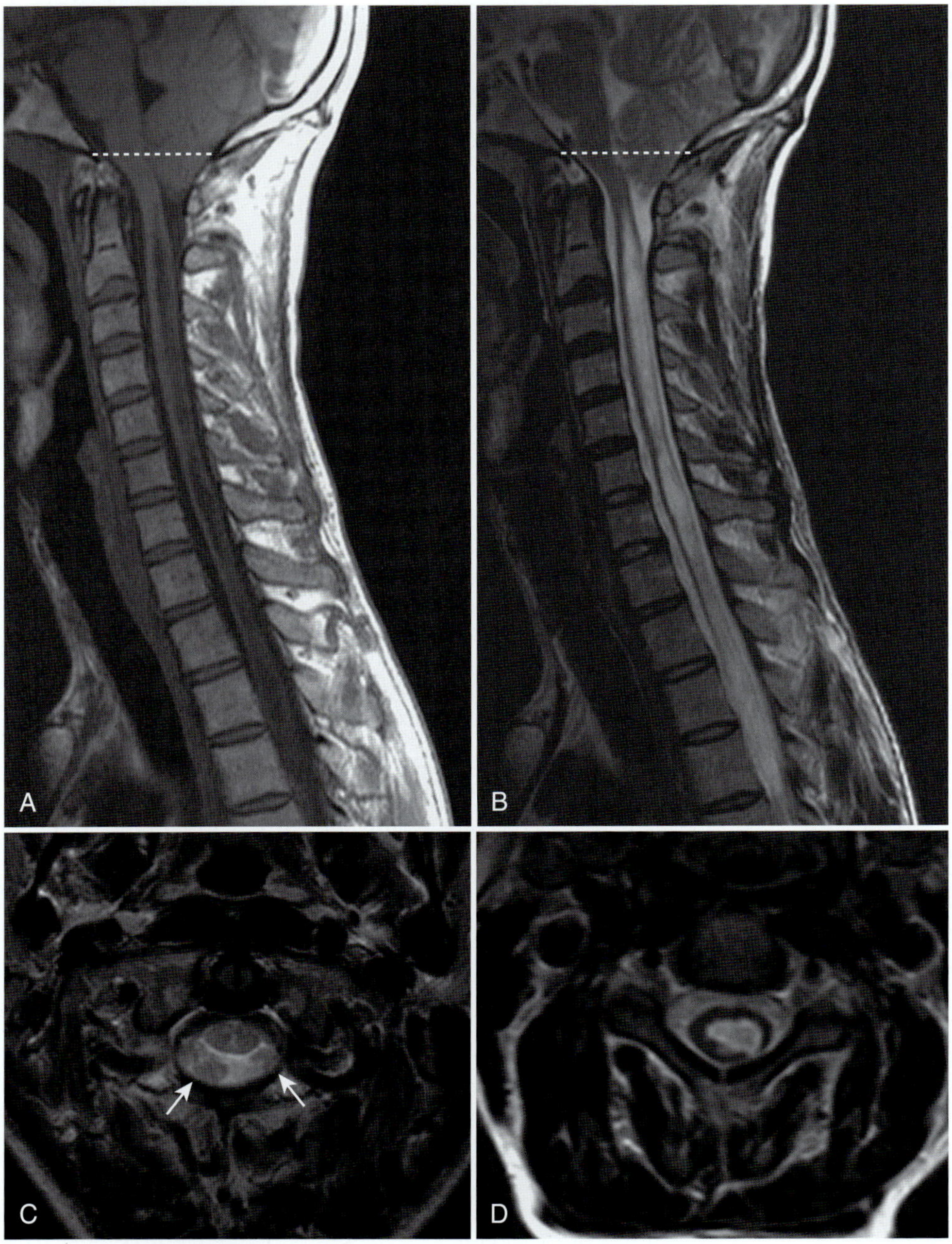

Figure 8.1 Sagittal T1W (**A**) and T2W (**B**) MR images of a patient with Arnold-Chiari malformation type I. The cerebellar tonsils protrude through the foramen magnum (*broken line*), and an associated syrinx is present. The fourth ventricle is normal, and there is no meningocele or other structural defect. (**C**), The herniation of the cerebellar tonsils (*white arrows*) is seen on the axial T2W MR image taken through the level of C1. (**D**), The syrinx is also well demonstrated on the axial T2W MR image taken through the midcervical spine.

CHAPTER 9

Arnold-Chiari Malformation Type II

DEFINITION

- Congenital malformation of the hindbrain almost always associated with concurrent meningomyelocele.

SIGNS AND SYMPTOMS

- The result of a neural tube defect.
- Manifests as:
  - Enlarging head size secondary to hydrocephalus in the neonate.
  - Hydrocephalus in children and adults.
- Lower extremity motor and sensory deficits.
- Sphincter dysfunction.
- Brainstem dysfunction.

DEMOGRAPHICS

- Incidence: Male = Female.
- Incidence: 0.4% per 1000 live births.
- Usually manifests at birth with concurrent meningomyelocele.
- If present in one child, later siblings have 6% risk of being affected.

IMAGING RECOMMENDATIONS

- MRI of brain and cervical spine.

IMAGING FINDINGS

- Infratentorial:
  - Tonsils and medulla below foramen magnum.
  - Fourth ventricle compressed and elongated.
  - Myelomeningocele and syringomyelia.
  - Enlarged foramen magnum, scalloping of clivus, and hyoplastic arch of C1.
  - Cervicomedullary kinking.
  - Morphologic abnormality of the cerebellum with dysplastic tentorium.
- Supratentorial:
  - Hydrocephalus.
  - Falx hypoplasia.
  - Callosal hypoplasia.

OTHER RECOMMENDED TESTING

- Evoked potential testing to quantify spinal cord and brainstem compromise.

DIFFERENTIAL DIAGNOSIS

- Arnold-Chiari malformation I.
- Congenital hydrocephalus.
- Low-pressure hydrocephalus.

TREATMENT

- Folate supplementation during pregnancy decreases risk.
- Posterior fossa decompression and decompression of the posterior arch of C1.
- Shunting to relieve hydrocephalus.
- Fetal meningomyelocele repair in severe cases that are diagnosed in utero by ultrasound may ameliorate severity of neurologic deficits.

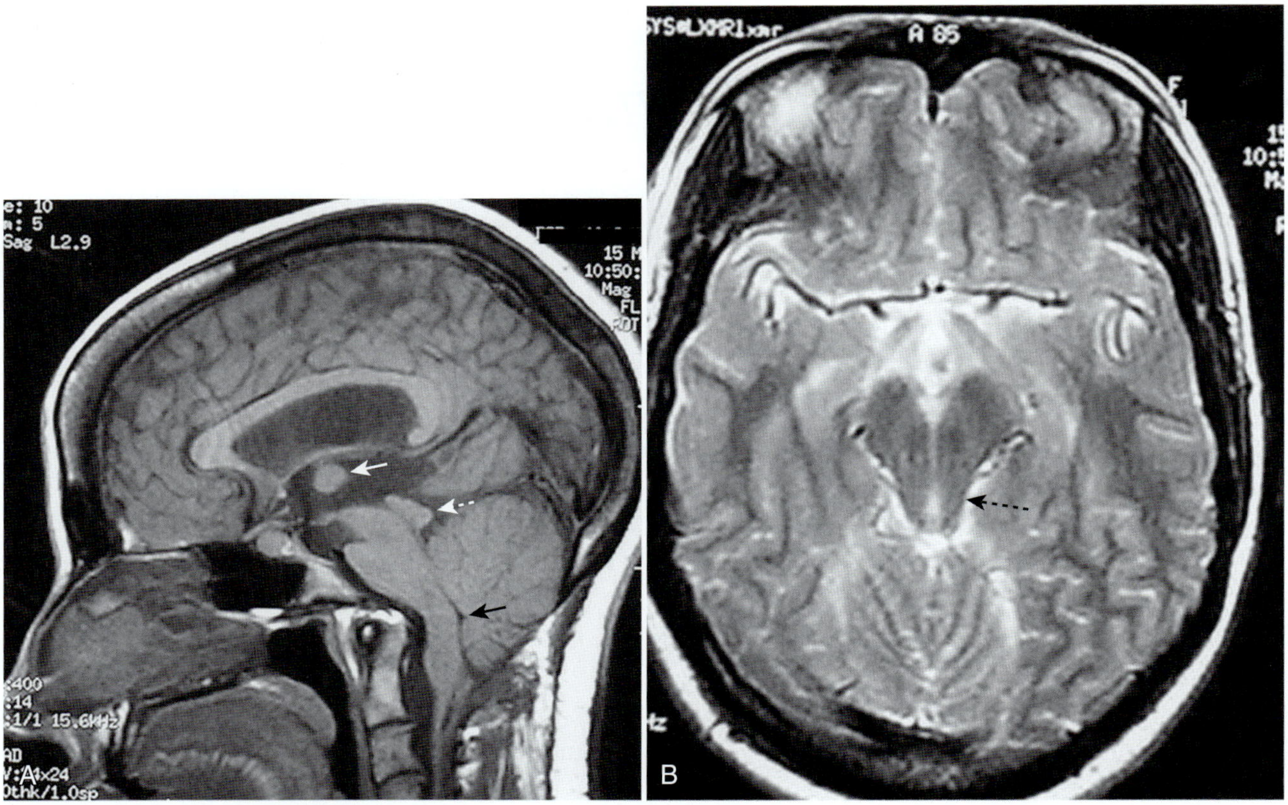

Figure 9.1 (**A**), Sagittal T1-weighted (T1W) MR image of an adult patient with Arnold-Chiari type II deformity. The posterior fossa is small with a widened foramen magnum. There is inferior displacement of the cerebellum and medulla with elongation of the pons and fourth ventricle (*black arrow*). The brainstem is kinked as it passes over the back of the odontoid. There is an enlarged massa intermedia (*white arrow*) and beaking of the tectum (*broken white arrow*). (**B**), The axial T2W MR image shows the small posterior fossa with beaking of the tectum (*broken black arrow*).

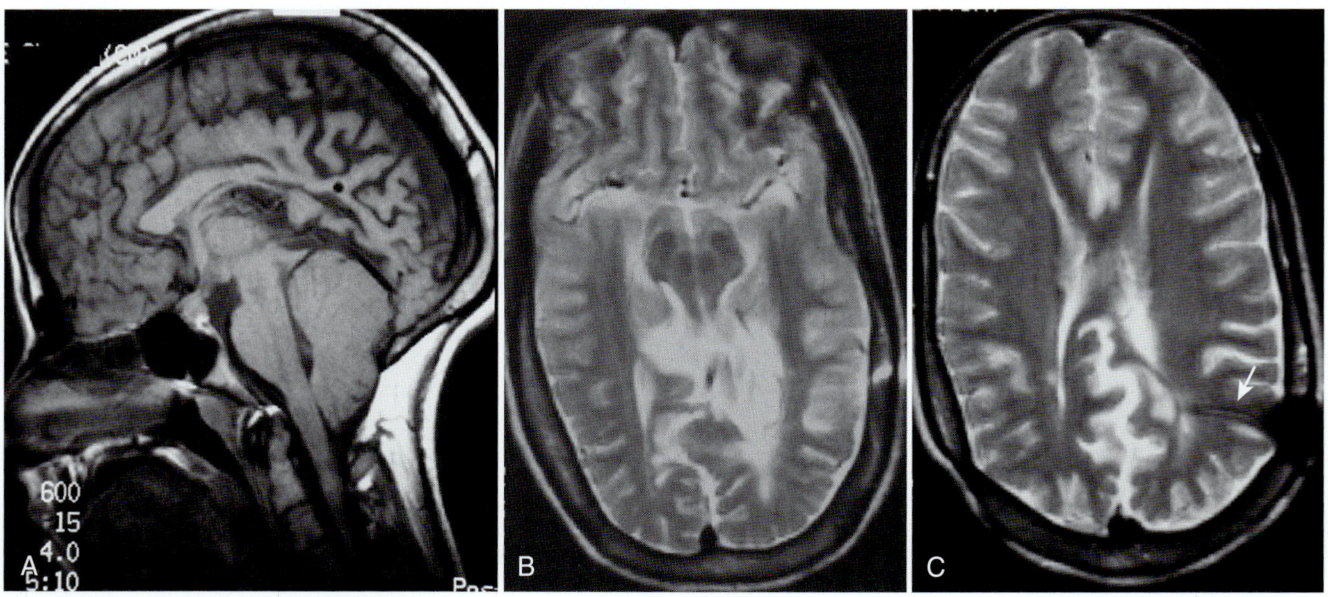

Figure 9.2 (**A**), Sagittal T1W MR image in another patient shows features similar to those in Figure 9.1, although there is less kinking of the brainstem. (**B** and **C**), The axial T2W MR images show the distortion of the occipital lobes, which is probably due to a combination of falx hypoplasia and the small posterior fossa. There is a ventricular shunt in situ (*white arrow*), but there is also some residual dilatation of the occipital horn of the lateral ventricle on the left side.

CHAPTER 10

Klippel-Feil Syndrome

DEFINITION

- Congenital cervical spine malformation characterized by abnormal segmentation and fusion of two or more spinal segments.

SIGNS AND SYMPTOMS

- Classic triad, consisting of short neck, low posterior hairline, and decreased range of motion of the cervical spine.
- Gradual onset of cervical myelopathy.
- Vocal impairment.
- Synkinesis or mirrored movements in the upper and, occasionally, lower extremities in approximately 20% of patients.

DEMOGRAPHICS

- Peak onset in second to third decade of life.
- Can manifest at any age.
- Occurs in 1 in 42,000 live births.
- Slight male preponderance.
- Increased incidence with fetal alcohol syndrome.

IMAGING RECOMMENDATIONS

- Radiography and CT to document vertebral alignment and bony anatomic abnormalities.
- MRI of cervical spine for neurologic symptoms.

IMAGING FINDINGS

- Fusion of two or more cervical segments:
  - C2 and C3 and lower cervical fusions are common.
  - Extensive fusions may extend into the upper thoracic spine.
  - Associated scoliosis.
- Omovertebral bones (scapula to vertebra): Best documented with CT.
- Cervical ribs.
- Hemivertebrae.
- Spinal stenosis and basilar impression.
- Syringomyelia (high signal intensity on sagittal and axial T2-weighted [T2W] MR images).
- Intervertebral disk extrusions.

OTHER RECOMMENDED TESTING

- Evoked potential testing to quantify spinal cord and brainstem compromise.
- Collagen vascular disease workup if juvenile rheumatoid arthritis or ankylosing spondylitis is suspected.

DIFFERENTIAL DIAGNOSIS

- Juvenile rheumatoid arthritis.
- Ankylosing spondylitis.
- Previous surgical fusion.
- Diskitis.

TREATMENT

- Avoid:
  - Activities that increase risk of cervical spine trauma, such as contact sports.
  - Extreme cervical spine positioning during anesthesia.
  - Therapeutic manipulation of the cervical spine.
- Modify activity to avoid overuse of the cervical spine.
- Bracing of the cervical spine.
- Surgical treatment indicated if neurologic symptoms progress.

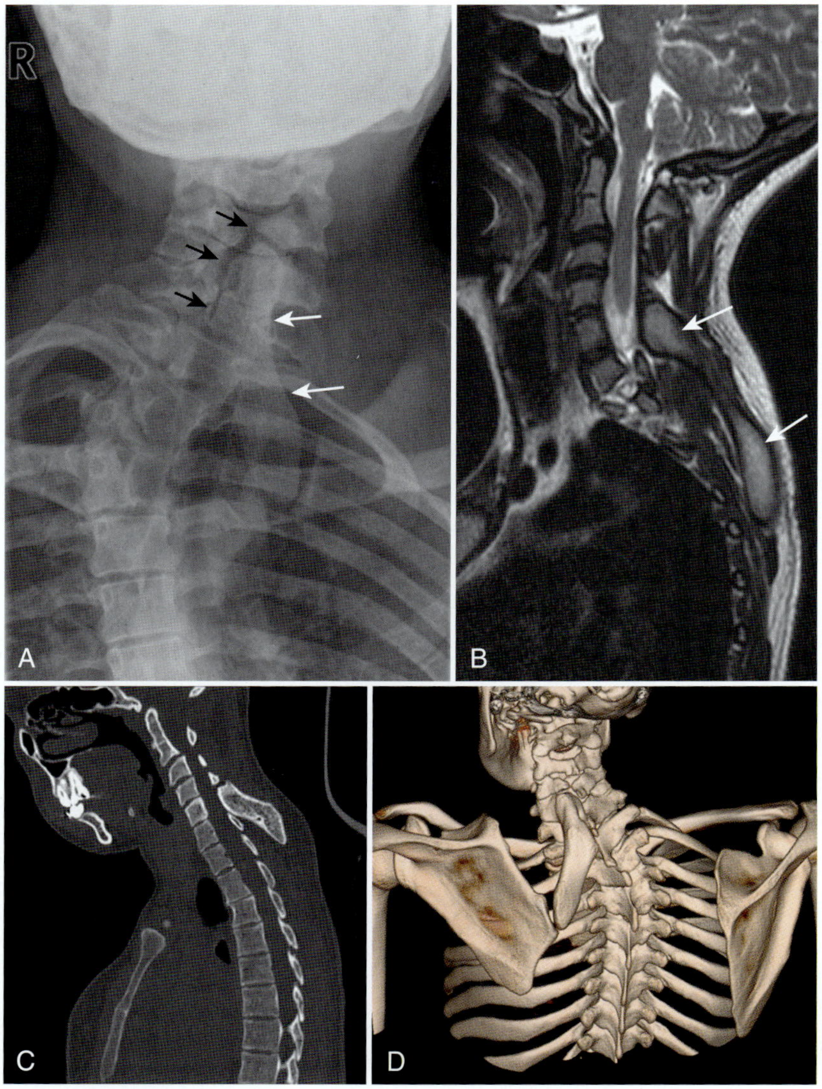

Figure 10.1 Female patient with Klippel-Feil Syndrome. (**A**), An AP radiograph demonstrates a scoliosis with osteogenic anomalies of the cervical and thoracic spine including several bifid spinous processes (*black arrows*). There is also a prominent omovertebral bar (*white arrows*), which articulates with the scapula. (**B**), The omovertebral bar is also seen on this sagittal T2W MR image (*white arrows*). There is no underlying neurologic abnormality. The bony anatomy and relationship of the omovertebral bar to the cervical spine and scapula are best demonstrated on the curved sagittal (**C**) and three-dimensional (**D**) CT scans.

CHAPTER 11

Atlanto-Occipital Abnormalities

DEFINITION

- Congenital anatomic variations of the craniovertebral junction.

SIGNS AND SYMPTOMS

- Gradual onset of cervical spine abnormalities related to instability.
- Posterior occipital headaches that are exacerbated with flexion and/or extension of the cervical spine.
  - May mimic basilar migraine.
- Cervical myelopathy.
- Sudden onset of quadriplegia may rarely occur after seemingly minor trauma.
- Lower cranial nerve abnormalities.
- Gait abnormalities including ataxic gait.
- Vascular symptomatology, including transient ischemic attacks, vertigo, and visual symptomatology, may accompany neurologic signs and symptoms.

DEMOGRAPHICS

- Onset of symptoms often occurs after cervical spine trauma.
- Incidence: Male = Female.

IMAGING RECOMMENDATIONS

- Cervical spine radiography to assess vertebral alignment, the odontoid peg, and the atlanto-occipital articulation.
- MRI for patients with neurologic deficit.
- CT for surgical planning to document anatomy of bony abnormalities.
- CT or MR angiography for vascular symptoms.

IMAGING FINDINGS

- Anterior arch of C1 or lateral masses fused to skull base.
- Frequent association with fusion of C2 and C3.
- High-lying odontoid process of C2, but platybasia and basilar impression are uncommon.
- Rarely, associated fusion of anterior arch of C1 with odontoid process of C2.
- Sagittal and axial T2-weighted (T2W) MR images will identify compression of the cervical cord.

OTHER RECOMMENDED TESTING

- Evoked potential testing to quantify spinal cord and brainstem compromise.

DIFFERENTIAL DIAGNOSIS

- Fracture and/or ligamentous injuries to this area.
- Erosion of the odontoid process by rheumatoid arthritis.
- Acquired basilar impression caused by upward displacement of the occipital condyles.
- Osteopenia secondary to hyperparathyroidism, Paget disease, rickets, or osteogenesis imperfecta.

TREATMENT

- Avoid:
  - Activities that increase the risk of cervical spine trauma, such as contact sports.
  - Extreme cervical spine positioning during anesthesia.
  - Therapeutic manipulation of the cervical spine.
- Modify activity to avoid overuse of cervical spine.
- Bracing of cervical spine.
- Surgical treatment indicated if neurologic symptoms progress.

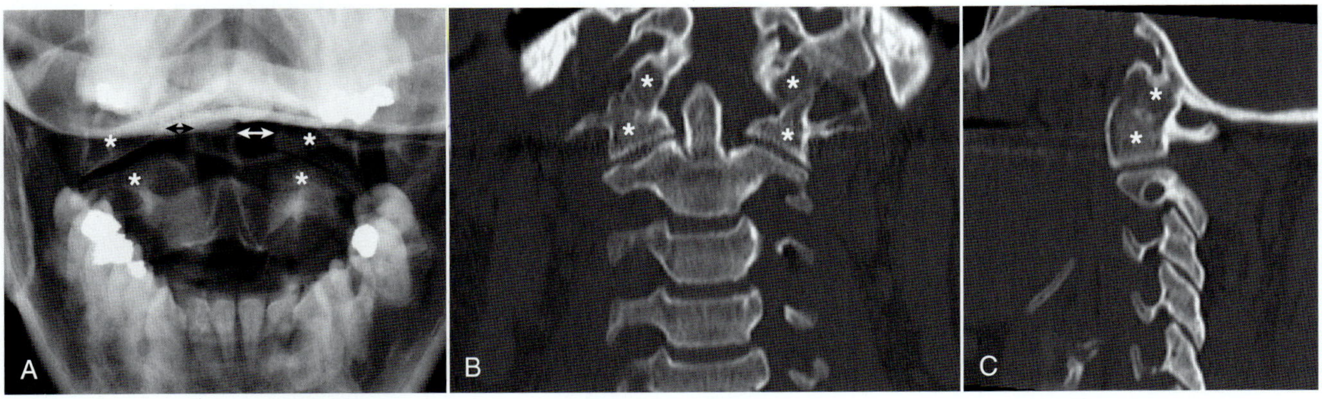

Figure 11.1 (**A**), AP radiograph of C1-C2 in a patient with neck pain. There is asymmetry of the articulation of the lateral masses of C1 and C2 (*asterisks*) as well as asymmetry of the articulation with the lateral masses of C1 and the odontoid peg (*double-ended arrows*). Congenital fusion of the lateral masses (*asterisks*) is demonstrated on the coronal (**B**), and parasagittal (**C**), CT scans.

CHAPTER 12

Hyperextension Injuries of the Cervical Spine

DEFINITION

- Fracture of the posterior elements due to forceful posterior displacement of the head and upper cervical spine, with concomitant disruption of the anterior and posterior longitudinal ligaments and, occasionally, displacement of disc fragments.

SIGNS AND SYMPTOMS

- Severe neck pain following extension trauma to the cervical spine.
- Transient and/or permanent neurologic deficits related to trauma to the cervical spinal cord.
- Symptoms secondary to trauma to the vertebral artery.
- Myelopathic signs and symptoms, especially if post-traumatic syrinx is present.

DEMOGRAPHICS

- Occurs after hyperextension forces are applied to the cervical spine, usually with some element of axial loading.
- Commonly occurs following motor vehicle accidents or sports injuries.

IMAGING RECOMMENDATIONS

- CT is usually the first-line investigation to identify bony injury.
- Three-view radiography if CT not immediately available or for minor injuries.
- MRI for neurologic symptoms and to assess soft tissue ligamentous injury.
- Flexion/extension views may be used to assess for instability in the absence of bony trauma.

IMAGING FINDINGS

- Hangman's fracture of C2 (unstable): Traumatic listhesis of C2 on C3 with bilateral pars interarticularis fractures that may involve the vertebral body.
- Extension teardrop fractures (stable): Small avulsion fractures of anteroinferior vertebral body, usually C2 (differentiate from calcification of anterior longitudinal ligament).
- Hyperextension-dislocation (unstable): Rupture of the anterior longitudinal ligament with minor retrolisthesis but often marked neurologic deficit, usually C4-C5 and C5-C6.
- Other fractures include spinous process fractures and fracture of the posterior arch of C1.
- T2-weighted (T2W) MR images best demonstrate high-signal intensity (SI) acute epidural and prevertebral hematomas.
- Cord contusions have high SI on T2W and gradient echo MR images.
- Bony and ligamentous injuries are assessed with a combination of T1W and T2W with fat saturation (or short T1 inversion recovery [STIR]) MR images.
- Sagittal T2W and axial T2W or gradient echo MR images to exclude traumatic disc herniation.

OTHER RECOMMENDED TESTING

- Angiography of the vertebral arteries to rule out dissection and/or post-traumatic aneurysm.

DIFFERENTIAL DIAGNOSIS

- Vertebral body fracture.
- Clay shoveler fracture due to sudden strong force applied to the ligamentum nuchae.
- Congenital midline cleft abnormality.

TREATMENT

- Immobilization of the cervical spine is the first line of treatment.
- Cervical spinal cord edema should be treated with high-dose corticosteroids.
- Compression of the cervical spinal cord and/or exiting nerve roots will often require emergency surgical decompression.

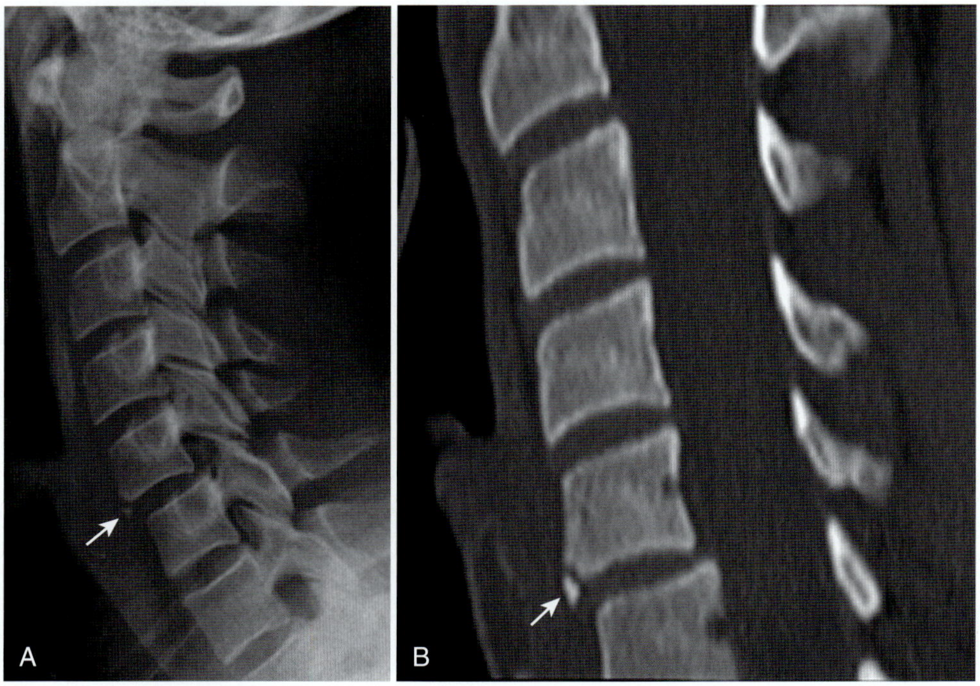

Figure 12.1 (**A**), Lateral radiograph of a patient with a hyperextension injury. There is a small extension teardrop fracture of the anteroinferior margin of C5 (*white arrow*), with minor anterior listhesis. (**B**), The sagittal CT scan also shows the teardrop fracture and anterior listhesis, but no other fractures were demonstrated. Flexion/extension radiographs showed no dynamic instability.

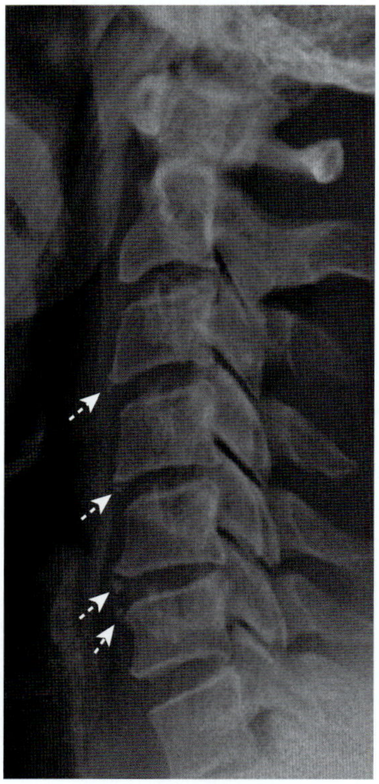

Figure 12.2 Lateral radiograph of a patient with simple axial pain. There are multiple small areas of calcification in the anterior longitudinal ligament (*broken white arrows*), which is associated with early features of disc degeneration and spondylosis. This appearance, when isolated, is important to distinguish from an extension teardrop fracture. If there is any doubt, MRI can be used to exclude ligamentous injury.

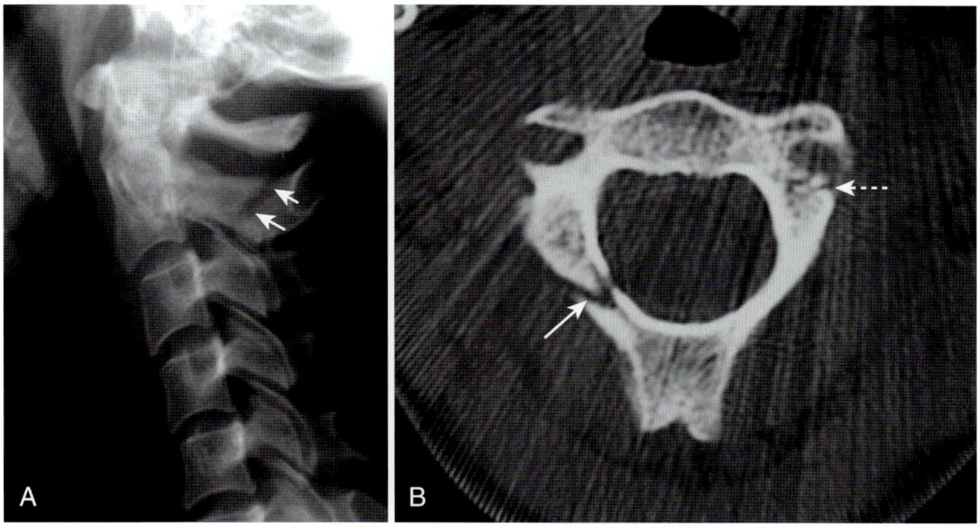

Figure 12.3 (**A**), Lateral radiograph of a patient who attempted suicide by hanging. There is a laminar fracture (*white arrows*), but no listhesis. (**B**), The axial CT scan shows the right-sided laminar fracture, and there is also an incomplete fracture of the base of the left pedicle adjacent to the foramen transversarium (*broken white arrow*). Although no other fractures were identified, the fracture was regarded as potentially unstable and was treated in halo fixation for 6 weeks.

CHAPTER 13

Hyperflexion Injuries of the Cervical Spine

DEFINITION

- Disruption of the posterior and capsular ligaments resulting in anterior subluxation of the vertebra due to extreme flexion forces placed on the cervical spine.

SIGNS AND SYMPTOMS

- Acute onset of neck pain following flexion injury.
- Associated neurologic deficits may be absent, subtle, or catastrophic.
- Myelopathic changes may be present and may be transient or permanent.

DEMOGRAPHICS

- Occurs after hyperflexion forces applied to the cervical spine, usually with some element of axial loading.
- Commonly occurs following motor vehicle accidents or sports injuries.

IMAGING RECOMMENDATIONS

- CT is usually the first-line investigation to identify bony injury.
- Three-view radiography if CT not immediately available or for minor injuries.
- MRI for neurologic symptoms and to assess soft tissue ligamentous injury.
- Flexion/extension views may be used to assess for instability in the absence of bony trauma.

IMAGING FINDINGS

- Odontoid peg fractures (unstable—types II and III).
- The most common type is type II at the base of the peg with a high incidence of non-union.
- Type III fractures extend into the vertebral body of C2, and non-union is less common.
- Forward listhesis is associated with instability.
- Facet dislocation:
  - Unilateral (stable): Minimal listhesis and usually no neurologic defect. May be associated with articular process fracture.
  - Bilateral (unstable): At least 50% listhesis with neurologic deficit and, often, articular process fractures.
- Flexion teardrop fractures (unstable): Lower cervical spine most commonly affected.
  - Widened interspinous distance with fractures through lamina and pars, large anteroinferior vertebral body fracture, and listhesis.
- Atlanto-occipital dislocation has a high incidence of mortality.
- T2-weighted (T2W) MR images best demonstrate high-signal-intensity acute epidural and prevertebral hematomas.
- Cord contusions have high signal intensity on T2W and gradient-echo MR images.
- Bony and ligamentous injuries are assessed with a combination of T1W and T2W fat saturation (or short T1 inversion recovery [STIR]) images.
- Sagittal T2W and axial T2W or gradient-echo MR images to exclude traumatic disc herniation.

OTHER RECOMMENDED TESTING

- Angiography of the vertebral arteries to rule out dissection and/or post-traumatic aneurysm.

DIFFERENTIAL DIAGNOSIS

- Cervical strain.
- Whiplash fracture associated with concurrent hyperextension injury commonly seen with acceleration/deceleration injuries.
- Flexion/rotation injury with associated fracture of cervical facets.
- Burst fracture.

TREATMENT

- Immobilization of the cervical spine is the first line of treatment.
- Cervical spinal cord edema should be treated with high-dose corticosteroids.
- Compression of the cervical spinal cord and/or exiting nerve roots will often require emergency surgical decompression.

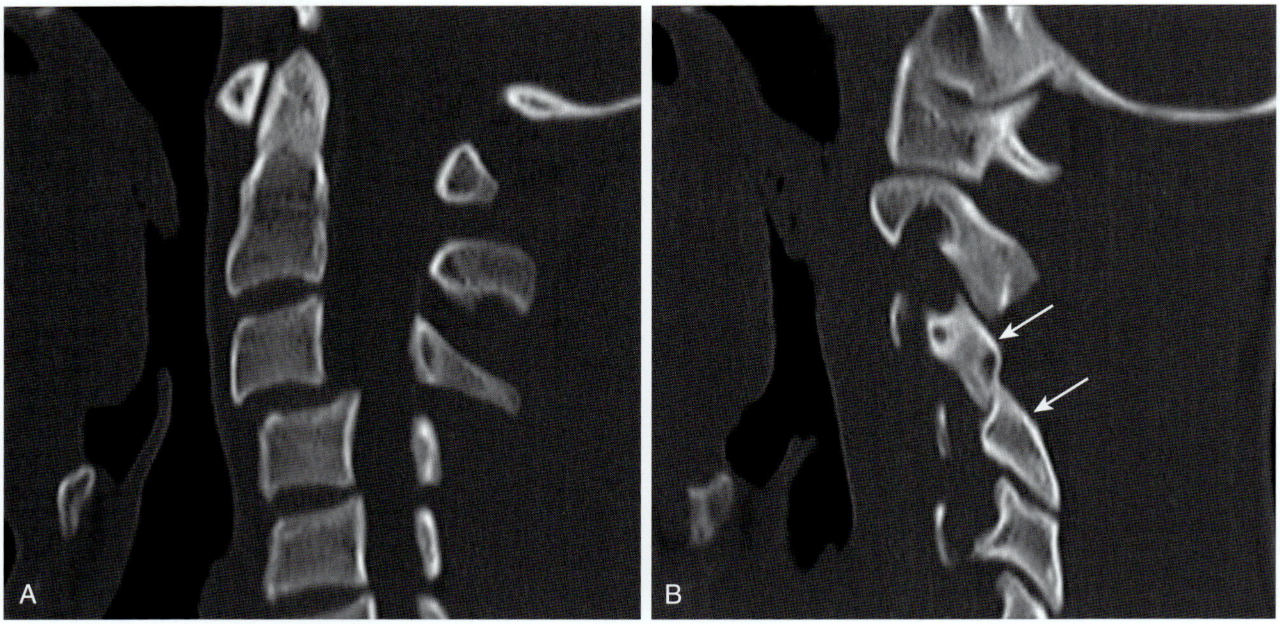

Figure 13.1 Patient with acute hyperflexion injury of the cervical spine. (**A**), Midline sagittal CT scan shows forward listhesis of C3 on C4. (**B**), Parasagittal CT scan shows unilateral facetal dislocation on the left side (*white arrows*). See also Figure 13.2.

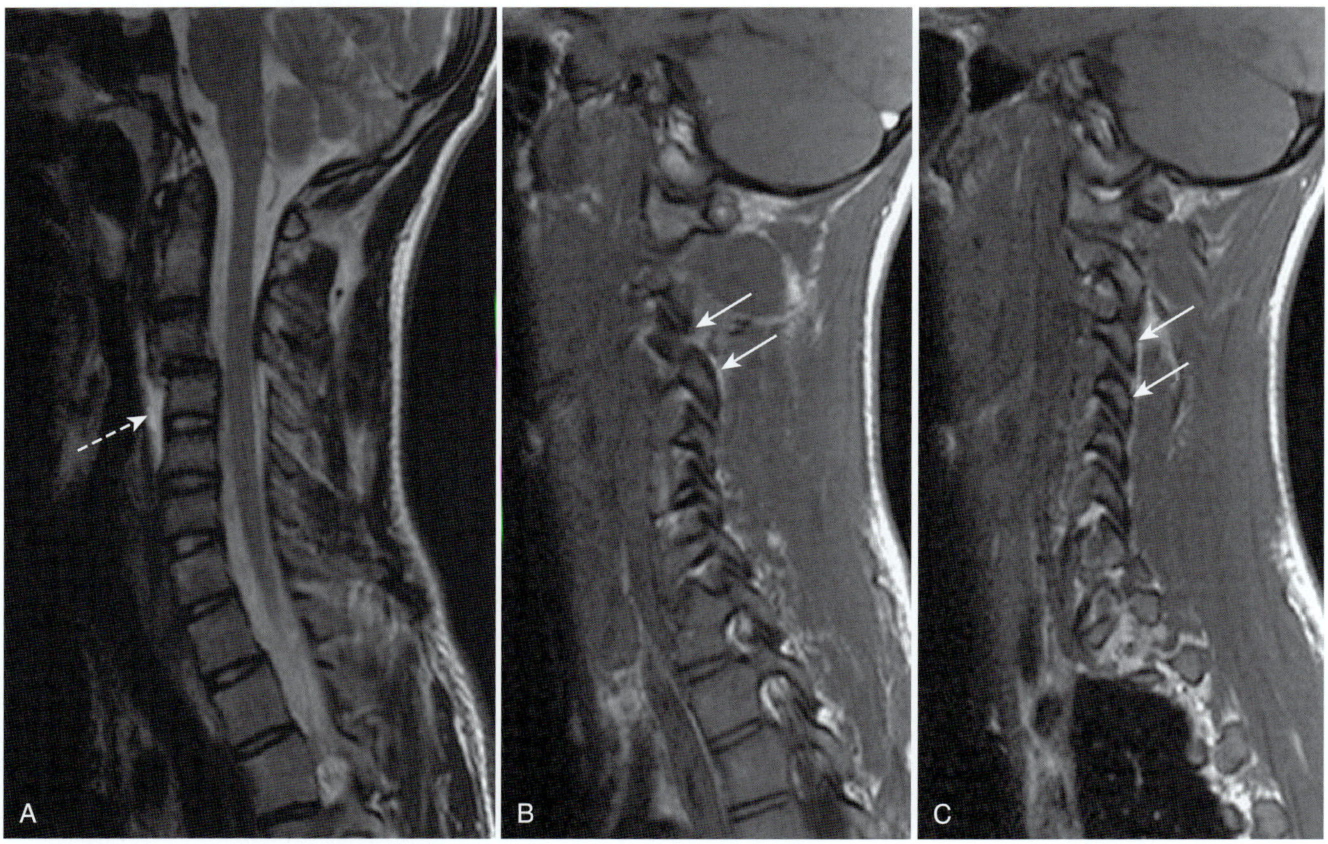

Figure 13.2 (**A**), Sagittal STIR MR image of the same patient as in Figure 13.1 shows the listhesis without cord compression or epidural hematoma, although there is a small prevertebral hematoma (*broken white arrow*). (**B**), Left parasagittal T1W MR image also demonstrates the facetal dislocation at C3-C4 (*white arrows*). (**C**), There is normal facet alignment on the right side.

CHAPTER 14

Degenerative Intervertebral Disc Disease of the Cervical Spine

DEFINITION

- Complex biochemical changes leading to morphologic and functional changes of the discovertebral complex due to degeneration of the intervertebral disc.

SIGNS AND SYMPTOMS

- Usually present as part of the normal aging process.
- Usually asymptomatic.
- May manifest as cervicalgia or radiculopathy after seemingly minor trauma.
- Neurologic findings may be normal or may be positive for sensory, motor, and/or reflex changes.
- Range of motion of the cervical spine may be decreased.
- Flexion, extension, rotation, or lateral bending may exacerbate symptomatology.

DEMOGRAPHICS

- Peak occurrence in the fourth through sixth decades of life.
- May occur at an earlier age following trauma.
- Incidence: Male = Female.
- Occurs in almost all patients by the sixth decade.
- There may be a genetic predisposition.

IMAGING RECOMMENDATIONS

- Routine imaging for cervicalgia alone is of limited value.
- MRI is the primary investigation of choice for patients with neurologic symptoms or "red flags."
- Radiographs are of limited value and required only in selected cases.

IMAGING FINDINGS

- Earliest signs are low signal intensity within the disc on T2-weighted (T2W) MRI due to disc dehydration.
- MRI or radiography will demonstrate progressive disc space narrowing.
- Modic vertebral end-plate changes may be seen on MRI: edema, fatty replacement, and sclerosis.
- Spondylosis frequently accompanies disc degeneration, with osteophytes, longitudinal ligament calcification, and uncovertebral hypertrophy.
- Facet arthropathy also occurs in association with disc degeneration.

OTHER RECOMMENDED TESTING

- Electromyography and nerve conduction velocity testing are indicated if radiculopathy is present.
- Provocative discography may serve as a useful diagnostic tool to determine whether a specific disc is serving as a nidus for the patient's pain.

DIFFERENTIAL DIAGNOSIS

- Discitis.
- Reiter syndrome.
- Hemodialysis spondyloarthropathy.

TREATMENT

- Conservative treatment consisting of local heat, cold, simple analgesics, and nonsteroidal anti-inflammatory agents will improve symptoms in many cases.
- Physical therapy, including gentle stretching, range-of-motion exercises, deep heat modalities, and stretch and spray, may be beneficial in selected patients.
- Epidural blocks will provide symptomatic relief if conservative therapy fails or if the pain is limiting activities of daily living.
- Osteopathic or chiropractic manipulation may provide symptomatic relief in selected patients.
- Surgery may be required in patients with persistent pain or progressive neurologic symptoms.

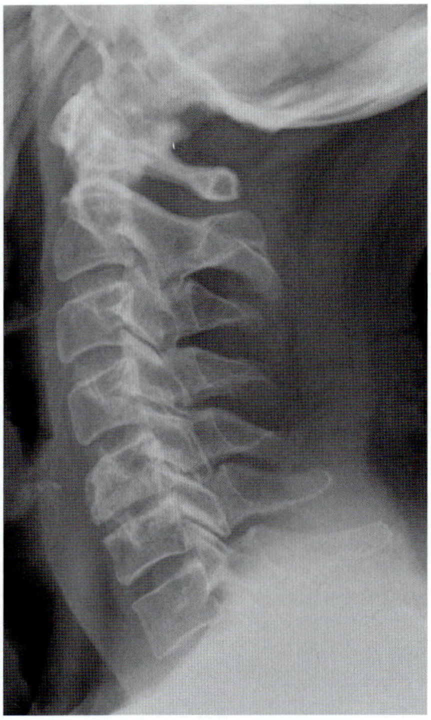

Figure 14.1 Lateral radiograph of a young man with neck pain. There is disc space narrowing at C5-C6 due to disc degeneration without other features of spondylosis.

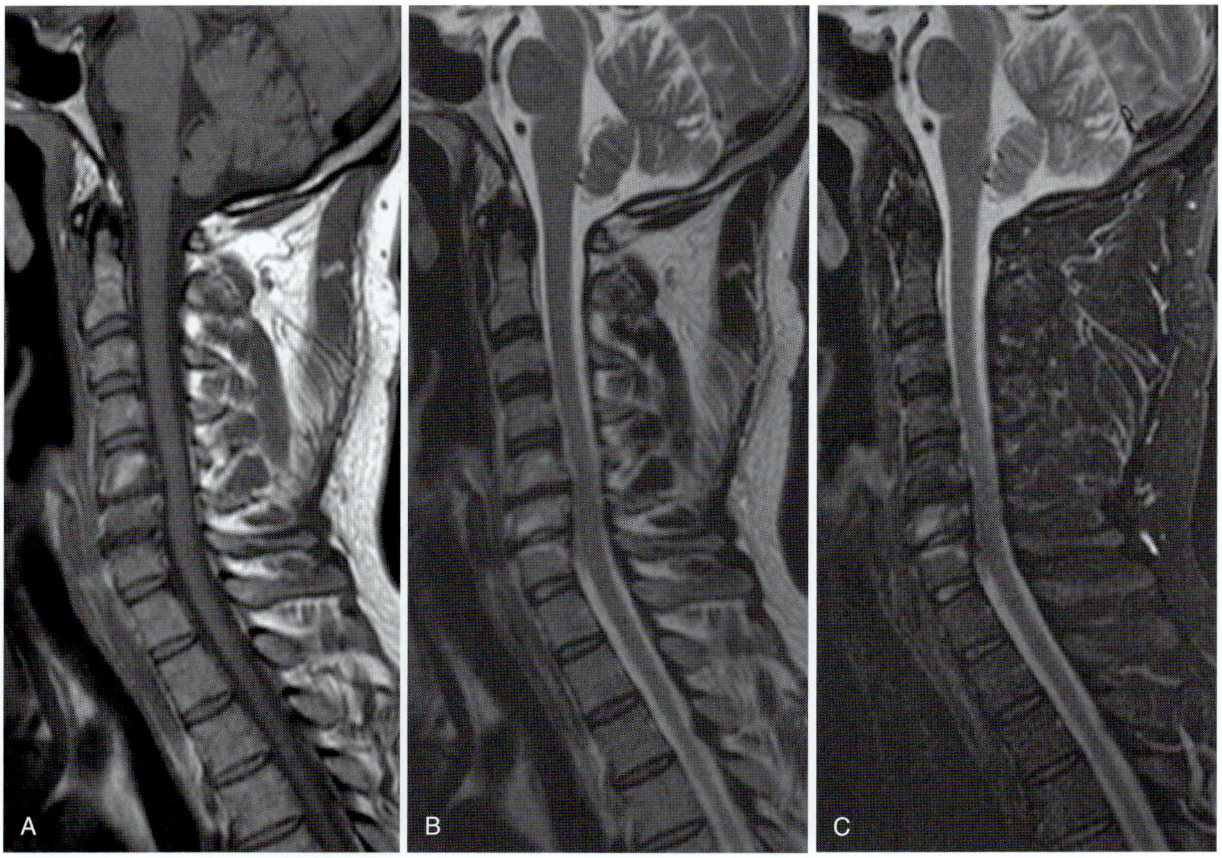

Figure 14.2 Sagittal T1W (**A**), T2W (**B**), and short T1 inversion recovery (STIR) (**C**), MR images of the cervical spine in a middle-aged woman with neck pain. The cervical intervertebral discs have low signal intensity on the T2W MR images because of disc dehydration (note the normal high signal intensity of the dorsal intervertebral discs). In addition, the discs at C5-C6 and C6-C7 are narrowed with a variety of fatty and edematous Modic changes in the vertebral end plates. There is an associated minor kyphosis. No disc protrusion or cord compression is demonstrated.

CHAPTER 15

Intervertebral Disc Bulging of the Cervical Spine

DEFINITION

- Nonfocal generalized extension of the intervertebral disc beyond the margins of the vertebra.

SIGNS AND SYMPTOMS

- Usually present as part of the normal aging process.
- Usually asymptomatic.
- May manifest as cervicalgia or radiculopathy after seemingly minor trauma.
- Neurologic findings may be normal or may be positive for sensory, motor, and/or reflex changes.
- Range of motion of the cervical spine may be decreased.
- Flexion, extension, rotation, or lateral bending may exacerbate symptomatology.

DEMOGRAPHICS

- May occur following acute trauma.
- Incidence increases with age.
- Repeated microtrauma to disc by repetitive activities may increase incidence.
- There may be a genetic predisposition.

IMAGING RECOMMENDATIONS

- Routine imaging for cervicalgia alone is of limited value.
- MRI is the primary investigation of choice for patients with neurologic symptoms or "red flags."
- CT myelography is an alternative when MRI is contraindicated and if there are neurologic symptoms.
- Radiographs are of limited value and required only in selected cases.

IMAGING FINDINGS

- The affected disc is usually degenerate and has low signal intensity on T2-weighted (T2W) MRI sequences.
- There may be associated changes characteristic of spondylosis.
- Chronic disc bulges may be difficult to distinguish from osteophytes (sometimes referred to as disc/osteophyte complex).
- Axial images may show compression of the thecal sac, effacement of the cerebrospinal fluid space, and compression and flattening of the spinal cord.
- Myelopathy is evident as a focal area of high signal intensity within the cord adjacent to the level of compression.

OTHER RECOMMENDED TESTING

- Electromyography and nerve conduction velocity testing are indicated if radiculopathy is present.
- Provocative discography may serve as a useful diagnostic tool to determine whether a specific disc is serving as a nidus for the pain.

DIFFERENTIAL DIAGNOSIS

- Disc protrusion.
- Ossification of the posterior longitudinal ligament (OPLL syndrome).
- Osteophyte of vertebral end plate.

TREATMENT

- Conservative treatment consisting of local heat, cold, simple analgesics, and nonsteroidal anti-inflammatory agents will improve symptoms in many cases,
- Physical therapy, including gentle stretching, range-of-motion exercises, deep heat modalities, and stretch and spray, may be beneficial in selected patients.
- Epidural blocks will provide symptomatic relief if conservative therapy fails or if the pain is limiting activities of daily living.
- Osteopathic or chiropractic manipulation may provide symptomatic relief in selected patients.
- Surgery may be required for persistent pain or progressive neurologic symptoms.

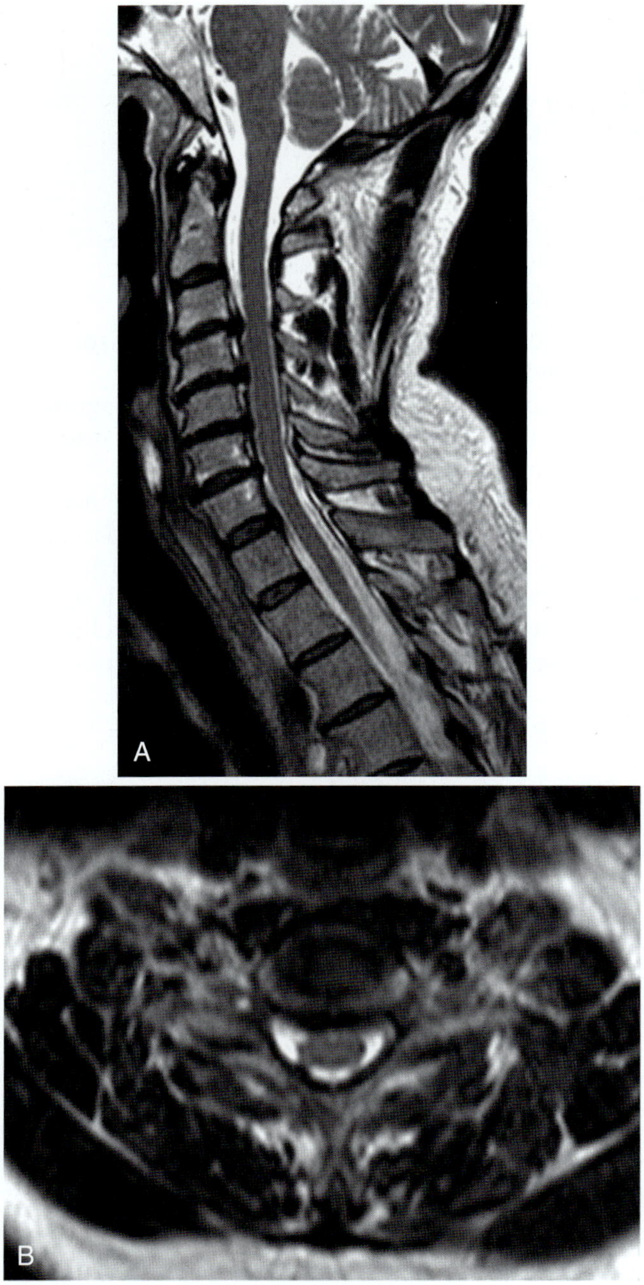

Figure 15.1 (**A**), Sagittal T2W MR image demonstrating multilevel disc degeneration with low–signal intensity discs. There is also multilevel disc bulging, and several of the disc bulges lie in contact with the anterior aspect of the cervical corc. (**B**), However, on the axial T2W MR image, there is no significant central canal stenosis or cord compression.

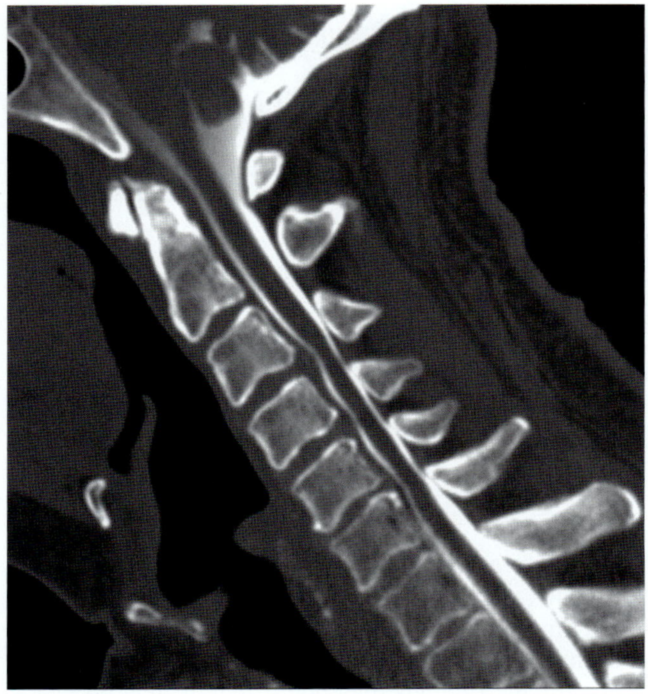

Figure 15.2 Sagittal CT myelogram demonstrating disc bulging that is most marked at the C3-C4 level.

CHAPTER 16

Intervertebral Disc Herniation of the Cervical Spine

DEFINITION

- Focal extension of the intervertebral disc of less than 50% of the disc circumference beyond the margins of the vertebra.

SIGNS AND SYMPTOMS

- Level, size and location—posterior, anterior, lateral, etc.—of disc herniation will determine the clinical presentation.
- Neck pain is the most common symptom.
- Decreased range of motion of the cervical spine with associated muscle spasm is also common.
- Pain may radiate in a dermatomal or nondermatomal pattern.
- Motor, sensory, and reflex changes may occur.
- Central disc herniation may cause compression of the cervical spinal cord with resultant cervical myelopathy.

DEMOGRAPHICS

- May occur following acute trauma.
- Incidence increases with age, and peak occurrence is between the fourth and fifth decades of life.
- Repeated microtrauma to disc by repetitive activities may increase incidence.
- There may be a genetic predisposition.
- Slight male preponderance.

IMAGING RECOMMENDATIONS

- MRI is the primary investigation of choice.
- CT is of limited value but may be used to demonstrate bony abnormalities such as uncovertebral osteophytes.
- CT myelography is an alternative when MRI is contraindicated.
- Radiographs are of limited value and required only in selected cases.

IMAGING FINDINGS

- Acute "soft" disc protrusion has high signal intensity (SI) on T2-weighted (T2W) sequences.
- Chronic "hard" disc protrusions have low SI on T2W sequences and are difficult to distinguish from osteophytes (sometimes referred to as disc/osteophyte complex).
- Axial images may show compression of the thecal sac, effacement of the cerebrospinal fluid space, and compression and flattening of the spinal cord.
- Myelopathy is evident as a focal area of high SI within the cord adjacent to the level of compression.
- Disc material may extend into the exit canal on axial images.
- MR myelography or CT myelography demonstrates the compression of the thecal sac and nerve root sleeve "cutoff."

OTHER RECOMMENDED TESTING

- Electromyography and nerve conduction velocity testing are indicated if radiculopathy is present.
- Provocative discography may serve as a useful diagnostic tool to determine whether a specific disc is serving as a nidus for the pain.

DIFFERENTIAL DIAGNOSIS

- Epidural abscess.
- Osteophyte of vertebral end plate.
- Epidural hematoma.
- Neoplasm.
- Ossification of the posterior longitudinal ligament (OPLL syndrome).

TREATMENT

- Conservative treatment, consisting of local heat, cold, simple analgesics, and nonsteroidal anti-inflammatory agents, will improve symptoms in many cases.
- Physical therapy, including gentle stretching, range-of-motion exercises, deep heat modalities, and stretch and spray, may be beneficial in selected patients.
- Epidural blocks will provide symptomatic relief if conservative therapy fails or the pain is limiting activities of daily living.
- Osteopathic or chiropractic manipulation may provide symptomatic relief in selected patients.
- Surgery may be required for persistent pain or progressive neurologic symptoms.

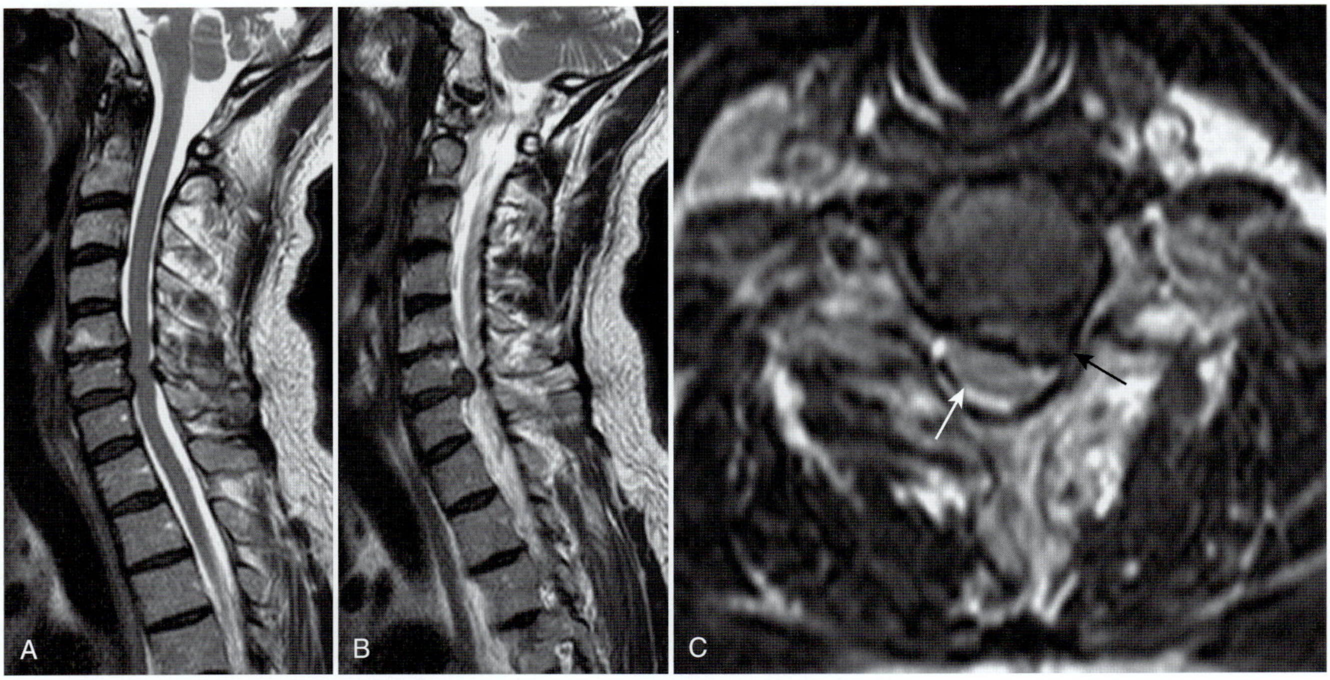

Figure 16.1 MR images of a patient with left-sided radicular symptoms. (**A**), The midline sagittal T2W MR image shows disc degeneration at C5-C6 with disc space narrowing. There is less marked disc narrowing at C6-C7, but there is also a posterior disc herniation, which is much more prominent on the parasagittal T2W MR image (**B**). (**C**), The axial T2W MR image demonstrates a large paracentral disc herniation (*black arrow*) that is compresing the cervical cord (*white arrow*).

CHAPTER 17

Facet Arthropathy of the Cervical Spine

DEFINITION

- Degenerative osteoarthritis of the synovium-lined zygapophyseal joints.

SIGNS AND SYMPTOMS

- May be asymptomatic.
- Onset may occur following seemingly minor trauma.
- Neck pain made worse with movement of the cervical spine.
- Worse after rest.
- Pain typically radiates into the shoulders and intrascapular region in a nondermatomal pattern.
- Pain can be made worse with axial loading combined with range of motion of the cervical spine.

DEMOGRAPHICS

- Incidence: Male = Female.
- Onset between the second and third decades of life.
- Universal finding after the fifth decade.
- Genetic predisposition possible.

IMAGING RECOMMENDATIONS

- Routine imaging for cervicalgia alone is of limited value.
- MRI is the primary investigation of choice for patients with neurologic symptoms or "red flags."
- Oblique radiographs or CT may be used in selective cases to identify the specific affected facet joint.

IMAGING FINDINGS

- Sclerosis and bony overgrowth of facets on radiography and CT.
- Secondary spondylolisthesis may develop.
- Low–signal intensity (SI) bony overgrowth, ligament hypertrophy, and ligament buckling are seen on sagittal and axial MR images.
- Joint effusions are occasionally seen with high SI on T2-weighted (T2W) MR images.

OTHER RECOMMENDED TESTING

- Intra-articular facet injection to ascertain whether a specific facet joint is the nidus of the pain.

DIFFERENTIAL DIAGNOSIS

- Inflammatory arthritides, especially rheumatoid arthritis.
- Septic facet joint.
- Healing facet joint fracture.
- Neoplasm.
- Paget disease.
- Myositis ossificans.

TREATMENT

- Conservative treatment consisting of local heat, cold, simple analgesics, and nonsteroidal anti-inflammatory agents will improve symptoms in many cases.
- Physical therapy, including gentle stretching, range-of-motion exercises, deep heat modalities, and stretch and spray, may be beneficial in selected patients.
- Facet blocks with local anesthetic and steroid will provide symptomatic relief if conservative therapy fails or the pain is limiting activities of daily living.
- Osteopathic or chiropractic manipulation may provide symptomatic relief in selected patients.
- Surgery may be required for persistent pain or progressive neurologic symptoms.

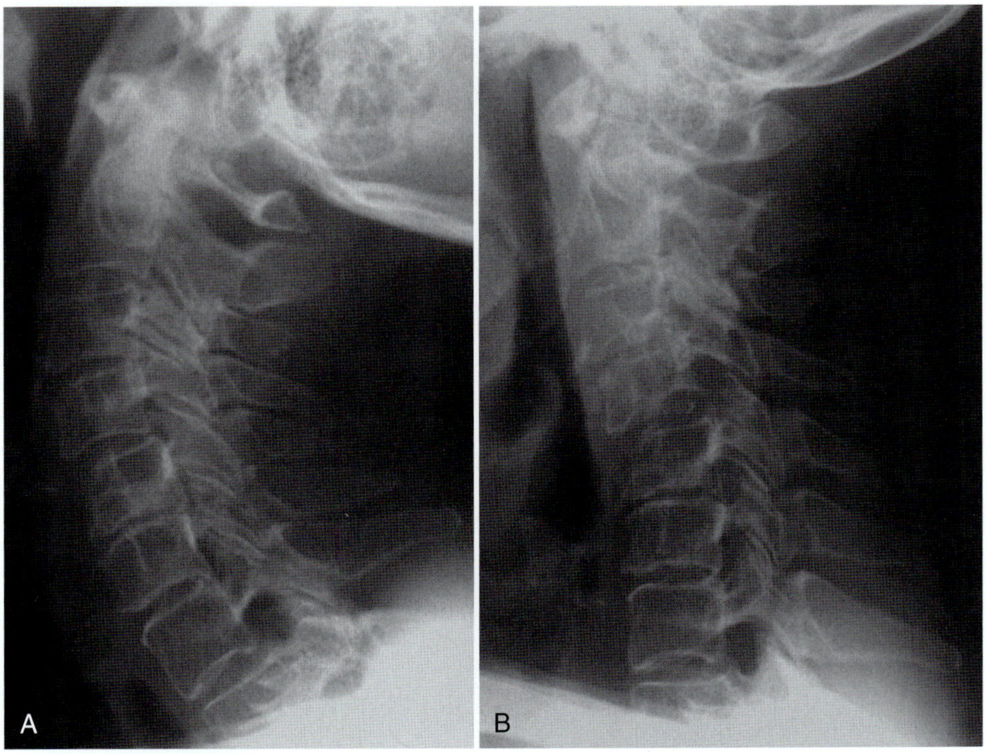

Figure 17.1 Lateral radiographs of the cervical spine in extension (**A**), and flexion (**B**). There is minor spondylolisthesis at C4-C5, which is accentuated in flexion because of instability secondary to facet arthropathy. Note also the disc degeneration with disc space narrowing at C5-C6.

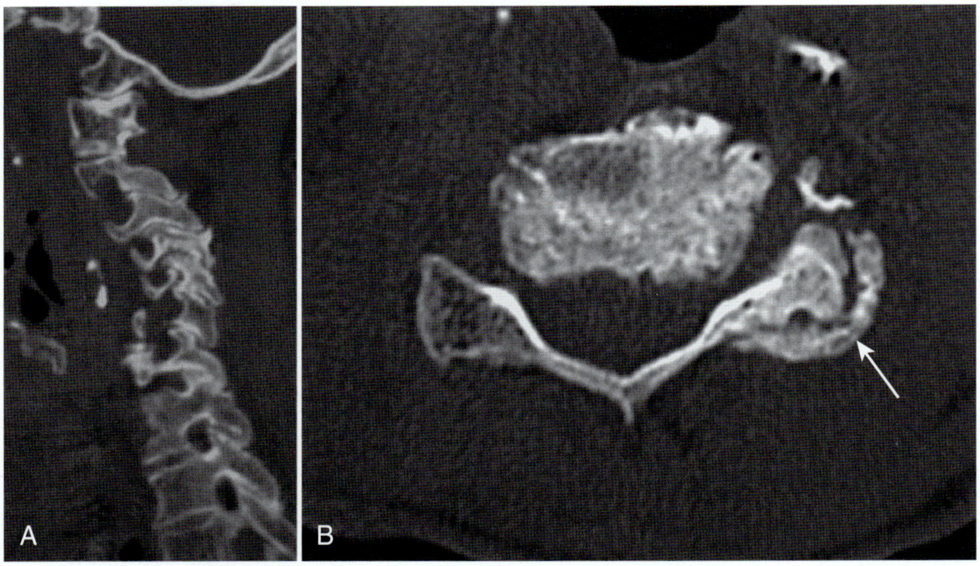

Figure 17.2 Sagittal (**A**), and axial (**B**), CT scans of the cervical spine in a patient with severe facet arthropathy. There are sclerosis and osteophyte formation. The bony overgrowth is best demonstrated on the axial scan (*white arrow*).

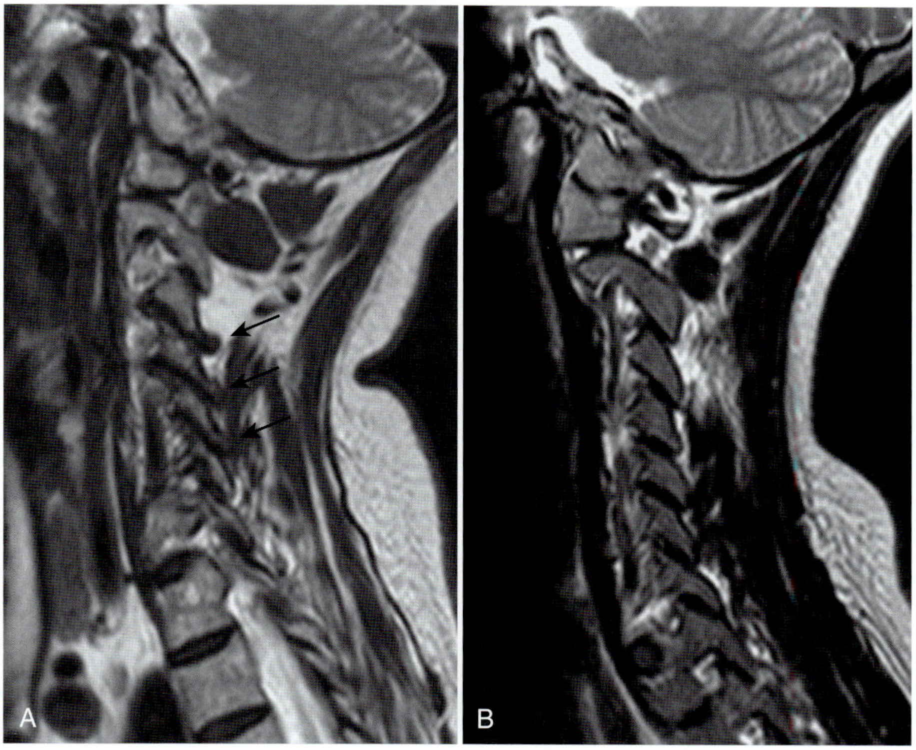

Figure 17.3 (**A**), Parasagittal T2W MR image of a patient with facet arthropathy. There is clear evidence of subchondral sclerosis, and osteophytes are present posteriorly (*black arrows*). (**B**), Compare **A**, with normal facet joints on this T2W MR image from another patient.

CHAPTER 18

Acquired Spinal Stenosis of the Cervical Spine

DEFINITION

- Narrowing of the cervical spinal canal and associated neuroforamina due to degenerative changes.

SIGNS AND SYMPTOMS

- In the absence of trauma, onset of symptoms is insidious.
- Gradual and subtle onset of cervical myelopathy.
- Neck pain with radicular and nonradicular radiation of pain.
- Upper extremity numbness, weakness, and reflex changes progressing to spastic paresis.
- Loss of proprioception and vibratory sensation.
- Ataxic, spastic gait.
- Hyperreflexia.
- Pathologic reflexes (e.g., Babinski reflex) present.
- Presence of Lhermitte sign.
- Bowel and bladder symptomatology.
- Central spinal cord fibers may be more severely affected, so that upper extremity symptoms are worse than lower extremity symptoms initially.
- More sudden onset of symptoms following trauma to the cervical spine.

DEMOGRAPHICS

- Peak age at onset in the fifth decade.
- Incidence: Male > Female.

IMAGING RECOMMENDATIONS

- MRI is the primary investigation of choice.
- CT myelography is an alternative when MRI is contraindicated.
- Radiographs are of limited value and required in only selected cases.

IMAGING FINDINGS

- Widespread spondylosis and disc degeneration.
- Cervical kyphosis and degenerative listhesis are common.
- Stenosis results from a combination of posterior disc/osteophyte complex, listhesis, and facet and ligamentous hypertrophy.
- Foraminal stenosis results from a combination of uncovertebral hypertrophy, lateral disc/osteophyte complex, and facet hypertrophy.
- Axial T2-weighted (T2W) MR images show effacement of the cerebrospinal fluid signal within the thecal sac, with compression and flattening of the spinal cord or narrowing of the exit foramen.
- Myelopathy is evident as a focal area of high signal intensity within the cord adjacent to the level of compression on T2W MR images.
- Chronic myelopathy may result in syrinx formation.

OTHER RECOMMENDED TESTING

- Electromyography and nerve conduction velocity testing are indicated if radiculopathy is present and to rule out amyotrophic lateral sclerosis.
- Evoked potential testing to quantify spinal cord compromise.

DIFFERENTIAL DIAGNOSIS

- Upper motor neuron disease (e.g., amyotrophic lateral sclerosis).
- Ossification of the posterior longitudinal ligament (OPLL syndrome).
- Syrinx.
- Multiple sclerosis.
- Neoplasms of the cervical spinal cord and/or surrounding structures.

TREATMENT

- Avoid:
  - Activities that increase risk of cervical spine trauma, such as contact sports.
  - Extreme cervical spine positioning during anesthesia.
  - Therapeutic manipulation of the cervical spine.
- Modify activity to avoid overuse of cervical spine.
- Conservative treatment consisting of local heat, cold, simple analgesics, and nonsteroidal anti-inflammatory agents will improve symptoms in many cases.

- Physical therapy, including gentle stretching and gentle range-of-motion exercises.
- Epidural blocks will provide symptomatic relief if conservative therapy fails or the pain is limiting activities of daily living.
- Cervical spine immobilization with a soft cervical collar.
- Surgical treatment indicated if neurologic symptoms progress.

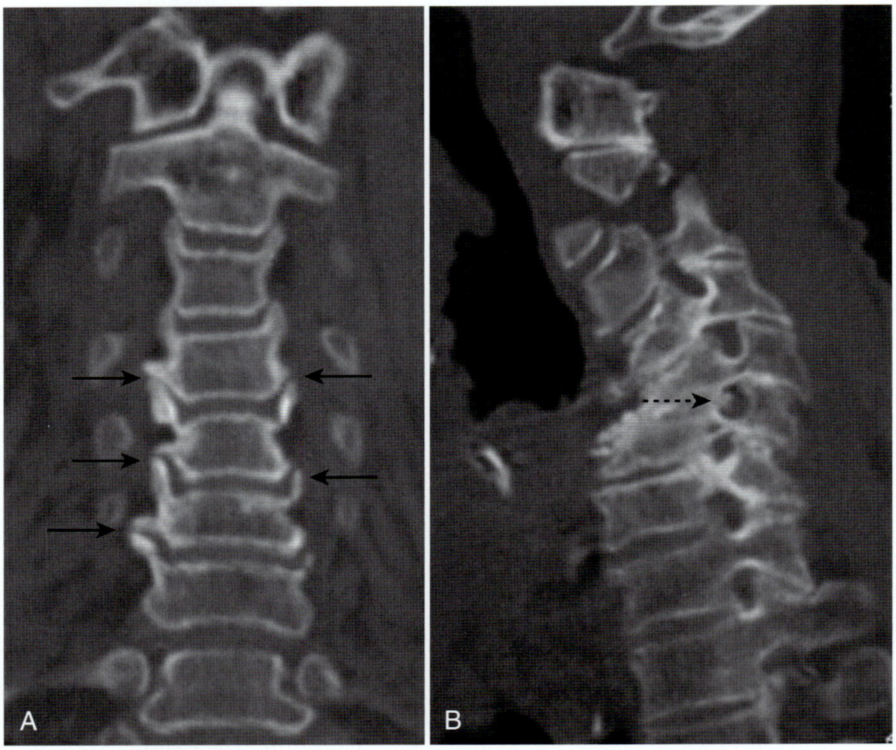

Figure 18.1 (**A**), Coronal CT scan demonstrating lateral uncovertebral osteophytes (*black arrows*). (**B**), Sagittal CT scan illustrating an osteophyte impinging the exit canal (*broken arrow*).

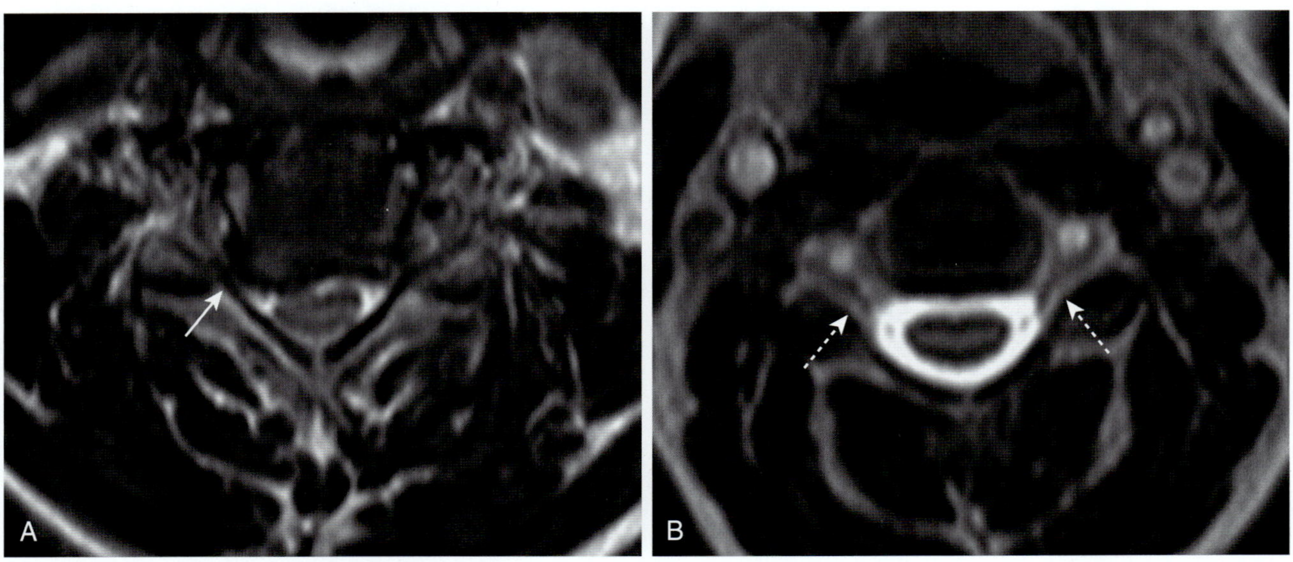

Figure 18.2 (**A**), Axial T2W MR image of bilateral foraminal stenosis that is most marked on the right side (*white arrow*). Compare with the axial T2W MR image (**B**), from a patient with normal exit canals (*broken white arrows*).

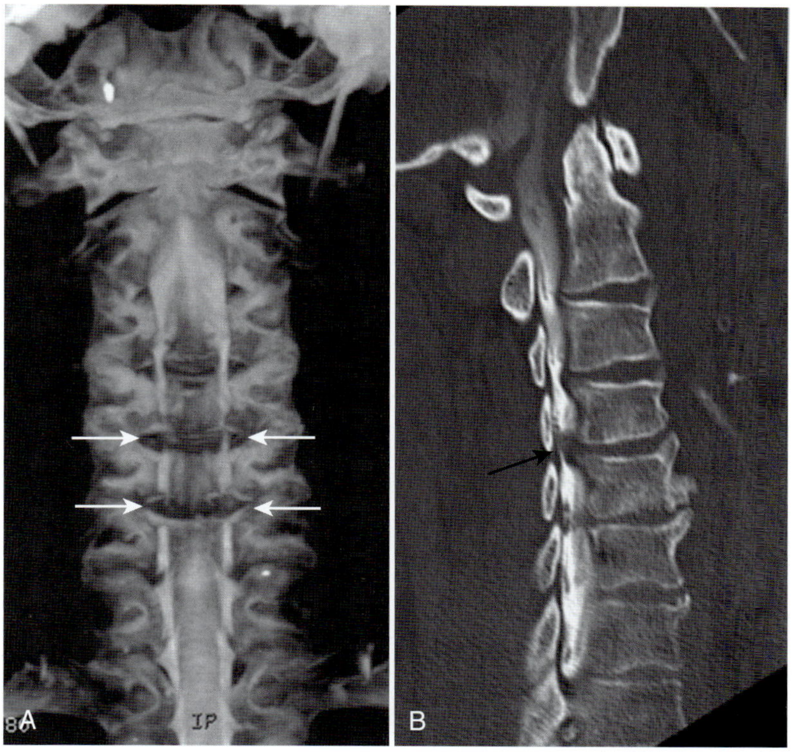

Figure 18.3 (A), Coronal CT myelogram demonstrating bilateral nerve root cutoff due to exit canal stenosis at two levels (*white arrows*). (B), The oblique sagittal image also shows the lateral disc/osteophyte complex (*black arrow*).

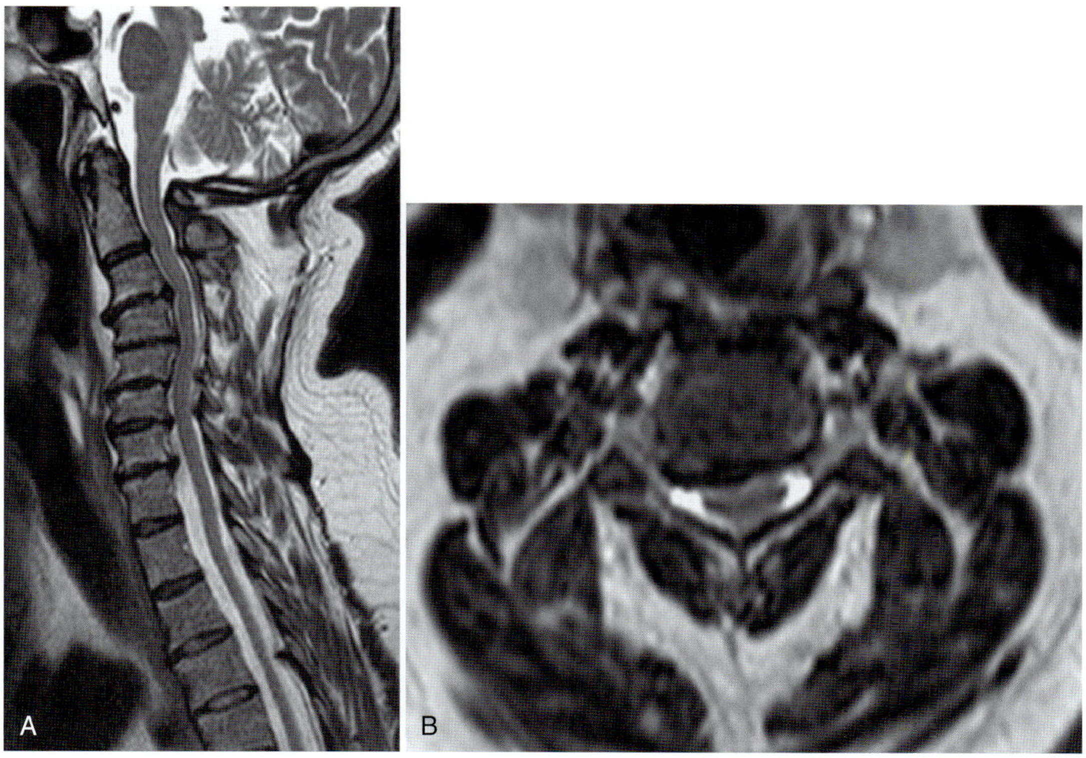

Figure 18.4 (A), Sagittal T2W MR image of a patient with cervical spondylosis and upper motor neuron symptoms. There are multilevel disc degeneration and spondylosis with multilevel disc bulging. There is associated kyphosis. (B), The axial T2W MR image demonstrates prominent central canal stenosis with flattening and compression of the cervical cord. However, there is no cord myelopathy present, and SI within the cervical cord is normal.

CHAPTER 19

OPLL Syndrome

DEFINITION

- Ossification within the posterior longitudinal ligament (PLL) related to an abnormal chromosome 6 XI collagen (alpha) 2 gene.

SIGNS AND SYMPTOMS

- Often an incidental finding in otherwise asymptomatic patients.
- In the absence of trauma, onset of symptoms is insidious.
- Gradual and subtle onset of cervical myelopathy.
- Neck pain with radicular and nonradicular radiation of pain.
- Upper extremity numbness, weakness, and reflex changes progressing to spastic paresis.
- Loss of proprioception and vibratory sensation.
- Ataxic, spastic gait.
- Hyperreflexia.
- Pathologic reflexes (e.g., Babinski reflex) present.
- Presence of Lhermitte sign.
- Bowel and bladder symptomatology.
- More sudden onset of symptoms following trauma to the cervical spine.

DEMOGRAPHICS

- Peak age at onset in the fifth decade of life.
- Incidence: Male > Female.
- Markedly higher incidence in Japanese persons.
- Overall higher incidence in non-Japanese Asians than in white persons.

IMAGING RECOMMENDATIONS

- Radiography and CT to document the extent of ligament ossification and bony central canal stenosis.
- MRI for symptoms of cervical stenosis and myelopathy.

IMAGING FINDINGS

- Dense ossified plaque of PLL.
- Occurs over several vertebral segments:
  - C3-C5 most common.
  - Thoracic spine may be involved.
- Ossification confined to posterior vertebral body wall or continuous across annulus of inter vertebral disc.
- Disc height preserved.
- Anterior osteophytes may be present.
- Ossification may involve other interspinal ligaments (e.g., ligamentum flavum).
- MRI:
  - Low-signal intensity (SI) ossification in PLL on T1-weighted (T1W) and T2W MR images.
  - Central canal stenosis.
  - Compression of the cervical cord.
  - Myelopathy with high SI within the cord on T2W MR images.

OTHER RECOMMENDED TESTING

- Electromyography and nerve conduction velocity testing are indicated if radiculopathy is present and to rule out amyotrophic lateral sclerosis.
- Evoked potential testing to quantify spinal cord compromise.

DIFFERENTIAL DIAGNOSIS

- Upper motor neuron disease (e.g., amyotrophic lateral sclerosis).
- Spondylosis.
- Calcified herniated cervical intervertebral disc.
- Syrinx.
- Multiple sclerosis.
- Meningioma.
- Other neoplasms of the cervical spinal cord and/or surrounding structures.
- Cervical epidural calcification due to hemodialysis.

TREATMENT

- Avoid:
  - Activities that increase the risk of cervical spine trauma, such as contact sports.
  - Extreme cervical spine positioning during anesthesia.
  - Therapeutic manipulation of the cervical spine.

- Modify activity to avoid overuse of the cervical spine.
- Conservative treatment consisting of local heat, cold, simple analgesics, and nonsteroidal anti-inflammatory agents will improve symptoms in many cases.
- Physical therapy, including gentle stretching and gentle range-of-motion exercises.
- Epidural blocks will provide symptomatic relief if conservative therapy fails or the pain is limiting activities of daily living.
- Cervical spine immobilization with a soft cervical collar.
- Surgical treatment indicated if neurologic symptoms progress or for critical cervical spinal stenosis (canal size of < 6 mm).

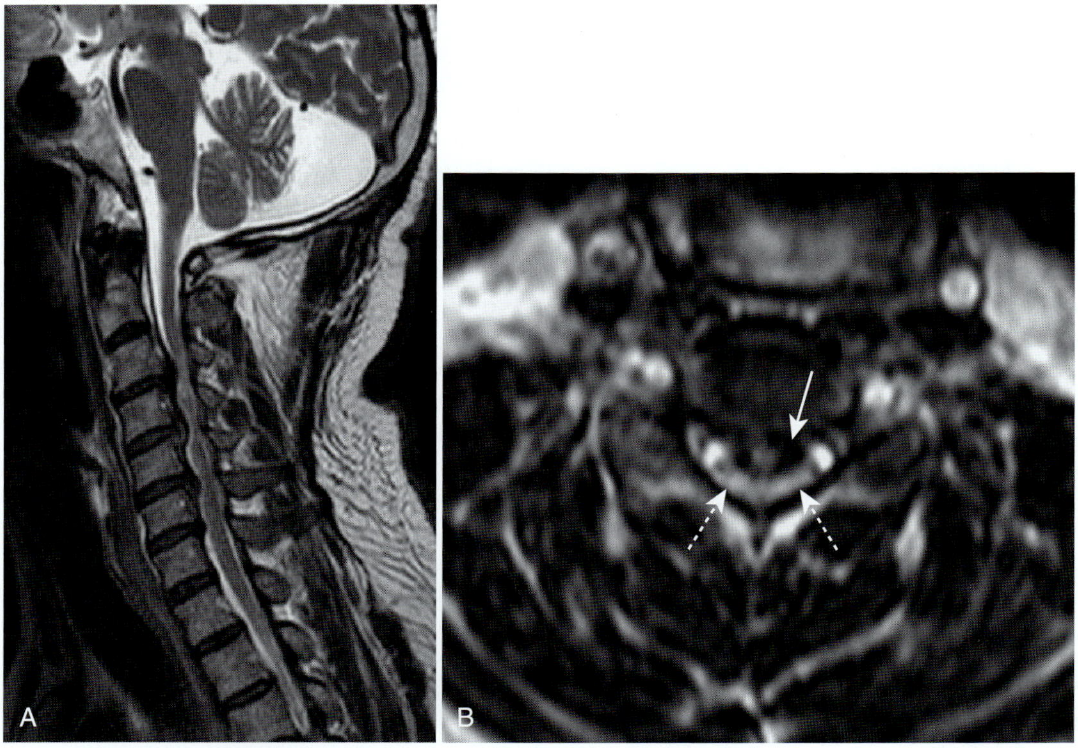

Figure 19.1 (**A**), An Asian patient with neck pain associated with leg weakness and upper motor neuron signs. The sagittal T2W MR image demonstrates flowing low-SI ossification along the posterior aspect of the C3 to C6 vertebral bodies due to OPLL. (**B**), The marked compression of the cervical cord is best appreciated on the axial T2W MR image. The prominent area of low-SI ossification (*white arrow*) is narrowing the cervical canal and flattening the cervical cord (*broken arrows*).

CHAPTER 20

Multiple Sclerosis of the Cervical Spinal Cord

DEFINITION

- An autoimmune disease that attacks the central nervous system with resultant sclerotic plaques scattered throughout the central nervous system; the cervical spinal cord is most commonly affected.

SIGNS AND SYMPTOMS

- Paresthesias.
- Motor and sensory symptoms mimicking radiculopathy and/or myelopathy.
- Often associated with optic neuritis.
- Hyperreflexia.
- Gait disturbance.
- Bowel and bladder symptomatology.
- High temperature can exacerbate symptoms (Uhthoff sign).
- Multiple sclerosis can manifest as essentially any neurologic sign or symptom.
- Natural history of the disease can vary from benign to a rapidly progressive disease with an extremely poor prognosis.

DEMOGRAPHICS

- Peak onset in the third to fourth decade of life but onset can occur at any age.
- Incidence: Female > Male.
- Higher incidence in patients of Western European origin.
- More common in the higher latitudes, with incidence of disease decreasing linearly as one moves toward the equator.
- Higher incidence in families.

IMAGING RECOMMENDATIONS

- MRI of the brain and cervical cord:
  - T1-weighted (T1W), T2W, and fluid attenuation and inversion recovery (FLAIR) sequences.
  - Occasionally a contrast agent is required.

IMAGING FINDINGS

- High-signal intensity (SI) plaques of demyelination on T2W MR images.
- Plaques are more conspicuous on FLAIR images.
- T1W imaging findings are often normal.
- Plaques are small, round, or ovoid and well defined.
- Plaques may enhance in early stages.
- No cord expansion.
- Combination of brain and spinal cord lesions increases specificity of diagnosis.

OTHER RECOMMENDED TESTING

- Electromyography and nerve conduction velocity testing are indicated if radiculopathy is present and to rule out amyotrophic lateral sclerosis.
- Evoked potential testing to quantify spinal cord compromise and cranial nerve deficits.

DIFFERENTIAL DIAGNOSIS

- Spinal cord ischemia and infarct.
- Idiopathic transverse myelitis.
- Spinal cord neoplasm.
- Syringomyelia.
- Acute disseminated encephalomyelitis (ADEM).

TREATMENT

- Systemic glucocorticoids.
- Interferon-β.
- Plasmapheresis.
- Glatiramer acetate
- Mitoxantrone.
- Natalizumab.
- Physical and occupational therapies.

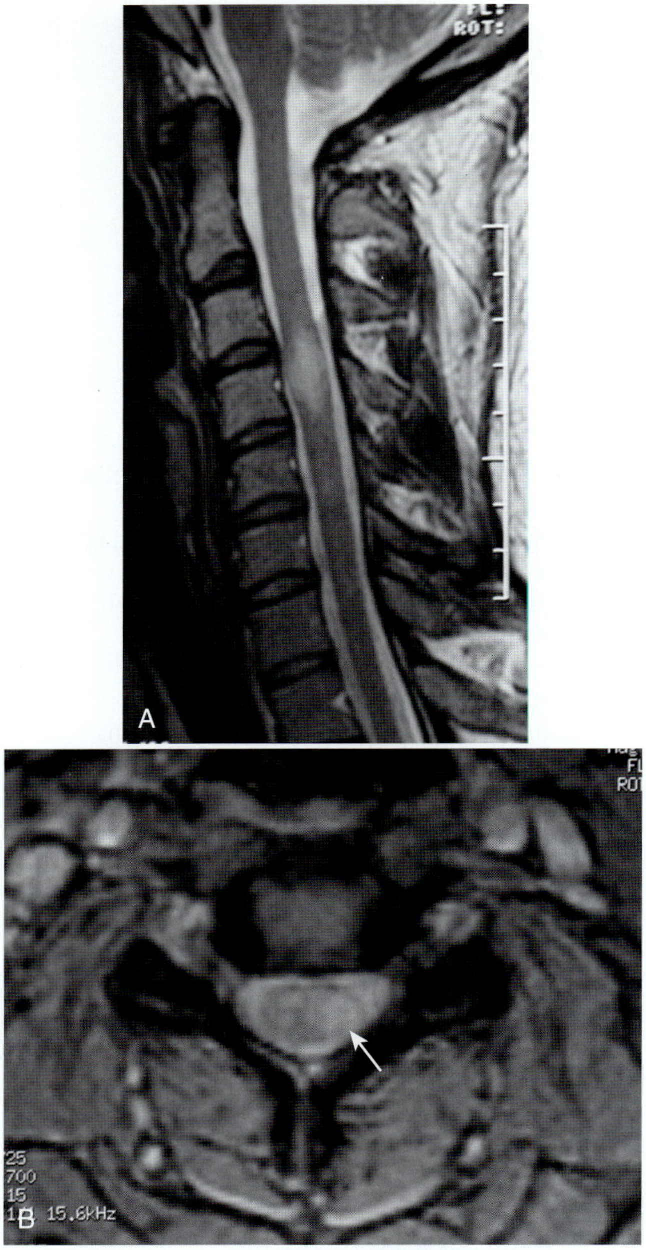

Figure 20.1 (**A**), Sagittal T2W MR image showing a well-defined ovoid area of increased SI within the cervical cord at the C4 level. The appearances are consistent with a multiple sclerosis plaque. (**B**), The plaque is also visible on the axial gradient echo image as an area of subtle increased SI to the left side of the cord (*white arrow*).

CHAPTER 21

Syringomyelia of the Cervical Spinal Cord

DEFINITION

- Idiopathic cystic dilatation of the spinal cord that may or may not communicate with the central canal of the spinal cord; also known as a syrinx.

SIGNS AND SYMPTOMS

- Pathopneumonic cloaklike pain with pain and temperature deficits in the presence of preserved proprioception and light touch.
- Weakness of the distal upper extremity.
- Gait disturbance.
- Pain resembling radicular pain.
- Spastic paraparesis.
- Cranial nerve deficits if brainstem is involved (syringobulbia).

DEMOGRAPHICS

- Onset in late childhood or early adulthood.
- Incidence: Male = Female.

IMAGING RECOMMENDATIONS

- MRI of cervical spine:
  - Include sagittal and axial T2-weighted (T2W) MR images.
- Post-contrast sequences (obtained after administration of a contrast agent) to exclude cord neoplasm.
- Extend MRI into thoracic spine or brain for large syrinx.

IMAGING FINDINGS

- High–signal intensity (SI), fluid-filled cavity within the cervical cord on T2W MR images.
  - Cavity is well defined.
  - Ovoid or tapering.
- Cord expansion and cord atrophy.
- No enhancement on post-contrast sequences except with associated cord neoplasms.

OTHER RECOMMENDED TESTING

- Electromyography and nerve conduction velocity testing are indicated if radiculopathy is present and to rule out amyotrophic lateral sclerosis.
- Evoked potential testing to quantify spinal cord compromise and cranial nerve deficits.

DIFFERENTIAL DIAGNOSIS

- Cystic spinal cord neoplasms.
- Myelomalacia.
- Ventriculus terminalis.

TREATMENT

- Small asymptomatic lesions are observed for progression.
- Surgical correction of associated bony abnormalities is indicated for more significant lesions.
- Drainage of the syrinx with an indwelling catheter if abnormal cerebrospinal fluid flow is a problem, because of the size of the syrinx relative to the spinal canal diameter.

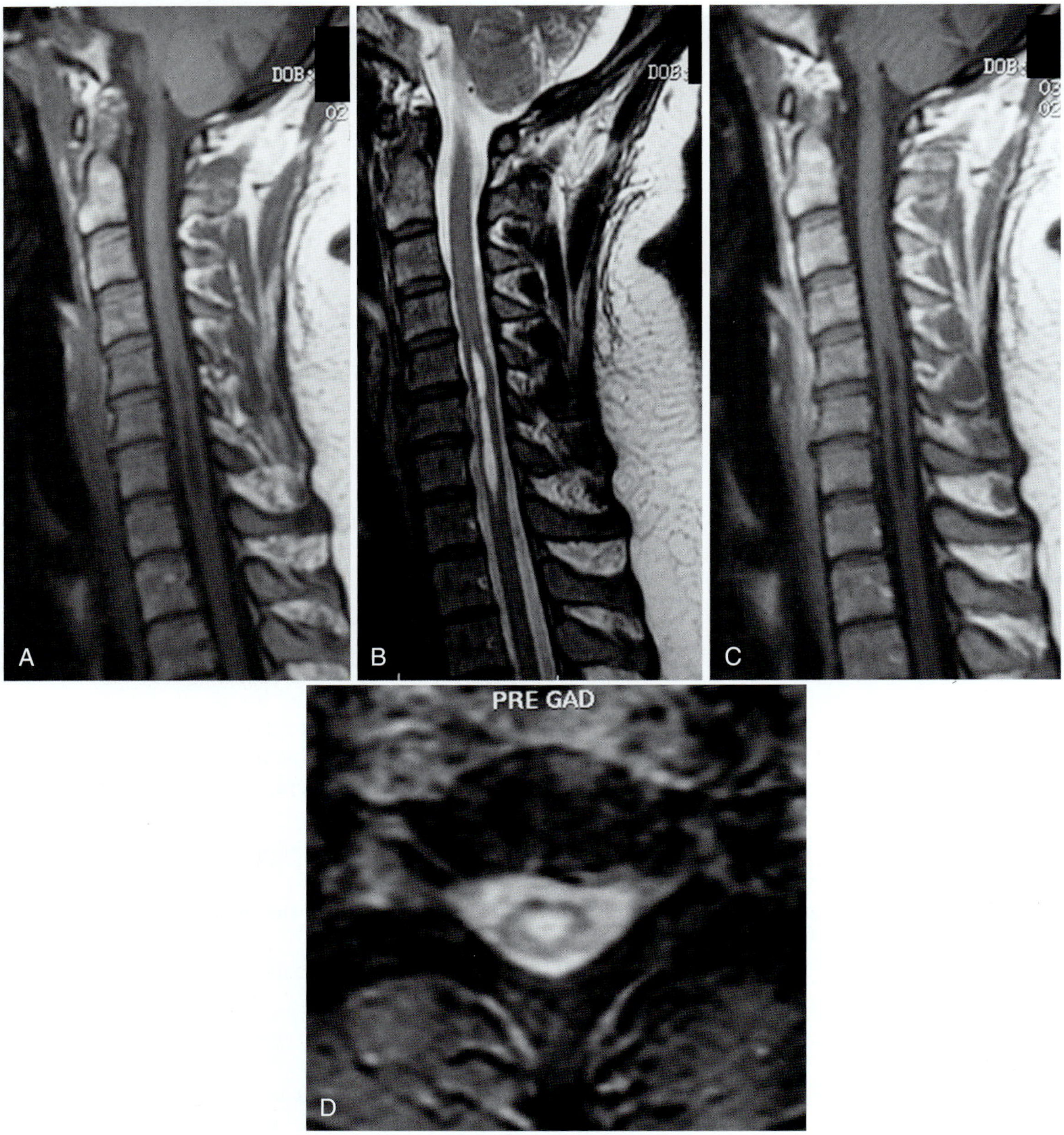

Figure 21.1 (**A**), Sagittal T1W MR image demonstrating a thin, low-SI cavity within the cervical cord at the C5-C7 level. (**B**), The cavity is filled with high-SI fluid on the sagittal T2W MR image. (**C**), There is no enhancement on the post-contrast sagittal T1W MR image, confirming the diagnosis of an idiopathic syrinx. There is no cord expansion in this case, but the axial gradient echo image (**D**), shows effacement of the anterior columns of the cord.

CHAPTER 22

Traumatic Syrinx of the Cervical Spinal Cord

DEFINITION

- Cystic dilatation of the spinal cord that may or may not communicate with the central canal of the spinal cord following trauma.

SIGNS AND SYMPTOMS

- Pathopneumonic cloaklike pain with pain and temperature deficits in the presence of preserved proprioception and light touch.
- Weakness of the distal upper extremity.
- Gait disturbance.
- Pain resembling radicular pain.
- Spastic paraparesis.
- Cranial nerve deficits if brainstem involved (syringobulbia).
- Symptoms may be worse with Valsalva maneuver.

DEMOGRAPHICS

- Following trauma.
- Incidence: Male > Female.

IMAGING RECOMMENDATIONS

- MRI of cervical spine:
  - Include sagittal and axial T2-weighted (T2W) MR images.
- Extend MRI into thoracic spine for large syrinx.
- CT to assess surgical bony fusion and failure of hardware.

IMAGING FINDINGS

- High-signal intensity (SI), fluid-filled cavity within the cervical cord on T2W MR images.
- Syrinx may be localized or may extend distally into the thoracic spine.
- Cord atrophy in association with cord injury.
- No enhancement on sequences obtained after administration of a contrast agent.
- Cord contusions occurring at the time of injury are poorly defined areas of high SI on T2 sequences.

OTHER RECOMMENDED TESTING

- Electromyography and nerve conduction velocity testing are indicated if radiculopathy is present and to rule out amyotrophic lateral sclerosis.
- Evoked potential testing to quantify spinal cord compromise and cranial nerve deficits.

DIFFERENTIAL DIAGNOSIS

- Cystic spinal cord neoplasms.
- Myelomalacia.
- Ventriculus terminalis.
- Multiple sclerosis.
- Associated possible association with Arnold-Chiari I malformation.

TREATMENT

- Small asymptomatic lesions are observed for progression.
- Surgical correction of associated bony abnormalities is indicated for more significant lesions.
- Removal of offending implanted surgical hardware.
- Drainage of the syrinx with an indwelling catheter if abnormal cerebrospinal fluid flow is a problem, because of the size of the syrinx relative to the spinal canal diameter.

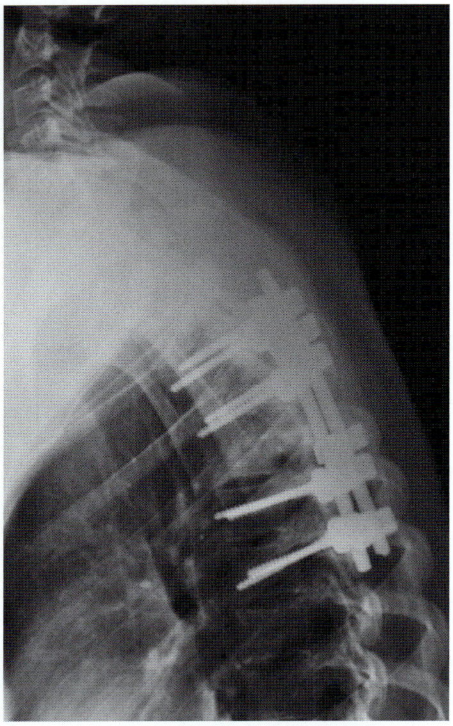

Figure 22.1 Radiographs of a young woman treated with spinal fixation of a traumatic unstable fracture of D5.

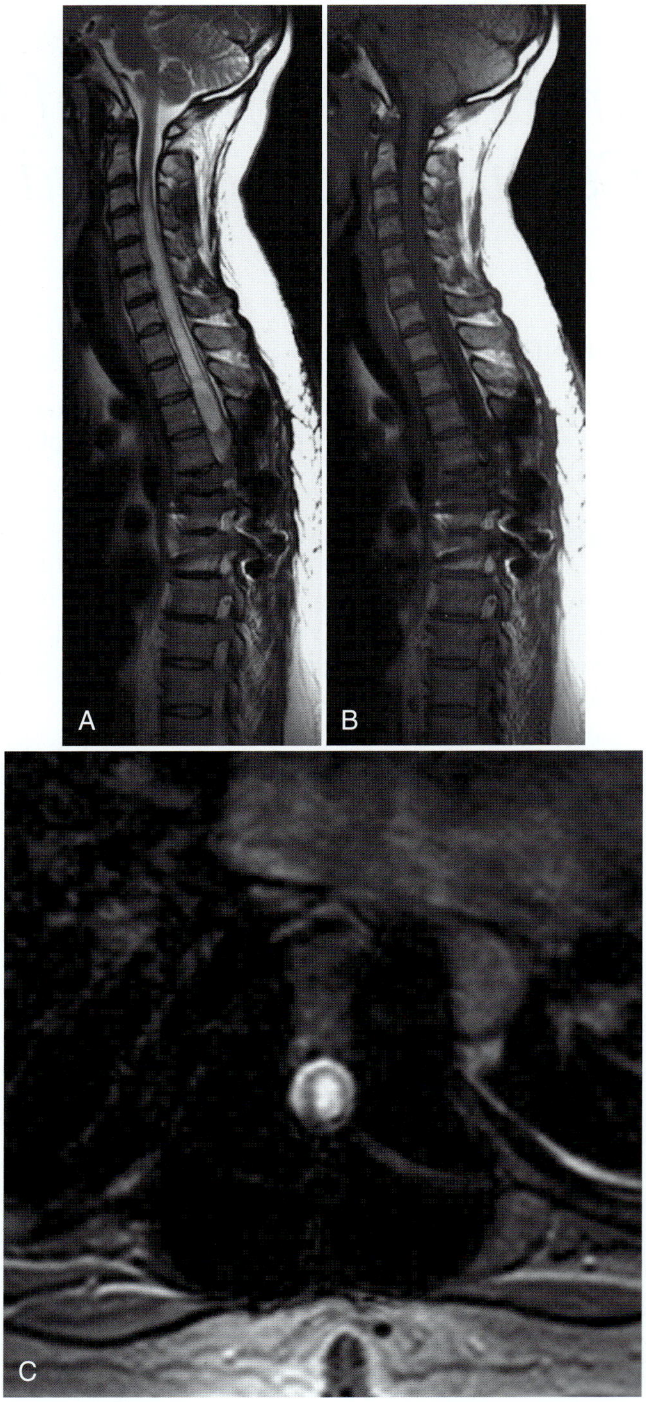

Figure 22.2 MRI was performed for progressive neurologic deficit. The sagittal T2W (**A**), T1W (**B**), and axial T2W (**C**) MR images demonstrate a large central syrinx extending proximally up to the C2-C3 level. There is marked cord expansion just above the fracture level. The spinal instrumentation is causing susceptibility artifact and obscuring parts of the image.

CHAPTER 23

Spontaneous Epidural Hematoma of the Cervical Spine

DEFINITION

- Spontaneous hemorrhage into the epidural space without significant antecedent trauma or medical procedure involving the epidural space.

SIGNS AND SYMPTOMS

- Acute onset of neck pain.
- Pain in radicular and nonradicular distribution.
- Rapidly progressive sensory, motor, and reflex changes progressing to myelopathy.
- Bowel and bladder symptomatology.
- May progress to paraparesis if left untreated, or occasionally may resolve without treatment.

DEMOGRAPHICS

- Bimodal age distribution in childhood and in the fifth and sixth decades of life:
  - Incidence in children: Male = Female.
  - Incidence in adults: Male > Female.
- Clinical outcome directly related to severity of symptoms and length of time to treatment.

IMAGING RECOMMENDATIONS

- MRI of cervical spine:
  - Combination of T1-weighted (T1W), T2W, and gradient echo sequences.

IMAGING FINDINGS

- Loculated collection in epidural space:
  - Anterior or posterior.
- May extend into neural foramina (this is not seen in subdural hematoma).
- Compression of thecal sac and cervical cord on axial images.
- MR signal intensity varies with age of hematoma as hemoglobin changes to deoxyhemoglobin and methemoglobin:
  - Acute: isointense to cord on T1W MR images and high signal intensity (SI) on T2W MR images.
  - Subacute: High SI on T1W and T2W MR images.
  - Chronic: Low SI on T1W MR images, and high SI on T2W MR images.
  - T2 effects are more pronounced on gradient echo imaging.

OTHER RECOMMENDED TESTING

- Laboratory testing for occult coagulopathy.

DIFFERENTIAL DIAGNOSIS

- Epidural abscess.
- Epidural neoplasm.
- Herniated intervertebral disc.

TREATMENT

- Immediate correction of underlying coagulopathy if present.
- Urgent decompressive laminectomy.
- Systemic glucocorticoids to treat spinal cord edema.

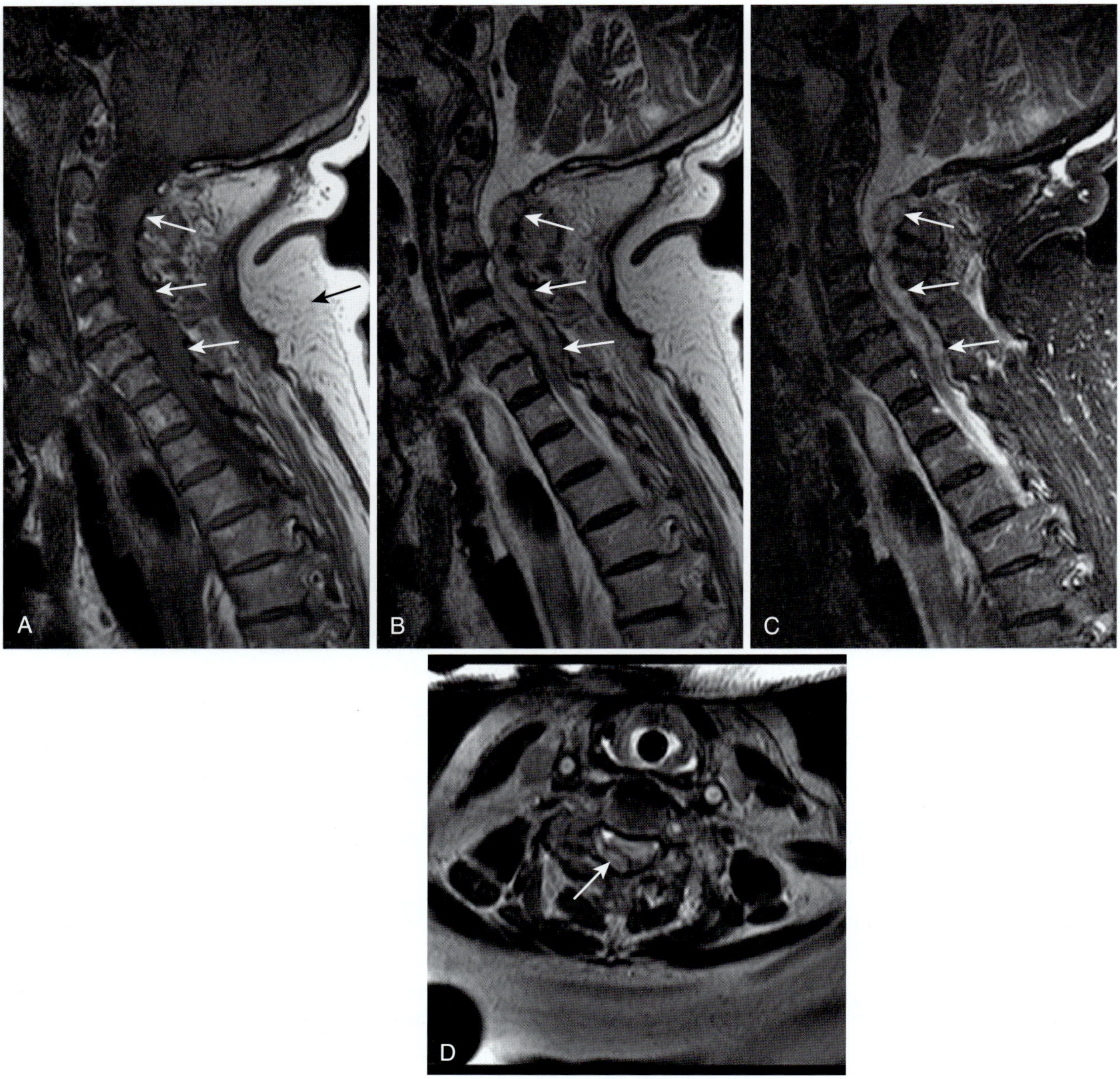

Figure 23.1 Sagittal T1W (**A**), T2W (**B**), and short T1 inversion recovery (STIR) (**C**), MR images of the cervical spine in an elderly woman who presented with progressive neurologic deficit following a minor fall, but with no evidence of bony injury on CT examination. There is an epidural hematoma in the posterior aspect of the spinal canal, extending down from the C1 to C6 level (*white arrows*). The hematoma has high SI on both T2W and STIR images. It also has high SI on the T1W MR image owing to deoxyhemoglobin, indicating a subacute hematoma. On the axial T2W MR image (**D**), the hematoma (*arrow*) displaces the spinal cord, and there is high SI within the cord because of myelopathy.

CHAPTER 24

Rheumatoid Arthritis of the Cervical Spine

DEFINITION

- Chronic, systemic autoimmune disease that causes inflammatory destruction to the spine, joints, and major organ systems of the body.

SIGNS AND SYMPTOMS

- Classic morning stiffness and gelling phenomenon.
- Pain worse in morning.
- Radiculopathy common as disease progresses in the cervical spine.
- High incidence of coexistent carpal tunnel syndrome and other entrapment neuropathies.
- Increased incidence of sudden C1-C2 subluxation in the absence of significant trauma.

DEMOGRAPHICS

- Affects all ages with peak incidence in the fourth to fifth decade of life.
- Incidence: Male > Female.

IMAGING RECOMMENDATIONS

- Flexion/extension radiographs to assess for C1-C2 instability and subaxial subluxation in symptomatic patients and prior to surgery.
- MRI for neurologic symptoms.

IMAGING FINDINGS

- Compression of brainstem and cervical cord due to:
  - Erosion of odontoid peg with mass effect from chronic pannus.
  - C1-C2 subluxation (> 3 mm).
  - Cranial settling.
- Intervertebral and facet erosions and sclerosis.
- Secondary subaxial spondylosis and instability with features of disc degeneration and spinal stenosis.
- There may be associated myelopathy and syrinx formation.
- Occasional cervical fusion (more common with juvenile inflammatory arthritis).

OTHER RECOMMENDED TESTING

- Electromyography and nerve conduction velocity testing to identify entrapment neuropathy.

DIFFERENTIAL DIAGNOSIS

- Seronegative spondyloarthropathies, including Reiter syndrome, psoriatic arthritis, and ankylosing spondylitis.
- Degenerative disc disease.
- Juvenile chronic arthritis.
- Infection.
- Hemodialysis arthropathy.

TREATMENT

- Disease-modifying agents, including gold salts, penicillamine, azathioprine, and cyclosporine A, can dramatically slow the progression of the disease, albeit not without side effects.
- Cytotoxic drugs, including methotrexate.
- Biologic agents, including interleukin and tumor necrosis factor-α.
- Salicylates, nonsteroidal anti-inflammatory agents, and corticosteroids.
- Physical and occupational therapies.
- Epidural blocks for symptomatic relief of radiculopathy.
- Early surgical treatment of entrapment neuropathies.
- Early stabilization of atlas and axis to avoid subluxation.

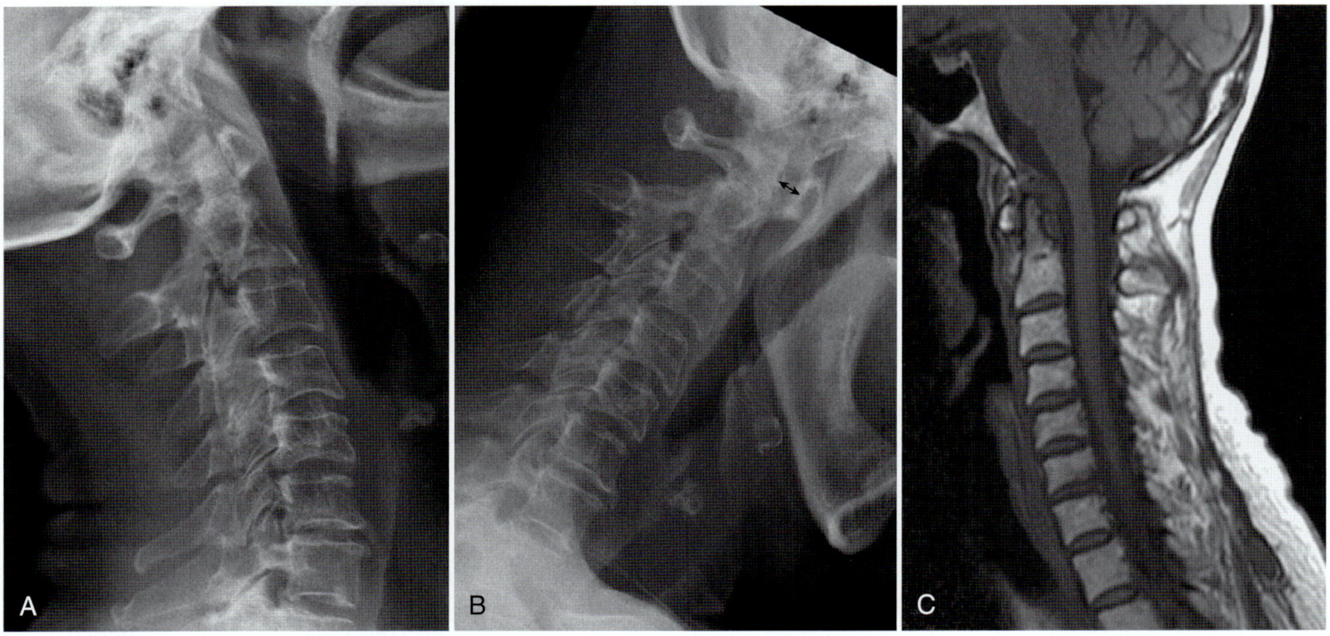

Figure 24.1 (**A**), Lateral radiograph of the cervical spine in extension shows normal C1-C2 alignment. (**B**), On cervical flexion, however, there is widening of the predental space due to C1-C2 instability (*double-headed arrow*). (**C**), The sagittal T1W MR image shows erosion of the dorsal aspect of the odontoid peg.

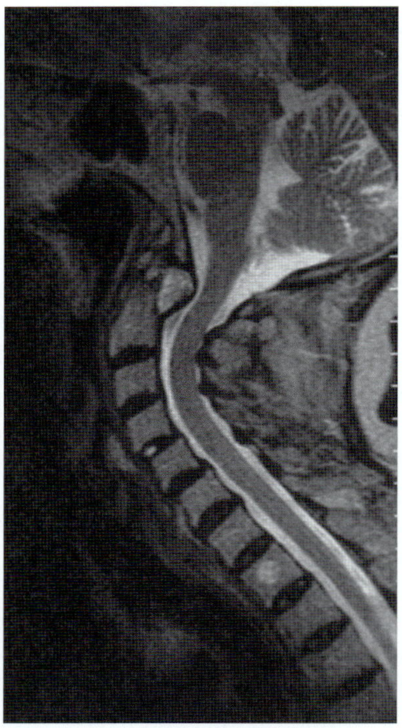

Figure 24.2 Sagittal T2W MR image demonstrating prominent high-SI rheumatoid synovitis and pannus formation arising posteriorly from the odontoid peg of the C2 vertebra, although there is no impingement on the cervical cord.

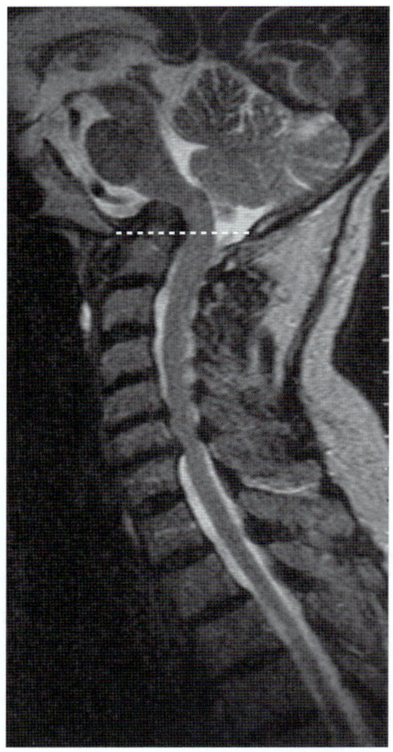

Figure 24.3 Sagittal T2W MR image of a patient with chronic rheumatoid arthritis with cranial settling. The odontoid peg projects through the foramen magnum (*dotted line*), and there is impingement of the brainstem.

CHAPTER 25

Anatomy: Special Imaging Considerations of the Thoracic Spine

OSSEOUS STRUCTURES

Thoracic Vertebrae. The thoracic vertebrae possess slightly triangular bodies with flat superior and inferior end plates and longer pedicles than the cervical vertebrae that cover the intervertebral foraminae. The thoracic transverse processes project posteroinferolaterally. Each thoracic vertebra articulates with a pair of ribs. Each rib end articulates with demifacets above and below the discs to form synovial costovertebral joints as well as the thoracic transverse processes to form costotransverse joints. The thoracic vertebrae possess longer laminae than the cervical vertebrae to form a wider spinal canal. They meet posteriorly to form long, inferiorly projecting spinous processes.

Thoracic Facet (Zygapophyseal) Joints. Synovial articulations formed between the inferior articular processes of the vertebra for which the joint is named, and the superior articular processes of the vertebra below. The articular surfaces are obliquely sagittal in orientation, thus preventing forward and lateral intervertebral translation. The facet joint capsules are tighter than those of the cervical facet joints and are innervated by the medial branches of the dorsal rami of the spinal nerves.

LIGAMENTS

Discs and Ligaments. Composed of a tough, complete annulus fibrosus that is attached to the adjacent end plates by Sharpey fibers. The central nucleus pulposus of the disc is a hydrated gel-like substance that may protrude into or through annular defects, resulting in disc herniations.

Longitudinal Ligaments. As in the cervical spine, the anterior and posterior longitudinal ligaments attach to the anterior and posterior surfaces of the vertebral bodies and annuli of the discs. They act to resist tension during flexion and extension.

Posterior Ligaments. The posterior elements are stabilized by a group of three ligaments. The ligamenta flava are composed of elastic collagen fibers that run the whole length of the spine, attaching to the internal surfaces of the laminae. The spinous processes are stabilized by the interspinous and supraspinous ligaments.

MUSCLES

The thoracic spine is supported by dorsal muscle groups consisting of the thoracic components of the longissimus and erector spinae thoracis muscles.

NEURAL STRUCTURES

The Spinal Nerves. As in the cervical spine, the spinal nerves are made up of a confluence of dorsal and ventral roots, each root being composed of smaller rootlets. The dorsal root contains a spinal ganglion located just proximal to the junction with the ventral root. The thoracic spinal nerves exit through the intervertebral foramina of the corresponding levels; for example, the T6 nerve passes through the T6 neural foramen.

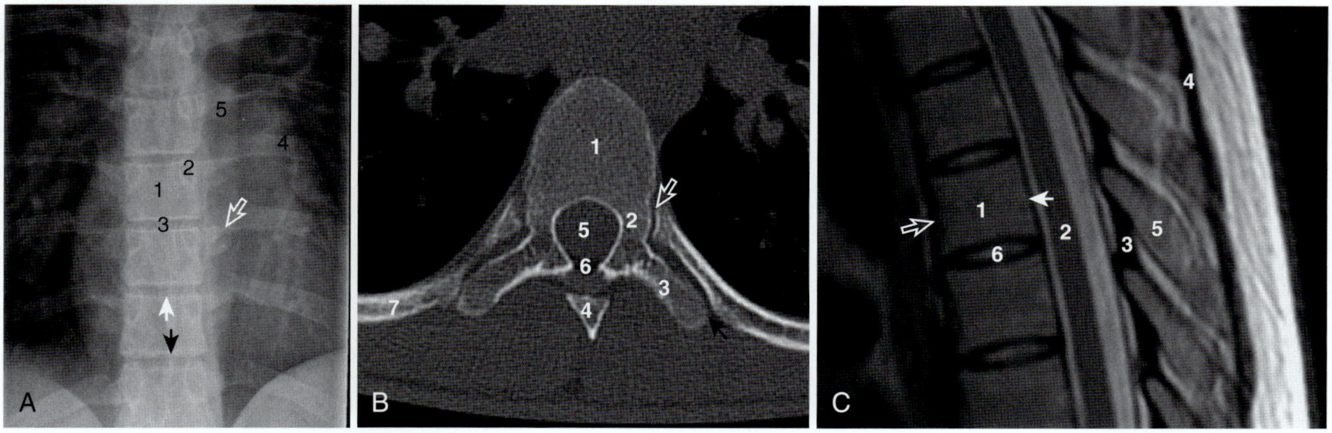

Figure 25.1 (**A**), Anteroposterior radiograph of the thoracic spine: 1, vertebral body; 2, pedicle; 3, disc space; 4, posterior rib; 5, transverse process; *open white arrow,* costotransverse joint; *white arrow,* superior end plate; *black arrow,* inferior end plate. (**B**), Axial CT scan of the thoracic spine: 1, vertebral body; 2, pedicle; 3, transverse process; 4, spinous process (level above); 5, thoracic cord within dural sac; 6, epidural fat; 7, posterior rib; *open white arrow,* costovertebral joint; *black arrow,* costotransverse joint. (**C**), Sagittal T2-weighted MR image of the thoracic spine: 1, vertebral body; 2, thoracic spinal cord; 3, ligamentum flavum; 4, supraspinous ligament; 5, spinous process; 6, intervertebral disc; *black arrow,* posterior longitudinal ligament; *open white arrow,* anterior longitudinal ligament.

CHAPTER 26

Intervertebral Disc Herniation of the Thoracic Spine

DEFINITION

- Focal extension of an intervertebral disc of less than 50% of the disc circumference beyond the margins of the vertebrae.

SIGNS AND SYMPTOMS

- Level, size and location (e.g., posterior, anterior, lateral) of disc herniation will determine the clinical presentation.
- Axial and radicular pain is the most common symptom.
- Decreased range of motion of the thoracic spine with associated muscle spasm is also common.
- Pain may radiate in a dermatomal or nondermatomal pattern.
- Pain may rarely manifest as subcostal or abdominal pain.
- Motor, sensory, and reflex changes may occur.
- Central disc herniation may cause compression of the thoracic spinal cord with resultant myelopathy.

DEMOGRAPHICS

- Adult population.
- Incidence: Male = Female.

IMAGING RECOMMENDATIONS

- MRI is the primary investigation of choice.
- CT is of limited value but may be used to identify chronic calcified disc protrusions prior to surgery.
- CT myelography is an alternative when MRI is contraindicated.
- Radiographs are of limited value and are required only in selected cases.

IMAGING FINDINGS

- Acute "soft" disc protrusions are high-signal intensity (SI) on T2-weighted (T2W) sequences.
- Chronic "hard" disc protrusions are low-SI on T2W sequences and may be calcified, a feature best confirmed by localized CT.
- Axial images may show compression of the thecal sac, effacement of the cerebrospinal fluid space, and compression and flattening of the spinal cord.
- Myelopathy is evident as a focal area of high SI within the cord adjacent to the level of compression.
- MR myelography sequences or CT myelography demonstrate the compression of the thecal sac.

OTHER RECOMMENDED TESTING

- Electromyography and nerve conduction testing are indicated if radiculopathy is present.
- Provocative discography may serve as a useful diagnostic tool to determine whether a specific disc is serving as a nidus for the pain.

DIFFERENTIAL DIAGNOSIS

- Epidural abscess.
- Epidural hematoma.
- Osteophyte.
- Neoplasm.

TREATMENT

- Conservative treatment consisting of local heat, cold, simple analgesics, and nonsteroidal anti-inflammatory agents will improve symptoms in many cases.
- Physical therapy, including gentle stretching, range-of-motion exercises, deep heat modalities, and stretch and spray, may be beneficial in selected patients.
- Epidural blocks will provide symptomatic relief if conservative therapy fails or if the pain is limiting activities of daily living.
- Osteopathic or chiropractic manipulation may provide symptomatic relief in selected patients.
- Surgery may be required for persistent pain or progressive neurologic symptoms.

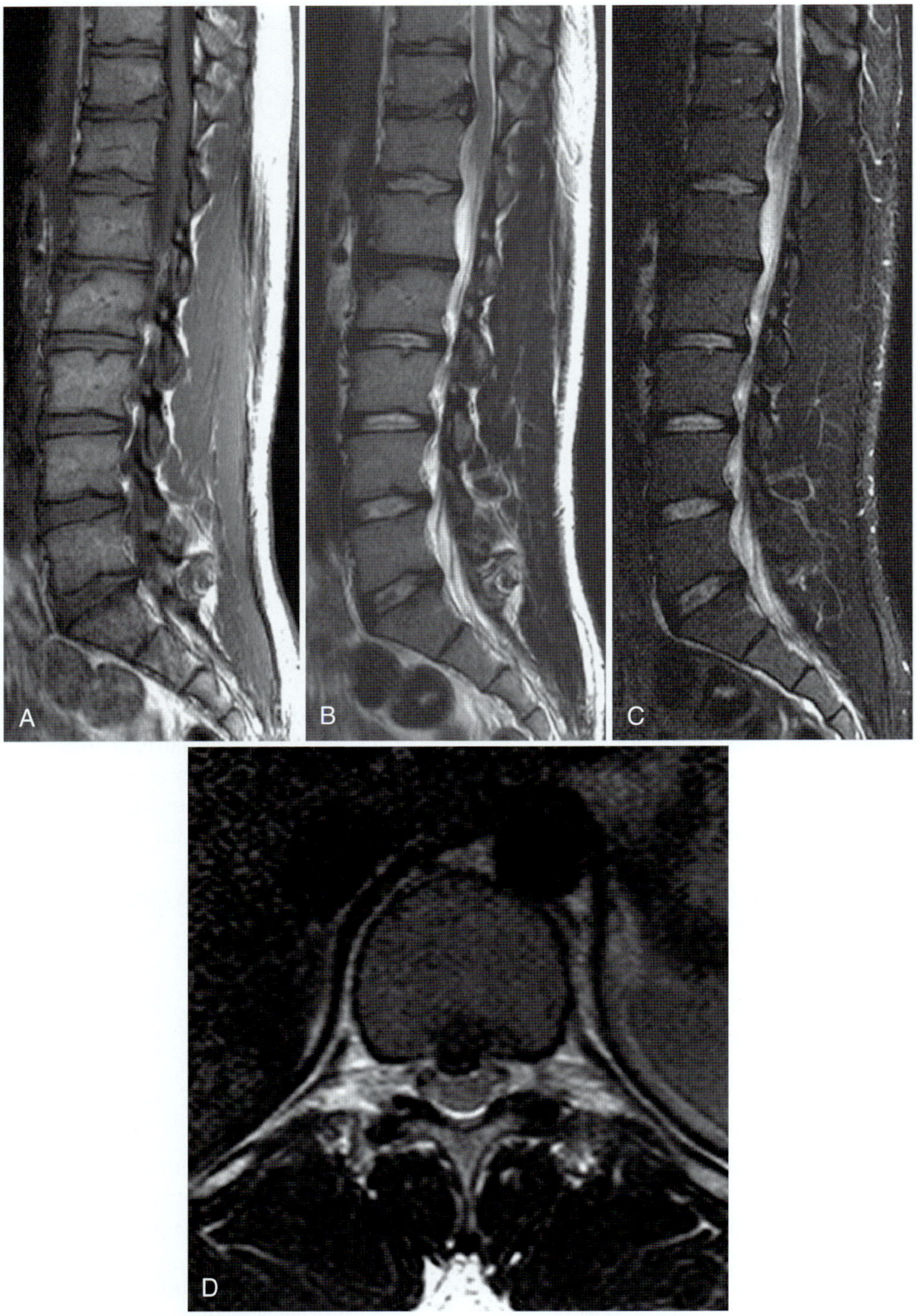

Figure 26.1 Sagittal T1W (**A**), T2W (**B**), and short T1 inversion recovery (STIR) (**C**) MR images and an axial T2W MR image (**D**) of a patient with a thoracic disc protrusion. There is a chronic bony defect of the posteroinferior margin of the T11 vertebra due to a posterior ring apophyseal avulsion, associated with a central disc protrusion. The disc protrusion is low-SI on the axial image and is causing compression of the conus medullaris. There is no associated myelopathy. The rest of the spine shows features of Scheuermann-type disease with formation of multiple Schmorl nodes and disc degeneration at L1-L2. These findings are of long standing, and there is no reactive marrow edema on the STIR images.

CHAPTER 27

Thoracic Anterior Vertebral Compression Fracture

DEFINITION

- Fracture of the thoracic vertebral body compressing the anterior portion of the body with relative sparing of the middle and posterior elements.

SIGNS AND SYMPTOMS

- Acute onset of localized back pain.
- Pain may radiate in a dermatomal or nondermatomal pattern.
- Myelopathy may be present.
- Bowel and bladder symptomatology with spinal cord compression.
- Previous dorsal kyphotic deformity may be clinically apparent.

DEMOGRAPHICS

- Bimodal distribution with young trauma victims and elderly patients with osteoporosis, especially postmenopausal women:
  - Incidence in patients with trauma: Male > Female.
  - Incidence in patients with osteoporosis: Female > Male.

IMAGING RECOMMENDATIONS

- Radiography is the first-line investigation to exclude vertebral fractures.
- MRI distinguishes between acute and chronic insufficiency fractures and pathologic fractures:
  - T1-weighted (T1W) and short T1 inversion recovery (STIR) or T2 with fat suppression (FST2W MR images) are the best sequences to assess bone marrow.
  - Diffusion-weighted imaging may help distinguish insufficiency from pathologic fractures.
- Traumatic fractures may require both CT and MRI to classify the fracture type, predict its stability, and exclude fractures at other levels.
- Isotope bone scanning is an alternative to MRI to identify recent fractures and also to assess the entire skeleton to exclude widespread metastatic disease.

IMAGING FINDINGS

- Anterior wedging of anterior vertebral body on lateral radiographs.
- Osteophyte formation and reparative bone formation suggest chronic fracture.
- MRI findings in acute fracture:
  - Diffuse marrow edema on STIR images that is confined to the vertebral body.
  - Linear high-signal intensity (SI) fracture cleft on STIR images which is low SI on T1W MR images.
- MRI findings in chronic fracture:
  - Return to normal fatty marrow SI on both T1W and STIR images.
- MRI findings in pathologic fracture:
  - Focal discrete high-SI lesion on STIR which is low SI on T1W MR images.
  - Involvement of posterior elements.
  - Cortical destruction and extraosseous soft tissue mass.
  - Buckling and destruction of posterior vertebral body wall.
  - Absence of fracture cleft.

OTHER RECOMMENDED TESTING

- In patients with osteoporosis, testing for hyperparathyroidism, panhypopituitarism, and sex hormone deficits.
- Electromyography and nerve conduction testing are indicated if radiculopathy is present.
- Evoked potential testing if myelopathy is present.

DIFFERENTIAL DIAGNOSIS

- Pathologic fracture due to tumor.
- Traumatic burst fractures of the vertebral body.
- Chance ("seat belt") fractures of the vertebral body.
- Scheuermann kyphosis.

TREATMENT

- Opioids for acute pain relief.
- Orthotic bracing.
- Epidural injections of local anesthetics, opioids, and/or corticosteroids for pain not relieved by opioids.
- Vertebroplasty and kyphoplasty.
- Bisphosphonates and calcitonin.

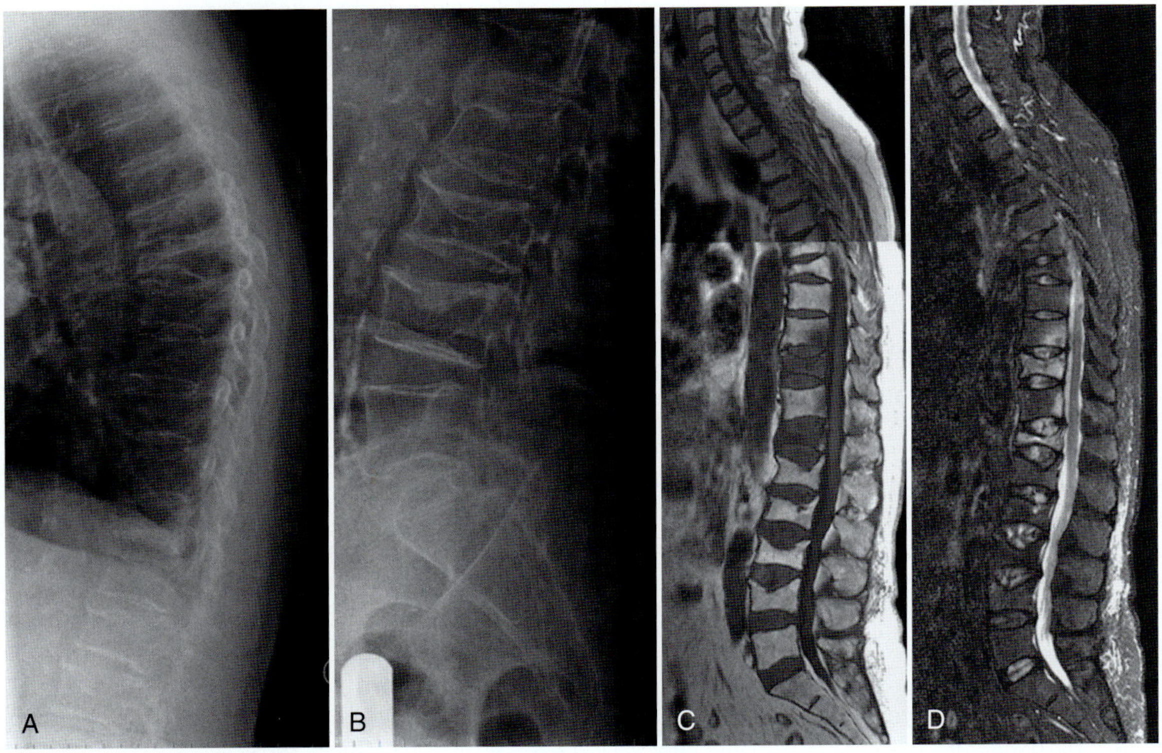

Figure 27.1 Lateral radiographs of the thoracic (**A**) and lumbar (**B**) spine demonstrate multilevel anterior vertebral body fractures. It is not possible to distinguish between acute and chronic fractures. The sagittal T1W (**C**) and STIR (**D**) MR images, however, visualize multiple anterior wedge fractures. The recent acute fractures have marrow edema, which are low SI on the T1W MR image and high SI on the STIR image. The chronic fractures have normal fatty marrow SI.

CHAPTER 28

Thoracic Lateral Vertebral Compression Fracture

DEFINITION

- Fracture of the thoracic vertebral body that compresses the lateral portion of the body with relative sparing of the posterior elements.

SIGNS AND SYMPTOMS

- Acute onset of localized back pain.
- Pain may radiate in a dermatomal or nondermatomal pattern.
- Myelopathy, although less common than with thoracic anterior vertebral compression fracture, may be present.
- Bowel and bladder symptomatology with spinal cord compression.
- Previous dorsal kyphotic deformity may be clinically apparent.

DEMOGRAPHICS

- Bimodal distribution, in young trauma victims and elderly patients with osteoporosis, especially postmenopausal women.
- Incidence in patients with trauma: Male > Female.
- Incidence in patients with osteoporosis: Female > Male.

IMAGING RECOMMENDATIONS

- Radiography is the first-line investigation to exclude vertebral fractures and assess vertebral alignment.
- MRI distinguishes between acute and chronic insufficiency fractures and pathologic fractures.
- Traumatic fractures may require both CT and MRI to classify the fracture type and predict stability and to exclude fractures at other levels.
- Isotope bone scanning is an alternative to MRI for identifying recent fractures and also assessing the entire skeleton to exclude metastases.

IMAGING FINDINGS

- Lateral wedging of vertebral body on AP radiographs:
  - Usually associated with some anterior body wedging.
  - Dramatic lateral wedging may indicate pathologic fracture.
- Scoliosis may be present as well as kyphosis.
- Prominent spondylosis with osteophytes most marked on the concave aspect of the scoliosis curve in chronic cases.
- MRI findings in acute fracture:
  - Diffuse marrow edema on short T1 inversion recovery (STIR) images confined to vertebral body.
  - Linear high-signal intensity (SI) fracture cleft on STIR images which is low SI on T1-weighted (T1W) MR images.
- MRI findings in chronic fracture:
  - Return to normal fatty marrow SI on both T1W and STIR images.
- MRI findings in pathologic fracture:
  - Focal discrete high-SI lesion on STIR images which is low SI on T1W MR images.
  - Involvement of posterior elements.
  - Cortical destruction and extraosseous soft tissue mass.
  - Buckling and destruction of posterior vertebral body wall.
  - Absence of fracture cleft.

OTHER RECOMMENDED TESTING

- In patients with osteoporosis, testing for hyperparathyroidism, panhypopituitarism, and sex hormone deficits.
- Electromyography and nerve conduction velocity testing are indicated if radiculopathy is present.
- Evoked potential testing if myelopathy present.

DIFFERENTIAL DIAGNOSIS

- Pathologic fracture due to tumor.
- Traumatic burst fractures of the vertebral body.
- Chance "seat belt" fractures of the vertebral body.
- Scheuermann kyphosis.

TREATMENT

- Opioids for acute pain relief.
- Orthotic bracing.
- Epidural injections of local anesthetics, opioids, and/or corticosteroids for pain not relieved by opioids.
- Vertebroplasty and kyphoplasty.
- Bisphosphonates and calcitonin.

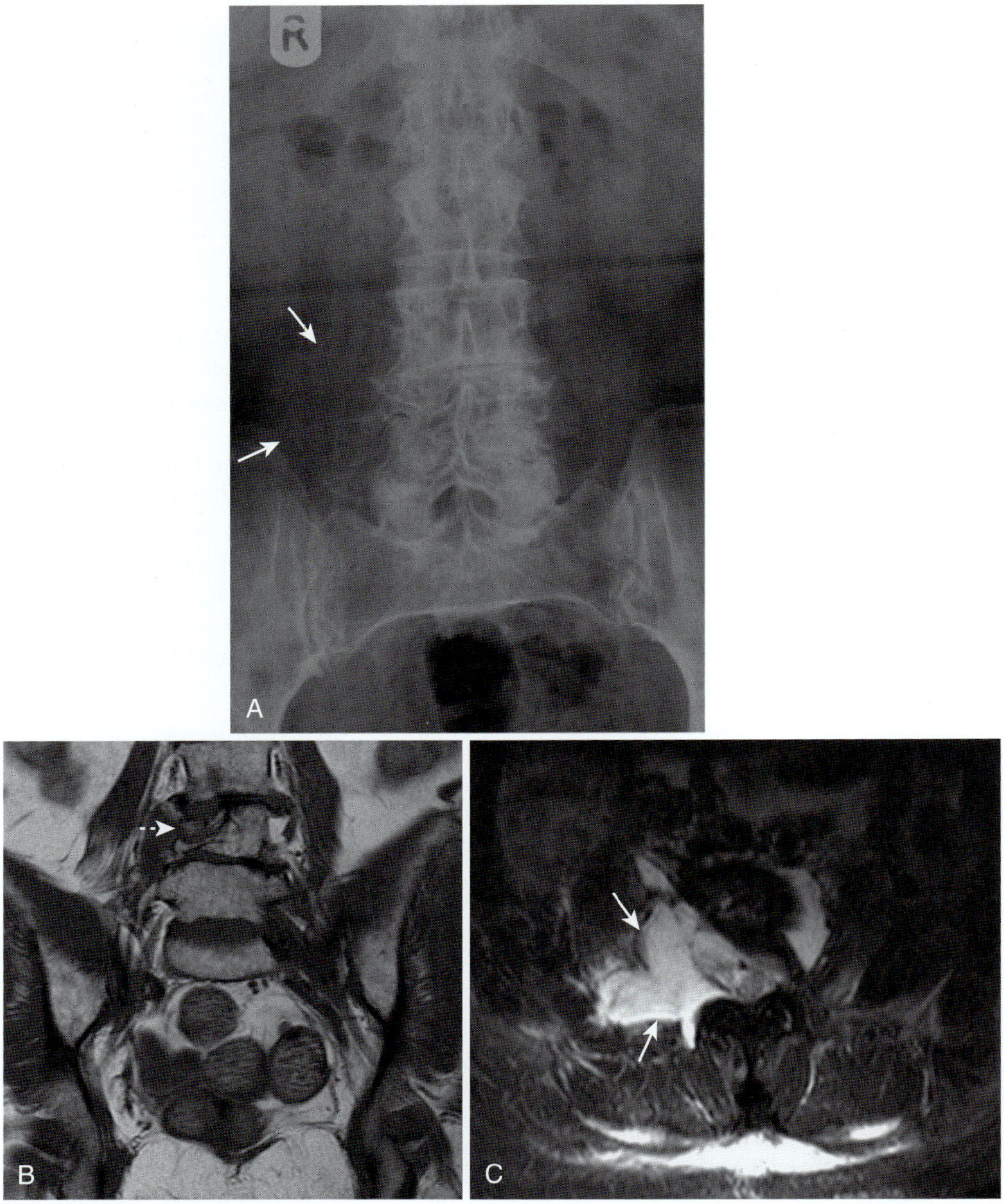

Figure 28.1 (**A**), AP radiograph of the lumbar spine in a patient with myeloma who had been previously treated with radiotherapy for an L4 deposit with extraosseous soft tissue tumor. There is a lateral compression fracture of the right side of the L4 vertebra. In addition, there is a thin shell of reparative bone formation around the pre-existing extraosseous tumor. (**B**), The coronal T1W MR image better demonstrates the lateral compression fracture. (**C**), The axial T2W with fat suppression (FST2W) MR image shows the high-SI fluid component of the extraosseous mass that is typical of treated myeloma.

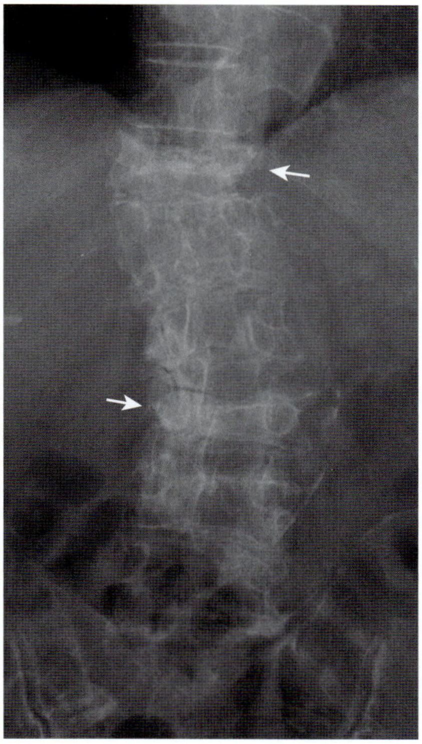

Figure 28.2 AP radiograph of an elderly woman with osteoporosis. Scoliosis is present, as well as vertebral compression factures that are more prominent on the concave aspects of the scoliosis at T11 and L3 (*white arrows*). The lateral compression fractures coexist with anterior wedge fractures and may be the result of scoliosis rather than the cause.

CHAPTER 29

Kümmel Disease

DEFINITION

- Delayed fracture and collapse of the thoracic vertebral body with persistent fracture cleft and adjacent avascular necrosis.

SIGNS AND SYMPTOMS

- Acute onset of localized back pain.
- Pain may radiate in a dermatomal or nondermatomal pattern.
- Myelopathy may be present.
- Bowel and bladder symptomatology with spinal cord compression.
- Previous thoracic kyphotic deformity from osteoporosis may be clinically apparent.

DEMOGRAPHICS

- Elderly patients with osteoporosis, especially postmenopausal women.
- Incidence in patients with osteoporosis: Female > Male.

IMAGING RECOMMENDATIONS

- Radiography to confirm or exclude the presence of vertebral fracture.
- MRI to assess age of fracture and distinguish pathologic fractures.

IMAGING FINDINGS

- Compression fracture of vertebral body.
- Gas may be seen within the fracture cleft on radiography and CT (intravertebral cleft sign).
- High-signal intensity (SI), fluid-filled fracture cleft may be present on short T1 inversion recovery (STIR) MR images.
- Gas or fluid in a fracture cleft is a specific sign of an insufficiency fracture and is not a feature of pathologic fracture.
- Other features are the same as those of simple insufficiency fractures.

OTHER RECOMMENDED TESTING

- In patients with osteoporosis, testing for hyperparathyroidism, panhypopituitarism, and sex hormone deficits.
- Electromyography and nerve conduction testing are indicated if radiculopathy is present.
- Evoked potential testing if myelopathy is present.

DIFFERENTIAL DIAGNOSIS

- Pathologic fracture due to tumor.
- Infection.
- Nontraumatic bone infarction.
- Neoplasm.

TREATMENT

- Opioids for acute pain relief.
- Orthotic bracing.
- Epidural injections of local anesthetics, opioids, and/or corticosteroids for pain not relieved by opioids.
- Vertebroplasty and kyphoplasty.
- Bisphosphonates and calcitonin if osteoporosis is present.

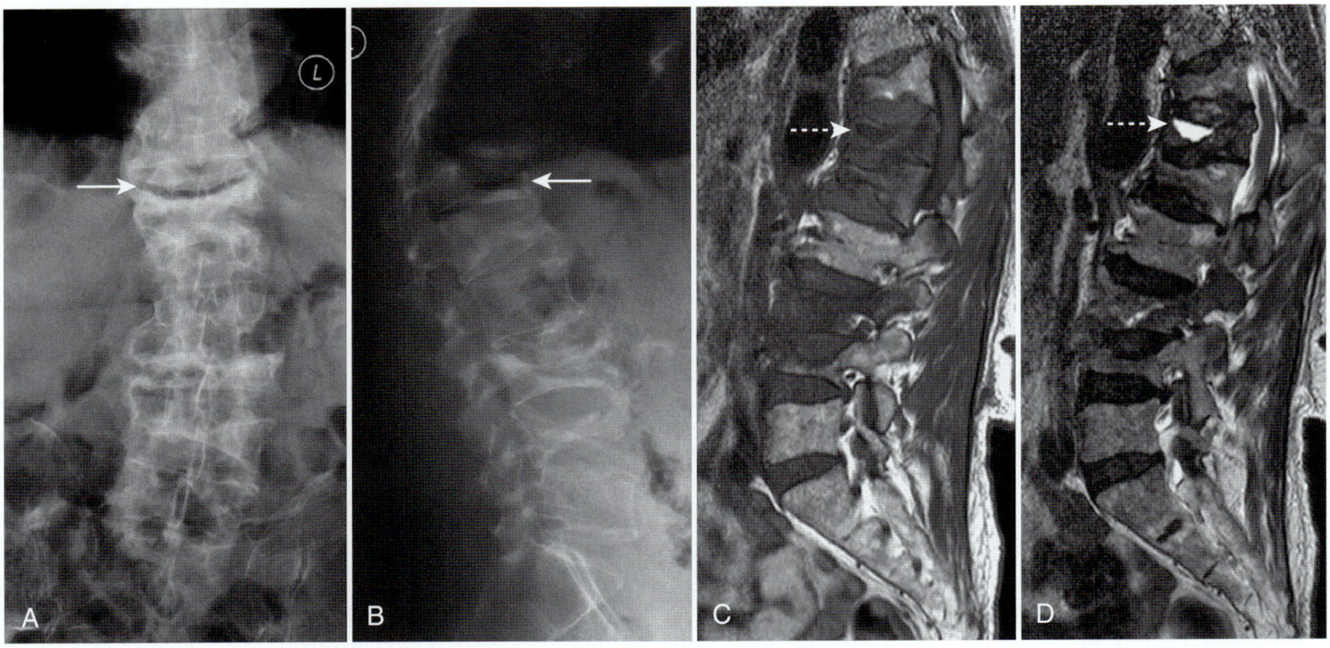

Figure 29.1 AP (**A**) and lateral (**B**) radiographs of the lower thoracic and lumbar spine in an elderly woman with multiple vertebral insufficiency fractures. The T12 vertebra has a lucent horizontal cleft (*white arrows*). (**C** and **D**), On MRI, the fracture cleft (*broken arrows*) is shown to be fluid filled, with low SI on the T1W MR image (**C**) and high SI on the T2W MR image (**D**).

CHAPTER 30

Complications of Vertebroplasty and Kyphoplasty

DEFINITION

- *Vertebroplasty* is defined as the injection of polymethylmethacrylate resin or another form of bone cement into the compressed vertebral body.
- *Kyphoplasty* is defined as the placement of a balloon into the compressed vertebral body with the goal of creating a cavity and restoring the vertebral body to its original height, followed by the injection of polymethylmethacrylate resin or other form of bone cement into the compressed vertebral body.

SIGNS AND SYMPTOMS

- Extravasation of bone cement, caused by improper needle placement, too large a volume of injectate, insufficient cement viscosity, or injection of cement at too high a pressure:
  - Acute onset of localized back pain, which is superimposed on the patient's preexisting compression fracture pain after extravasation of bone cement into the vertebral canal or neural foramina.
  - Pain may radiate in a dermatomal or nondermatomal pattern.
  - Myelopathy may be present if there is significant compression of the spinal cord.
  - Bowel and bladder symptomatology with spinal cord compression.
  - Previous thoracic kyphotic deformity from osteoporosis may be clinically apparent.
- Embolization of bone cement and/or fat caused by intravascular needle placement, too large a volume of injectate, insufficient cement viscosity, or injection of cement at too high a pressure:
  - Acute onset of shortness of breath if cement is carried into pulmonary circulation.
  - Chest pain.
  - Rarely, acute cardiopulmonary failure.
- Vertebral osteomyelitis is a rare, potential late complication that is caused by failure to use intraoperative antibiotics, compromise of the patient's immune system, or improper sterile technique:
  - Late onset of back pain following vertebroplasty or kyphoplasty.
  - Elevations of erythrocyte sedimentation rate and white blood cell count.
  - Fever and sepsis.

DEMOGRAPHICS

- Elderly patients with osteoporosis, especially postmenopausal women.
- Incidence in patients with osteoporosis: Female > Male.
- Incidence in patients with preexisting pulmonary disease at greater risk for clinically significant embolic complications.

IMAGING RECOMMENDATIONS

- Imaging investigations are recommended only for symptomatic cement leakage.
- Radiography and CT of spine or chest for cement leakage or embolus.
- MRI for spinal infection or cord injury resulting from incorrect needle placement.

IMAGING FINDINGS

- Localized cement leak:
  - Cement within basivertebral veins, in the epidural space, around the nerve root sleeve, or within the intervertebral disk.
  - Rarely, cement may leak around the descending aorta.
  - Cement casts may occur around the posterior needle track.
- Cement emboli:
  - Rounded areas of cement density within peripheral pulmonary arteries on radiography or CT.
- Spinal infection, which is evaluated by MRI:
  - On short T1 inversion recovery (STIR) images, high signal intensity (SI) around the cement within the vertebral body.
  - Erosion of the vertebral endplate and extension into disk space.
  - Cortical destruction.
  - Paravertebral or epidural soft tissue mass and abscess formation.

OTHER RECOMMENDED TESTING

- In patients with osteoporosis, testing for hyperparathyroidism, panhypopituitarism, and sex hormone deficits.
- Electromyography and nerve conduction testing are indicated if radiculopathy is present.
- Evoked potential testing if myelopathy is present.
- Erythrocyte sedimentation rate, C-reactive protein, and white blood cell count measurements if osteomyelitis is being considered.
- Bone biopsy and culture if osteomyelitis is being considered.

DIFFERENTIAL DIAGNOSIS

- Extravasation of bone cement:
  - Migration of bone fragments into the spinal canal or neural foramina.
  - Osteophyte.
- Embolization of bone cement:
  - Phlebolith.
  - Pulmonary embolus.
  - Calcified pulmonary granuloma.
- Vertebral osteomyelitis:
  - Neoplasm.
  - Kummel disease.

TREATMENT

- If no significant neural compromise or cardiopulmonary embarrassment, treat symptomatically.
- Opioids for acute pain relief if no neurologic deficit.
- Orthotic bracing if no neurologic deficit.
- Epidural injections of local anesthetics, opioids, and/or corticosteroids for pain not relieved by opioids if no there is neurologic deficit and osteomyelitis has been ruled out.
- If untreated osteomyelitis has been ruled out, vertebroplasty and kyphoplasty of other compression fractures may be contributing to the pain and functional disability.
- Bisphosphonates and calcitonin if osteoporosis is present.

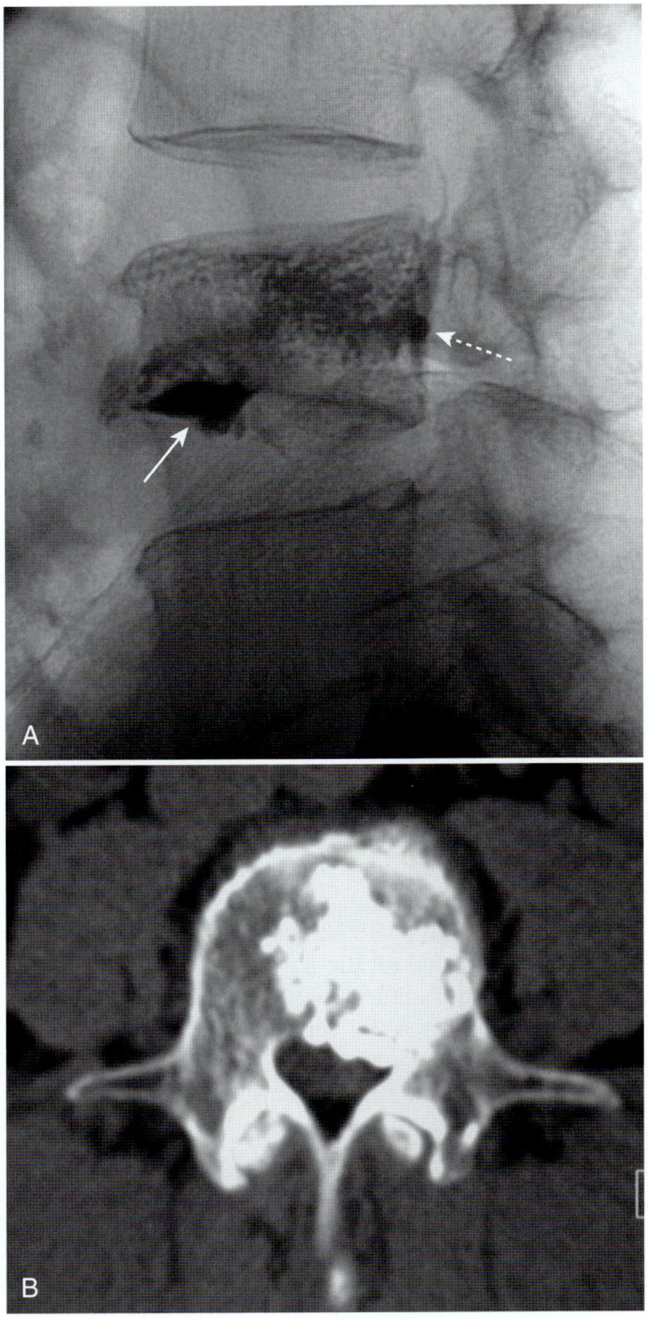

Figure 30.1 (A), Fluoroscopic image acquired during vertebroplasty showing intradiskal leakage of cement (*arrow*). More significant is the cement filling the basivertebral vein (*broken arrow*). The patient complained of nerve root pain after the procedure. (B), The CT scan shows cement within the basivertebral veins and within the lateral recess on the left side compressing the traversing nerve root.

CHAPTER 31

Costovertebral Joint Abnormalities

DEFINITION

- Pain and dysfunction of the costovertebral joint due to arthritis, neoplasm, and/or trauma.

SIGNS AND SYMPTOMS

- May mimic pain of pulmonary origin.
- Patient attempts to splint the affected joint or joints by splinting that area of the back to avoid flexion, extension, and lateral bending of the spine.
- Patient may retract the scapulas in an effort to gain relief from the pain emanating from this joint.
- The costovertebral joint may be tender to palpation and may feel hot and swollen if acutely inflamed.
- Patient may also complain of a "clicking" sensation with movement of the joint.

DEMOGRAPHICS

- Incidence: Male = Female.
- Common in patients with ankylosing spondylitis and Reiter syndrome.
- Also seen in patients with rheumatoid arthritis and psoriatic arthritis.

IMAGING RECOMMENDATIONS

- Radiographic findings are often normal in early disease.
- MRI is the primary investigation for early disease:
  - T1-weighted (T1W) MR images and short T1 inversion recovery (STIR) or T2W with fat suppression (FST2W) images to detect marrow edema.
- Isotope bone scanning may be useful for localized pain when MRI findings are normal.
- CT may be useful to characterize abnormalities identified on isotope bone scans.

IMAGING FINDINGS

- Marrow edema adjacent to costovertebral joints on parasagittal STIR MR images in early or active inflammatory spondylarthropathy.
- Ankylosis of the costovertebral joint is present on radiography or CT in established ankylosing spondylitis. This is invariably accompanied by more widespread spinal involvement.
- Sclerosis and osteophyte formation occur with degenerative osteoarthritis of the costovertebral joint, best demonstrated on CT.

OTHER RECOMMENDED TESTING

- Electromyography and nerve conduction velocity testing to rule out radiculopathy and/or peripheral neuropathy.
- Serum amylase measurement to rule out pancreatitis.
- Serum glucose measurement to rule out diabetic truncal neuropathy.

DIFFERENTIAL DIAGNOSIS

- Posterior pulmonary abnormalities, including pneumonia, abscess, embolus, and infarct.
- Neoplasm of vertebral body.
- Vertebral compression fracture.
- Kummel disease.
- Osteomyelitis of vertebral body.
- Pancreatitis.
- Diabetic truncal neuropathy.

TREATMENT

- Simple analgesics and nonsteroidal anti-inflammatory agents for mild to moderate pain.
- Injection of the offending costovertebral joint or joints with local anesthetic and corticosteroid.
- Local superficial heat modalities, including silica gel–filled (Hydrocollator) packs and radiant heat.
- Topical lidocaine transdermal patches.

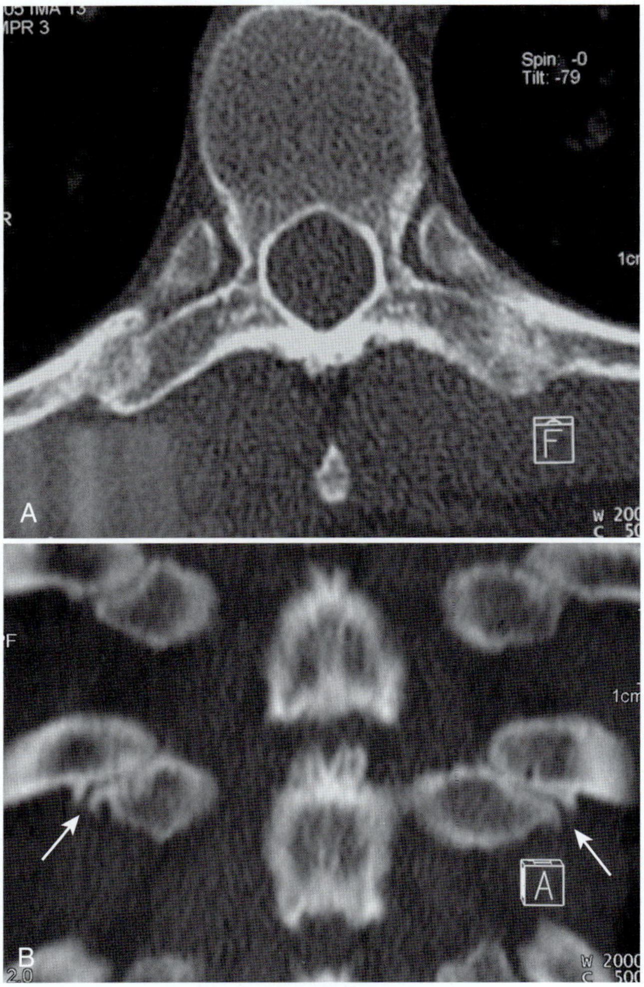

Figure 31.1 Young woman with vague nonspecific mid- dorsal pain. MRI findings were normal, and isotope bone scanning showed minor localized parasagittal increased uptake in the dorsal spine. (**A**), Axial CT shows loss of definition of the costovertebral joints bilaterally with minor sclerosis. (**B**), The coronal reconstruction images show early osteophyte formation (*arrows*) consistent with costovertebral osteoarthritis.

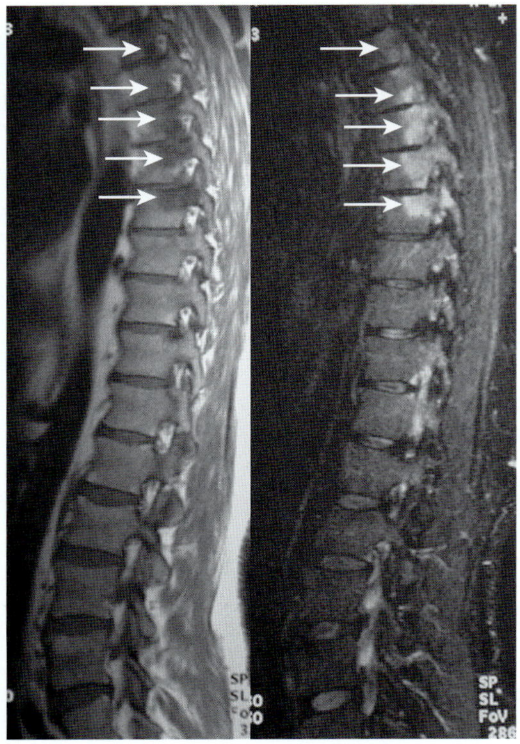

Figure 31.2 Sagittal T1W (*left*) and STIR (*right*) MR images of early ankylosing spondylitis in a young man with confirmed sacroiliitis. Marrow edema due to inflammatory changes is adjacent to the costovertebral joints of the lower dorsal spine; the edema has low signal intensity (SI) on the T1W MR images (**A**) (*white arrows*) and high SI on the STIR MR images (**B**) (*white arrows*).

CHAPTER 32

Idiopathic Scoliosis

DEFINITION

- Lateral curvature with varying degrees of rotation of the spine, usually in an S shape, without apparent underlying neuromuscular or bony abnormalities.

SIGNS AND SYMPTOMS

- Often asymptomatic, with the patient seeking medical attention because of cosmetic deformity or functional disability.
- May be painful with activity or during growth spurts.
- Pain may be secondary to development of degenerative disk disease, osteoporotic fractures, and degenerative arthritis of the facet joints and sacroiliac joints.
- Pain may be due to spondylolysis, especially at L5.
- Respiratory compromise may occur as scoliosis worsens.

DEMOGRAPHICS

- Age at onset is usual during adolescence, less common during early childhood, and rare in infancy.
- Female incidence seven times greater than male incidence.
- Strong familial incidence.
- Curvature often worsens during growth spurts.
- Increased incidence of syrinx in patients with levoscoliosis.

IMAGING RECOMMENDATIONS

- Radiography:
  - Assess degrees of scoliosis and kyphosis.
  - Identify osteogenic abnormality.
  - Obtain lateral flexion views to assess reducibility.
  - Monitor progression of scoliosis.
- MRI:
  - Identify features of occult spinal dysraphism prior to corrective surgery.
- CT:
  - Occasionally required if osteogenic abnormality present.

IMAGING FINDINGS

- Radiography:
  - Rotational deformity.
  - Cobb angle measured on AP radiographs.
  - Congenital hemivertebrae and other deformities may be seen in osteogenic scoliosis.
- MRI:
  - Findings usually normal.
  - MRI features of occult spinal dysraphism include:
    - Chiari malformation.
    - Diastematomyelia.
    - Syringomyelia.
    - Tethered cord.
    - Cord lipoma.
    - Bifid spinous processes.

OTHER RECOMMENDED TESTING

- Electromyography, nerve conduction velocity testing, and muscle biopsy to rule out neuromuscular disease.

DIFFERENTIAL DIAGNOSIS

- Scoliosis secondary to tumor, which usually manifests as a short painful curve.
- Scoliosis due to neuromuscular disease, which usually manifests as an elongated single thoracolumbar curve.
- Scoliosis secondary to infection, which usually manifests as a short painful curve.
- Scoliosis secondary to bony trauma, which usually manifests as a short painful curve with fractures evident on imaging.
- Scoliosis associated with congenital abnormalities, including Marfan syndrome, Ehlers-Danlos syndrome, osteogenesis imperfecta, neurofibromatosis, and certain types of dwarfism.
- Scheuermann disease, which manifests as kyphosis and characteristic end-plate changes.

TREATMENT

- Mild cases with curvature of less than 25 degrees are treated with watchful waiting.
- Orthotic bracing is the first step in the absence of neural compromise.
- Fusion with instrumentation to help straighten and stabilize progression of the disease in more severe cases.

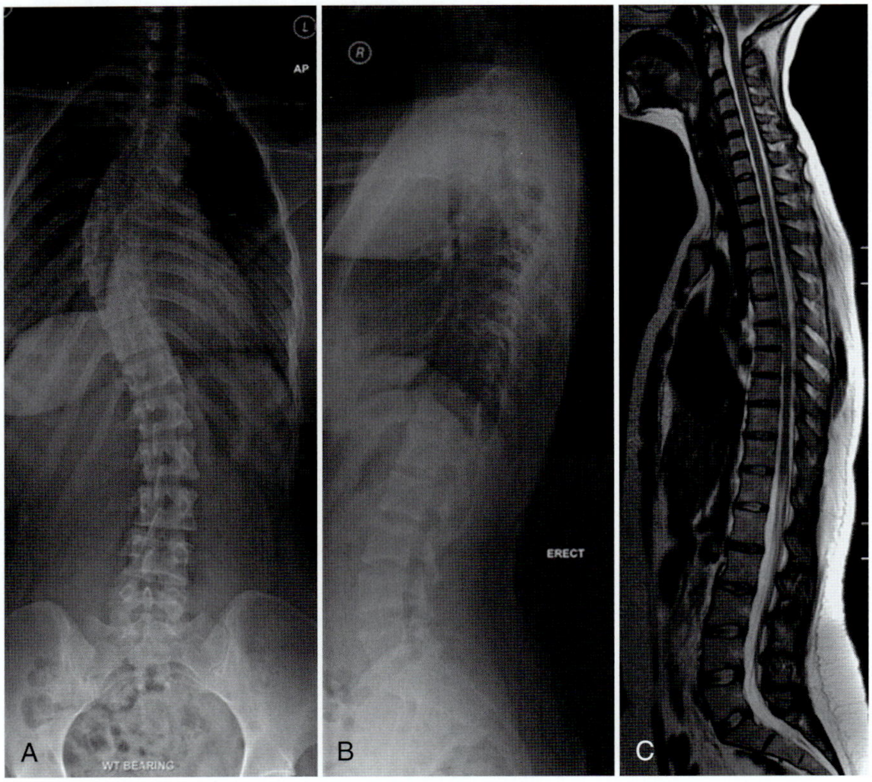

Figure 32.1 AP (**A**) and lateral (**B**) radiographs of a young patient with idiopathic juvenile scoliosis. The primary curve is centered in the dorsal spine convex to the right side. There is no osteogenic abnormality. (**C**), Sagittal T2-weighted (T2W) MR image with curved reconstruction shows the entire cord in profile. There is no Chiari malformation, tethered cord, or other feature of occult spinal dysraphism.

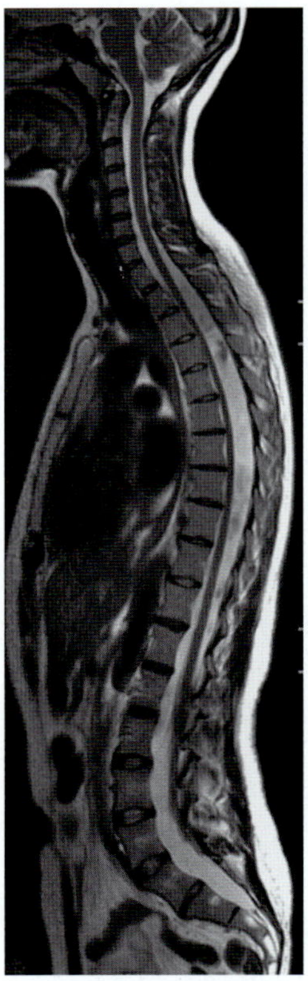

Figure 32.2 Sagittal T2W MR image with curved reconstruction from another patient with idiopathic juvenile scoliosis, demonstrating a capacious spinal canal due to dural ectasia. The dorsal cord appears rather atrophic, but no other cord abnormality was found on axial imaging. (Note the presence of flow artifacts posterior to the cord in the dorsal spine.)

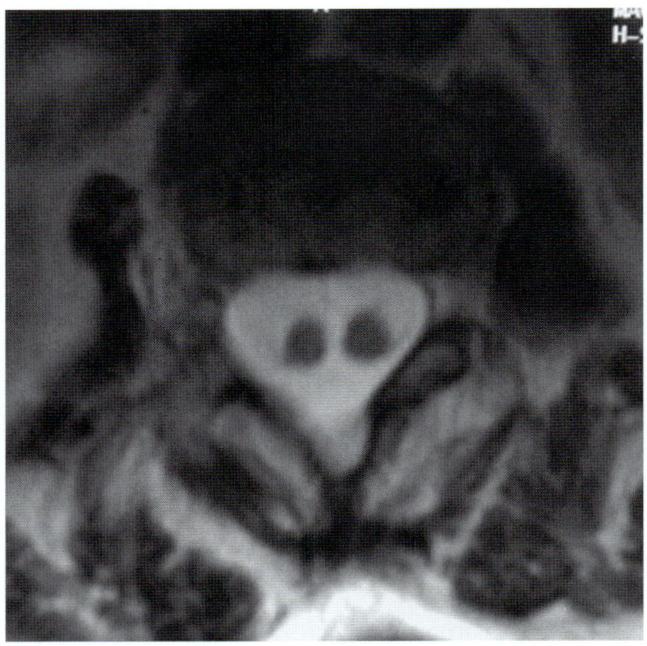

Figure 32.3 Axial T2W MR image of a patient with osteogenic scoliosis and multiple vertebral anomalies. Diastematomyelia (split cord) is present without an intervening fibrous or bony septum.

CHAPTER 33

Idiopathic Kyphosis

DEFINITION

- Curvature of the dorsal spine without underlying structural abnormality.

SIGNS AND SYMPTOMS

- Dorsal kyphosis located primarily in the upper vertebrae.
- More flexibility in the early stages of the disease.
- Straight curvature without scoliosis.
- Pain with activity in some patients because of muscle deconditioning.

DEMOGRAPHICS

- Most common in adolescents.
- Incidence: Female > Male.
- Coexistent degenerative disc disease of upper thoracic segments common.

IMAGING RECOMMENDATIONS

- Radiography and MRI to exclude structural causes of kyphosis.

IMAGING FINDINGS

- Kyphosis greater than 40 to 50 degrees.
- Absence of scoliosis and structural abnormalities.
- Increasing prevalence of disc degeneration and spondylosis in older patients.

OTHER RECOMMENDED TESTING

- Rule out osteoporosis in perimenopausal women and all men suffering from dorsal kyphosis, with laboratory testing for hyperparathyroidism, panhypopituitarism, and sex hormone deficits.
- Electromyography and nerve conduction testing are indicated if radiculopathy is present.
- Evoked potential testing if myelopathy is present.

DIFFERENTIAL DIAGNOSIS

- Scheuermann kyphosis.
- Post-traumatic kyphosis.
- Congenital kyphosis.
- Kyphosis due to anterior vertebral compression fractures.
- Ankylosing spondylitis.
- Infection.
- Neuromuscular disease.

TREATMENT

- Exercise and postural training.
- Orthotic bracing.
- Local injections and epidural nerve blocks with local anesthetic and corticosteroids for symptomatic relief.

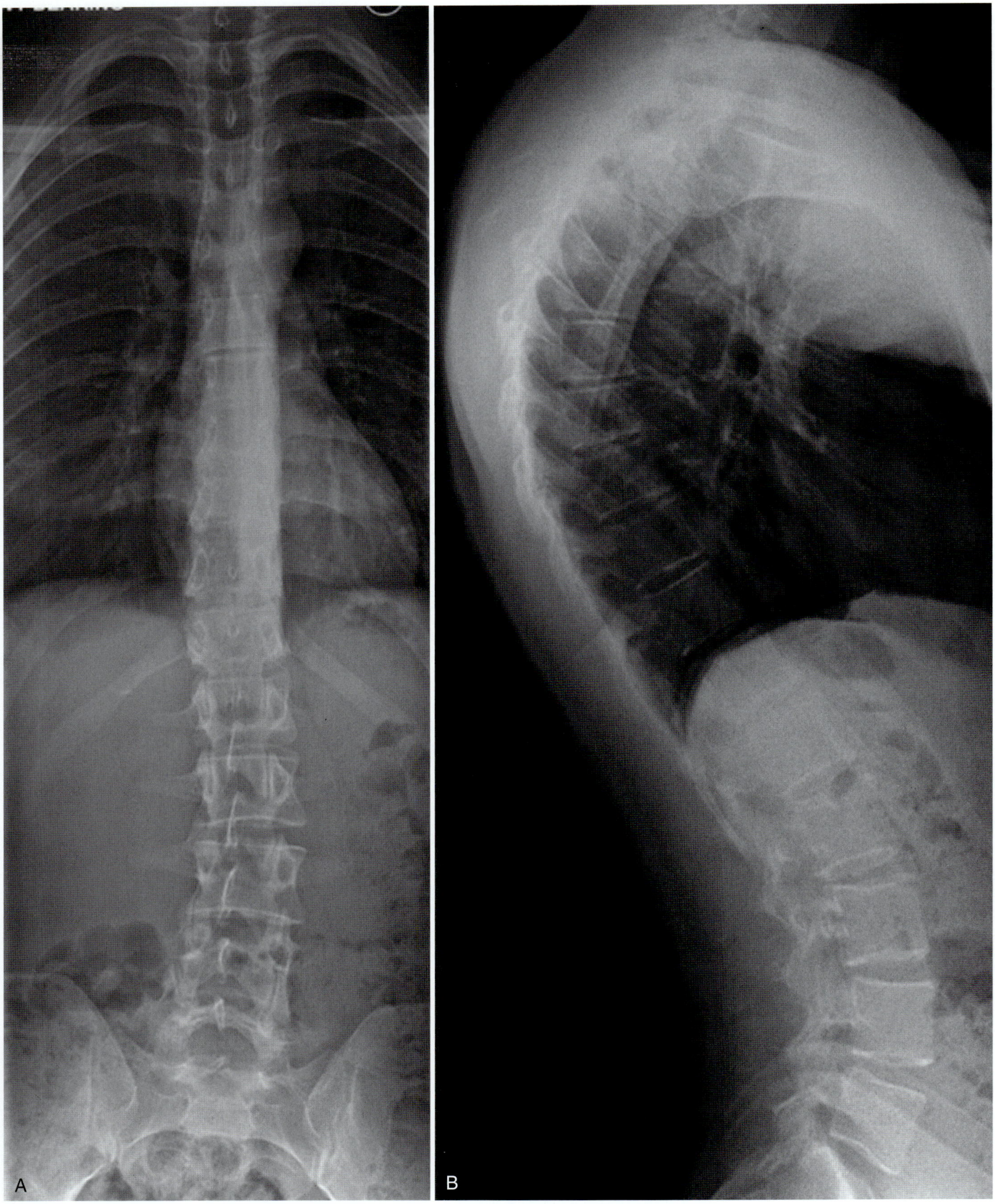

Figure 33.1 AP (A) and lateral (B) radiographs of an 18-year-old male patient with a kyphosis of 60 degrees, without associated Scheuermann disease or other structural abnormality. There is no associated scoliosis.

CHAPTER 34

Schmorl's Node

DEFINITION

- Superior or inferior herniation of the intervertebral disc through a weakened vertebral body end plate, resulting in an irregular node within the affected vertebral body.

SIGNS AND SYMPTOMS

- Sudden onset of localized, nonradiating, midline pain.
- Pain is aching and deep.
- Often asymptomatic.

DEMOGRAPHICS

- Most common in adolescents and young adults.
- Incidence: Male > Female.
- Often an incidental finding during spine imaging.
- Most commonly manifests clinically after axial loading.

IMAGING RECOMMENDATIONS

- Radiography or MRI.

IMAGING FINDINGS

- Localized area of cartilaginous disc herniation through the vertebral end plate (VEP) on MRI.
- Associated with accelerated disc space narrowing and disc degeneration.
- Multiple Schmorl nodes may occur without other features of Scheuermann disease.
- Acute traumatic Schmorl node formation may be associated with marrow edema on short T1 inversion recovery (STIR) MR images.
- Causes include Scheuermann disease, trauma, osteoporosis, hyperparathyroidism, and disc degeneration.
- Occasionally, infection and metastatic disease based on the VEP can mimic a Schmorl node.

OTHER RECOMMENDED TESTING

- Osteoporosis screening.
- In patients with osteoporosis, testing for hyperparathyroidism, panhypopituitarism, and sex hormone deficits.

DIFFERENTIAL DIAGNOSIS

- Acute vertebral compression fracture.
- Neoplasms, including metastatic lesions.
- Diskitis.
- Bone island.
- Limbus vertebrae.
- Type II VEP changes.
- Focal fatty marrow syndrome.

TREATMENT

- Conservative therapy consisting of local heat, simple analgesics, and nonsteroidal anti-inflammatory agents.
- Opioids are reserved for acute pain relief in patients for whom conservative therapy fails.
- Short-term orthotic bracing.
- Epidural injections of local anesthetics, opioids, and/or corticosteroids for pain not relieved by opioids.
- Treatment of underlying osteoporosis if present.

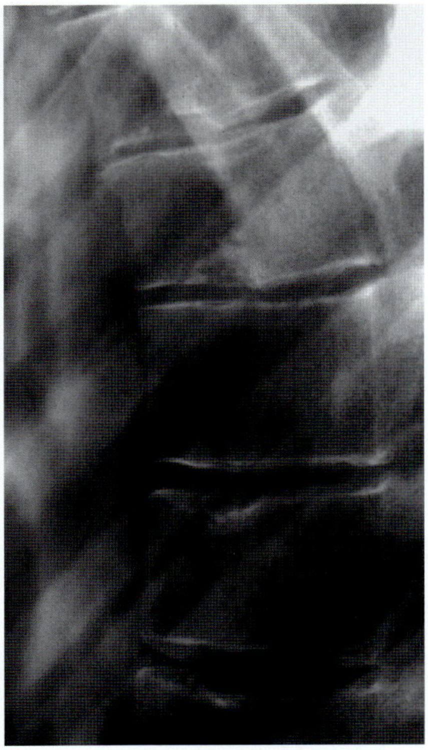

Figure 34.1 Lateral radiograph demonstrating small cartilaginous Schmorl nodes in the VEP.

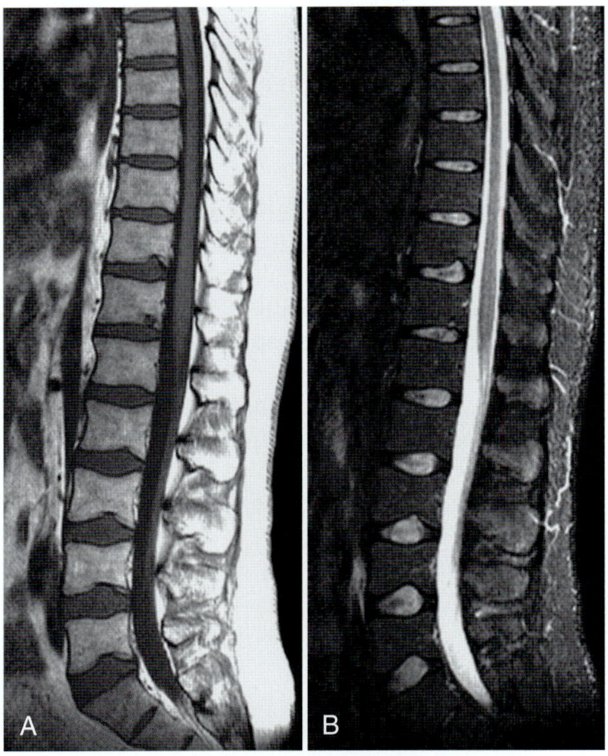

Figure 34.2 Sagittal T1-weighted (T1W) (**A**) and STIR (**B**) MR images of a localized Schmorl node in T11 and T12, with further nodes in the lower lumbar spine. The normal discal cartilage extends into the nodes, and there are no other features of Scheuermann disease.

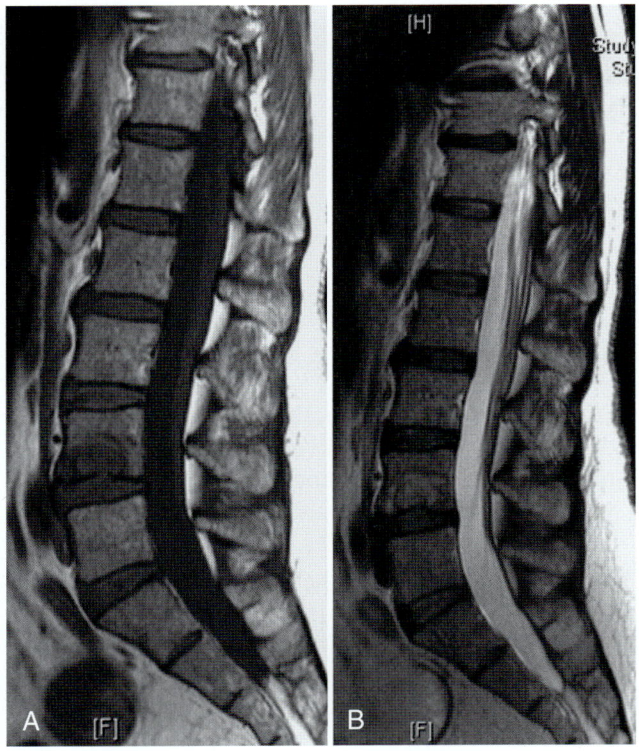

Figure 34.3 Sagittal T1W (**A**) and T2W (**B**) MR images of a solitary metastasis in a patient with non–small cell carcinoma of the lung. The metastasis is based on the inferior VEP of L4 and mimics a Schmorl node.

CHAPTER 35

Scheuermann Disease

DEFINITION

- Progressive kyphosis due to anterior wedging of vertebral bodies as a result of multiple Schmorl nodes.

SIGNS AND SYMPTOMS

- Sudden onset of localized, nonradiating thoracic midline pain.
- Pain aching and deep in character.
- Pain made worse by activity.
- Kyphosis is progressive.
- If kyphosis is significant, radiculopathy and/or myelopathy may be present.
- Fatigue may be present.

DEMOGRAPHICS

- Most common in adolescents.
- Most common in thoracic spine.
- Incidence: Male > Female.
- Familial tendency possible.
- May be caused by repetitive skeletal trauma in skeletally immature individuals, for example, from gymnastics and weight lifting.

IMAGING RECOMMENDATIONS

- Radiography or MRI.

IMAGING FINDINGS

- Sorenson criteria:
  - Wedging of more than 5 degrees of three or more contiguous vertebral bodies.
  - Kyphosis greater than 40 degrees.
- Secondary signs:
  - Vertebral end-plate irregularity and Schmorl node formation.
  - Disk space narrowing and disc degeneration.
  - Scoliosis.
- Lesser degrees of abnormality that do not fulfill Sorensen criteria are frequently encountered.
- Anterior Schmorl nodes may mimic traumatic ring apophyseal avulsion.
- Lumbar spine involvement is associated with pars stress fractures.

OTHER RECOMMENDED TESTING

- Osteoporosis screening.
- In patients with osteoporosis, testing for hyperparathyroidism, panhypopituitarism, and sex hormone deficits.
- Tuberculosis screening.
- Electromyography and nerve conduction velocity testing to rule out neuromuscular disease.
- Laboratory testing to rule out ankylosis spondylitis.

DIFFERENTIAL DIAGNOSIS

- Acute vertebral compression fracture.
- Neoplasm, including metastatic lesions.
- Pott's disease.
- Congenital kyphosis.
- Postural kyphosis.
- Neuromuscular disease.
- Osteogenesis imperfecta tarda.
- Spranger-Weidemann syndrome.

TREATMENT

- Conservative therapy consisting of local heat, simple analgesics, and nonsteroidal anti-inflammatory agents.
- Opioids are reserved for acute pain relief in those patients for whom conservative therapy fails.
- Orthotic bracing.
- Epidural injections of local anesthetics, opioids, and/or corticosteroids for pain not relieved by opioids.
- Treatment of underlying osteoporosis if present.
- Surgical stabilization of the spine if neurologic symptoms progress.

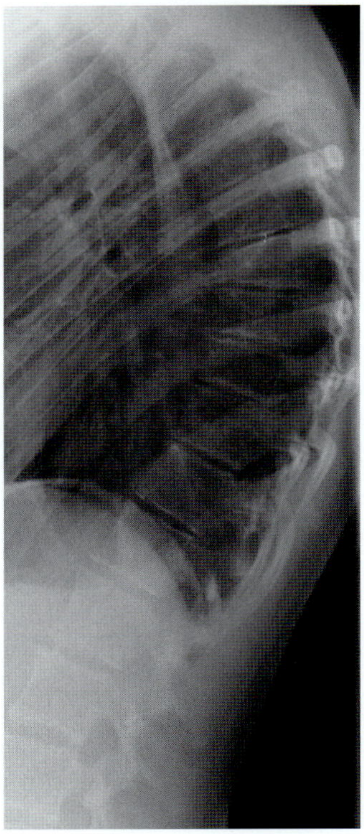

Figure 35.1 Lateral radiograph of an adolescent with kyphosis. There is anterior wedging of the T7 vertebral body and multilevel disk space narrowing and vertebral end-plate irregularity.

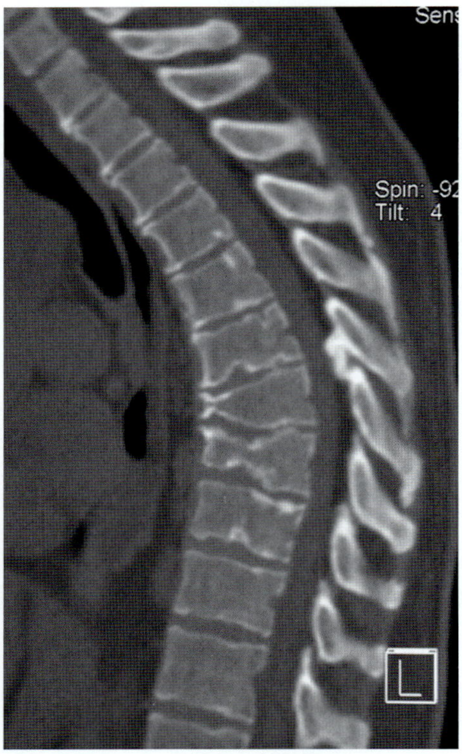

Figure 35.2 CT scan of a different patient with similar changes: vertebral wedging, kyphosis, vertebral end-plate irregularity, and secondary disk degeneration.

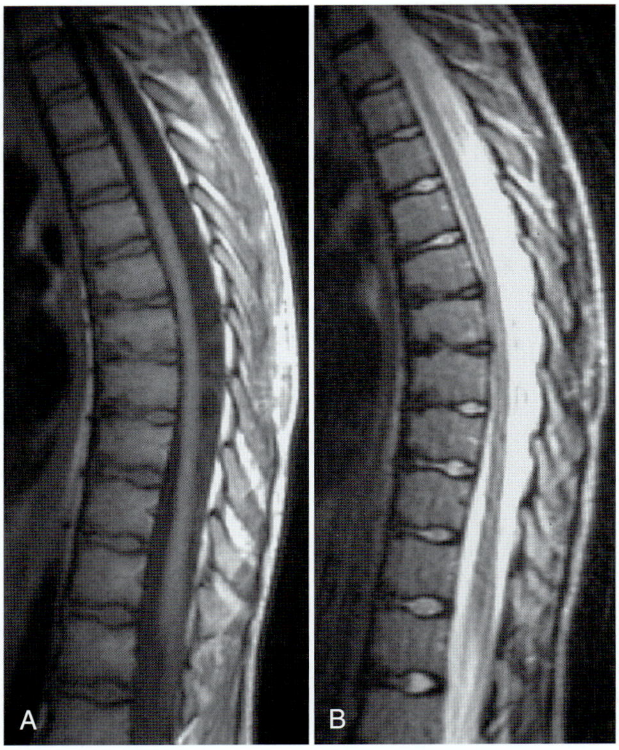

Figure 35.3 T1-weighted (T1W) (**A**) and T2W (**B**) MR images of an adolescent with vague back pain. There is minor kyphosis, multilevel anterior Schmorl node formation, and disk degeneration. These findings do not completely fulfill the Sorenson criteria for Scheuermann disease.

CHAPTER 36

DISH Syndrome

DEFINITION

- Diffuse idiopathic skeletal hyperostosis characterized by flowing ossification of the anterior longitudinal ligament.

SIGNS AND SYMPTOMS

- Often an incidental finding in otherwise asymptomatic patients.
- In the absence of trauma, onset of symptoms is insidious.
- Patient may complain of spinal stiffness.
- Patient may complain of decreased spinal range of motion.
- Symptoms worse in the morning, with cold exposure, or with periods of prolonged inactivity.
- Anterior osteophytes may cause dysphagia and respiratory embarrassment.
- Associated tendonitis often present.

DEMOGRAPHICS

- Onset in the fifth decade of life.
- Incidence: Male > Female.
- Marked increase of incidence in white persons.
- Uncommon in Asians.

IMAGING RECOMMENDATIONS

- Conventional radiographs are usually diagnostic.
- MRI or CT is usually indicated only for complications.
- Barium swallow study for patients with dysphagia.

IMAGING FINDINGS

- Bridging osteophyte formation or large claw osteophytes across three or more contiguous vertebral segments.
- Disk height is usually preserved.
- Absence of syndesmophytes, but ribbon-like pattern in the dorsal spine may mimic ankylosing spondylitis.
- Dorsal spine is most frequently involved, but disease may extend into cervical or lumbar spine.
- Entheseal new bone formation at other skeletal sites.

OTHER RECOMMENDED TESTING

- Laboratory screening for ankylosing spondylitis.

DIFFERENTIAL DIAGNOSIS

- Spondylosis.
- Epidural calcification due to hemodialysis.
- Ankylosing spondylitis.
- Reiter syndrome.
- Psoriatic arthritis.

TREATMENT

- Conservative treatment consisting of local heat, simple analgesics, and nonsteroidal anti-inflammatory agents will improve symptoms in many cases.
- Physical therapy, including gentle stretching and gentle range-of-motion exercises.
- Epidural blocks will provide symptomatic relief if conservative therapy fails or if the pain is limiting activities of daily living.
- Treatment of associated tendonitis to avoid functional disability.
- Surgical excision of any osteophytes compromising the esophagus or trachea.

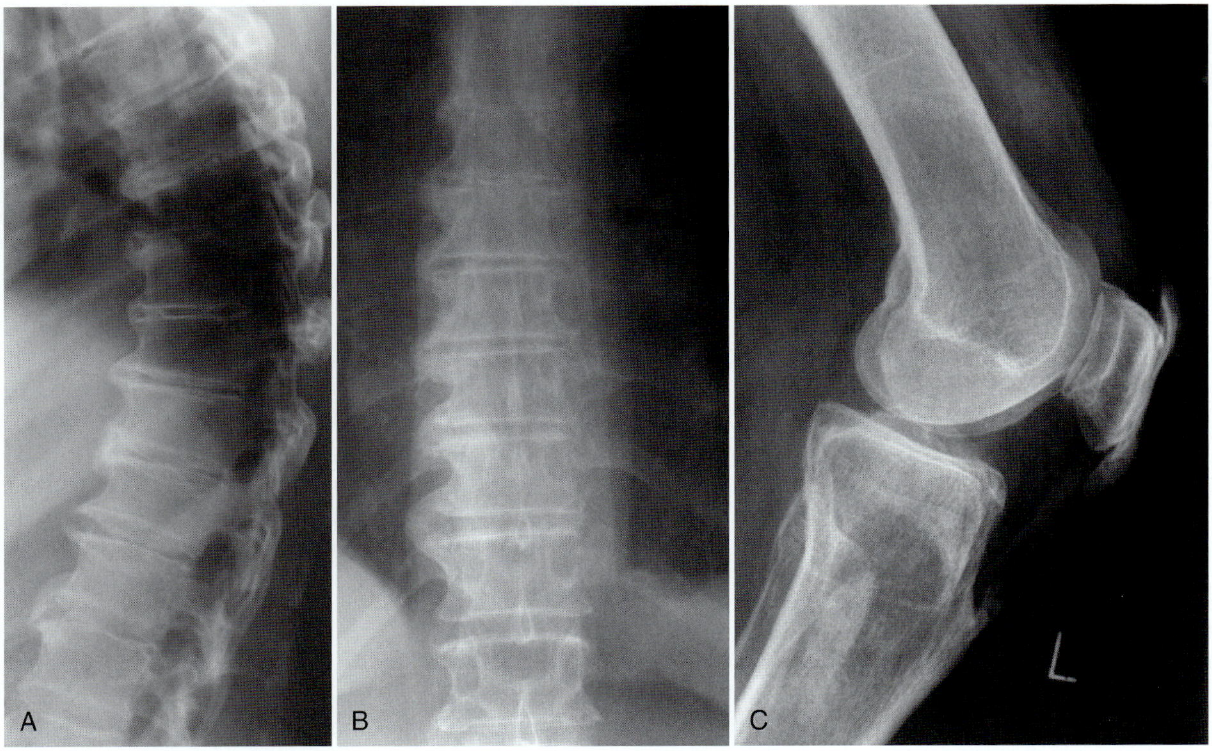

Figure 36.1 Lateral (**A**) and AP (**B**) radiographs of the lower dorsal spine of a middle-aged man with DISH syndrome. Profuse claw osteophyte and bridging ossification are present at multiple contiguous vertebral levels. Disk height is generally well preserved. (**C**), The lateral radiograph of the knee in the same patient demonstrates prominent entheseal new bone formation, which is a hallmark of the widespread skeletal involvement in DISH syndrome.

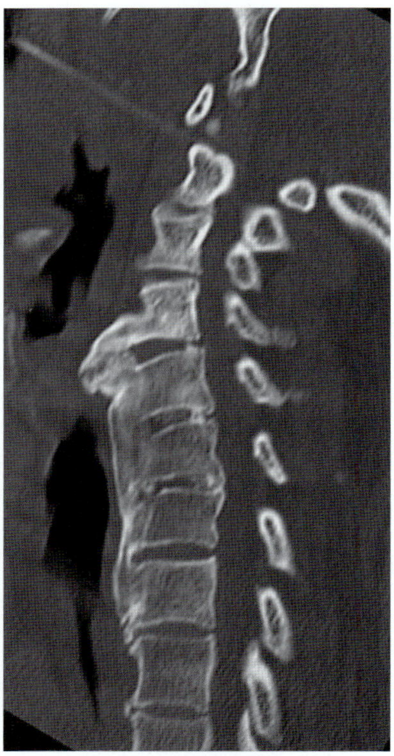

Figure 36.2 Sagittal CT scan of a patient with DISH syndrome of the cervical and upper thoracic spine. There is extensive anterior bridging ossification with large claw osteophytes at C4-C5.

CHAPTER 37

Multiple Sclerosis of the Thoracic Spinal Cord

DEFINITION

- An autoimmune disease that attacks the central nervous system, with resultant sclerotic plaques scattered throughout the central nervous system and the thoracic spinal cord commonly affected.

SIGNS AND SYMPTOMS

- Paresthesias.
- Motor and sensory symptoms mimicking radiculopathy and/or myelopathy.
- Often associated with optic neuritis.
- Hyperreflexia.
- Gait disturbance.
- Bowel and bladder symptomatology.
- High temperature can exacerbate symptoms (Uhthoff sign).
- Multiple sclerosis can manifest as essentially any neurologic sign or symptom.
- Natural history of the disease can vary from benign to a rapidly progressive disease with an extremely poor prognosis.

DEMOGRAPHICS

- Peak onset in third to fourth decades of life, but can occur at any age.
- Incidence: Female > Male.
- Higher incidence in patients of Western European origin.
- More common in the higher latitudes, with incidence of disease decreasing linearly as one moves toward the equator.
- Increased incidence in families.

IMAGING RECOMMENDATIONS

- MRI:
  - Include brain and cervical cord.
  - T1-weighted (T1W), T2W, and fluid-attenuated inversion recovery (FLAIR) sequences.
  - Administration of high doses of a contrast agent with MR imaging may increase conspicuity of lesions.

IMAGING FINDINGS

- High-signal intensity (SI) plaques of demyelination on T2W MR images.
- Plaques are more conspicuous on FLAIR images.
- T1W MR images are often normal.
- Plaques are small, round, or ovoid and are well defined.
- Plaques may enhance with contrast agent in early stages.
- More extensive confluent lesions may occur.
- No cord expansion.
- Combination of brain and spinal cord lesions increases specificity of diagnosis.

OTHER RECOMMENDED TESTING

- Electromyography and nerve conduction velocity testing are indicated if radiculopathy is present and to rule out amyotrophic lateral sclerosis.
- Evoked potential testing to quantify spinal cord compromise and cranial nerve deficits.

DIFFERENTIAL DIAGNOSIS

- Spinal cord ischemia and infarct.
- Idiopathic transverse myelitis.
- Spinal cord neoplasm.
- Syringomyelia.
- Acute disseminated encephalomyelitis (ADEM).

TREATMENT

- Systemic glucocorticoids.
- Interferon-β
- Plasmapheresis.
- Glatiramer acetate.
- Mitoxantrone.
- Natalizumab.
- Physical and occupational therapies.

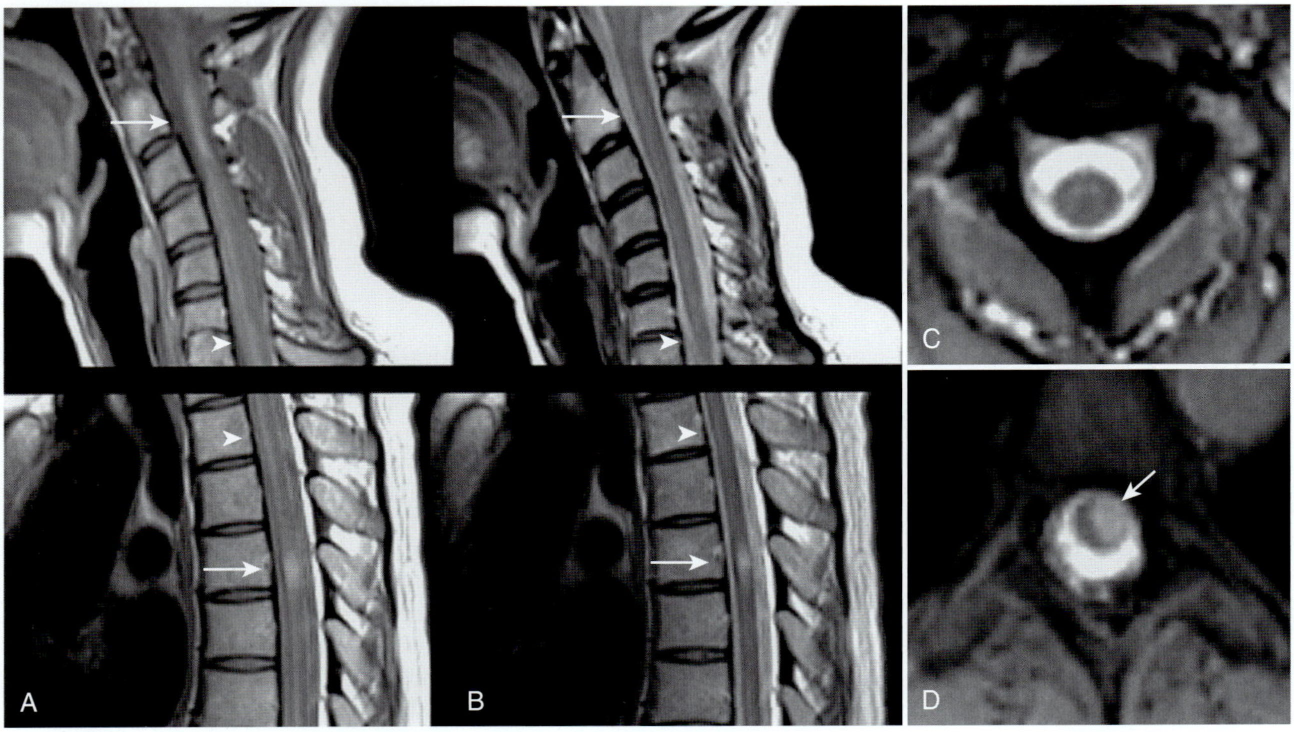

Figure 37.1 Sagittal intermediate TE (**A**, *top and bottom*) and T2W (**B**, *top and bottom*) dual echo MR images of a patient with multiple sclerosis. There are both focal (*arrows*) and diffuse (*arrowheads*) areas of demyelination. The diffuse lesions are more easily appreciated on the intermediate TE MR images. Axial T2W gradient echo images in a different subject show the normal appearance of the cord (**C**) and a focal demyelination plaque of the thoracic cord (**D**). Note that the plaque (*arrow*) occupies the lateral aspect of the cord and does not spare the gray matter. There is no cord expansion. *(From Bot JC, Barkhof F: Spinal-cord MRI in multiple sclerosis: Conventional and nonconventional MR techniques. Neuroimaging Clin N Am 2009;19:81-99.)*

CHAPTER 38

Idiopathic Transverse Myelitis

DEFINITION

- An acute inflammatory disorder, often associated with previous viral infection or vaccination, that results in perivascular inflammation of both halves of the spinal cord, causing bilateral autonomic, sensory, and motor dysfunction.

SIGNS AND SYMPTOMS

- Prodrome with generalized myalgias and aching, often occurring after a viral illness and rarely after vaccination.
- Rapid onset of neurologic symptoms over a period of days.
- Sensory deficits with clearly defined neurologic level.
- Ascending paresthesias.
- Constricting, bandlike paresthesias.
- Motor and sensory symptoms mimicking radiculopathy and/or myelopathy.
- Initially manifests as hyporeflexia and hypotonia progressing to varying degrees of spasticity and hyperreflexia.
- Paraparesis and quadriparesis progressing to paraplegia and quadriplegia in severe cases.
- Bowel and bladder symptomatology.
- Cranial nerves always spared.
- Natural history of the disease can vary from benign to a rapidly progressive disease with an extremely poor prognosis.

DEMOGRAPHICS

- Bimodal onset in patients 10 through 19 and 30 through 39 years of age, but can occur at any age.
- Incidence: Female = Male.
- No ethnic predilection.
- The more rapid the onset and the more severe the neurologic deficit, the worse the prognosis.

IMAGING RECOMMENDATIONS

- MRI:
  - T2-weighted (T2W) and/or fluid-attenuated inversion recovery (FLAIR) sequences.
  - Imaging after administration of a contrast agent (post-contrast imaging).
  - Diffusion-weighted imaging.

IMAGING FINDINGS

- High–signal intensity (SI) foci within the spinal cord on T2W MR images.
  - Enhancement on post-contrast images.
- Typically confined to four spinal levels.
- More extensive changes have been designated as longitudinal transverse myelitis.
- Later, cord atrophy may be seen.

OTHER RECOMMENDED TESTING

- Electromyography and nerve conduction velocity testing are indicated if radiculopathy is present and to rule out amyotrophic lateral sclerosis.
- Evoked potential testing to quantify spinal cord compromise and to identify cranial nerve deficits more likely associated with multiple sclerosis.

DIFFERENTIAL DIAGNOSIS

- Multiple sclerosis.
- Spinal cord ischemia and infarct.
- Spinal cord neoplasm.
- Syringomyelia.
- Acute disseminated encephalomyelitis (ADEM).

TREATMENT

- Systemic glucocorticoids.
- Physical and occupational therapies.
- Aggressive pain control with the use of simple analgesics, nonsteroidal anti-inflammatory agents, opioids, and adjuvant analgesics, including gabapentin, antidepressants, anticonvulsants, and membrane stabilizers.

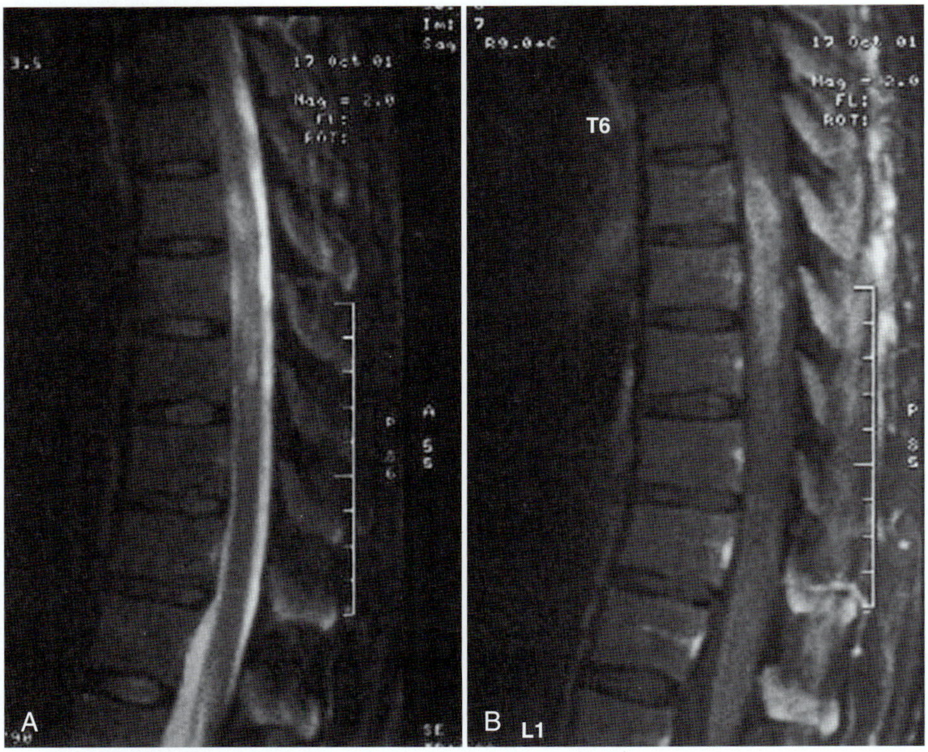

Figure 38.1 (**A**), Sagittal T2W with fat suppressicn (FST2W) MR image of a patient with acute transverse myelitis showing a focal high-SI lesion extending from T7 to T9. (**B**), The area of demyelination enhances on the post-contrast FST1W MR image. *(From Chan KH, Tsang KL, Fong GC, et al: Idiopathic severe recurrent transverse myelitis: A restricted variant of neuromyelitis optica. Clin Neurol Neurosurg 2005;107:132-135.)*

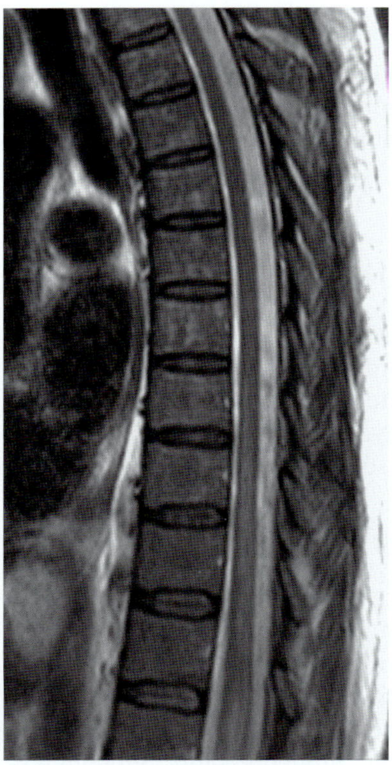

Figure 38.2 Sagittal T2W MR image of a different patient with transverse myelitis demonstrating more diffuse linear increased high SI throughout the lower dorsal cord.

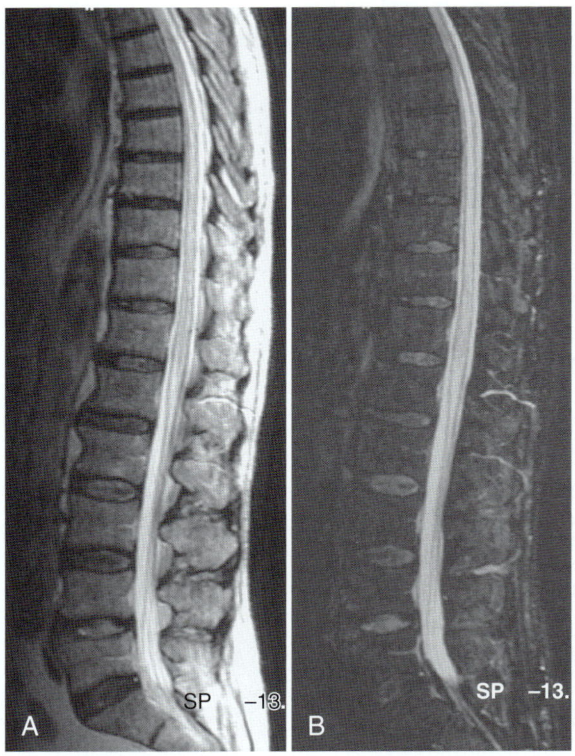

Figure 38.3 Sagittal T2W (**A**) and short T1 inversion recovery (STIR) (**B**) MR images in a patient with an acute spinal cord infarct. There is diffuse increased SI throughout the dorsal spinal cord. This appearance can also be seen with multiple sclerosis, longitudinal transverse myelitis, and ADEM.

CHAPTER 39

Guillain-Barré Syndrome

DEFINITION

- An acute inflammatory disorder, often associated with previous viral infection or vaccination, that results in acute demyelination of the nerve roots, peripheral nerves, and cranial nerves.

SIGNS AND SYMPTOMS

- Onset with distal paresthesias and autonomic dysfunction, often occurring after viral illness and rarely after vaccination.
- Rapid onset of neurologic symptoms of characteristic ascending paralysis.
- Neurologic deficits are usually bilateral and symmetrical.
- Ascending paralysis may involve brainstem, with cranial nerve deficits and respiratory paralysis.
- Facial nerve the most commonly affected.
- Sensory loss less severe relative to motor and autonomic deficits.
- Clinical nadir at 3½ to 4 weeks.

DEMOGRAPHICS

- Peak occurrence in children and young adults, but can occur at any age.
- Incidence: Female = Male.
- Common cause of paralysis in Western countries, with incidence of 1.5 cases per 100,000.
- 50% of patients still have symptoms at 1 year.
- Permanent neurologic deficits in 10% of patients.
- 7% to 8% of patients may experience relapse.

IMAGING RECOMMENDATIONS

- Imaging not indicated initially. Diagnosis is made by cerebrospinal fluid analysis, electromyography, and so on.
- MRI may be used to exclude other causes of neurologic dysfunction.

IMAGING FINDINGS

- MRI findings in the spinal cord are usually normal.
- There is some evidence that enhancement of the cauda equina and lumbosacral nerve roots may be seen in Guillain-Barré syndrome.

OTHER RECOMMENDED TESTING

- Cerebrospinal fluid analysis.
- Electromyography and nerve conduction velocity testing are indicated if radiculopathy is present and to rule out amyotrophic lateral sclerosis and inflammatory muscle disease.
- Evoked potential testing to quantify spinal cord compromise and to identify cranial nerve deficits more likely associated with multiple sclerosis.
- Laboratory workup for collagen vascular diseases.
- Muscle biopsy.

DIFFERENTIAL DIAGNOSIS

- Multiple sclerosis.
- Idiopathic acute transverse myelitis.
- Spinal cord ischemia and infarct.
- Spinal cord neoplasm.
- Syringomyelia.
- Acute disseminated encephalomyelitis (ADEM).
- Miller Fischer syndrome.
- Tick paralysis.
- Meningitis.
- Chronic polyneuropathies, including Charcot-Marie-Tooth disease.
- Polyarteritis nodosa.

TREATMENT

- Gamma globulin.
- Plasmapheresis.
- Aggressive pain control with the use of simple analgesics, nonsteroidal anti-inflammatory agents, opioids, and adjuvant analgesics, including gabapentin, antidepressants, anticonvulsants, and membrane stabilizers.
- Physical and occupational therapy.

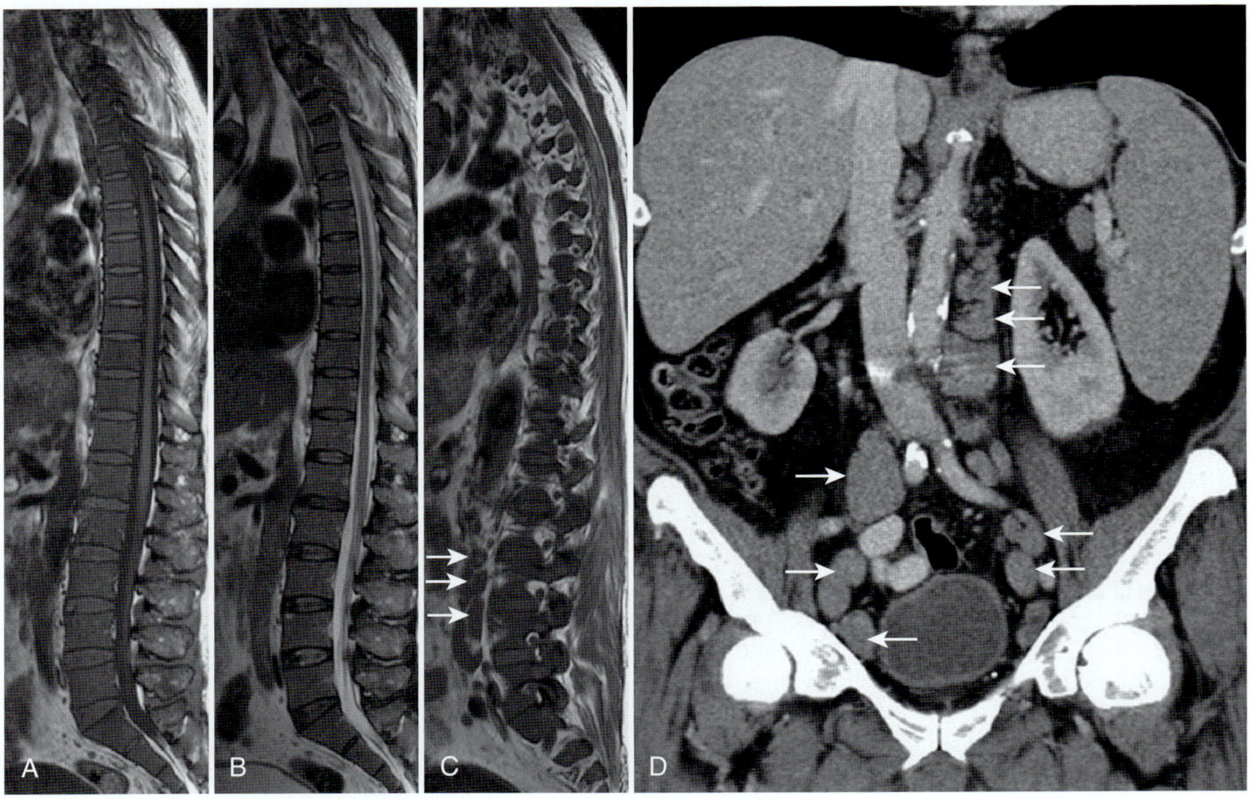

Figure 39.1 Patient being treated for presumed Guillain-Barré syndrome. Sagittal T1-weighted (T1W) (**A**) and T2W (**B**) MR images demonstrate a normal spinal cord. However, lymphadenopathy is present on the parasagittal T1W MR image (**C**) (*arrows*). (**D**), Staging CT scan shows extensive retroperitoneal and pelvic lymphadenopathy (*arrows*). The patient was diagnosed as having lymphoma with paraneoplastic syndrome.

CHAPTER 40

Hemangioma of the Thoracic Spine

DEFINITION

- Benign, slow-growing tumor of vascular origin, usually confined to the vertebral body but occasionally extending epidurally with resultant spinal cord compression.

SIGNS AND SYMPTOMS

- Often an incidental finding during other diagnostic imaging.
- More aggressive hemangiomas may cause severe dorsal spine pain.
- Occasionally, acute onset of back pain follows hemangioma-induced collapse of a vertebral body.
- With epidural extension, signs and symptoms of radiculopathy and myelopathy may occur.

DEMOGRAPHICS

- Most common spinal axis tumor.
- Peak occurrence in middle-aged women.
- Rare autosomal dominant familial occurrence with associated cerebral cavernous arteriovenous malformations.
- Most lesions confined to the vertebral body.
- 25% to 30% of thoracic hemangiomas are multiple.
- Thoracic lesions tend to be more aggressive than lesions involving the lumbar and cervical spine.

IMAGING RECOMMENDATIONS

- MRI is most sensitive modality for detection of hemangiomas.
- CT may aid characterization for lesion that appears indeterminate on MRI.
- Radiographs demonstrate only large hemangiomas.

IMAGING FINDINGS

- MRI:
  - High signal intensity (SI) of the fatty component on T1-weighted (T1W) and T2W MR images.
  - Lesions may have low SI on short T1 inversion recovery (STIR) MR images because of fat suppression.
  - High SI occurs on STIR MR images if there is a prominent vascular component.
- Hemangiomas are usually rounded and confined to the vertebral body.
- Posterior elements are less frequently involved.
- Paravertebral soft tissue extension and vertebral fracture may be seen with aggressive lesions.
- CT demonstrates the characteristic vertical trabecular pattern of hemangiomas. This pattern is also seen on radiographs of larger lesions.

OTHER RECOMMENDED TESTING

- Osteoporosis screening if compression fracture is present.
- Electromyography and nerve conduction velocity testing are indicated if radiculopathy is present.
- Evoked potential testing if myelopathy is present to quantify extent of spinal cord compromise.
- Bence Jones protein analysis for multiple myeloma if diagnosis is in question.

DIFFERENTIAL DIAGNOSIS

- Metastatic disease involving vertebral body.
- Vertebral compression fracture.
- Focal fatty marrow.
- Paget disease.
- Degenerative end plates Modic type II.
- Radiation treatment involving thoracic vertebra.

TREATMENT

- Serial neurologic and radiographic monitoring of asymptomatic patients.
- More aggressive monitoring for patients with axial pain ascribed to hemangioma.
- Intralesional injection of alcohol.
- Vertebroplasty.
- Kyphoplasty.
- Radiation therapy for more aggressive lesions.

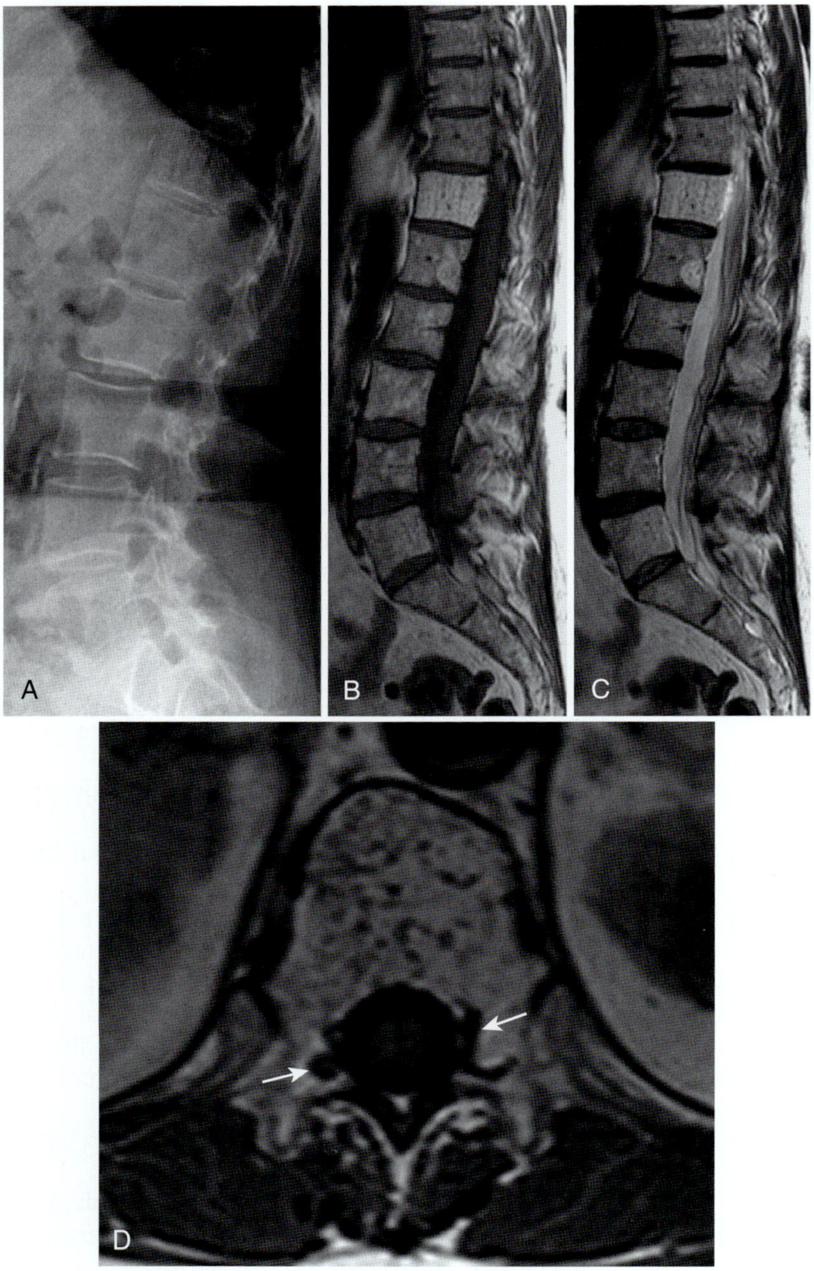

Figure 40.1 Lateral radiograph (**A**) of a patient with a large hemangioma of the T12 vertebral body. There is a typical pattern of coarse vertical trabeculation within the affected vertebra. The sagittal T1W (**B**) and T2W (**C**) MR images show the predominantly fatty content as high SI on both pulse sequences. A second, smaller hemangioma is present in the L1 vertebral body. The low-SI vertical trabeculae are best appreciated on the T1W axial image (**D**), with rounded areas of low SI giving a "polka dot" appearance. Note also the large feeding vessels (*white arrows*).

CHAPTER 41

Schwannoma of the Thoracic Spine

DEFINITION

- Slow-growing, benign, dumbbell-shaped neoplasm of the nerve sheath, most often arising from a single fascicle, that occurs most commonly in dorsal spinal nerve roots and rarely may undergo malignant degeneration.

SIGNS AND SYMPTOMS

- Most often manifests as radicular symptoms.
- Pain often very neuritic in nature.
- Pain often exacerbated with movement of affected spinal segment.
- Untreated or rapidly growing schwannomas may cause spinal cord compression with resultant myelopathy.
- More aggressive schwannomas may cause severe dorsal spine pain.

DEMOGRAPHICS

- Peak occurrence between the third and sixth decades of life.
- Incidence: Male = Female.
- No ethnic predilection.
- Increased incidence in patients with neurofibromatosis type II.
- Increased incidence in patients with Carney complex.

IMAGING RECOMMENDATIONS

- MRI is the primary imaging modality.
- Radiographic findings are often normal.
- CT myelography is alternative if MRI is contraindicated.

IMAGING FINDINGS

- Radiographs may show scalloping of the vertebral body or pedicle and widening of the exit canal.
- Rounded or bilobed extradural mass that may have both intraspinal and extraspinal involvement.
- The involved nerve is contiguous with the mass.
- Masses have intermediate signal intensity (SI) on T1-weighted (T1W) MR images and high SI on T2W or short T1 inversion recovery (STIR) MR images.
- Contrast enhancement is typical. A "target" sign is more suggestive of neurofibroma.
- Ancient schwannomas may undergo cystic degeneration.

OTHER RECOMMENDED TESTING

- Electromyography and nerve conduction velocity testing are indicated if radiculopathy is present.
- Evoked potential testing if myelopathy is present, to quantify extent of spinal cord compromise.
- Echocardiogram if atrial myxoma associated with Carney complex is being considered.

DIFFERENTIAL DIAGNOSIS

- Neurofibroma.
- Extruded disk fragments.
- Meningioma.
- Myxopapillary ependymoma.
- Meningocele.

TREATMENT

- Surgical resection of tumor and associated nerve root.
- Radiation therapy for malignant degeneration.

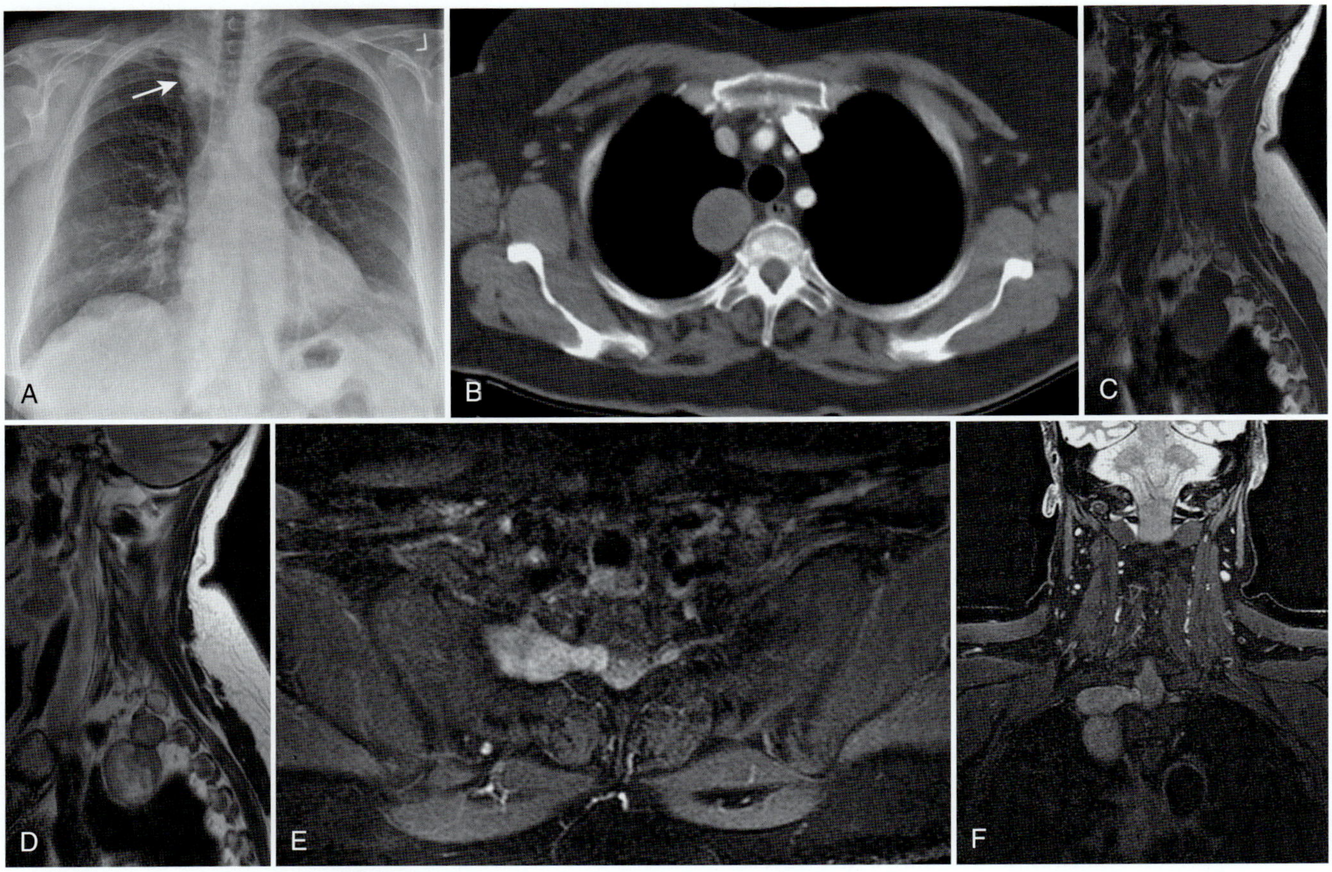

Figure 41.1 (A), Chest radiograph showing a right paratracheal mass (*white arrow*). (B), CT scan of the chest demonstrates a well-defined rounded posterior mediastinal mass. The mass is bilobed on the sagittal T1W (C) and T2W (D) MR images, a feature that is highly suspicious for a nerve sheath tumor. Axial (E) and coronal (F) STIR images demonstrate extension of the mass into the exit foramen of the spinal canal, confirming the diagrosis of a nerve sheath tumor.

CHAPTER 42

Epidural Lipomatosis of the Thoracic Spine

DEFINITION

- Gradual increase in the amount of epidural fat, most commonly associated with excessive endogenous or exogenous glucocorticoids, that can result in compression of the spinal cord and exiting nerve roots.

SIGNS AND SYMPTOMS

- Most often manifests as weakness.
- Radicular symptoms often present.
- Back pain.
- Altered reflexes.
- Gait abnormalities.
- Left untreated, may cause spinal cord compression with resultant myelopathy.

DEMOGRAPHICS

- Peak occurrence in mid-fourth decade of life.
- Incidence: Male > Female.
- No ethnic predilection.
- Increased incidence in patients with Cushing disease.
- Increased incidence in patients taking exogenous steroids.
- Increased incidence in patients with endogenous obesity.

IMAGING RECOMMENDATIONS

- MRI is the primary imaging modality.
- CT is an alternative to MRI.

IMAGING FINDINGS

- Intraspinal fat signal intensity (SI) tissue in the epidural space on MRI. (Low-density fat tissue see on CT.)
- Usually located posterior to the thecal sac.
- Compression of the thecal sac with obliteration of the cerebrospinal fluid space.
- Spinal stenosis is often aggravated by the presence of associated degenerative processes, such as disc bulging and ligament hypertrophy.
- Cord compression may lead to development of syrinx.
- Lumbar lipomatosis may cause symptomatic stenosis.

OTHER RECOMMENDED TESTING

- Electromyography and nerve conduction velocity testing are indicated if radiculopathy is present.
- Evoked potential testing is indicated if myelopathy is present, to quantify extent of spinal cord compromise.
- Laboratory evaluation for Cushing disease and other endocrinopathies.

DIFFERENTIAL DIAGNOSIS

- Epidural abscess.
- Epidural hematoma.
- Epidural metastasis.
- Lymphoma.
- Spinal angiolipoma.

TREATMENT

- Weight loss for endogenous obesity.
- Discontinuation of exogenous steroids.
- Correction of underlying endocrinopathies.
- Surgical decompression of area of spine that is compromised.

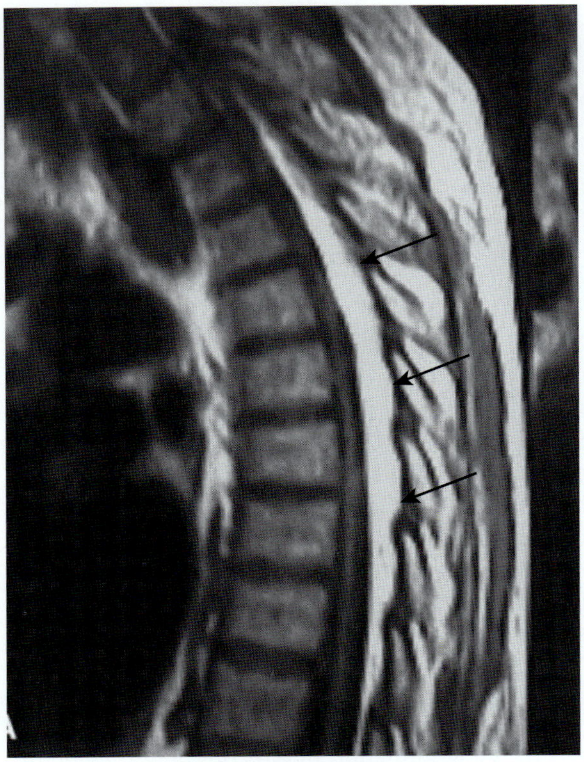

Figure 42.1 Sagittal T1-weighted (T1W) MR image of a patient with a 15-year history of progressive right lower extremity stiffness and weakness. There is excessive high-SI epidural fat posteriorly (*arrows*), which is compressing the spinal cord. *(From Citow JS, Kranzler L: Thoracic epidural lipmatosis with associated syrinx: Case report. Surg Neurol 2000;53:589-591.)*

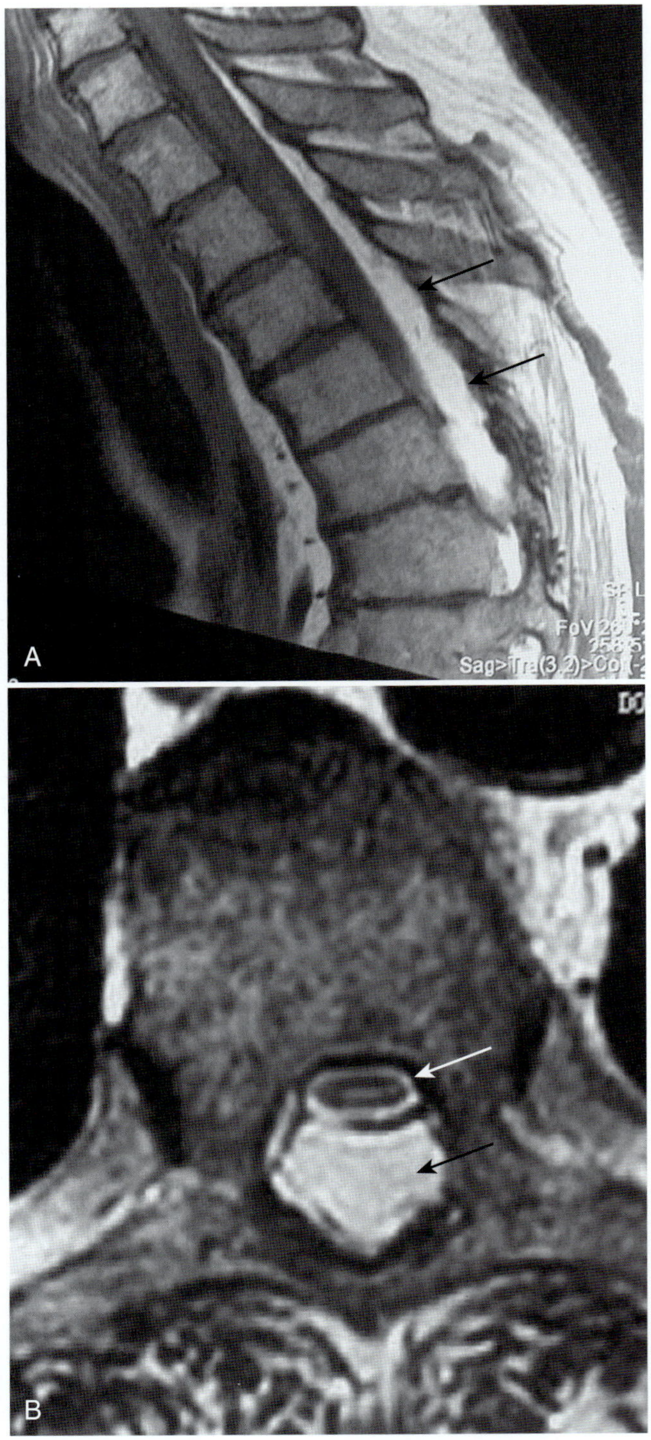

Figure 42.2 (**A**), Sagittal T1W MR image with lipomatosis of the upper thoracic region (*arrows*). (**B**), The axial T1W MR image shows the fatty tissue (*black arrow*) compressing the thecal sac and spinal cord (*white arrow*). *(From Al-Khawaja D, Seex K, Eslick GD: Spinal epidural lipomatosis: A brief review. J Clin Neurosci 2008;15:1323-1326.)*

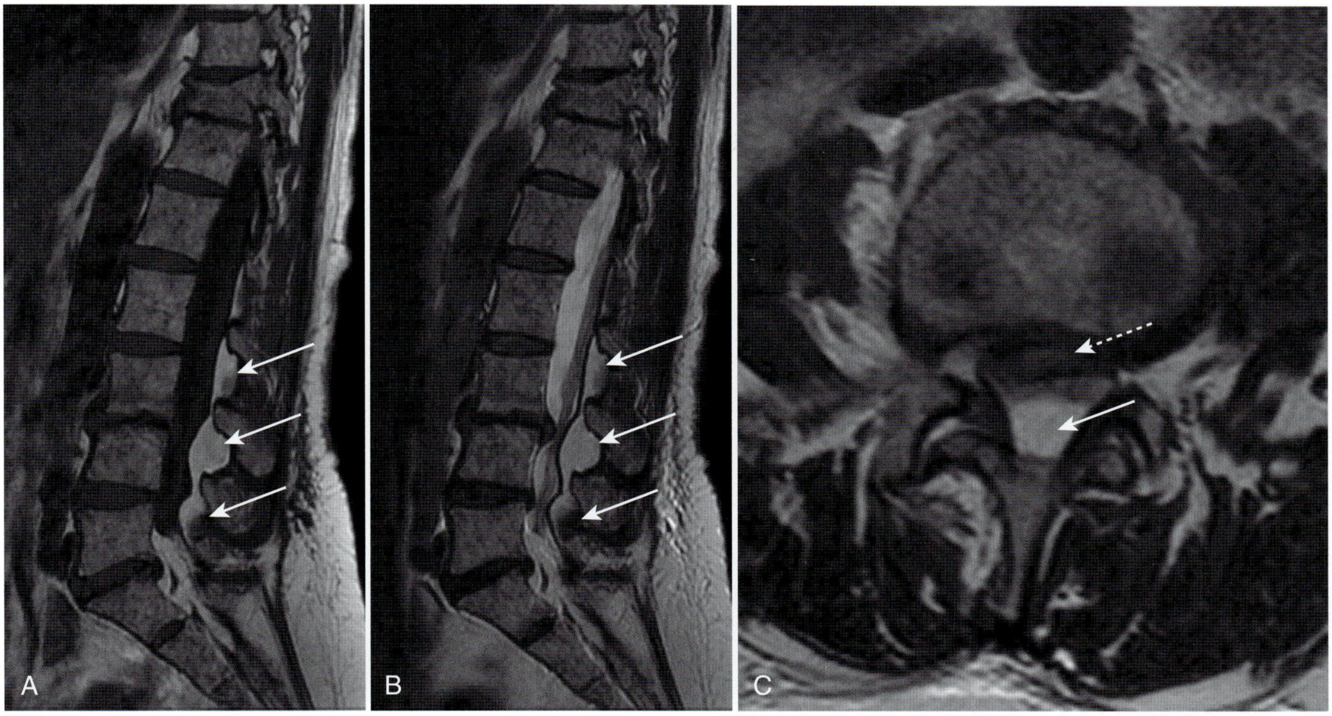

Figure 42.3 Sagittal T1W (**A**) and T2W (**B**) MR images of the lumbar spine with high-SI epidural lipomatosis (*arrows*). (**C**), The axial T2W MR image shows the degree of spinal stenosis, with the thecal sac compressed between the high-SI lipomatosis posteriorly (*solid arrow*) and the low-SI degenerated disc bulge anteriorly (*broken arrow*).

CHAPTER 43

Meningioma of the Thoracic Spine

DEFINITION

- Slow-growing benign neoplasm arising from the dura mater that may rarely become aggressive, compressing rather than invading neural structures.

SIGNS AND SYMPTOMS

- Most often manifests as dorsal spine pain.
- Radicular signs and symptoms common.
- Pain often very neuritic in nature.
- Pain often exacerbated with movement of affected spinal segment.
- Untreated or rapidly growing meningiomas may cause spinal cord compression with resultant myelopathy.

DEMOGRAPHICS

- Peak occurrence in fifth to sixth decade of life.
- Incidence: Female > Male.
- No ethnic predilection.
- Genetic predisposition in women.
- Increased incidence in patients with neurofibromatosis type II.
- Increased incidence in patients with previous irradiation to the spine.

IMAGING RECOMMENDATIONS

- MRI is the primary imaging modality.
- Radiographic findings are often normal.
- CT myelography is alternative if MRI is contraindicated.

IMAGING FINDINGS

- Radiographs may show scalloping of the vertebral body.
- Ovoid intradural, extra-axial soft tissue mass.
- Compression or displacement of the spinal cord or cauda equina.
- Masses are intermediate–signal intensity (SI) on T1-weighted (T1W) MR images and high-SI on T2W MR images.
- Uniform contrast enhancement is typical, although central necrosis may be seen.

OTHER RECOMMENDED TESTING

- Electromyography and nerve conduction velocity testing are indicated if radiculopathy is present.
- Evoked potential testing if myelopathy is present to quantify extent of spinal cord compromise.

DIFFERENTIAL DIAGNOSIS

- Schwannoma.
- Chordoma.
- Cyst.
- Lymphoma.
- Paraganglioma.
- Metastatic lesions.
- Myxopapillary ependymoma.
- Meningocele.

TREATMENT

- Surgical resection of tumor.

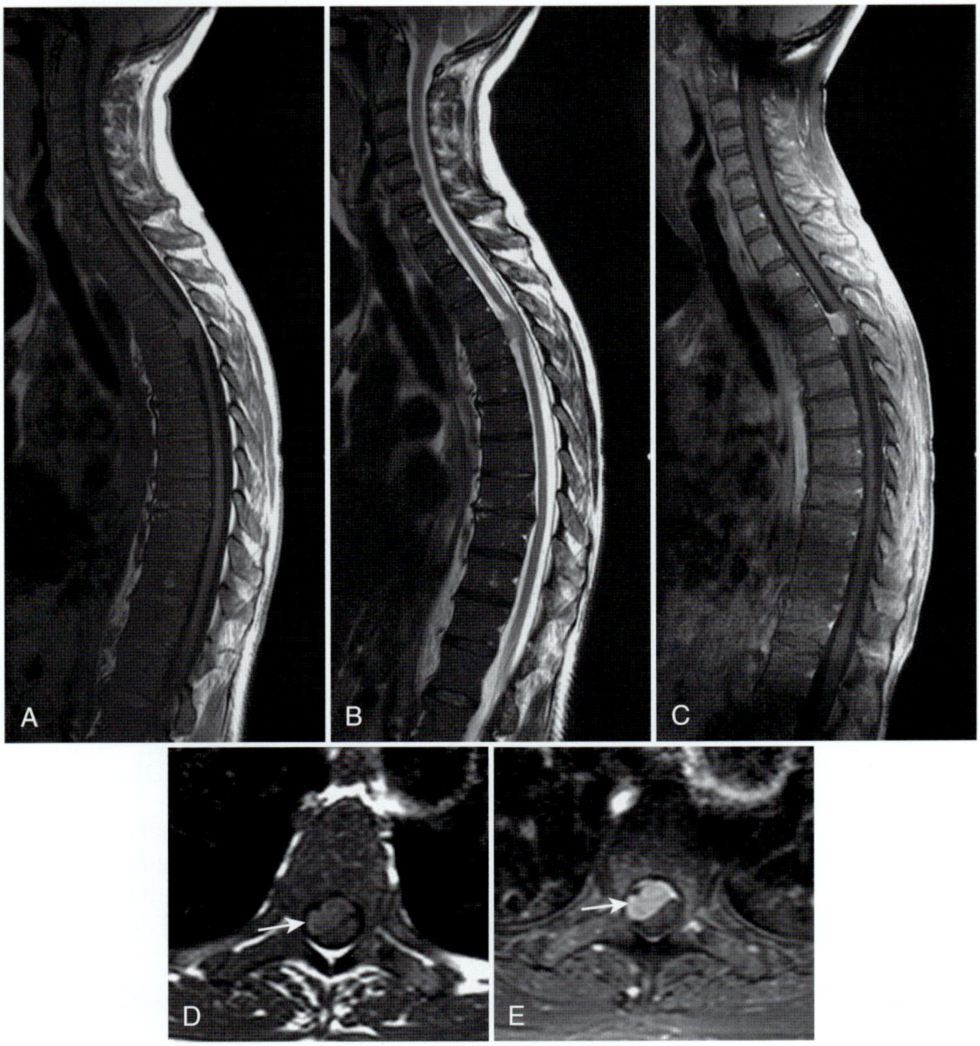

Figure 43.1 MRI in woman with slowly progressive neurologic deficit of the lower limbs and upper motor neuron signs. There is a rounded soft tissue mass anterior to the spinal cord that is intermediate-SI on both the T1W (**A**) and T2W (**B**) MR images. The mass enhances markedly on the post-contrast (obtained after administration of a contrast agent) T1W with fat suppression (FST1W) MR image (**C**). The axial pre-contrast T1W MR image (**D**) and post-contrast FST1W MR image (**E**) show the extent of enhancement (*arrows*) and the degree of cord compression.

CHAPTER 44

Anatomy: Special Imaging Considerations of the Lumbar Spine

OSSEOUS STRUCTURES

Lumbar Vertebrae. The lumbar vertebral bodies are rounded and box-shaped, with cylindrical pedicles bridging the neural exit foraminae. The transverse processes are thicker and straighter than in the thoracic spine and bear attachment to the psoas muscle. The superior and inferior articular processes arise at the bases of the pedicles and are separated by an area known as the *pars interarticularis*. The lumbar facet joints are almost sagittally oriented at L1, becoming more coronally oriented at L5-S1 and thus resisting forward vertebral translation.

Lumbar Intervertebral Discs. The lumbar discs are much thicker than thoracic discs and contain a large volume of nucleus pulposus, which is contained by a tough, circumferential annulus fibrosis. The annulus attaches to the vertebral end plates via Sharpey fibers, as in the thoracic and cervical spine. Because of the increased nuclear volume and axial loading in the lumbar spine, degenerative annular fissures are more common, often leading to nuclear herniation.

Lumbar Facet (Zygapophyseal) Joints. These synovial articulations are formed between the inferior articular process of the vertebra for which the joint is named and the superior articular process of the vertebra below it. The articular surfaces are obliquely sagittal in orientation in the upper lumbar levels, becoming more coronally oriented toward the L5-S1 level. The facet joint capsules are tighter than those of the cervical facet joints and are innervated by the medial branches of the dorsal rami of the spinal nerves. The medial branches pass over the posterior surfaces of the bases of the transverse processes.

LIGAMENTS

Longitudinal Ligaments. As in the cervical and thoracic spine, the anterior and posterior longitudinal ligaments attach to the anterior and posterior surfaces of the vertebral bodies and annuli of the discs. They act to preserve the lumbar lordosis and vertebral body alignment.

Iliolumbar Ligaments. Thick ligaments that arise from the tips of the L5 transverse processes and project laterally, inserting on the posterosuperior iliac spines.

Posterior Ligament. The posterior elements are stabilized by a group of three ligaments. The ligamenta flava are composed of elastic collagen fibers that run the whole length of the spine, attaching to the internal surfaces of the laminae. The spinous processes are stabilized by the interspinous and supraspinous ligaments.

MUSCLES

The dorsal lumbar spinal musculature is composed of three groups: the short intersegmental muscles, the polysegmental muscles of the multifidus, and the lumbar components of the longissimus and iliocostalis muscles.

NERVES

The lumbar spinal nerves are formed from the fusion of a dorsal and ventral root and are numbered according to the vertebral pedicles beneath which they exit. Each spinal nerve possesses a dural sheath, which arises just lateral to the opening of the neural exit foramen. The lumbar dorsal root ganglia lie within the exit foramina.

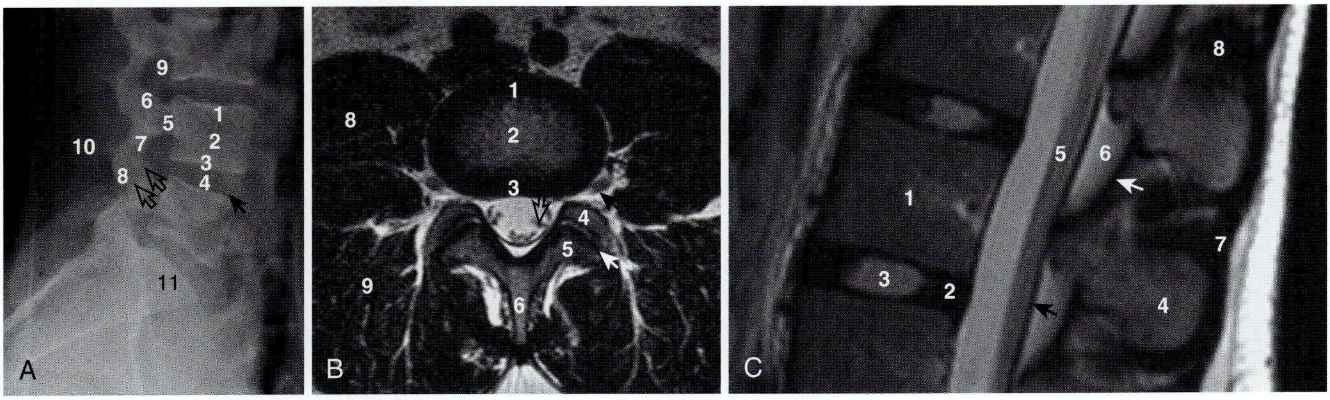

Figure 44.1 (**A**), Lateral radiograph of the lumbar spine: 1, superior end plate of L4; 2, vertebral body; 3, inferior end plate of L4; 4, L4-L5 disc space; 5, pedicle; 6, superior articular process; 7, pars interarticularis; 8, inferior articular process; 9, intervertebral (neural exit) foramen; 10, spinous process of L4; 11, superior end plate of S1; *open black arrows,* L3-L4 facet joint. (**B**), Axial T2-weighted MR image through the L3-L4 disc: 1, anterior annulus fibrosus; 2, nucleus pulposus; 3, posterior annulus fibrosus; 4, superior articular process of L4; 5, inferior articular process of L3; 6, spinous process of L3; 7, posterior epidural fat; 8, right psoas major muscle; 9, right erector spinae muscle; *black arrow,* left L3 nerve root; *black open arrow,* spinal nerve roots of cauda equina; *white arrow,* left L3-L4 facet joint. (**C**), Sagittal T2-weighted MR image of the lumbar spine: 1, vertebral body; 2, posterior annulus fibrosus; 3, nucleus pulposus; 4, spinous process; 5, cauda equina; 6, epidural fat; 7, supraspinous ligament; 8, interspinous ligament; *white arrow,* ligamentum flavum; *black arrow,* dural sac.

CHAPTER 45

Spondylolysis of the Lumbar Spine

DEFINITION

- Defect in the pars interarticularis that is believed to be either developmental or the result of a stress fracture secondary to repetitive trauma during a growth spurt of the immature skeleton.

SIGNS AND SYMPTOMS

- Established pars defects may be asymptomatic.
- Low back pain worse in extension.
- Hamstring tightness.
- Usually no history of trauma.
- Neurologic findings may be normal or may be positive for sensory, motor, and/or reflex changes.
- Range of motion of the lumbar spine may be decreased because of spasm.
- Flexion, extension, rotation, or lateral bending may exacerbate symptomatology.

DEMOGRAPHICS

- Peak occurrence in the second decade of life.
- Developmental defects occur in first decade of life.
- Increased incidence in young patients who participate in vigorous athletic training.
- Incidence: Male > Female.
- Unhealed defects may progress to lytic (isthmic) spondylolisthesis.
- There is a genetic predisposition.
- Increased incidence in Marfan syndrome, osteogenesis imperfecta, and osteopetrosis.

IMAGING RECOMMENDATIONS

- Radiographs:
  - Diagnosis of established pars defects.
  - Monitoring the development of secondary spondylolisthesis.
  - Not sensitive for acute stress fractures.
- MRI:
  - Detection and grading of acute stress fractures.
  - Assessing spondylolisthesis with associated neurology.
- CT:
  - Monitoring bony healing of acute stress fractures.
- Isotope bone scanning with single-photon emission CT (SPECT)
  - Alternative to MRI for acute stress fractures.

IMAGING FINDINGS

- Radiographs:
  - Defect in pars (Scotty dog appearance on oblique views).
- MRI:
  - Marrow edema in pars on short T1 inversion recovery (STIR) MR images in acute stress fracture.
  - Defect in bony cortex on T1-weighted (T1W) MR images.
  - Fatty marrow replacement in chronic defects.
- CT:
  - Fracture with "incomplete ring" sign.
  - Incomplete fractures may be seen in the early stages.
- Secondary spondylolisthesis:
  - Stenosis of exit canals.
  - Absence of central stenosis.
  - Associated disc degeneration.

OTHER RECOMMENDED TESTING

- Electromyography and nerve conduction velocity testing are indicated if radiculopathy is present.

DIFFERENTIAL DIAGNOSIS

- Stress fractures of other posterior elements.
- Osteoid osteoma and other primary bone tumors.
- Degenerative spondylolisthesis in adults.
- Pathologic or insufficiency fracture of pedicle in adults.

TREATMENT

- Modification of exercise regimen.
- Conservative treatment consisting of local heat, cold, simple analgesics, and nonsteroidal anti-inflammatory agents will improve symptoms in many cases.
- Physical therapy, including gentle stretching, range-of-motion exercises, deep heat modalities, and strengthening exercises, may be beneficial in selected patients.

- Epidural blocks will provide symptomatic relief if conservative therapy fails or the pain is limiting activities of daily living.
- Osteopathic or chiropractic manipulation may provide symptomatic relief in selected patients.
- Orthotic back brace for acute stress fractures.
- Surgery may be required with persistent pain or progressive neurologic symptoms.

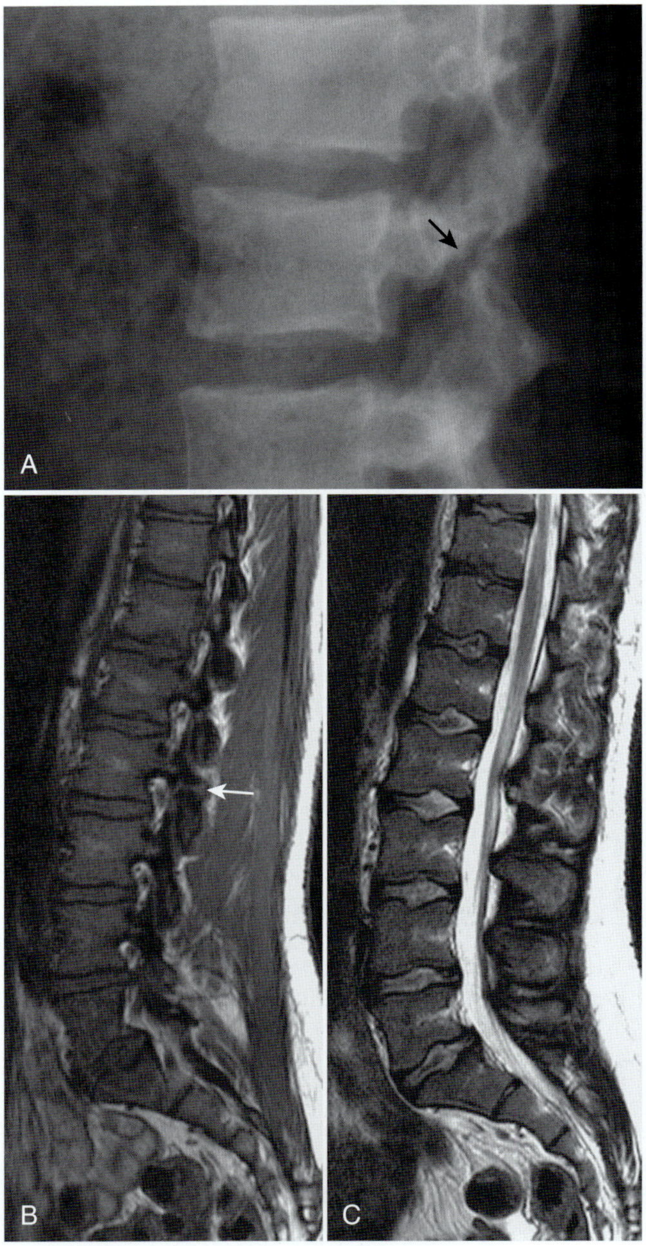

Figure 45.1 (**A**), Lateral radiograph of a juvenile with extension back pain and an obvious lysis at the L2 level (*black arrow*). Isolated L2 lysis is unusual; most cases affect L4 and L5. (**B**), The parasagittal T1W MR image also clearly demonstrates the lysis (*white arrow*). (**C**), The midline sagittal T2W MR image shows multilevel Schmorl node formation and disc degeneration consistent with the lumbar form of Scheuermann disease, which is often associated with spondylolysis.

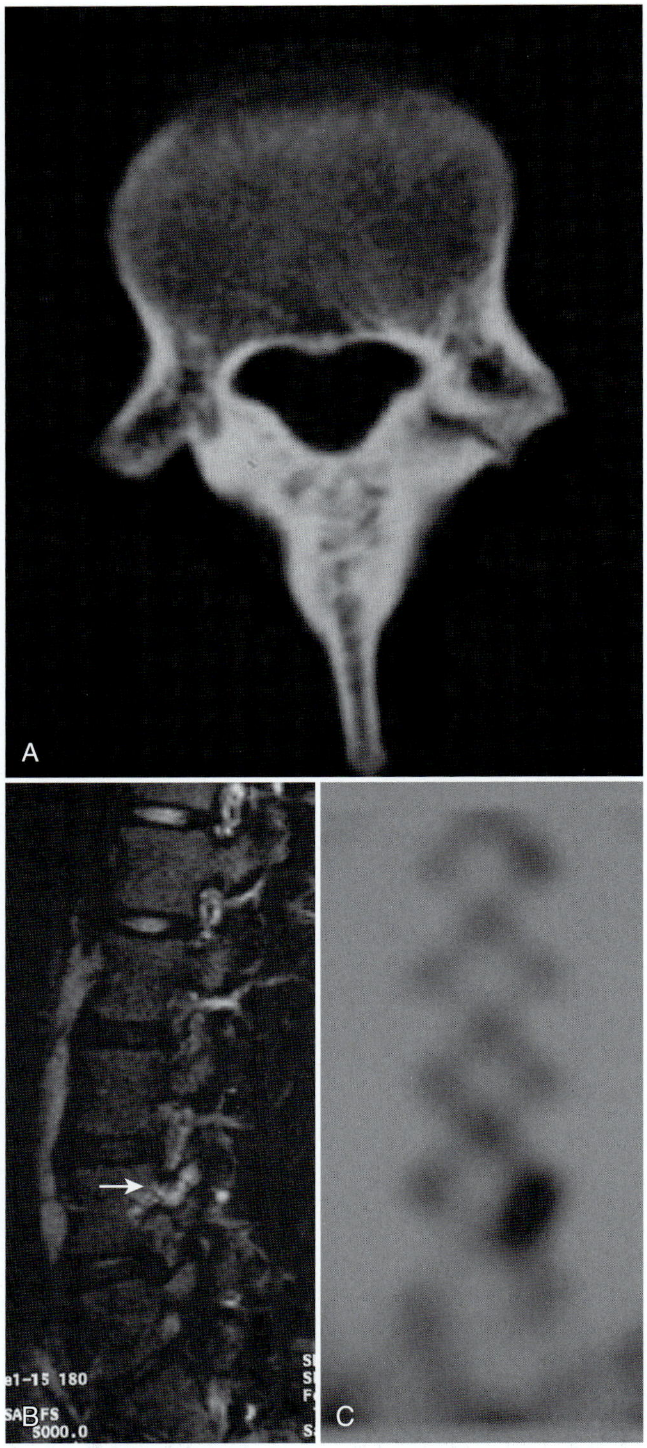

Figure 45.2 (**A**), Oblique axial CT scan demonstrating the incomplete ring sign due to a left-sided spondylolysis at L4. There are bone marrow edema (*white arrow*) in the adjacent pedicle on the sagittal STIR MR image (**B**) and increased uptake on the SPECT scan (**C**), indicating that this is an acute stress fracture.

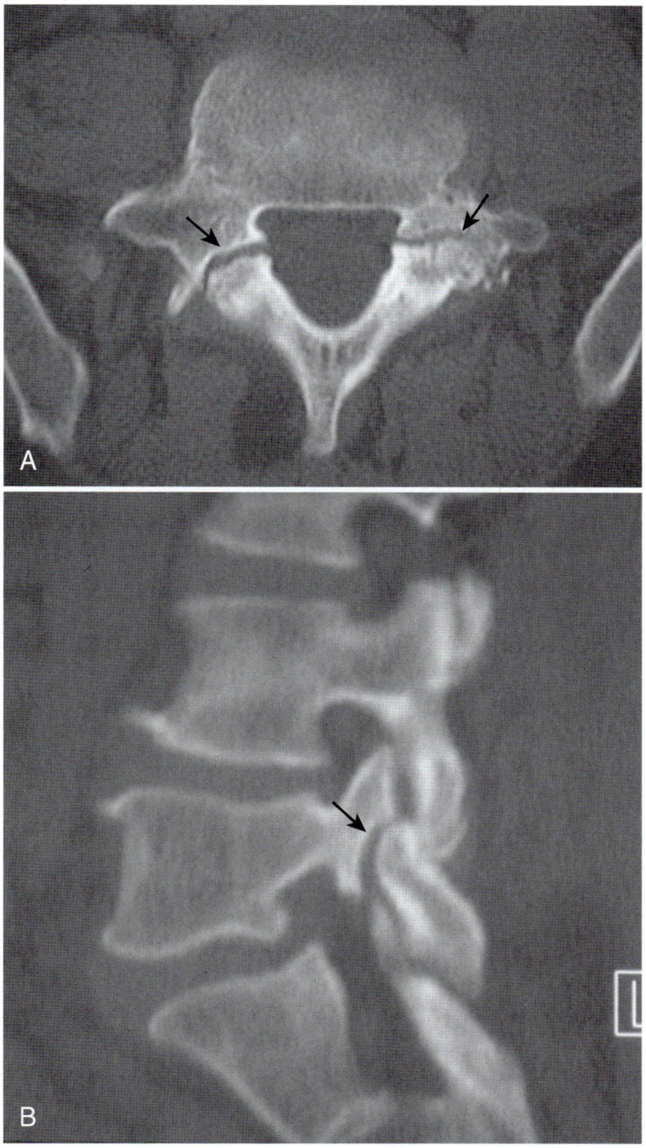

Figure 45.3 Oblique axial (**A**) and sagittal (**B**) CT scans of chronic bilateral L5 pars defects with smooth sclerotic and partly fragmented fracture margins (*black arrows*). There was no marrow edema on STIR MR images.

CHAPTER 46

Degenerative Spondylolisthesis of the Lumbar Spine

DEFINITION

- Slippage of one adjacent vertebral body relative to another adjacent vertebral body, which is usually either due to degenerative changes of the intervertebral disc and facet joints (degenerative spondylolisthesis) or secondary to spondylolysis (lytic spondylolisthesis).

SIGNS AND SYMPTOMS

- Often asymptomatic.
- May manifest as radiculopathy after seemingly minor trauma.
- Neurologic findings may be normal or may be positive for sensory, motor, and/or reflex changes.
- Neurogenic claudication may often be present secondary to relative spinal stenosis caused by slippage of vertebral bodies.
- Range of motion of the lumbar spine may be decreased due to spasm.
- Flexion, extension, rotation, or lateral bending may exacerbate symptomatology.

DEMOGRAPHICS

- Peak occurrence in the fifth and sixth decades of life.
- Most common causes are degenerative facet disease and spondylolysis.
- May occur at an earlier age after trauma.
- Incidence: Female > male.
- Most commonly occurs at L4-L5 and L5-S1.
- More common after spinal surgery.

IMAGING RECOMMENDATIONS

- Radiographs to assess vertebral alignment:
  - Flexion/extension radiographs may be used to identify instability.
- MRI to assess spinal stenosis.
- CT is alternative when MRI is contraindicated

IMAGING FINDINGS

- Listhesis:
  - Based on degree of slip:
    Grade I: < 25%.
    Grade II: 25%-50%.
    Grade III: 50%-75%.
    Grade IV: > 75%.
  - Slip is usually anterior but may be posterior.
- Central stenosis:
  - Effacement of the cerebrospinal fluid space and the cauda equina on T2-weighted (T2W) MR images.
  - Obliteration of fat in the lateral recess on T1W MR images.
  - Disc bulging, facet osteoarthritis, and ligament hypertrophy.
  - Usually due to degenerative listhesis.
  - Uncommon with lytic spondylolisthesis.
- Foraminal stenosis:
  - Obliteration of epidural fat around nerve root in exit canal.
  - Loss of height of exit canal due to disc degeneration.
  - Disc bulging, facet osteoarthritis, and lateral osteophyte formation.
  - Occurs in both degenerative and lytic spondylolisthesis.
- Associated disc degeneration, facet arthropathy, and so on.

OTHER RECOMMENDED TESTING

- Electromyography and nerve conduction testing are indicated if radiculopathy is present.
- Evoked potential testing is indicated if myelopathy present.

DIFFERENTIAL DIAGNOSIS

- Displaced vertebral body fracture.

TREATMENT

- Modification of exercise regimen.
- Conservative treatment consisting of local heat, cold, simple analgesics, and nonsteroidal anti-inflammatory agents will improve symptoms in many cases.
- Physical therapy, including gentle stretching, range-of-motion exercises, deep heat modalities, and strengthening exercises, may be beneficial in selected patients.
- Epidural blocks will provide symptomatic relief if conservative therapy fails or the pain is limiting activities of daily living.
- Osteopathic or chiropractic manipulation may provide symptomatic relief in selected patients.
- Orthotic back brace.
- Surgery may be required in patients with persistent pain or progressive neurologic symptoms.

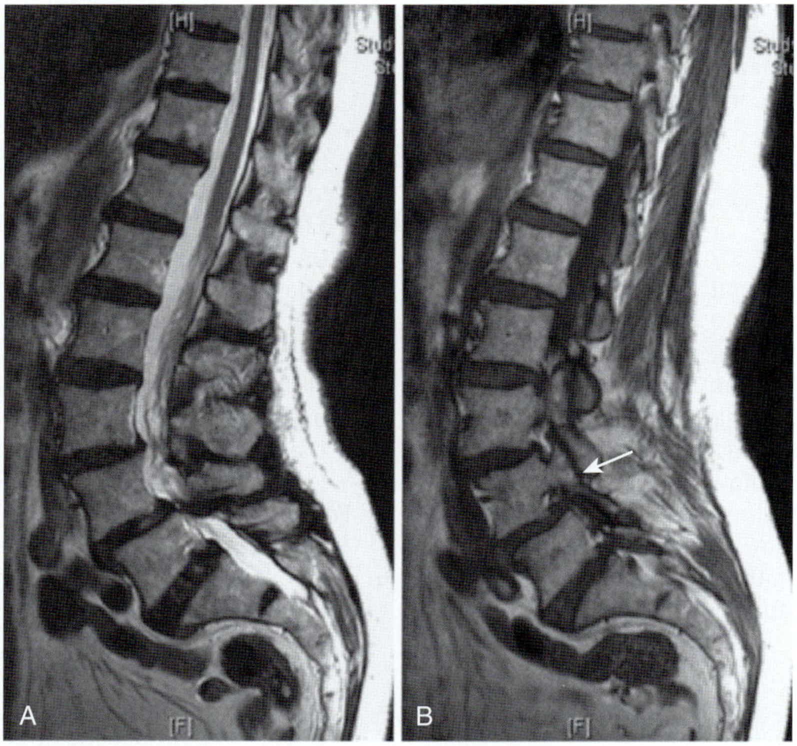

Figure 46.1 (A), Sagittal T2W MR image of grade I degenerative spondylolisthesis at L4-L5 with associated central spinal canal stenosis. Note also the widespread disc degeneration. (B), The parasagittal T1W MR image shows an intact pars interarticularis at L4 (*black arrow*).

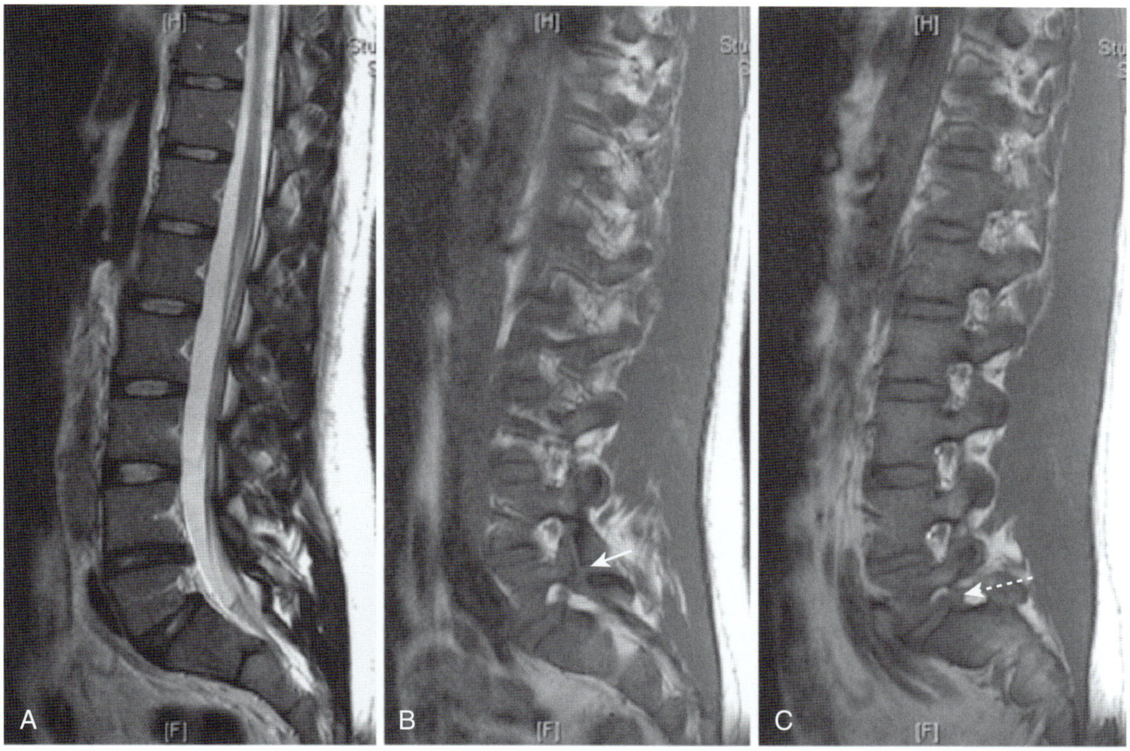

Figure 46.2 (**A**), Sagittal T2W MR image of lytic spondylolisthesis at L5-S1 with associated disc degeneration and disc bulging at L4-L5. There is no central spinal canal stenosis. (**B** and **C**), The parasagittal T1W MR images demonstrate the pars defect (*black arrow*) and the associated foraminal stenosis with early compression of the exiting nerve root (*broken arrow*).

CHAPTER 47

Bulging Intervertebral Disc of the Lumbar Spine

DEFINITION

- Nonfocal generalized extension of the intervertebral disc beyond the margins of the vertebra.

SIGNS AND SYMPTOMS

- Usually present as part of the normal aging process.
- Usually asymptomatic.
- May manifest as lumbago or radiculopathy after seemingly minor trauma.
- Neurologic findings may be normal or may be positive for sensory, motor, and/or reflex changes.
- Range of motion of the lumbar spine may be decreased.
- Flexion, extension, rotation, or lateral bending may exacerbate symptomatology.

DEMOGRAPHICS

- May occur following acute trauma.
- Incidence increases with age.
- Repeated microtrauma to disc by repetitive activities may increase incidence.
- There may be a genetic predisposition.

IMAGING RECOMMENDATIONS

- Imaging not routinely indicated for mechanical back pain without "red flags."
- MRI is the primary investigation for assessing intervertebral discs.
- CT is an alternative when MRI is contraindicated.
- Discography to identify discogenic pain.
- Radiography demonstrates only disc space narrowing.

IMAGING FINDINGS

- Disc degeneration with low–signal intensity (SI) disc on T2-weighted (T2W) MR images and loss of disc height.
- Diffuse bulging of the discs beyond the margin of the vertebral bodies.
- Posterior discs are normally concave, except for the:
  - L4-L5 disc, which is normally flat.
  - L5-S1 disc, which may be slightly convex.
- Spondylosis with osteophytosis may be associated with disc bulging.
- Disc bulging may contribute to spinal stenosis.

OTHER RECOMMENDED TESTING

- Electromyography and nerve conduction velocity testing are indicated if radiculopathy is present.
- Provocative discography may serve as a useful diagnostic tool to determine whether a specific disc is serving as a nidus for the pain.

DIFFERENTIAL DIAGNOSIS

- Disc protrusion.
- Ossification of the posterior longitudinal ligament (OPLL).
- Osteophyte of vertebral end plate.

TREATMENT

- Conservative treatment consisting of local heat, cold, simple analgesics, and nonsteroidal anti-inflammatory agents will improve symptoms in many cases.
- Physical therapy, including gentle stretching, range-of-motion exercises, deep heat modalities, and stretch and spray, may be beneficial in selected patients.
- Epidural blocks will provide symptomatic relief if conservative therapy fails or the pain is limiting activities of daily living.
- Osteopathic or chiropractic manipulation may provide symptomatic relief in selected patients.
- Surgery may be required in patients with persistent pain or progressive neurologic symptoms.

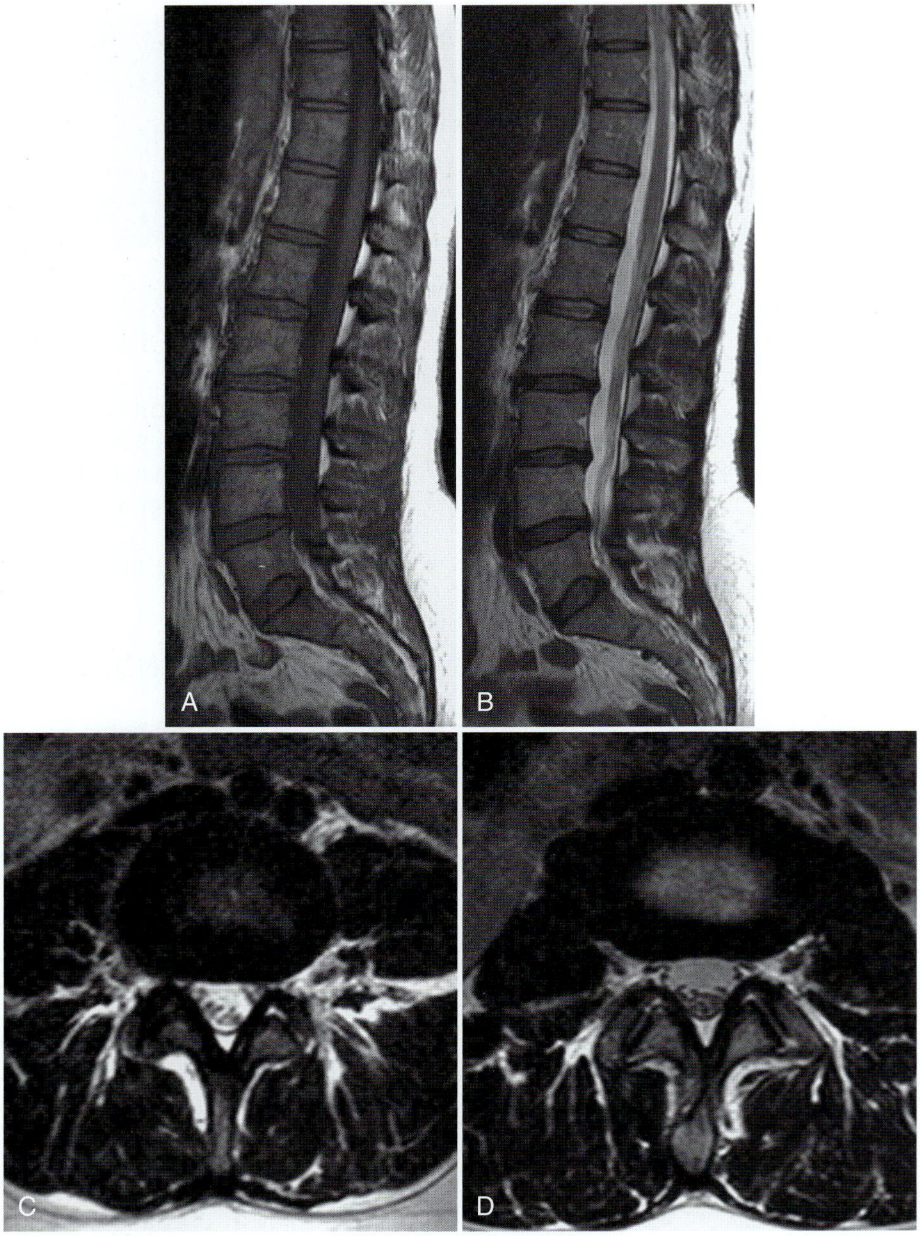

Figure 47.1 Sagittal T1W (**A**) and T2W (**B**) MR images of the lumbar spine. The SI of the intervertebral discs is normal on the T1W MR images, but there is disc space narrowing at L2-L3 and L3-L4. The T2W MR images shows early loss of disc hydration with low-SI changes at L2-L3, L3-L4, and L4-L5. In addition, there is bulging of the posterior discs beyond the posterior margin vertebral body wall at these three levels, which is most markec at L3-L4. (**C**), An axial T2W MR images shows that the posterior margin of the disc is flat, but without significant narrowing of the lateral recesses and with no compression of the thecal sac. (**D**), An axial T2W MR images of a normal L3-L4 disc shows that the posterior margin of the disc should be slightly concave.

CHAPTER 48

Degenerative Intervertebral Disk Disease of the Lumbar Spine

DEFINITION

- Complex biochemical changes leading to morphologic and functional changes of the discovertebral complex due to degeneration of the intervertebral disk.

SIGNS AND SYMPTOMS

- Usually present as part of the normal aging process.
- Usually asymptomatic.
- May manifest as lumbago or radiculopathy after seemingly minor trauma.
- Neurologic findings may be normal or may be positive for sensory, motor, and/or reflex changes.
- Range of motion of the lumbar spine may be decreased.
- Flexion, extension, rotation, or lateral bending may exacerbate symptomatology.

DEMOGRAPHICS

- Peak occurrence in the fourth through six decades of life.
- May occur at an earlier age following trauma.
- Incidence: Male = Female.
- Occurs in almost all patients by the sixth decade.
- There may be a genetic predisposition.

IMAGING RECOMMENDATIONS

- Imaging is not routinely indicated for mechanical back pain without "red flags."
- MRI is the primary investigation for assessing intervertebral disks.
- Discography to identify discogenic pain.
- CT is an alternative when MRI is contraindicated.
- Radiography demonstrates only disk space narrowing.

IMAGING FINDINGS

- Loss of signal intensity (SI) of the nucleus pulposus on T2-weighted (T2W) MR images.
- Loss of disk height.
- Intradiscal gas may be seen as an area of very low SI within the disc but is better appreciated on CT.
- Secondary vertebral end-plate changes of Modic:
  - Type I: Marrow.
  - Type II: Fatty replacement.
  - Type III: Bony sclerosis.
  - Often a combination of end-plate changes is present.
- Increased SI and discovertebral erosion on T2W MR images may also mimic disk space infection.
- Frequently associated with spondylosis with osteophytosis.

OTHER RECOMMENDED TESTING

- Electromyography and nerve conduction velocity testing are indicated if radiculopathy is present.
- Provocative diskography may serve as a useful diagnostic tool to determine whether a specific disc is serving as a nidus for the pain.

DIFFERENTIAL DIAGNOSIS

- Diskitis.
- Reiter syndrome.
- Hemodialysis spondyloarthropathy.

TREATMENT

- Conservative treatment consisting of local heat, cold, simple analgesics, and nonsteroidal anti-inflammatory agents will improve symptoms in many cases.
- Physical therapy, including gentle stretching, range-of-motion exercises, deep heat modalities, and stretch and spray, may be beneficial in selected patients.
- Epidural blocks will provide symptomatic relief if conservative therapy fails or the pain is limiting activities of daily living.
- Osteopathic or chiropractic manipulation may provide symptomatic relief in selected patients.
- Surgery may be required for persistent pain or progressive neurologic symptoms.

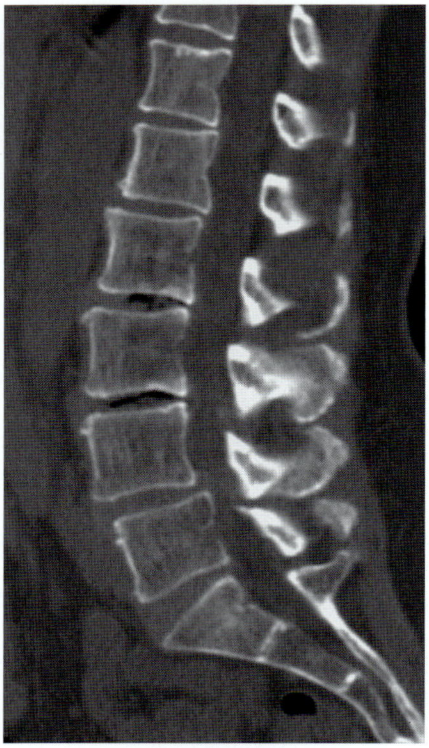

Figure 48.1 Sagittal CT scan demonstrating narrowing of several intervertebral disks with intradiscal gas at L2-L3 and L3-L4 due to disk degeneration. There is minor degenerative spondylolisthesis at L4-L5.

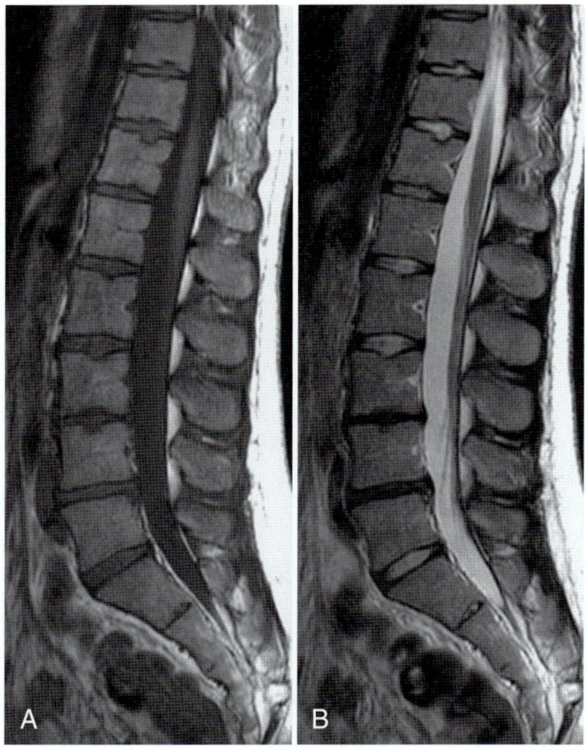

Figure 48.2 Sagittal T1W MR image showing disk space narrowing at L3-L4 and L4-L5 (**A**), with low-SI within the affected disks on the T2W MR image (**B**). There are no associated Modic vertebral end-plate changes. Schmorl node formation is present at other levels without associated disk degeneration.

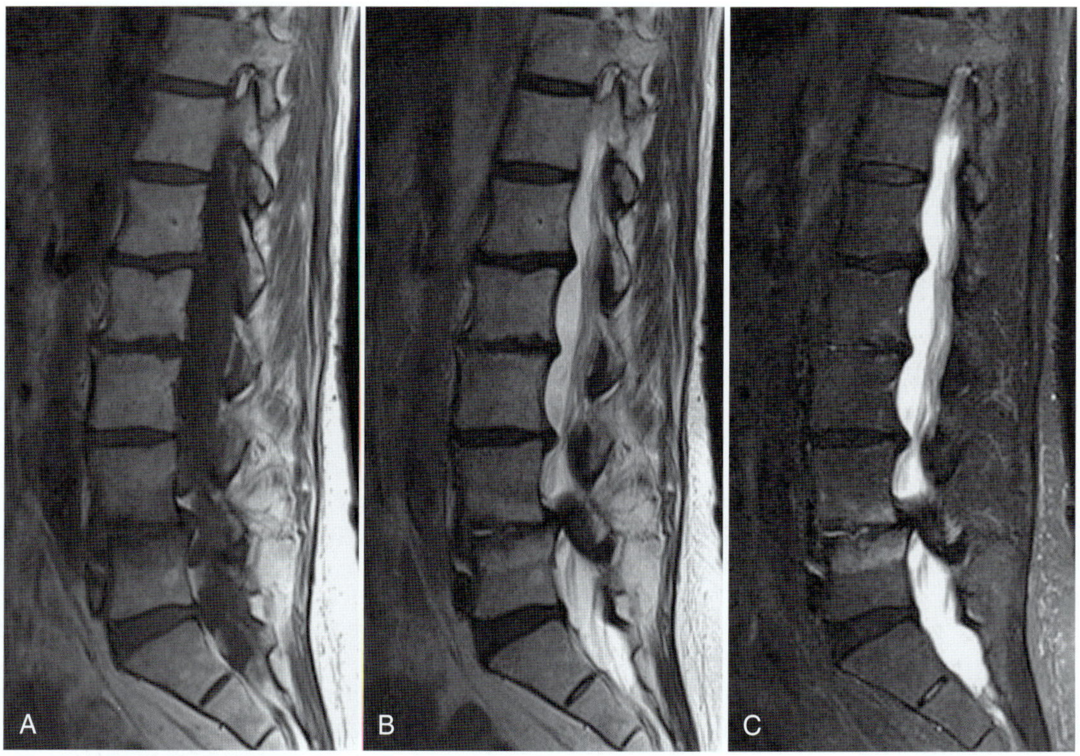

Figure 48.3 Sagittal T1W (**A**), T2W (**B**), and short T1 inversion recovery (STIR) (**C**) MR images in a patient with severe disk degeneration at L4-L5. There are disk narrowing and discovertebral erosion. High SI within the disk is apparent on the T2W and STIR images. There are Modic type I changes with vertebral end-plate edema, which has low SI on the T1W MR image and high SI on the T2W and STIR images. These features mimic disk space infection, but there are no paravertebral inflammatory changes. Multilevel disk degeneration and disk bulging are present at the other lumbar levels.

CHAPTER 49

Annular Fissure of the Lumbar Intervertebral Disk

DEFINITION

- Disruption of the concentric, vertically oriented collagen fibers of the intervertebral disk due to repetitive stress and trauma.

SIGNS AND SYMPTOMS

- Usually present as part of the normal aging process.
- Usually asymptomatic.
- May manifest as lumbago or radiculopathy after seemingly minor trauma.
- Neurologic findings may be normal or may be positive for sensory, motor, and/or reflex changes.
- Range of motion of the lumbar spine may be decreased.
- Flexion, extension, rotation, or lateral bending may exacerbate symptomatology.

DEMOGRAPHICS

- Peak occurrence in the fourth through six decades of life.
- May occur at an earlier age following trauma.
- Incidence: Male = Female.
- Occurs in almost all patients by the sixth decade.
- There may be a genetic predisposition.

IMAGING RECOMMENDATIONS

- Imaging not routinely indicated for mechanical back pain without "red flags."
- MRI is primary investigation for assessing intervertebral disks.
- Diskography to identify discogenic pain.
- CT does not demonstrate annular fissures without combined diskography.
- Radiography demonstrates only disk space narrowing.

IMAGING FINDINGS

- High-signal intensity (SI) fissure in annulus on T2-weighted (T2W) MR images: High-intensity zone (HIZ).
- Presence of HIZ does not correlate with low back pain.
- Disk may be otherwise normal.
- Fissure in isolation without disk protrusion will not efface lumbar nerve roots on MRI.

OTHER RECOMMENDED TESTING

- Electromyography and nerve conduction velocity testing are indicated if radiculopathy is present.
- Provocative diskography may serve as a useful diagnostic tool to determine whether a specific disk is serving as a nidus for the pain.

DIFFERENTIAL DIAGNOSIS

- Diskitis.
- Focal herniated disk.
- Focal fat deposition.

TREATMENT

- Conservative treatment consisting of local heat, cold, simple analgesics, and nonsteroidal anti-inflammatory agents will improve symptoms in many cases.
- Physical therapy, including gentle stretching, range-of-motion exercises, deep heat modalities, and stretch and spray, may be beneficial in selected patients.
- Epidural blocks will provide symptomatic relief if conservative therapy fails or the pain is limiting activities of daily living.
- Osteopathic or chiropractic manipulation may provide symptomatic relief in selected patients.
- Surgery may be required for persistent pain or progressive neurologic symptoms.

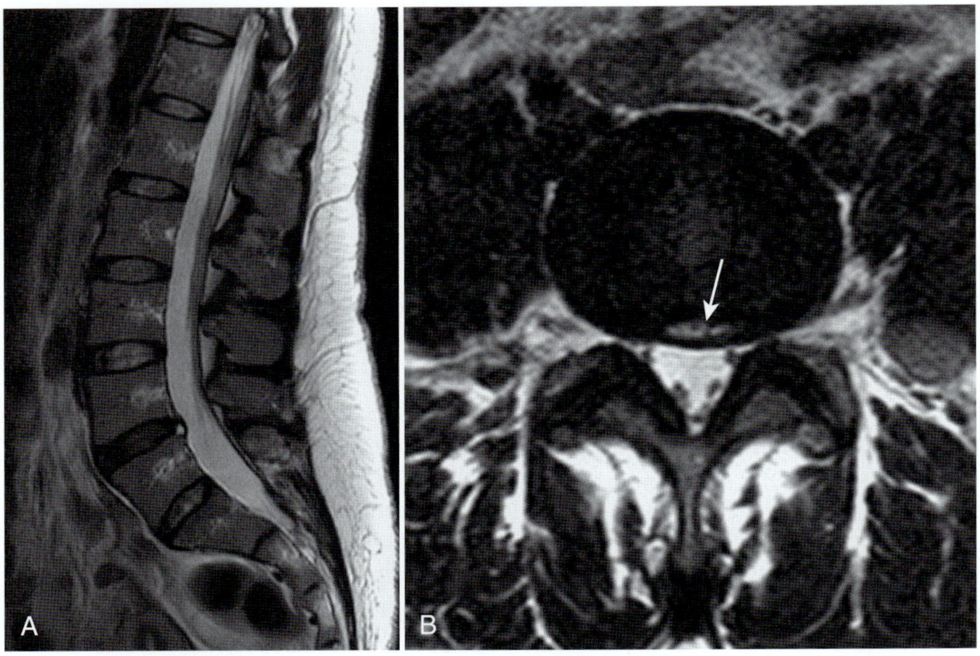

Figure 49.1 (**A**), Sagittal T2W MR image demonstrating early low-SI disk degeneration in the L4-L5 disk. There is a small focal high-SI zone at the posterior margin of the disk, which represents an annular fissure. (**B**), The fissure can also be seen on the axial T2W MR image (*white arrow*).

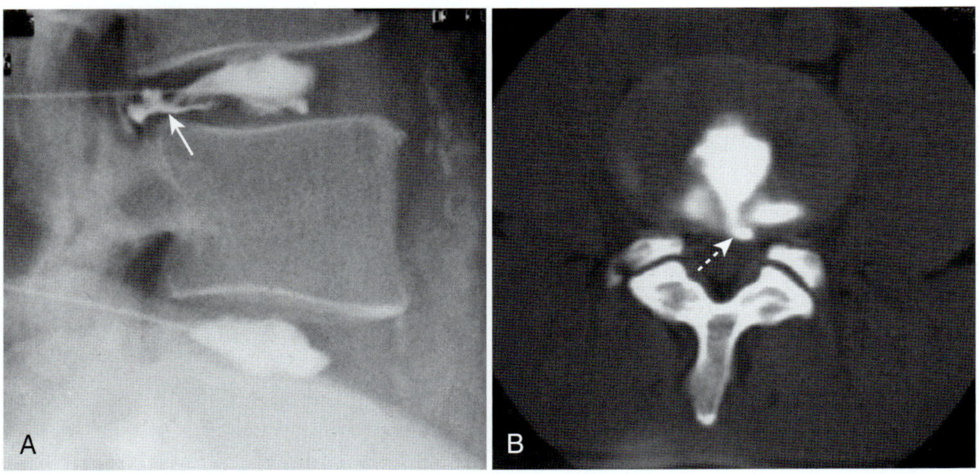

Figure 49.2 (**A**), Diskogram demonstrating an annular fissure extending from the nucleus pulposus to the posterior disk margin (*white arrow*). (**B**), The same appearance is seen on a CT diskogram, with high-density contrast medium extending into a posterior annular fissure (*broken arrow*).

CHAPTER 50

Intervertebral Disk Herniation of the Lumbar Spine

DEFINITION

- Focal extension of the intervertebral disk of less than 50% of the disk circumference beyond the margins of the vertebra.

SIGNS AND SYMPTOMS

- Level, size and location (e.g., posterior, anterior, lateral) of disk herniation will determine the clinical presentation.
- Back and lumbar radicular pain the most common symptom.
- Decreased range of motion of the lumbar spine with associated muscle spasm also common.
- Pain may radiate in a dermatomal or nondermatomal pattern.
- Motor, sensory, and reflex changes may occur.
- Central disk herniation may cause compression of the lumbar spinal cord with resultant lumbar myelopathy.

DEMOGRAPHICS

- May occur following acute trauma.
- Incidence increases with age, with peak occurrence between the fourth and fifth decades of life.
- Repeated microtrauma to disk by repetitive activities may increase incidence.
- There may be a genetic predisposition.
- Slight male preponderance.

IMAGING RECOMMENDATIONS

- MRI is the primary investigation for sciatica:
  - Usually performed after 6 weeks of conservative therapy.
  - Early imaging for neurologic deficit.
- CT is an alternative when MRI is contraindicated.
- Radiography demonstrates only disk space narrowing.

IMAGING FINDINGS

- Prolapsed intervertebral disk (PID):
  - Protrusion: Contained by posterior longitudinal ligament (PLL).
  - Extrusion: Ruptured through PLL.
  - Sequestration: Separated disk fragment that may migrate.
- Acute PID: High signal intensity (SI) on T2-weighted (T2W) MR images.
- Chronic PID: Low SI on T2W MR images.
- Location:
  - Central: Compression of thecal sac.
  - Paracentral: Compression of traversing nerve root in lateral recess.
- Nerve root swelling and perineural enhancement on images obtained after admnistration of a contrast agent.

OTHER RECOMMENDED TESTING

- Electromyography and nerve conduction velocity testing are indicated if radiculopathy is present.
- Provocative diskography may serve as a useful diagnostic tool to determine whether a specific disk is serving as a nidus for the pain.

DIFFERENTIAL DIAGNOSIS

- Epidural abscess.
- Osteophyte of vertebral end plate.
- Epidural hematoma.
- Neoplasm.
- Schwannoma.

TREATMENT

- Conservative treatment consisting of local heat, cold, simple analgesics, and nonsteroidal anti-inflammatory agents will improve symptoms in many cases.
- Physical therapy, including gentle stretching, range-of-motion exercises, deep heat modalities, and stretch and spray, may be beneficial in selected patients.
- Epidural blocks will provide symptomatic relief if conservative therapy fails or the pain is limiting activities of daily living.
- Osteopathic or chiropractic manipulation may provide symptomatic relief in selected patients.
- Surgery may be required for persistent pain or progressive neurologic symptoms.

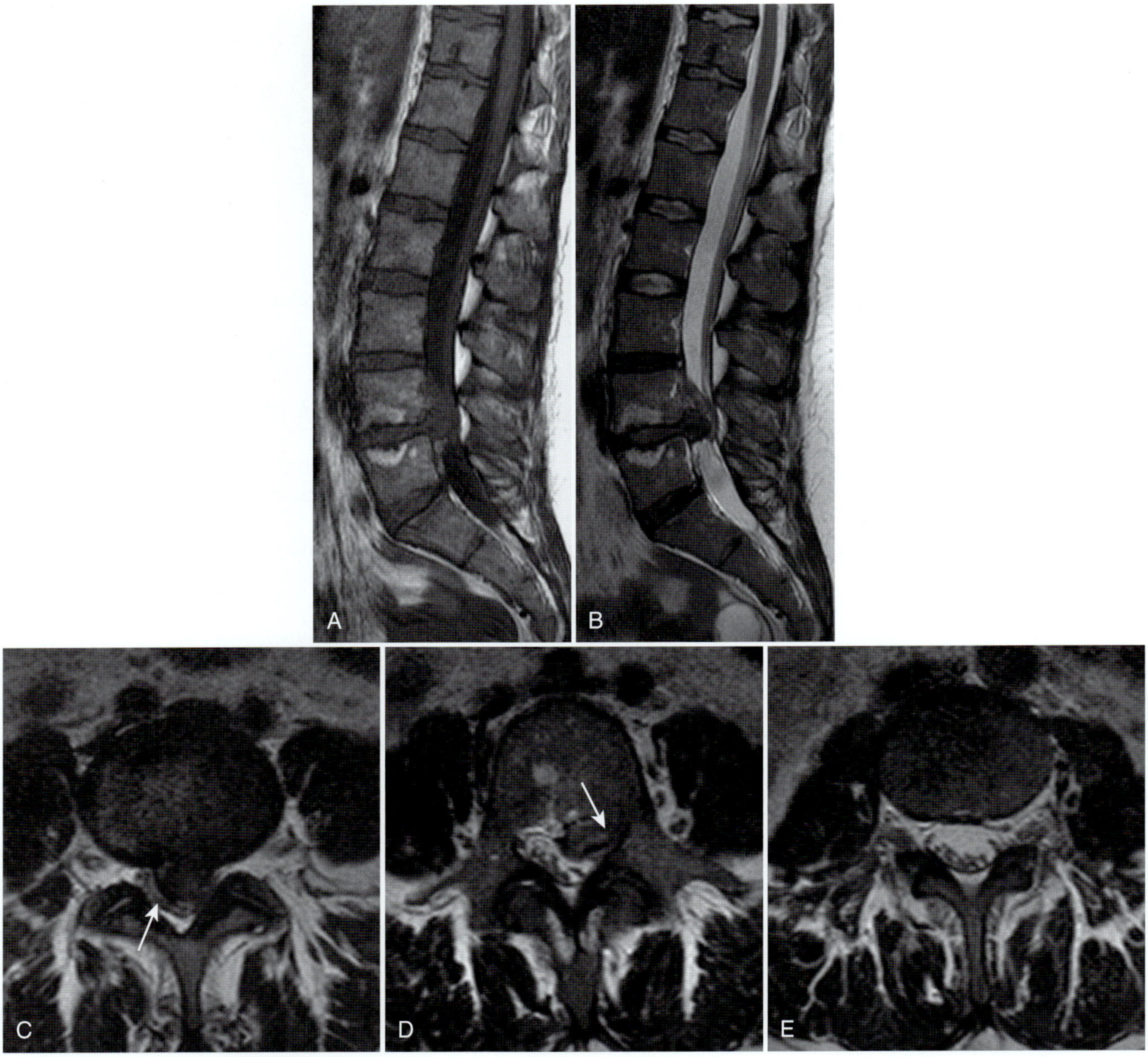

Figure 50.1 Sagittal T1W (**A**) and T2W (**B**) MR images of a young woman with cauda equina syndrome and radicular left leg pain. There is a large disk extrusion at the L4-L5 level, which has intermediate SI on both the T1W and T2W MR images. (**C**), An axial T2W MR image shows compression of the thecal sac, which is displaced to the right (*white arrow*). (**D**), More proximally, the disc protrusion obliterates the traversing nerve root within the lateral recess (*black arrow*). Compare with the normal appearance of the thecal sac at the L3-L4 level (**E**).

CHAPTER 51

Foraminal Intervertebral Disk Herniation of the Lumbar Spine

DEFINITION

- Focal extension of extruded intervertebral disk material into the neural foramina.

SIGNS AND SYMPTOMS

- Level and size of disk herniation will determine the clinical presentation.
- Severe lumbar radicular pain is the most common symptom.
- Decreased range of motion of the lumbar spine with associated muscle spasm also common.
- Pain may radiate in a dermatomal or, less commonly, nondermatomal pattern.
- Motor, sensory, and reflex changes may occur.
- Result of femoral stretch test often positive.
- Valsalva maneuver often worsens radicular symptomatology.

DEMOGRAPHICS

- Much less common than other types of lumbar disk herniation.
- May occur following acute trauma.
- Incidence increases with age, with peak occurrence between the fifth and seventh decades of life.
- Repeated microtrauma to disk by repetitive activities may increase incidence.
- There may be a genetic predisposition.
- Incidence: Male = Female.
- No ethnic or racial predilection.

IMAGING RECOMMENDATIONS

- MRI is the primary investigation for sciatica:
  - Usually performed after 6 weeks of conservative therapy.
  - Early imaging for neurologic deficit.
- CT is an alternative when MRI is contraindicated.
- Radiography demonstrates only disk space narrowing.

IMAGING FINDINGS

- Acute prolapsed intervertebral disk (PID): High signal intensity (SI) on T2-weighted (T2W) MR images.
- Chronic PID: Low SI on T2W MR images.
- Location:
  - Lateral: Within exit canal.
  - Far lateral: Outside confines of exit canal.
- Compression of the exiting nerve root.
- Nerve root swelling and perineural enhancement on images obtained after administration of a contrast agent.

OTHER RECOMMENDED TESTING

- Electromyography and nerve conduction velocity testing are indicated if radiculopathy is present.
- Provocative discography may serve as a useful diagnostic tool to determine whether a specific disk is serving as a nidus for the pain.
- Diagnostic selective nerve root block may serve as a useful diagnostic tool to determine whether a specific disk is serving as a nidus for the pain.

DIFFERENTIAL DIAGNOSIS

- Osteophyte of vertebral end plate.
- Nerve root sleeve cyst or diverticulum.
- Facet osteophyte.
- Neoplasm.
- Schwannoma.

TREATMENT

- Conservative treatment consisting of local heat, cold, simple analgesics, and nonsteroidal anti-inflammatory agents will improve symptoms in many cases.
- Physical therapy, including gentle stretching, range-of-motion exercises, deep heat modalities, and stretch and spray, may be beneficial in selected patients.
- Epidural blocks will provide symptomatic relief if conservative therapy fails or the pain is limiting activities of daily living.
- Selective nerve root blocks may provide symptomatic relief if conservative therapy fails or the pain is limiting activities of daily living.
- Osteopathic or chiropractic manipulation may provide symptomatic relief in selected patients.
- Surgery may be required for persistent pain or progressive neurologic symptoms.

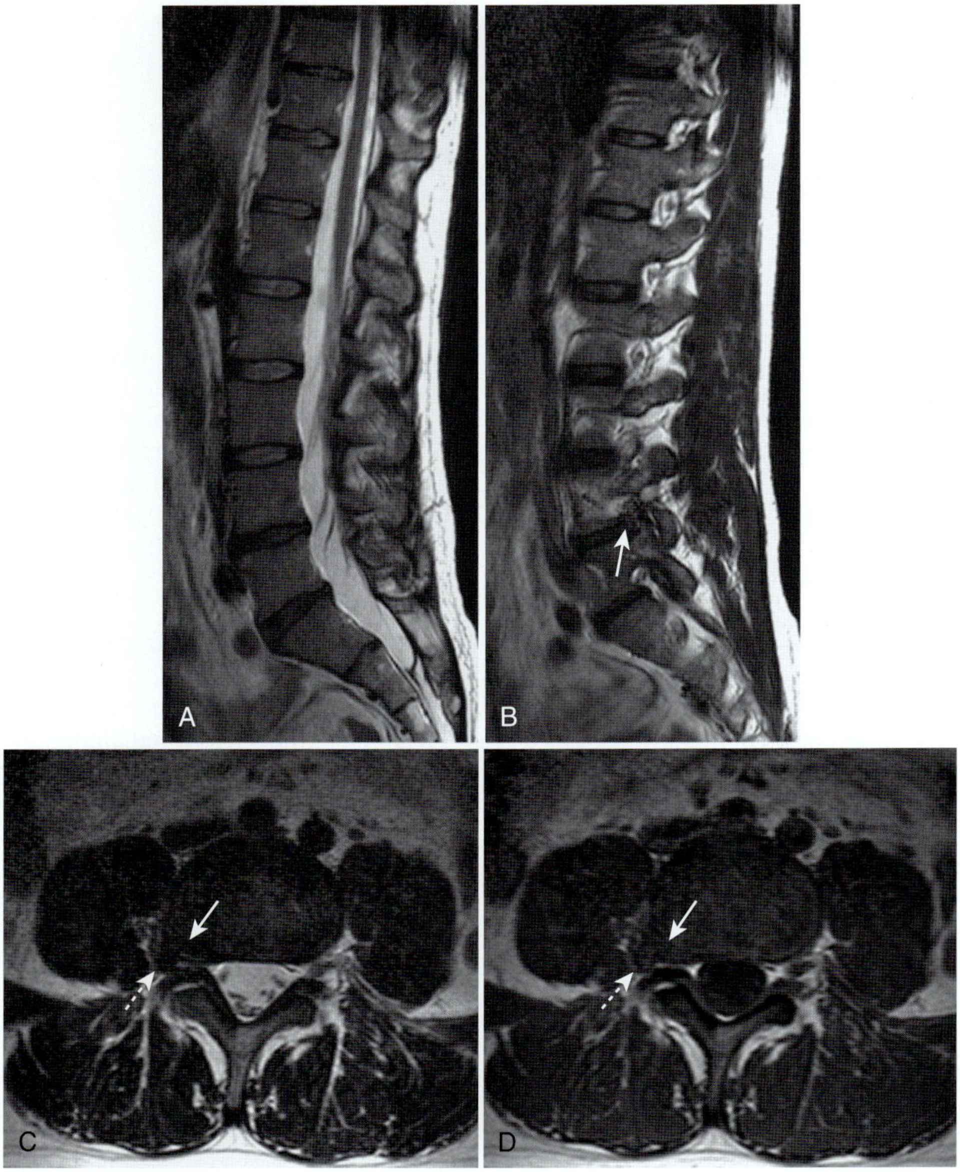

Figure 51.1 (**A**), Midline sagittal T2W MR image demonstrating early disk degeneration at the lower two lumbar levels with low-SI discs and minor bulging. (**B**), Parasagittal T2W MR image shows disk material within the exit canal displacing the nerve root (*white arrow*). The lateral disk protrusion is more easily appreciated on the axial T2W (**C**) and T1W (**D**) images, on which the disk herniation (*white arrow*) is displacing the exiting nerve root (*broken arrow*), which is swollen. Compare with the left side, which has clearly defined fat planes around the exiting nerve root; the fat planes are obliterated on the side of the disk protrusion.

CHAPTER 52

Tarlov Perineural Root Sleeve Cyst

DEFINITION

- Focal dilatation of the arachnoid and dura mater of the spinal posterior nerve root sheath that may be progressive.

SIGNS AND SYMPTOMS

- Level and size of cyst will determine the clinical presentation.
- Most are asymptomatic until size reaches critical proportions.
- Lumbar radicular pain is most common symptom.
- Back and/or sacral pain is also common.
- Bowel and/or bladder symptomatology may be seen with larger cysts.
- Pain may radiate in a dermatomal or, less commonly, nondermatomal pattern.
- Motor, sensory, and reflex changes may occur.
- Valsalva maneuver often worsens radicular symptomatology.
- Bending forward often worsens radicular symptomatology.

DEMOGRAPHICS

- Peak incidence between third and fourth decades of life.
- Incidence: Male = Female.
- No ethnic or racial predilection.

IMAGING RECOMMENDATIONS

- Radiography:
  - Not routinely indicated for radicular symptoms.
- MRI.
- CT myelography:
  - When MRI is contraindicated.

IMAGING FINDINGS

- Fluid-filled rounded "cysts" adjacent to nerve roots:
  - Low signal intensity (SI) on T1-weighted (T1W) and high SI on T2W MR images.
  - Found in exit foramina or sacral canal.
- Most common in lower lumbar spine, but may be encountered in dorsal spine.
- Usually small (5-10 mm in size).
- Frequently multiple.

OTHER RECOMMENDED TESTING

- Electromyography and nerve conduction velocity testing are indicated if radiculopathy is present.
- Diagnostic selective nerve root block may serve as a useful diagnostic tool to determine whether a specific disc is serving as a nidus for the pain.

DIFFERENTIAL DIAGNOSIS

- Schwannoma.
- Intraforaminal intervertebral disc herniation.
- Meningocele.
- Synovial cyst of the facet joint.
- Spinal nerve root avulsion.
- Neoplasm.

TREATMENT

- Conservative treatment consisting of local heat, cold, simple analgesics, and nonsteroidal anti-inflammatory agents will improve symptoms in many cases.
- Physical therapy, including gentle stretching, range-of-motion exercises, deep heat modalities, and stretch and spray, may be beneficial in selected patients.
- Epidural blocks will provide symptomatic relief if conservative therapy fails or the pain is limiting activities of daily living.
- Selective nerve root blocks may provide symptomatic relief if conservative therapy fails or the pain is limiting activities of daily living.
- Surgery may be required for persistent pain or progressive neurologic symptoms.

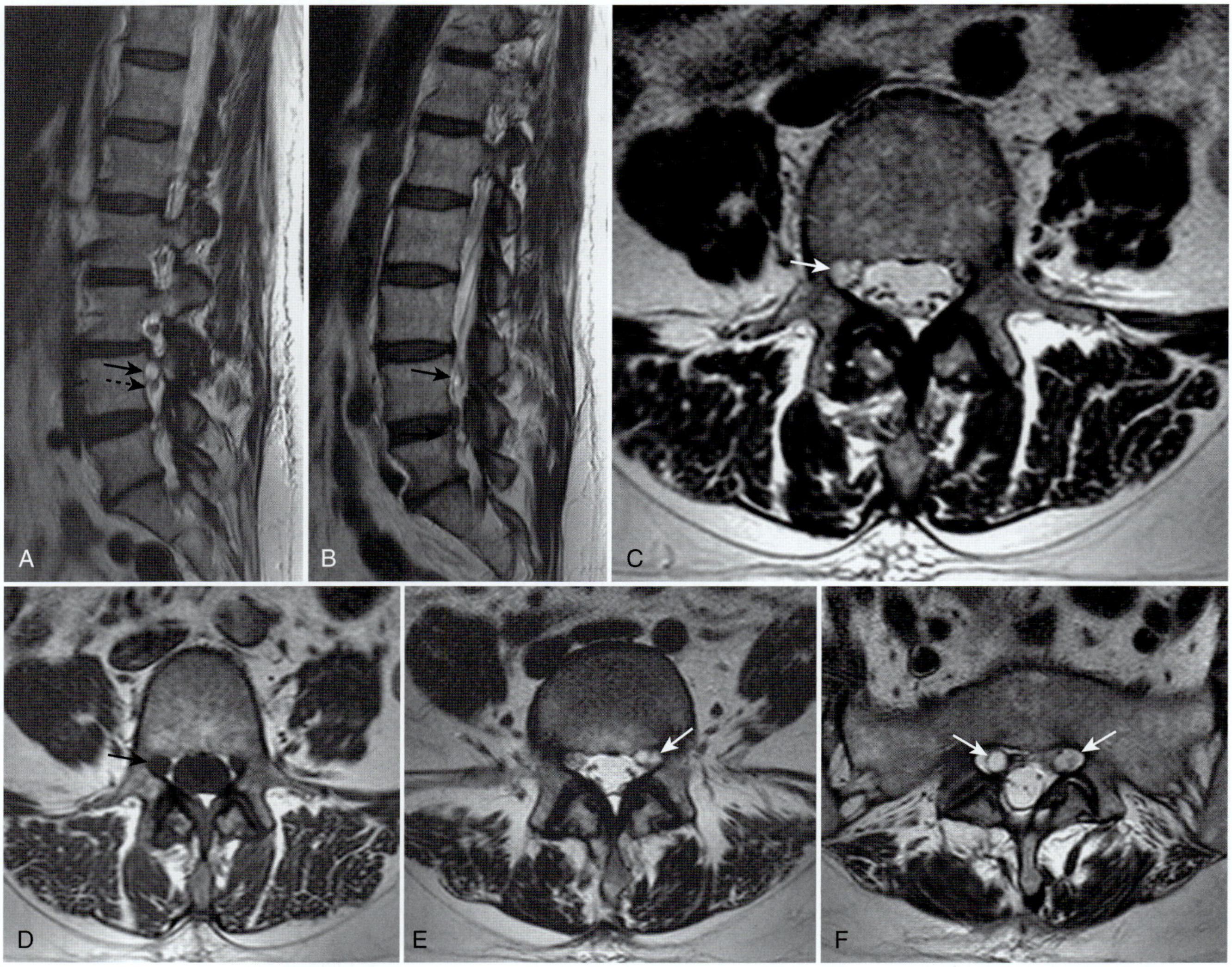

Figure 52.1 Patient with multiple Tarlov cysts in the lumbar sacral spine. (**A**), A right-sided parasagittal T2W MR image shows a high-SI cyst within the exit canal at the L4-L5 level (*solid black arrow*) adjacent to the exiting nerve root (*broken black arrow*). (**B**), Two additional Tarlov cysts can be seen on a left-sided parasagittal T2W MR image (*black arrows*). (**C**), An axial T2W MR image shows the high-SI cyst at L4-L5 (*white arrow*), which has low SI on the T1W MR image (**D**) (*black arrow*). Additional cysts are shown on T2W MR images on the left side, at the L5 level (**E**) and within the sacral canal bilaterally (**F**) (*white arrows*).

CHAPTER 53

Acquired Spinal Stenosis of the Lumbar Spine

DEFINITION

- Narrowing of the lumbar spinal canal and associated neuroforamina due to degenerative changes.

SIGNS AND SYMPTOMS

- In the absence of trauma, onset of symptoms is insidious.
- Gradual and subtle onset of lumbar myelopathy.
- Neurogenic claudication.
- Back pain with radicular and nonradicular radiation of pain.
- Lower extremity numbness, weakness, and reflex changes progressing to spastic paresis.
- Loss of proprioception and vibratory sensation.
- Ataxic, spastic gait.
- Hyperreflexia.
- Pathologic reflexes (e.g., Babinski reflex) present.
- Bowel and bladder symptomatology.
- More sudden onset of symptoms following trauma to the lumbar spine.

DEMOGRAPHICS

- Peak age at onset in the fifth and sixth decades of life.
- Incidence: Male = Female.
- Congenitally shortened pedicles increase incidence.

IMAGING RECOMMENDATIONS

- Radiographs to assess vertebral alignment:
  - Flexion/extension radiographs may be used to identify instability.
- MRI is the primary investigation for neurogenic claudication.
- CT is an alternative when MRI is contraindicated.

IMAGING FINDINGS

- Central stenosis:
  - Effacement of the cerebrospinal fluid (CSF) space and the cauda equina on T2-weighted (T2W) MR images.
  - Obliteration of fat in the lateral recess on T1W MR images.
  - Trefoil shape of canal on axial imaging.
  - Disk bulging, facet osteoarthritis (OA), and ligament hypertrophy.
  - Associated disc degeneration and spondylosis.
  - Lateral recess stenosis may occur in isolation.
  - No validated method for grading stenosis because imaging does not correlate with symptomatology.
- Foraminal stenosis:
  - Obliteration of epidural fat around nerve root in exit canal.
  - Loss of height of exit canal due to disk degeneration.
  - Disk bulging, facet OA, and lateral osteophyte formation.
- Acute focal disk protrusions do not typically cause neurogenic claudication.

OTHER RECOMMENDED TESTING

- Electromyography and nerve conduction velocity testing are indicated if radiculopathy is present and to rule out amyotrophic lateral sclerosis.
- Evoked potential testing to quantify spinal cord compromise.

DIFFERENTIAL DIAGNOSIS

- Multiple sclerosis.
- Neoplasm of the lumbar spinal cord and/or surrounding structures.
- Diskitis.
- Herniation of the lumbar disc.
- Epidural hematoma.
- Paget disease.

TREATMENT

- Avoid:
  - Activities that increase risk of lumbar spine trauma, such as contact sports.
  - Extreme lumbar spine positioning during anesthesia.
  - Therapeutic manipulation of the lumbar spine.
- Modify activity to avoid overuse of lumbar spine.

- Conservative treatment consisting of local heat, cold, simple analgesics, and nonsteroidal anti-inflammatory agents will improve symptoms in many cases.
- Physical therapy, including gentle stretching and gentle range-of-motion exercises.
- Epidural blocks will provide symptomatic relief if conservative therapy fails or the pain is limiting activities of daily living.
- Surgical treatment indicated if neurologic symptoms progress.

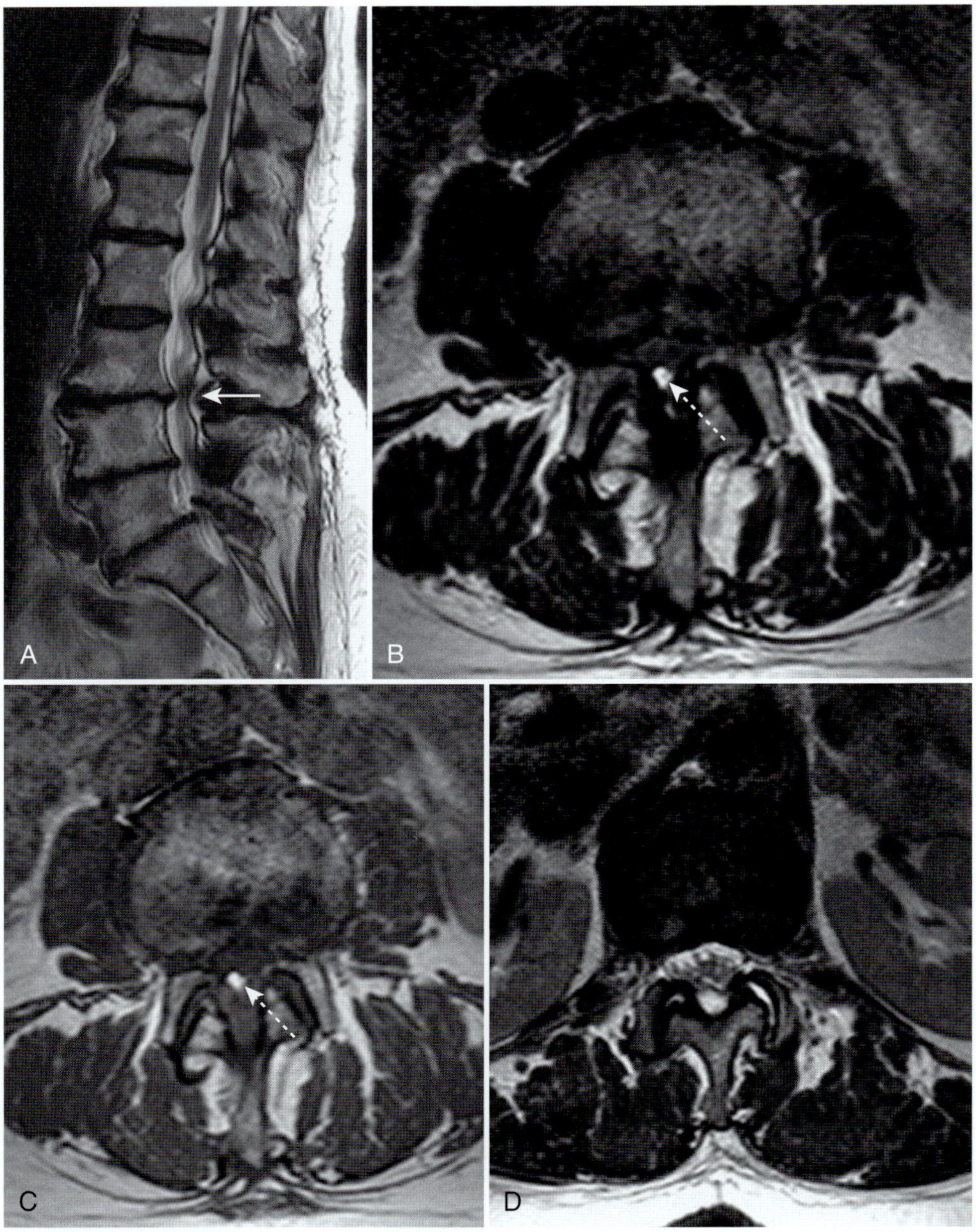

Figure 53.1 (**A**), Sagittal T2W MR image of a patient with established spondylosis and disk degeneration in combination with facet OA. There is multilevel disk bulging, resulting in central canal stenosis that is most marked at the L3-L4 level with crowding of the nerve roots (*white arrow*). The severity of stenosis is best appreciated on the axial T2W (**B**) and T1W (**C**) images, which show complete obliteration of the CSF space. The small focus of high signal intensity (SI) in the posterior canal (*broken arrow*) is due to normal fat within the canal. (**D**), Compare the d ameter of the canal on an axial T2W image at the L1-L2 level with preservation of the CSF space around the cauda equina.

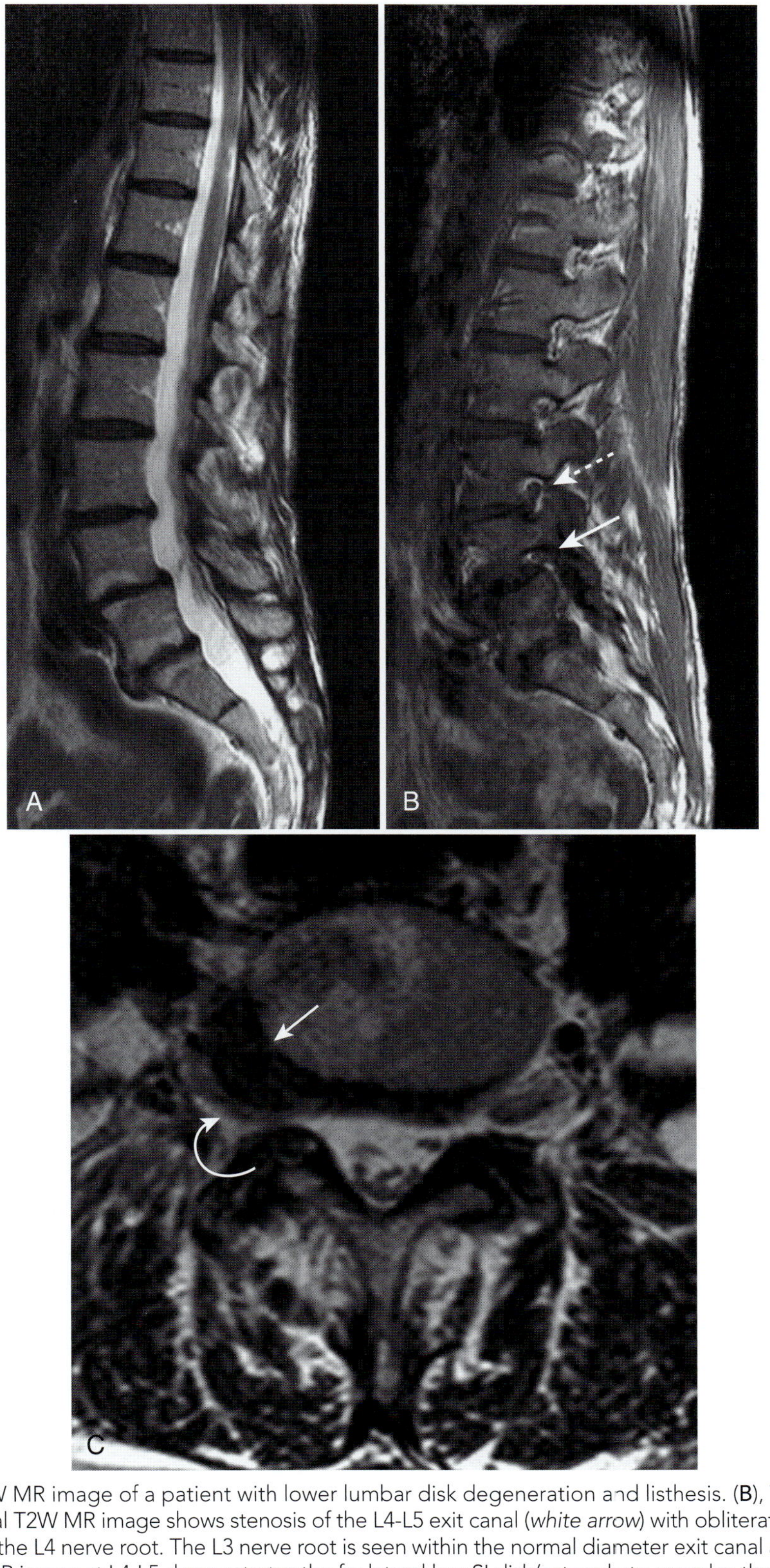

Fig 53.2 (A), Sagittal T2W MR image of a patient with lower lumbar disk degeneration and listhesis. (B), There is no central canal stenosis, but the parasagittal T2W MR image shows stenosis of the L4-L5 exit canal (*white arrow*) with obliteration of the epidural fat planes and compression of the L4 nerve root. The L3 nerve root is seen within the normal diameter exit canal at the level above (*broken arrow*). (C), The axial T2W MR image at L4-L5 demonstrates the far lateral low-SI disk/osteophyte complex that is compressing the exiting L4 nerve root (*curved arrow*).

CHAPTER 54

Ossification Ligamentum Flavum

DEFINITION

- Idiopathic ossification of the ligamentum flavum.

SIGNS AND SYMPTOMS

- Usually asymptomatic.
- Onset of symptoms is insidious.
- Gradual and subtle onset of lumbar myelopathy.
- Back pain with radicular and nonradicular radiation of pain.
- Lower extremity numbness, weakness, and reflex changes progressing to spastic paresis.
- Loss of proprioception and vibratory sensation.
- Ataxic, spastic gait.
- Hyperreflexia.
- Pathologic reflexes (e.g., Babinski reflex) present.
- Bowel and bladder symptomatology.
- More sudden onset of symptoms following trauma to the lumbar spine.

DEMOGRAPHICS

- Peak age at onset in the fourth to sixth decade of life.
- Incidence: Male > Female.
- Symptomatic presentation more common in Japanese and North African persons.

IMAGING RECOMMENDATIONS

- Radiography or CT for identification of ligament calcification and ossification.
- MRI to assess associated spinal stenosis and neural compression.

IMAGING FINDINGS

- Calcification and ossification within the ligamentum flavum.
- Low-signal intensity (SI) thickening of the ligament on MRI pulse sequences.
- Other degenerative features may be present.
  - Facet osteoarthritis.
  - Discal degeneration.
  - Spondylosis.

OTHER RECOMMENDED TESTING

- Electromyography and nerve conduction velocity testing are indicated if radiculopathy is present and to rule out amyotrophic lateral sclerosis.
- Evoked potential testing to quantify spinal cord compromise.
- Laboratory testing to rule out calcium pyrophosphate dihydrate (CPPD) deposition disease.

DIFFERENTIAL DIAGNOSIS

- CPPD disease.
- Neoplasm of the lumbar spinal cord and/or surrounding structures.
- Meningioma.
- Facet arthropathy.

TREATMENT

- Avoid:
  - Activities that increase the risk of lumbar spine trauma, such as contact sports.
  - Extreme lumbar spine positioning during anesthesia.
  - Therapeutic manipulation of the lumbar spine.
- Modify activity to avoid overuse of the lumbar spine.
- Conservative treatment consisting of local heat, cold, simple analgesics, and nonsteroidal anti-inflammatory agents will improve symptoms in many cases.
- Physical therapy, including gentle stretching and gentle range-of-motion exercises.
- Epidural blocks will provide symptomatic relief if conservative therapy fails or the pain is limiting activities of daily living.
- Surgical treatment indicated if neurologic symptoms progress.

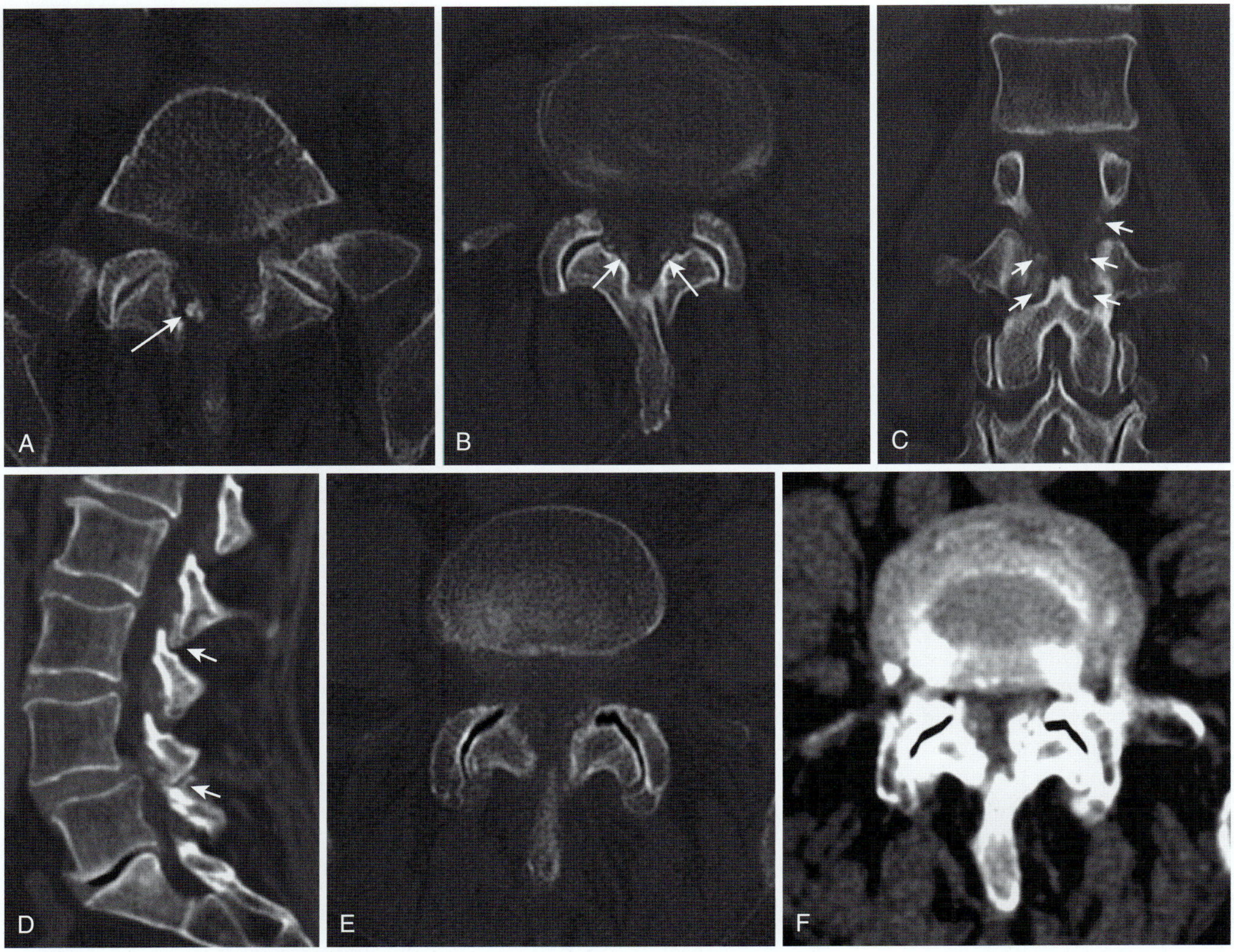

Figure 54.1 Elderly woman with back pain and symptoms of spinal stenosis. (**A** and **B**), The axial CT scans show areas of focal calcification and ossification within the thickened ligamentum flavum at several levels in the lumbar spine. This is also evident on the coronal (**C**) and sagittal (**D**) scans (*white arrows*). In this case the process is primarily degenerative, with associated facet osteoarthritis visible on an axial section at L4-L5 (**E**), along with bony facet overgrowth and intra-articular gas. There is also disc degeneration, with intradiscal gas at L5-S1 and degenerative listhesis at L4-L5 (**D**). The stenosis at L4-L5 is best appreciated on the axial soft tissue window (**F**).

CHAPTER 55

Facet Arthropathy of the Lumbar Spine

DEFINITION

- Degenerative osteoarthritis of the synovium-lined zygapophyseal joints.

SIGNS AND SYMPTOMS

- May be asymptomatic.
- Onset may occur following seemingly minor trauma.
- Back pain made worse with movement of lumbar spine.
- Worse after rest.
- Pain typically radiates into the low back and buttocks in a nondermatomal pattern.
- Pain can be made worse with axial loading combined with range of motion of the lumbar spine.

DEMOGRAPHICS

- Incidence: Male = Female.
- Onset in second and third decades of life.
- Universal finding after fifth decade.
- There may be a genetic predisposition.

IMAGING RECOMMENDATIONS

- Imaging not routinely indicated for mechanical back pain without "red flags."
- MRI and CT both demonstrate facet osteoarthritis (OA).
- CT may be combined with guided facet joint injection.
- Radiographs are less sensitive for early facet OA.

IMAGING FINDINGS

- Bony overgrowth of facet joints with bony sclerosis.
- Low-signal intensity (SI) thickening of joint capsule and ligament hypertrophy.
- Facet joint effusions.
- Intra-articular gas on radiography or CT.
- Facet subluxation associated with spondylolisthesis.

OTHER RECOMMENDED TESTING

- Intra-articular facet injection to determine whether a specific facet joint is the nidus of the pain.

DIFFERENTIAL DIAGNOSIS

- Inflammatory arthritides, especially rheumatoid arthritis.
- Septic facet joint.
- Healing facet joint fracture.
- Neoplasm.
- Paget disease.
- Myositis ossificans.

TREATMENT

- Conservative treatment consisting of local heat, cold, simple analgesics, and nonsteroidal anti-inflammatory agents will improve symptoms in many cases.
- Physical therapy, including gentle stretching, range-of-motion exercises, deep heat modalities, and stretch and spray, may be beneficial in selected patients.
- Facet blocks with local anesthetic and steroid will provide symptomatic relief if conservative therapy fails or the pain is limiting activities of daily living.
- Osteopathic or chiropractic manipulation may provide symptomatic relief in selected patients.
- Surgery may be required for persistent pain or progressive neurologic symptoms.

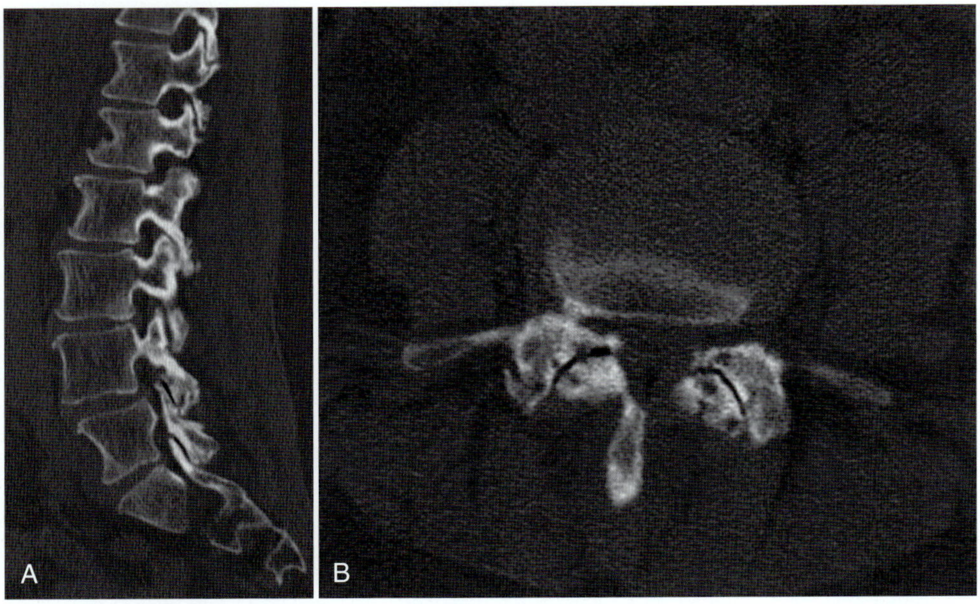

Figure 55.1 Sagittal (**A**) and axial (**B**) CT scans of the lumbar spine with widespread facet OA. The L4-L5 level is most affected, with subchondral sclerosis and cyst formation. There is bony overgrowth, and gas is present within the joint line.

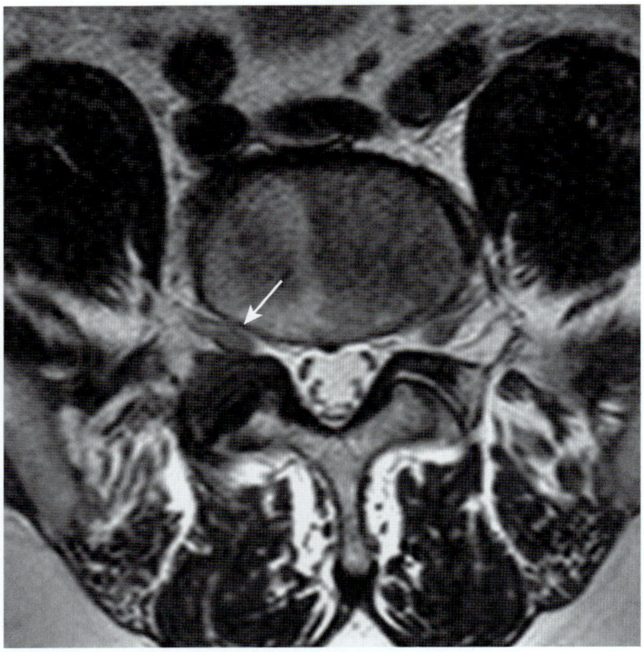

Figure 55.2 Axial T2-weighted (T2W) MR image of unilateral right-sided facet OA, with ligament hypertrophy and bony overgrowth. There is early compromise of the exiting nerve root within the neural foramen (*white arrow*).

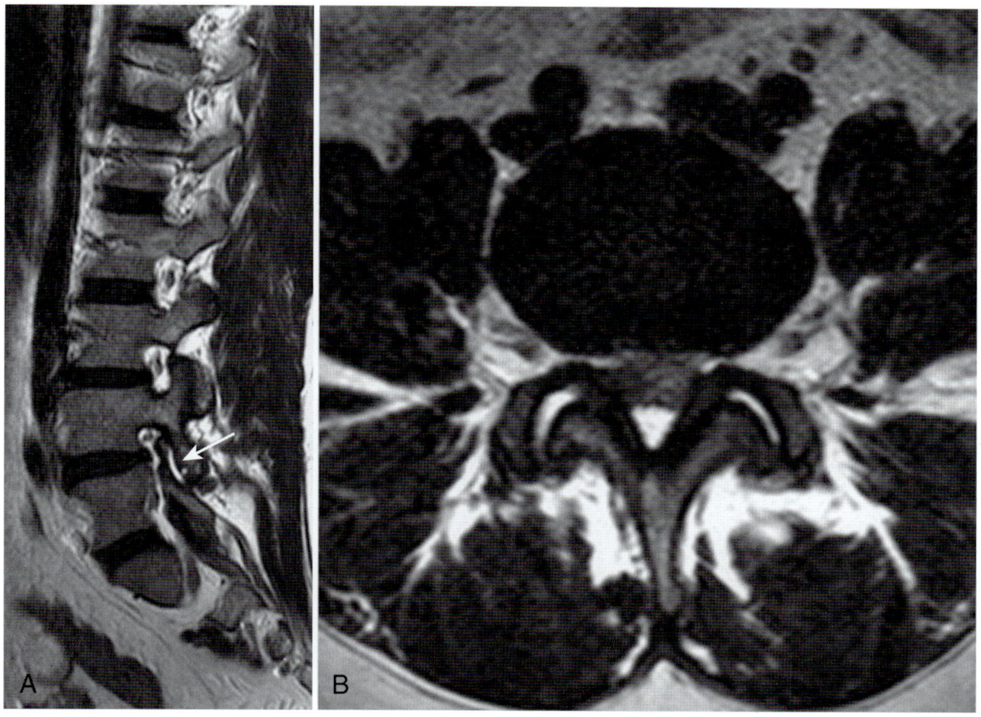

Figure 55.3 (A), Bilateral facet joint effusions with a high-SI effusion in the L4-L5 facet on this sagittal T2W MR image (*white arrow*). (B), The effusions are also visible on this axial T2W MR image, and there is central canal stenosis secondary to the associated ligament hypertrophy.

CHAPTER 56

Seronegative Spondyloarthropathy

DEFINITION

- Inflammatory destructive arthritis involving the spine and sacroiliac joints in the absence of rheumatoid factor and the presence of an elevated erythrocyte sedimentation rate.
- Most common causes include ankylosing spondylitis, enteropathic spondyloarthropathy, psoriasis, and Reiter disease.
- The sacroiliac joint features of ankylosing spondylitis are described in Chapter 135.

SIGNS AND SYMPTOMS

- Most common presentation is low back pain that is worse in the morning.
- Fatigue.
- Low-grade fever.
- Decreased range of motion of the spine and sacroiliac joints.
- Coexisting uveitis, iritis, and conjunctivitis.
- Heel pain and plantar fasciitis are common findings, especially in reactive arthritis.
- Onset of symptoms may appear to occur after seemingly minor trauma.
- Pathologic spine fractures are common occurrences.
- May be characterized by exacerbations and remissions.

DEMOGRAPHICS

- Incidence: Male > Female.
- Onset between the second and third decades of life.
- High incidence of HLA-B27 haplotype in patients with seronegative spondyloarthropathy.

IMAGING RECOMMENDATIONS

- Radiography of lumbar spine and sacroiliac joints (SIJs).
- MRI of lumbar spine and SIJs for early disease if radiographic findings are normal.
- CT is useful for detection of fractures in areas of bony ankylosis.

IMAGING FINDINGS

- Ankylosing spondylitis:
  - Syndesmophyte formation and discovertebral erosion.
  - Romanus lesion:
    "Shiny corner" sign on radiographs.
    High signal intensity (SI) on short T1 inversion recovery (STIR) MR images due to reactive edema.
  - Inflammatory arthritis of facets joint and costovertebral joint:
    Reactive edema on STIR images.
  - Eventual ankylosis:
    Bamboo spine and "trolley track" sign.
  - Osteoporosis.
  - SIJ and dorsolumbar involvement initially. May progress to involve entire spine.
  - Enteropathic spondyloarthropathy has the same radiologic features.
- Psoriasis/Reiter disease:
  - Mixed pattern including:
    Syndesmophytes.
    More prominent osteophytes.
  - Distribution may be asymmetrical.
- Often limited to the lumbar spine and lower dorsal spine.

OTHER RECOMMENDED TESTING

- HLA-B27 testing in all patients in whom seronegative spondyloarthropathy is suspected.
- Erythrocyte sedimentation rate measurement in all patients in whom seronegative spondyloarthropathy is suspected.

DIFFERENTIAL DIAGNOSIS

- Inflammatory arthritides, especially rheumatoid arthritis.
- Septic sacroiliac joint.
- Healing sacroiliac joint fracture.
- DISH (diffuse idiopathic skeletal hyperostosis) syndrome.

- Chronic juvenile arthritis.
- Retinoid therapy.
- Neoplasm.

TREATMENT

- Conservative treatment consisting of local heat, cold, simple analgesics, and nonsteroidal anti-inflammatory agents will improve symptoms in many cases.
- Physical therapy, including gentle stretching, range-of-motion exercises, deep heat modalities, and stretch and spray, may be beneficial in selected patients.
- Injections of symptomatic joints with local anesthetic and steroid will provide symptomatic relief if conservative therapy fails or the pain is limiting activities of daily living.
- Disease-modifying drugs such as methotrexate and sulfasalazine.
- Surgery may be required for persistent pain or progressive neurologic symptoms.

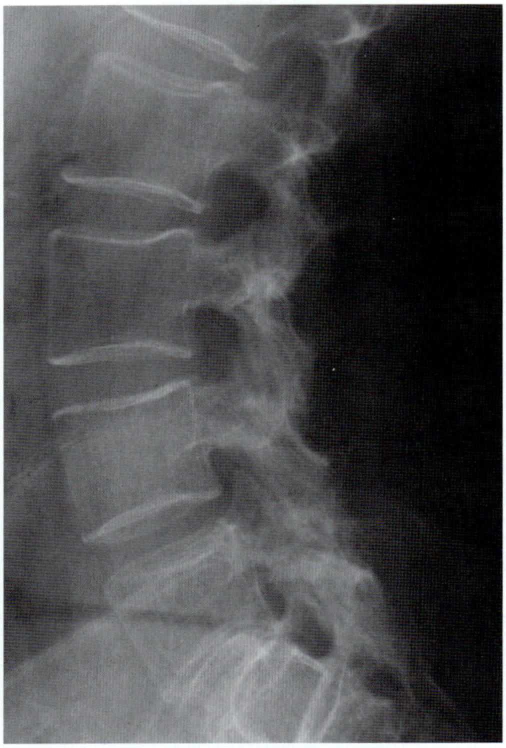

Figure 56.1 Lateral radiograph of the lumbar spine with squaring of the vertebral bodies, which is typical of early ankylosing spondylitis. There are also generalized osteopenia and early inflammatory arthropathy of the lower facet joints.

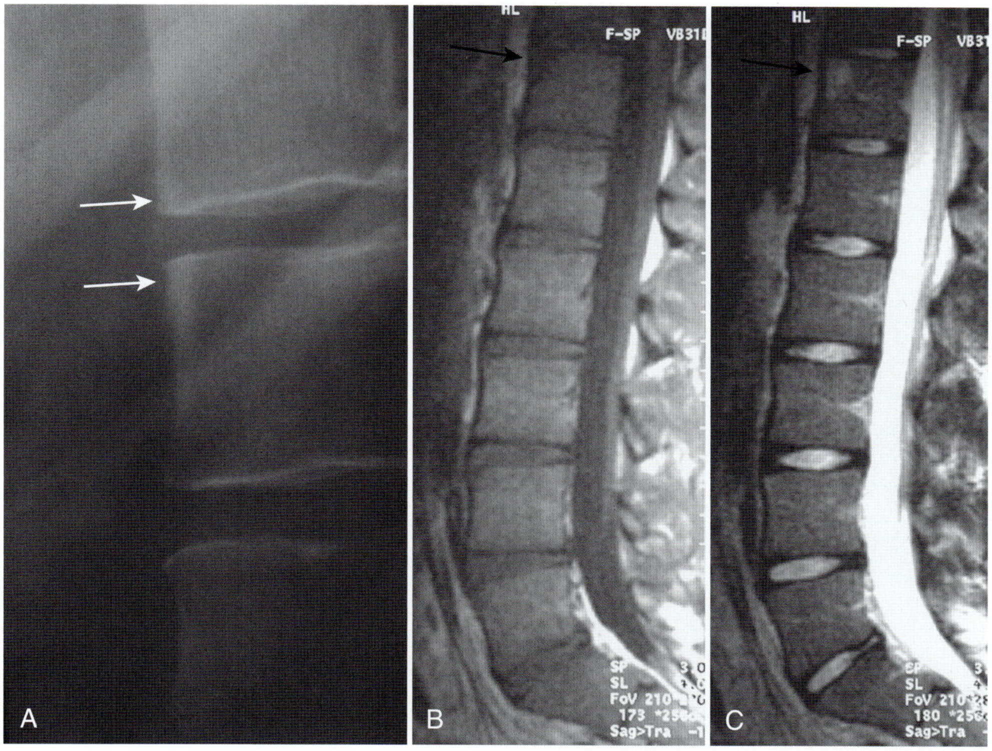

Figure 56.2 (**A**), Lateral radiograph demonstrating Romanus lesions in early ankylosing spondylitis, with sclerosis of the anterior margins of adjacent vertebral bodies (*white arrows*) due to reactive osteitis. (**B** and **C**), Sagittal MR images demonstrate the same type of lesion in a different patient with an edematous response that has low SI on the T1-weighted (T1W) MR image (**B**) (*black arrow*) and high SI on the STIR image (**C**) (*black arrow*).

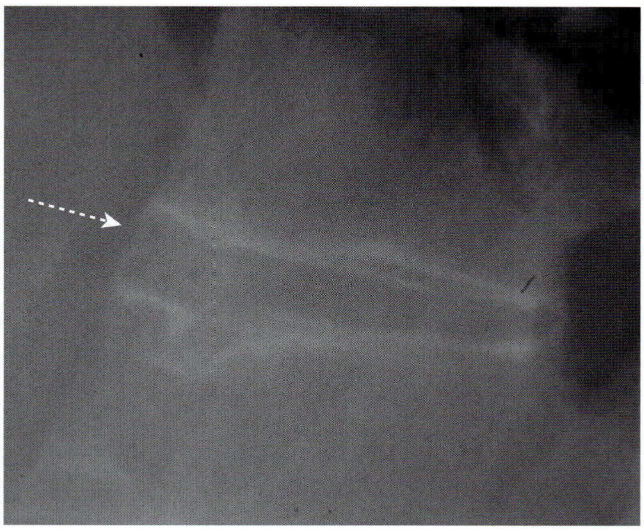

Figure 56.3 Lateral radiograph demonstrating syndesmophyte formation with calcification of the outer fibers of the annulus fibrosus, which extends across adjacent vertebral bodies (*arrow*). There is also a discovertebral erosion that mimics a Schmorl node.

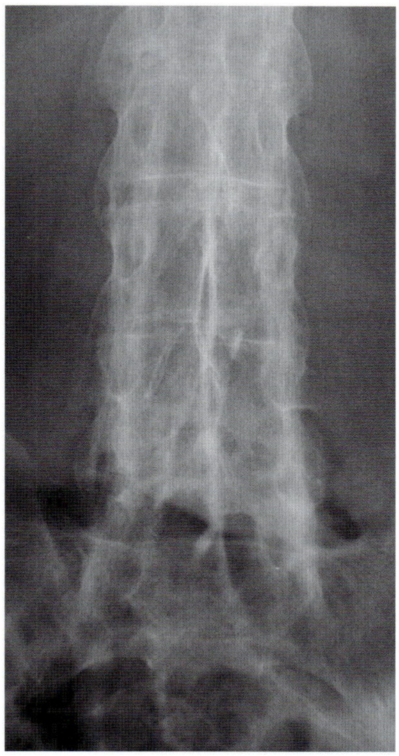

Figure 56.4 AP radiograph of established ankylosing spondylitis. The "trolley track" sign results from bilateral ankylosis of the facet joints and ossification of the interspinous and supraspinous ligaments.

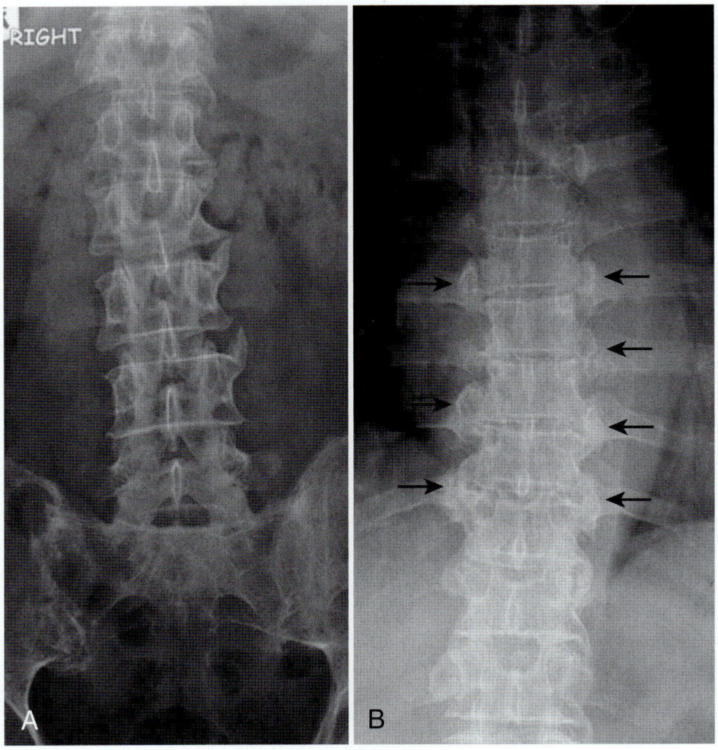

Figure 56.5 AP radiographs of the lumbar (**A**) and dorsal (**B**) spine in a patient with psoriatic arthritis and associated spondyloarthropathy. There is bilateral sacroiliitis with ankylosis. Asymmetrical osteophytes are affecting the left side of the mid and upper lumbar spine. There is also proliferative bone formation in multiple costovertebral joints in the dorsal spine (*black arrows*).

CHAPTER 57

Bacterial Diskitis and Osteomyelitis of the Lumbar Spine

DEFINITION

- Diskitis and osteomyelitis due to a suppurative bacterial infection of the intervertebral disk and vertebral body.

SIGNS AND SYMPTOMS

- Acute onset of localized back pain.
- Back pain may be quite focal or localized.
- Vertebral collapse with acute pain not an uncommon sequela of infection.
- Fever that may be fulminant or subtle.
- Night sweats.
- Pain may radiate in a dermatomal or nondermatomal pattern.
- Myelopathy may be present.
- Bowel and bladder symptomatology with spinal cord compression.

DEMOGRAPHICS

- Bimodal age distribution, with children and elderly patients most commonly affected.
- Incidence: Male > Female.
- Increased incidence in patients with chronic diseases, such as diabetes, or immunocompromised states (e.g., human immunodeficiency virus, cancer).
- Increased incidence in intravenous drug abusers.
- *Staphylococcus aureus* the most common pathogen.
- *Escherichia coli* the most common gram-negative pathogen.
- *Salmonella* the most common pathogen in patients with sickle cell disease.
- Recurrent disease not uncommon, especially in immunocompromised patients.
- Postoperative infection following disk surgery, etc.

IMAGING RECOMMENDATIONS

- MRI is the primary investigation for suspected spinal infection.
- Radiographs are insensitive for early disease.
- CT is an alternative when MRI is contraindicated.
- CT- or fluoroscopy-guided biopsy.

IMAGING FINDINGS

- Infective process starts at vertebral end plate (VEP) and rapidly involves the disk space.
- Erosion of VEP occurs early and is best seen on T1-weighted (T1W) MR images.
- High signal intensity (SI) in the disk on T2W MR images with enhancement on images obtained after administration of a contrast agent (post-contrast images).
- Pronounced reactive marrow edema in adjacent vertebral bodies progressing to sclerosis.
- Paravertebral soft tissue mass with developing abscess:
  - Fluid component is high-SI on T2W MR images and without enhancement on post-contrast images.
  - Granulation tissue enhances on post-contrast images.
- Epidural abscess may compress the thecal sac and cauda equina.
- Healing phase:
  - Abscesses and granulation tissue resolve with reduced enhancement in the disk space and paravertebral soft tissues.
  - Progressive bony sclerosis and ankylosis may occur.

OTHER RECOMMENDED TESTING

- White blood cell count, erythrocyte sedimentation rate, and C-reactive protein determinations in all patients in whom osteomyelitis of the spine is suspected.
- Blood and urine cultures in all patients in whom osteomyelitis of the spine is suspected.
- Electromyography and nerve conduction velocity testing are indicated if radiculopathy is present.
- Evoked potential testing if myelopathy is present.

DIFFERENTIAL DIAGNOSIS

- Pathologic fracture due to tumor.
- Traumatic burst fractures of the vertebral body.
- Pott's disease.
- Degenerative end-plate changes.
- Chronic hemodialysis spondyloarthropathy.
- Charcot disease of the spine.

TREATMENT

- Aggressive antibiotic therapy.
- Opioids for acute pain relief.
- Orthotic bracing.
- Emergency surgical decompression and drainage of abscess.

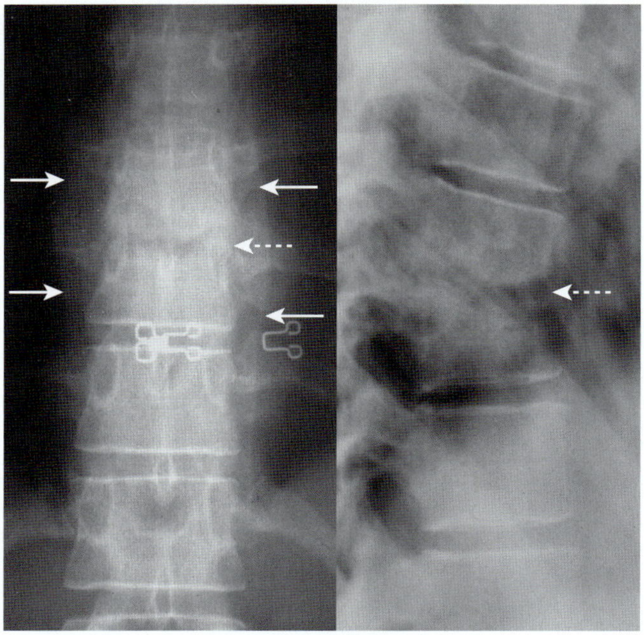

Figure 57.1 AP and lateral radiographs of discitis of the dorsal spine. A paravertebral soft tissue mass is present (*white arrows*), and there is loss of definition of the VEP's with bone erosion (*broken arrows*).

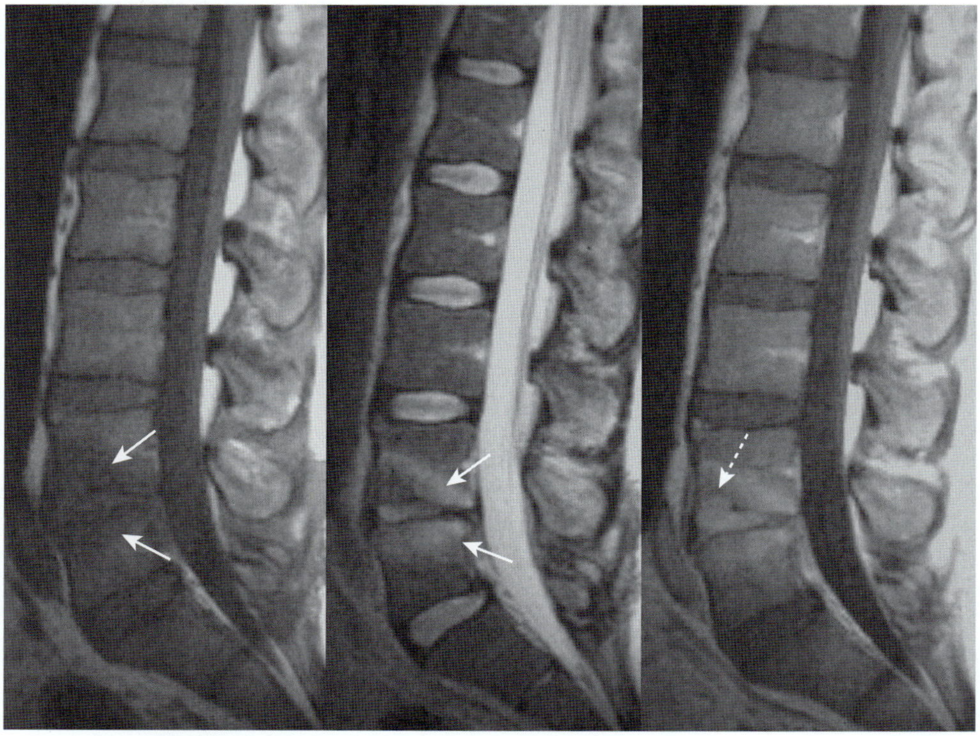

Figure 57.2 Early diskitis demonstrated on sagittal T1W MR image (*left*), T2W MR image (*center*), and post-contrast T1W MR image with fat saturation (*right*). There is low-SI vertebral edema on the T1W MR images, on either side of the disk space (*black arrows*), with loss of definition of the VEPs. The marrow edema has high SI on the T2W MR images (*white arrows*), and there is also high SI within the narrowed disk space. The areas of reactive edema enhance on the post-contrast image, and a diskovertebral erosion is more clearly seen (*broken white arrow*).

CHAPTER 58

Pott's Disease

DEFINITION

- Osteomyelitis due to a granulomatous tubercular infection of the vertebral body and surrounding soft tissue, often with gibbus formation.

SIGNS AND SYMPTOMS

- Gradual onset of localized back pain.
- Back pain may be quite focal or localized.
- Vertebral collapse with acute pain not an uncommon sequela of infection.
- Fever that may be subtle.
- Night sweats.
- Pain may radiate in a dermatomal or nondermatomal pattern.
- Myelopathy may be present.
- Bowel and bladder symptomatology with spinal cord compression.

DEMOGRAPHICS

- Most common in fifth and sixth decades of life.
- Incidence: Male = Female.
- Increased incidence in patients with chronic diseases, such as diabetes, and in immunocompromised states (e.g., human immunodeficiency virus or cancer).
- Diagnosis often delayed.

IMAGING RECOMMENDATIONS

- Radiography:
  - Chest radiograph should be included if there is suspicion of tuberculosis of the spine.
- MRI:
  - Coronal imaging in addition to routine sagittal and axial imaging may be useful to identify psoas abscesses.

IMAGING FINDINGS

- Disk involvement is most common pattern:
  - Erosion of vertebral end plates similar to that seen in diskitis.
  - In African American patients, posterior elements may be involved.
- Bony destruction and vertebral collapse leading to kyphotic angulation.
- Early subligamentous spread to involve adjacent vertebral levels.
- Soft tissue abscesses may be extensive.
- Late disease:
  - Reactive bony sclerosis.
  - Bony ankylosis.
  - Calcified soft tissue abscesses.

OTHER RECOMMENDED TESTING

- Chest radiograph for granulomatous disease.
- White blood cell count with special attention to monocyte count, erythrocyte sedimentation rate, and C-reactive protein determinations for all patients in whom osteomyelitis of the spine is suspected.
- Sputum and urine cultures for *Mycobacterium* for all patients in whom tubercular osteomyelitis of the spine is suspected.
- Electromyography and nerve conduction velocity testing are indicated if radiculopathy present.
- Evoked potential testing if myelopathy present.

DIFFERENTIAL DIAGNOSIS

- Pathologic fracture because of tumor.
- Pyogenic bacterial osteomyelitis of the lumbar spine.
- Fungal spondylitis.

TREATMENT

- Aggressive antibiotic therapy.
- Opioids for acute pain relief.
- Orthotic bracing.
- Emergency surgical decompression and drainage of abscesses.

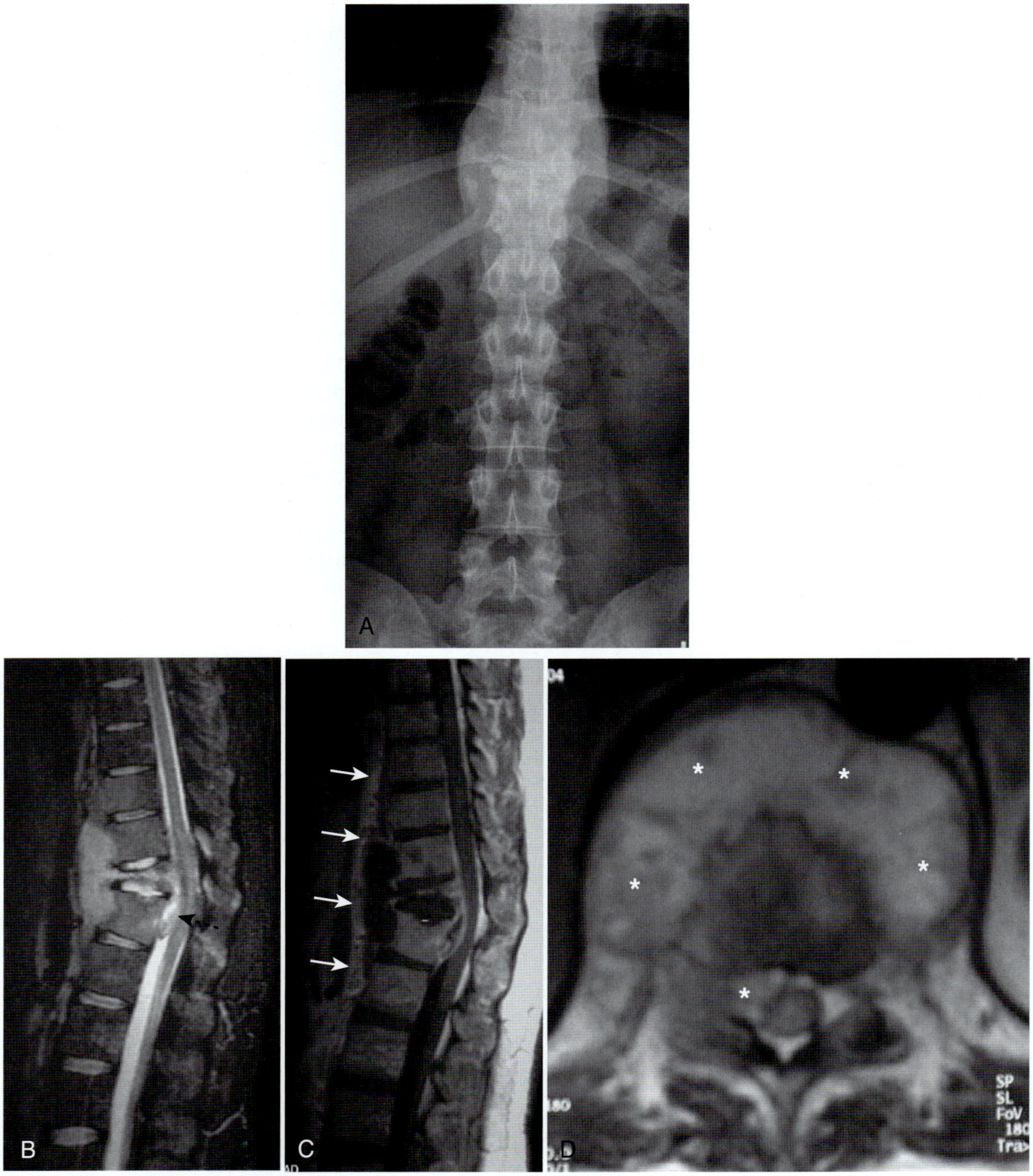

Figure 58.1 (**A**), AP radiograph demonstrating a paravertebral soft tissue mass in the lower dorsal region with collapse of the T11 vertebral body. (**B**), The sagittal T2-weighted (T2W) MR image confirms the vertebral collapse with fluid signal intensity (SI) in the adjacent disc spaces. There is a large anterior high-SI paravertebral soft tissue abscess. There is also an epidural abscess extending behind the T12 vertebra and compressing the spinal cord (*broken arrow*). (**C**), The nonenhancing fluid collections are seen on the T1W MR image obtained after administration of a contrast agent, which also shows extensive enhancing soft tissue inflammatory disease (*white arrows*). The prominent superior and inferior spread is typical of TB. The large abscess collection is also seen on the axial T2W MR image (**D**) (*asterisks*).

CHAPTER 59

Paraspinal Abscess

DEFINITION

- Infection of the soft tissues surrounding the spine due to a suppurative bacterial or mycobacterial infection with phlegmon formation.

SIGNS AND SYMPTOMS

- Acute onset of localized back pain with bacterial infection.
- Gradual onset of localized back pain with *Mycobacterium* infection.
- Back pain may be quite focal or localized in nature.
- Fever that may be fulminant or subtle.
- Night sweats.
- Pain may radiate in a dermatomal or nondermatomal pattern.
- Myelopathy may be present.
- Bowel and bladder symptomatology with spinal cord compression.

DEMOGRAPHICS

- All ages, but most common in the fifth and sixth decades of life.
- Incidence: Male > Female.
- Increased incidence in patients with chronic diseases such as diabetes, and in immunocompromised states (e.g., human immunodeficiency virus or cancer).
- Increased incidence in intravenous drug abusers.
- *Staphylococcus aureus* is the most common pathogen.
- *Escherichia coli* is the most common gram-negative pathogen.
- Fungal infection is quite rare in immunocompetent patients.

IMAGING RECOMMENDATIONS

- Radiography.
- MRI is primary investigation for assessing soft tissues:
  - Coronal images to assess extensive collections.
- US for superficial soft tissue abscesses and to guide drainage procedures.
- CT is alternative to CT for psoas abscesses and to guide drainage procedures.

IMAGING FINDINGS

- High-signal intensity (SI) fluid collections on T2-weighted (T2W) MR images:
  - Often within paraspinal muscles.
- Peripheral enhancement in areas of reactive granulation tissue on post-contrast (obtained after administration of a contrast agent) MR images.
- May be associated with intervertebral disc space infection.
- Tubercular abscesses may eventually calcify.

OTHER RECOMMENDED TESTING

- White blood cell count, erythrocyte sedimentation rate, and C-reactive protein determinations in all patients in whom paraspinal abscess is suspected.
- Blood and urine cultures in all patients in whom bacterial paraspinal abscess is suspected.
- Chest radiograph and urine and sputum cultures for *Mycobacterium* in all patients in whom tubercular paraspinal abscess is suspected.
- Electromyography and nerve conduction velocity testing are indicated if radiculopathy is present.
- Evoked potential testing if myelopathy present.

DIFFERENTIAL DIAGNOSIS

- Pathologic fracture due to tumor.
- Neoplasm.
- Retroperitoneal hematoma.
- Extramedullary hematopoiesis.

TREATMENT

- Aggressive antibiotic or anti-*Mycobacterium* therapy as indicated.
- Opioids for acute pain relief.
- Percutaneous catheter drainage of phlegmon.
- Emergency surgical decompression and drainage of abscesses.

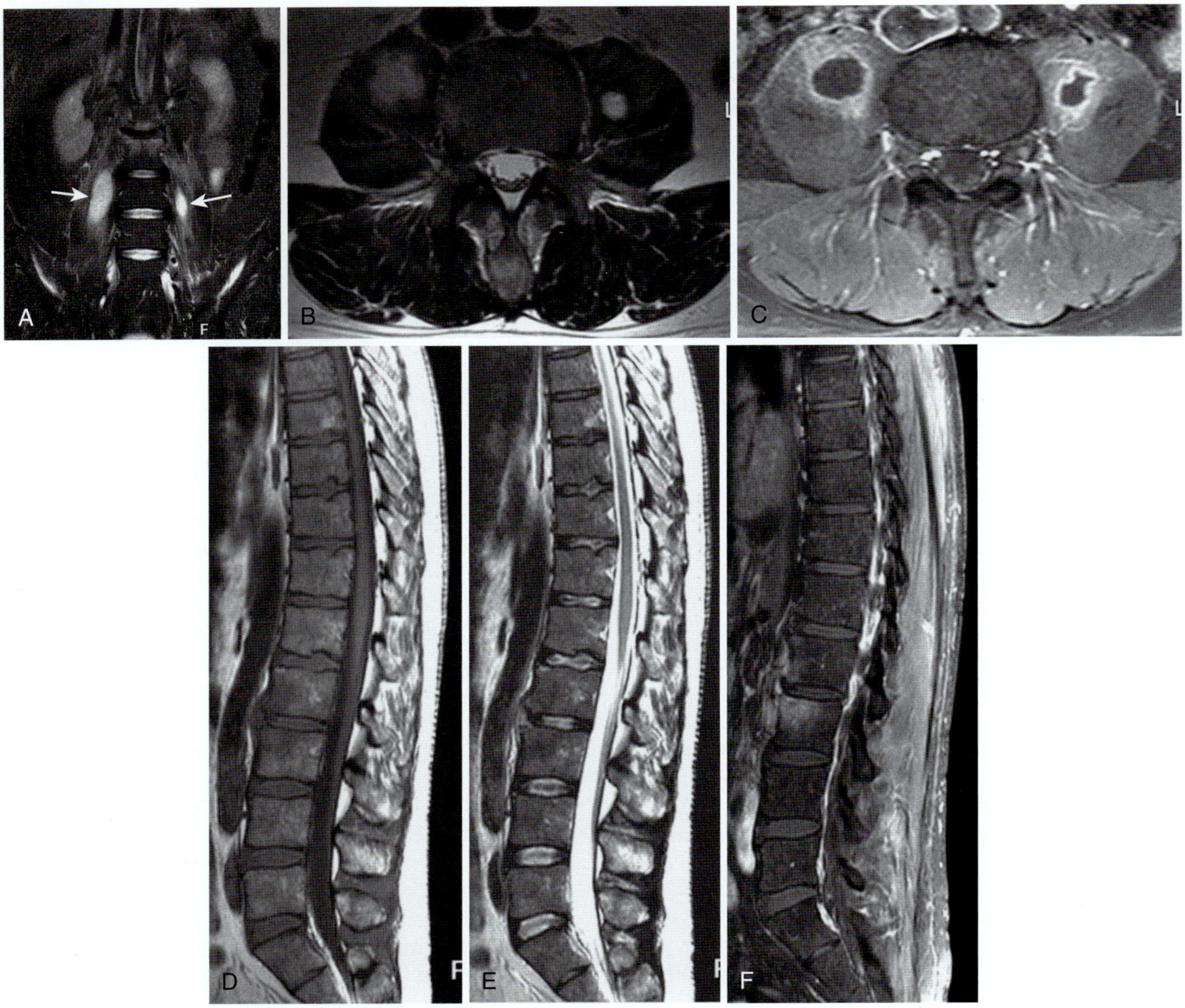

Figure 59.1 (**A**), Coronal short T1 inversion recovery (STIR) MR image demonstrating bilateral high-SI psoas abscesses (*white arrows*). The abscesses are also high SI on the axial T2W MR image (**B**), and low SI with enhancing peripheral granulation tissue on the axial post-contrast T1W with fat suppression (FST1W) MR image (**C**). (**D**), The sagittal T1W MR image demonstrates subtle erosion of the anterior margins of the vertebral bodies at the L2-L3 level with a small anterior mass. (**E**), On a sagittal T2W MR image there is a small focus of high SI in the outer margin of the disc. (**F**), The post-contrast FST1W MR image also shows enhancement in the upper anterior portion of the L3 vertebral body, which is due to osteitis. These appearances are in keeping with disc space infection, which is the source of origin for the psoas abscesses.

CHAPTER 60

Epidural Abscess

DEFINITION

- Infection of the epidural space due to a suppurative bacterial or mycobacterial infection with phlegmon formation.

SIGNS AND SYMPTOMS

- Acute onset of localized back pain with bacterial infection.
- Gradual onset of localized back pain with *Mycobacterium* infection.
- Back pain may be quite focal or localized.
- Fever that may be fulminant or subtle.
- Night sweats.
- Pain may radiate in a dermatomal or nondermatomal pattern.
- Myelopathy may be present.
- Bowel and bladder symptomatology with spinal cord compression.

DEMOGRAPHICS

- All ages, but most common in the sixth and seventh decades of life.
- Incidence: Male > Female.
- Increased incidence in patients with chronic diseases, such as diabetes, or immunocompromised states (e.g., human immunodeficiency virus, cancer).
- Increased incidence in intravenous drug abusers.
- *Staphylococcus aureus* the most common pathogen.
- *Escherichia coli* the most common gram-negative pathogen.
- Fungal infection relatively rare in immunocompetent patients.

IMAGING RECOMMENDATIONS

- MRI is the primary investigation for suspected epidural infection.
- Radiography and CT may provide limited information when MRI is contraindicated.

IMAGING FINDINGS

- High-signal intensity (SI) fluid collection within the epidural space on T2-weighted (T2W) MR images.
- Low-SI fluid on T1W MR images.
- On images obtained after administration of a contrast agent (post-contrast images):
  - Nonenhancement of abscess.
  - Peripheral enhancement of phlegmon.
- Compression of the thecal sac and cauda equina with effacement of cerebrospinal fluid space.
- Associated disc space infection and paraspinal abscess.

OTHER RECOMMENDED TESTING

- White blood cell count, erythrocyte sedimentation rate, and C-reactive protein determinations in all patients in whom paraspinal abscess is suspected.
- Blood and urine cultures in all patients in whom bacterial paraspinal abscess is suspected.
- Chest radiographs and urine and sputum cultures for *Mycobacterium* in all patients in whom tubercular paraspinal abscess is suspected.
- Electromyography and nerve conduction testing is indicated if radiculopathy is present.
- Evoked potential testing if myelopathy is present.

DIFFERENTIAL DIAGNOSIS

- Pathologic fracture due to tumor.
- Metastatic disease involving the epidural space.
- Epidural hematoma.
- Extruded disc fragment.
- Epidural lipomatosis.

TREATMENT

- Aggressive antibiotic or anti-*Mycobacterium* therapy as indicated.
- Opioids for acute pain relief.
- Emergency surgical decompression and drainage of abscess.

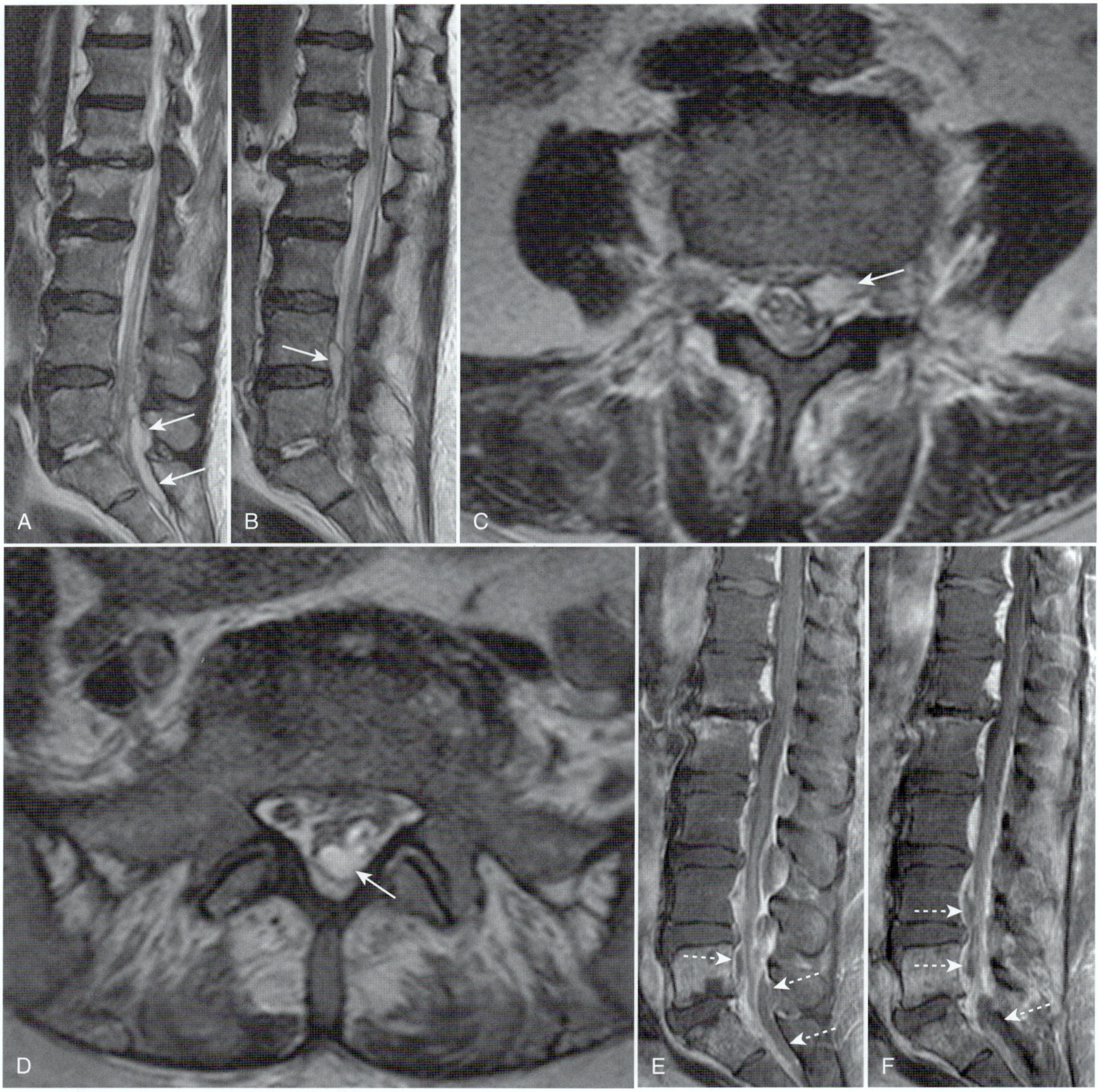

Figure 60.1 Sagittal (**A** and **B**) and axial (**C** and **D**) T2W MR images of discitis at the L5-S1 disc level showing high-SI fluid within the disc. There are high-SI fluid collections (*white arrows*) in the epidural space consistent with abscesses. The sagittal post-contrast T1W MR images with fat saturation (FST1W) (**E** and **F**) show the abscesses as low-SI areas with only peripheral enhancement (*broken white arrows*).

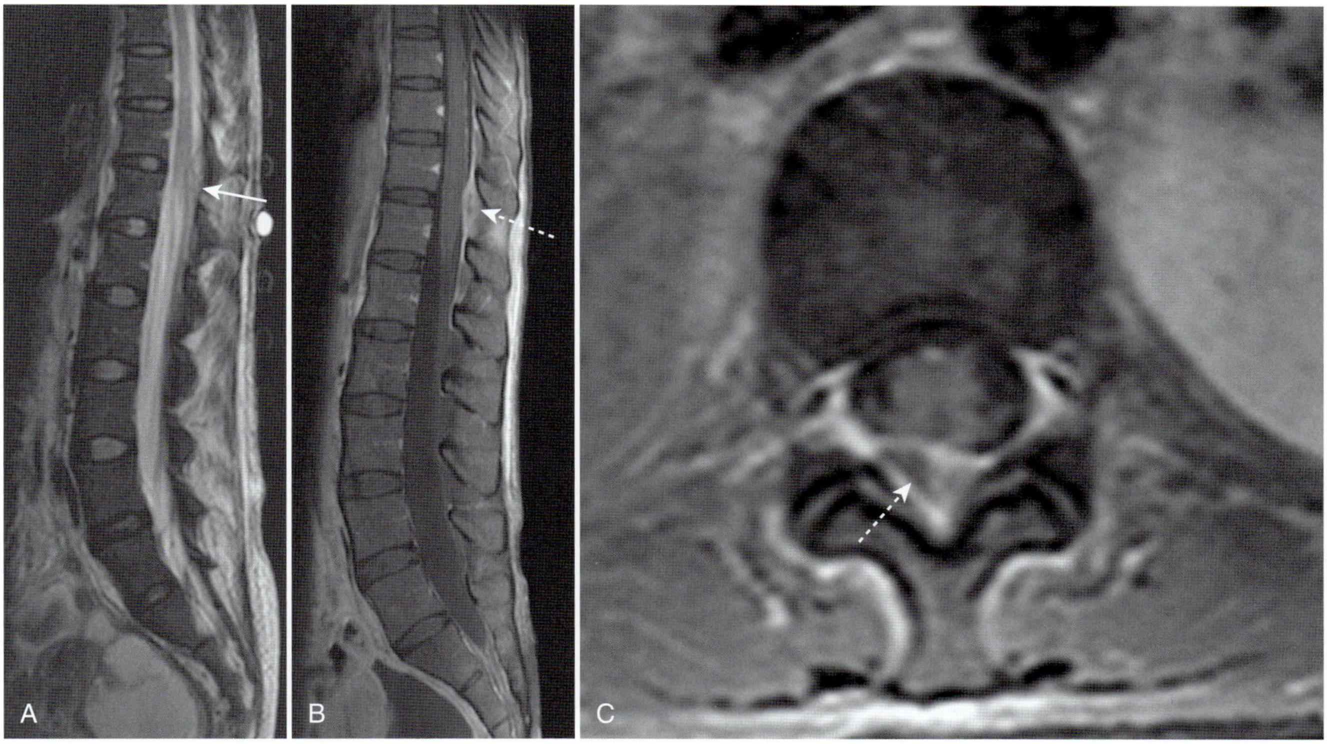

Figure 60.2 Sagittal T2W MR image (**A**) of a patient with sepsis after receiving an epidural anesthetic. There is a subtle epidural mass posterior to the cord (*white arrow*) at the level of the epidural puncture. The sagittal (**B**) and axial (**C**) post-contrast FST1W MR images show the mass as an area of low-SI, nonenhancing fluid with an enhancing peripheral rim (*broken arrow*). The appearances are consistent with a small epidural abscess. The symptoms responded to simple antibiotic therapy.

CHAPTER 61

Septic Facet Joint Arthritis

DEFINITION

- Facet joint infection due to a suppurative bacterial infection.

SIGNS AND SYMPTOMS

- Acute onset of localized back pain.
- Back pain may be quite focal or localized.
- Fever that may be fulminant or subtle.
- Night sweats.
- Pain may radiate in a dermatomal or nondermatomal pattern.
- Myelopathy may be present.
- Bowel and bladder symptomatology with spinal cord compression.

DEMOGRAPHICS

- Peak incidence in the fifth and sixth decades of life.
- Incidence: Male > Female.
- Increased incidence in patients with chronic diseases, such as diabetes, and in immunocompromised states (e.g., human immunodeficiency and cancer).
- Increased incidence in intravenous drug abusers.
- *Staphylococcus aureus* the most common pathogen.

IMAGING RECOMMENDATIONS

- MRI is primary investigation.
- US may be useful to detect superficial soft tissue fluid collections and guide diagnostic aspiration.
- CT may be helpful to assess extent of bony destruction.

IMAGING FINDINGS

- Prominent high-signal intensity (SI) effusions within facet joint on T2-weighted (T2W) MR images.
- Reactive marrow edema in adjacent facets on short T1 inversion recovery (STIR) images.
- Enhancement and thickening of synovium on post-contrast (obtained after administration of a contrast agent) MR images.
- Juxta-articular soft tissue inflammatory changes and abscess formation.
- Bony destruction.
- May eventually lead to ankylosis.

OTHER RECOMMENDED TESTING

- White blood cell count, erythrocyte sedimentation rate, and C-reactive protein determinations in all patients in whom osteomyelitis of the spine is suspected.
- Blood and urine cultures in all patients in whom osteomyelitis of the spine is suspected.
- Electromyography and nerve conduction velocity testing are indicated if radiculopathy present.
- Evoked potential testing if myelopathy present.

DIFFERENTIAL DIAGNOSIS

- Pathologic fracture due to tumor.
- Facet joint arthritis.
- Metastatic disease involving the facet joint.
- Facet joint synovial cyst.
- Rheumatoid arthritis.

TREATMENT

- Aggressive antibiotic therapy.
- Opioids for acute pain relief.
- Orthotic bracing.
- Emergency surgical decompression and drainage of abscess.

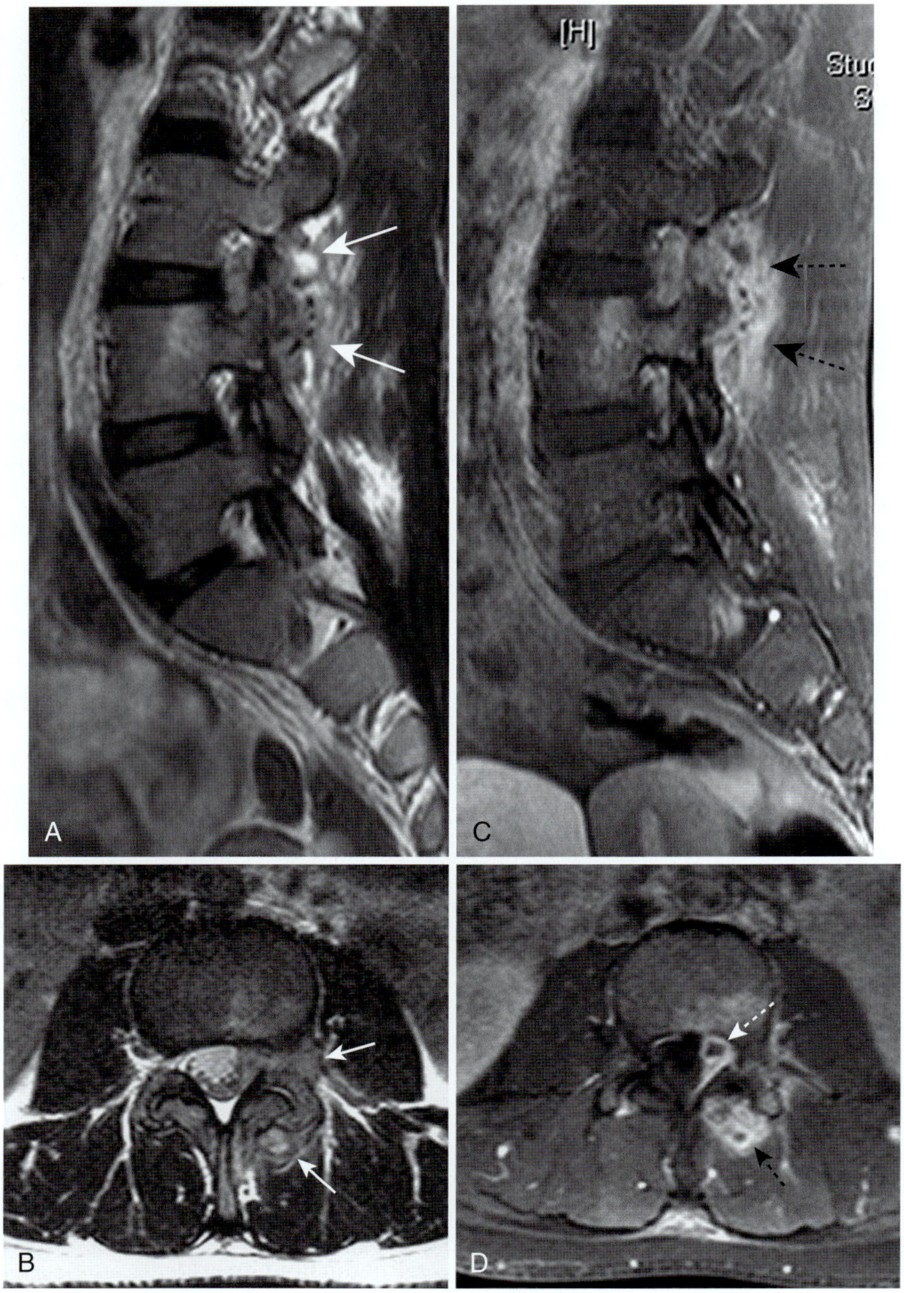

Figure 61.1 Sagittal (**A**) and axial (**B**) T2W MR images of a woman with low back pain, fever, and elevated CRP due to septic facet arthritis. There is bony destruction of the L3-L4 facet joint with posterior inflammatory tissue and small pockets of high-SI fluid collections (*black arrows*). There is also inflammatory tissue within the exit foramen (*white arrow*). The post-contrast sagittal (**C**) and axial (**D**) T1W with fat suppression (FST1W) MR images show enhancing inflammatory tissue with pockets of nonenhancing, low-SI fluid (*broken black arrows*), and a small epidural abscess compressing the thecal sac (*broken white arrow*).

CHAPTER 62

Spontaneous Epidural Hematoma of the Lumbar Spine

DEFINITION

- Spontaneous hemorrhage into the epidural space without significant antecedent trauma or medical procedure involving the epidural space.

SIGNS AND SYMPTOMS

- Acute onset of back pain.
- Pain in radicular and nonradicular distributions.
- Rapidly progressive sensory, motor, and reflex changes progressing to myelopathy/cauda equina syndrome.
- Bowel and bladder symptomatology.
- If left untreated may progress to paraparesis, or occasionally may resolve without treatment.

DEMOGRAPHICS

- Bimodal age distribution, in childhood and between the fifth and sixth decades of life.
- Incidence:
  - Children: Male = Female.
  - Adults: Male > Female.
- Clinical outcome directly related to severity of symptoms and length of time to treatment.

IMAGING RECOMMENDATIONS

- MRI.
- CT:
  - Alternative if MRI contraindicated.
  - CT myelography may be contraindicated in patients taking anticoagulants.

IMAGING FINDINGS

- Lenticular mass compressing the thecal sac.
- Variable signal intensity (SI), depending on the age of the blood products within the hematoma.
- Enhancement of the periphery of the hematoma on images obtained after administration of contrast agent (post-contrast).
- No central enhancement.
- Myelopathy of spinal cord or conus.

OTHER RECOMMENDED TESTING

- Laboratory testing for occult coagulopathy.

DIFFERENTIAL DIAGNOSIS

- Epidural abscess.
- Epidural neoplasm.
- Herniated intervertebral disc.

TREATMENT

- Immediate correction of underlying coagulopathy if present.
- Urgent decompressive laminectomy.
- Systemic glucocorticoids to treat spinal cord edema.

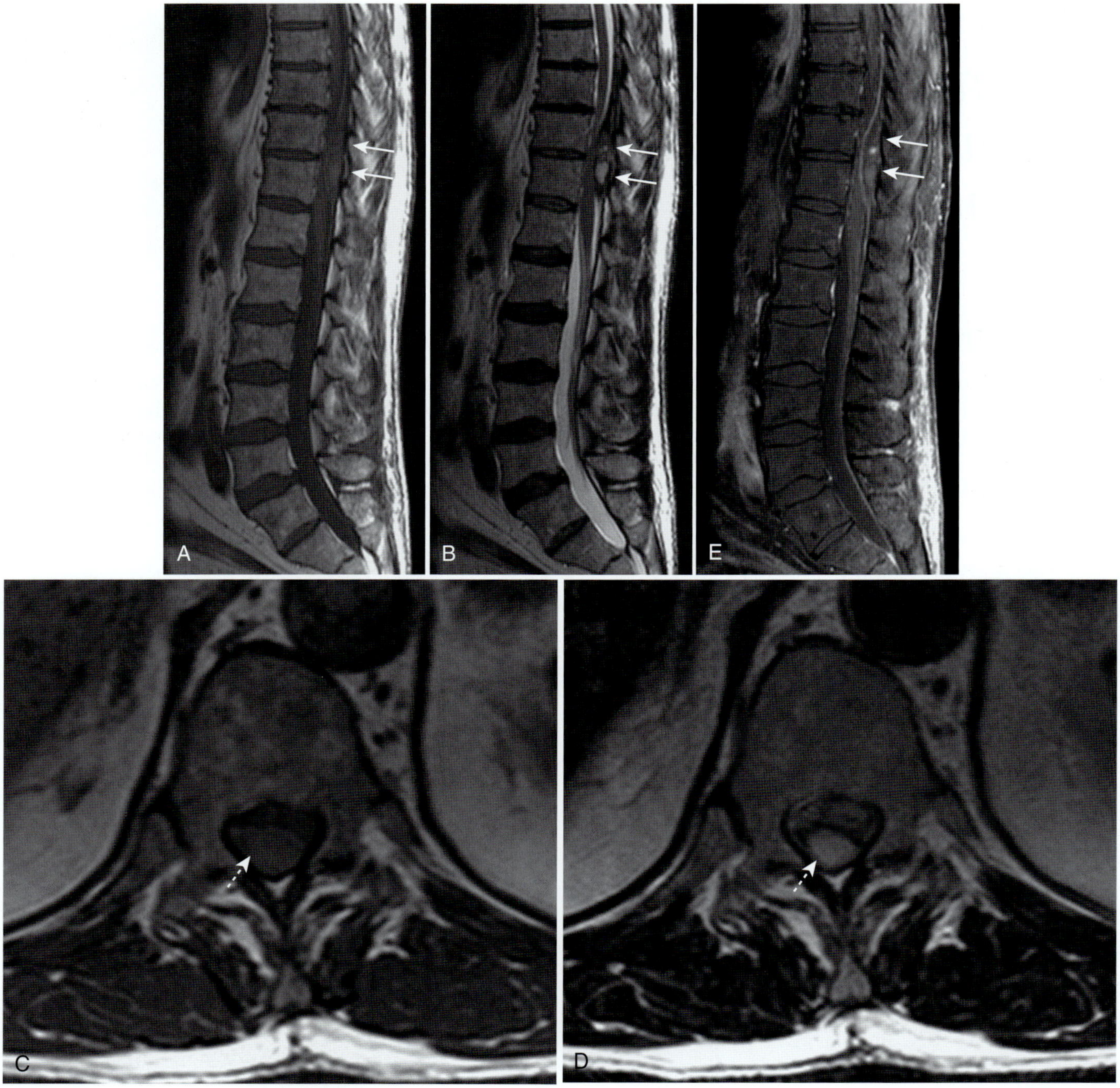

Figure 62.1 Sagittal T1-weighted (T1W) (**A**) and T2W (**B**) MR images in a patient undergoing warfarin therapy who presented with gradual onset of leg weakness. There is a lenticular mass within the posterior aspect of the spinal canal at the T10-T12 levels (*white arrows*). The mass has a low-SI periphery on the T2W MR image, with areas of variable high SI centrally that also show some moderately increased SI on the T1W MR image. These appearances are consistent with a subacute epidural hematoma with blood products of varying ages. The axial T1W (**C**) and T2W (**D**) MR images show the same signal characteristics within the hematoma (*broken white arrows*), and the spinal cord is compressed anteriorly. Early increased SI within the cord due to early myelomalacia is visible on the T2W MR image. (**E**) The sagittal post-contrast T1W with fat suppression (FST1W) MR image shows minor peripheral enhancement, but no central enhancement (*white arrows*).

CHAPTER 63

Subdural Hematoma

DEFINITION

- Hemorrhage into the space between the dura and arachnoid, often following a lumbar puncture or epidural block, or occurring spontaneously in patients with coagulopathy.

SIGNS AND SYMPTOMS

- Acute onset of back pain.
- Pain in radicular and nonradicular distributions.
- Rapidly progressive sensory, motor, and reflex changes progressing to myelopathy/cauda equine syndrome.
- Bowel and bladder symptomatology.
- If left untreated may progress to paraparesis, or occasionally may resolve without treatment.

DEMOGRAPHICS

- All ages.
- Incidence: Male = Female.
- Clinical outcome directly related to severity of symptoms and length of time to treatment.

IMAGING RECOMMENDATIONS

- MRI.

IMAGING FINDINGS

- Fluid confined within the subdural space and compressing the thecal sac.
- Hemorrhage may be of varying signal intensity (SI), depending on the age of the hematoma.
  - Typically high SI on T2-weighted (T2W) MR images.
  - Intermediate or high SI on T1W MR images.

OTHER RECOMMENDED TESTING

- Laboratory testing for occult coagulopathy.

DIFFERENTIAL DIAGNOSIS

- Subdural abscess.
- Epidural hematoma.
- Epidural abscess.
- Epidural neoplasm.
- Cerebrospinal fluid (CSF) leakage syndrome.
- Spinal meningitis.

TREATMENT

- Immediate correction of underlying coagulopathy if present.
- Urgent decompressive laminectomy.
- Systemic glucocorticoids to treat spinal cord edema.

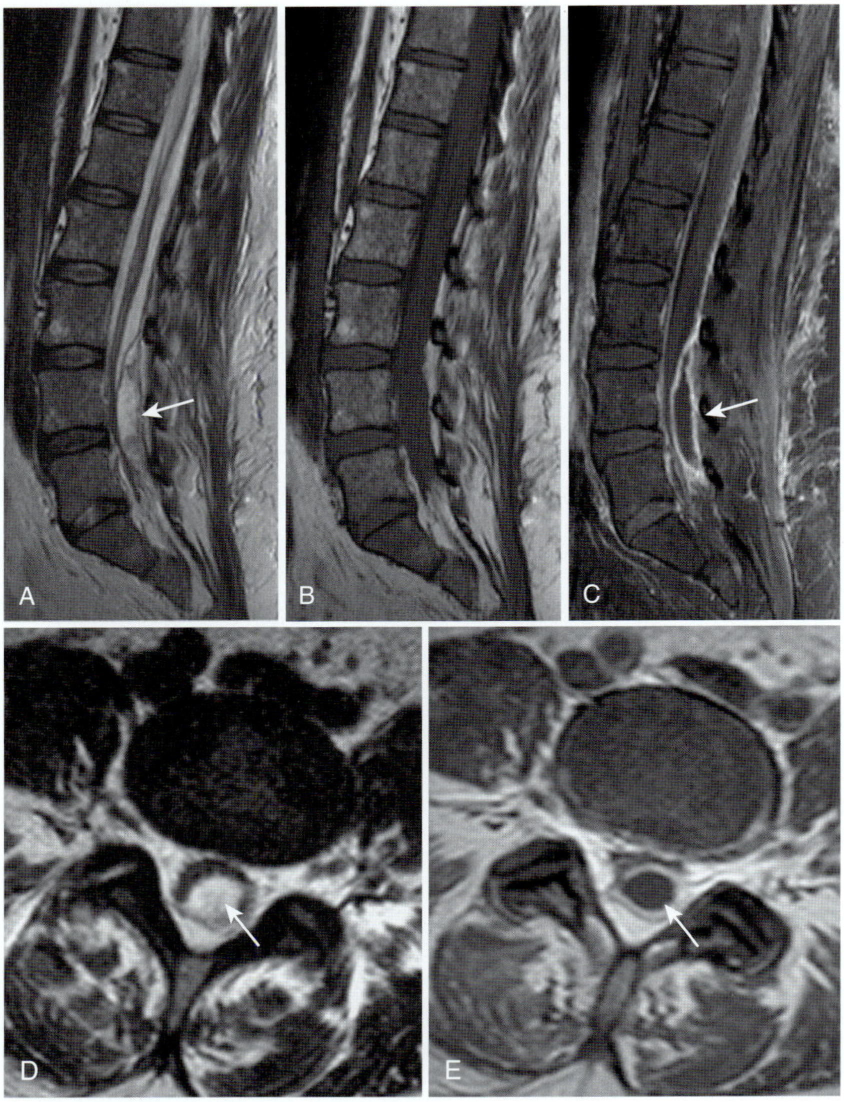

Figure 63.1 A middle-aged patient undergoing diskectomy at L5-S1 experienced injury to the thecal sac during surgery, followed by onset of cauda equina symptoms over the following 48 hours. (**A**), The sagittal T2W MR image shows a lenticular, heterogeneous, high-SI hematoma extending from L3 to S1 and confined to the subdural space (*white arrow*). (**B**), The hematoma is largely isointense with CSF on the T1W MR image. (**C**), There is peripheral enhancement on the sagittal T1W with fat suppression (FST1W) post-contrast (obtained after administration of a contrast agent) image (*white arrow*). (**D**), The compression of the thecal sac by the hematoma is best visualized on the axial T2W MR image (*black arrow*).

CHAPTER 64

Conjoined Nerve Roots

DEFINITION

- An anomalous enlarged nerve root sleeve containing two nerve roots.

SIGNS AND SYMPTOMS

- Usually an asymptomatic finding on spine imaging or at the time of spine surgery.
- Level of conjoined nerve root determines the clinical presentation.
- Lumbar radicular pain the most common symptom.
- Motor, sensory, and reflex changes may occur.

DEMOGRAPHICS

- Present in 1% to 2% of patients.
- Incidence higher in patients with congenital spinal stenosis.
- Incidence: Male = Female.
- No ethnic or racial predilection.

IMAGING RECOMMENDATIONS

- Imaging not routinely recommended.
- MRI to identify other causes of radicular pain.

IMAGING FINDINGS

- Axial T1-weighted (T1W) and T2W MR images:
  - Fusion of ipsilateral nerve roots of adjacent levels.
  - Asymmetry of nerve roots within lateral recesses.
  - Apparent thickening of involved nerve roots.
- Sagittal MR image findings are often normal.

OTHER RECOMMENDED TESTING

- Electromyography and nerve conduction velocity testing are indicated if radiculopathy present.
- Provocative discography may serve as a useful diagnostic tool to determine whether a specific disk is serving as a nidus for the pain and to identify the presence of conjoined nerve roots in a confusing diagnosis.

DIFFERENTIAL DIAGNOSIS

- Osteophyte of vertebral end plate.
- Nerve root sleeve cyst or diverticulum.
- Facet osteophyte.
- Neoplasm.
- Schwannoma.

TREATMENT

- Conservative treatment consisting of local heat, cold, simple analgesics, and nonsteroidal anti-inflammatory agents will improve symptoms in many cases.
- Physical therapy, including gentle stretching, range-of-motion exercises, deep heat modalities, and stretch and spray, may be beneficial in selected patients.
- Epidural blocks will provide symptomatic relief if conservative therapy fails or the pain is limiting activities of daily living.
- Selective nerve root blocks may provide symptomatic relieve if conservative therapy fails or the pain is limiting activities of daily living.
- Osteopathic or chiropractic manipulation may provide symptomatic relief in selected patients.
- Surgery may be required for persistent pain or progressive neurologic symptoms.

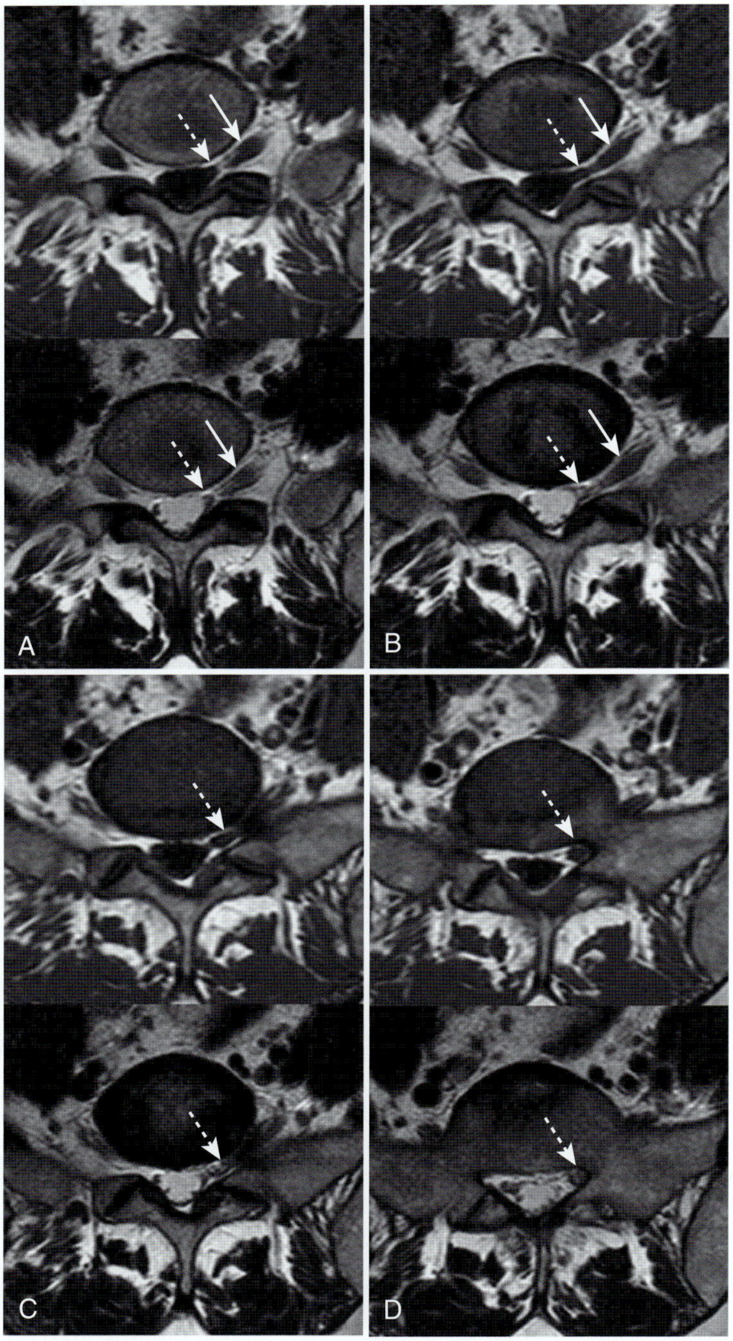

Figure 64.1 (A to D), Consecutive axial T1W and T2W MR images. The left L5 (*white arrows*) and left S1 (*broken white arrows*) nerve roots are conjoined. They lie much closer together in the lateral recess and exit canal than the L5 and S1 nerve roots on the right. The exit canal is a little narrowed on the left side, a feature that is far more likely to the source of root symptoms than the conjoined roots.

CHAPTER 65

Ventriculus Terminalis

DEFINITION

- Small cystic dilatation of the terminal spinal cord located between the tip of the conus medullaris and the origin of the filum terminale.

SIGNS AND SYMPTOMS

- Usually asymptomatic.
- Back pain with radicular and nonradicular radiation of pain occasionally present.
- Rarely, lower extremity numbness, weakness, and reflex changes progressing to spastic paresis.
- Loss of proprioception and vibratory sensation.
- Ataxic, spastic gait.
- Hyperreflexia.
- Pathologic reflexes (e.g., Babinski reflex) present.
- Bowel and bladder symptomatology.
- More sudden onset of symptoms following trauma to the distal spinal cord.

DEMOGRAPHICS

- Identified in all age groups, but more common in children.
- Incidence: Male = Female.

IMAGING RECOMMENDATIONS

- MRI.

IMAGING FINDINGS

- Focal cystic lesion in conus medullaris or filum terminale:
  - Low signal intensity (SI) on T1-weighted (T1W) MR images.
  - High SI on T2W MR images (equivalent to cerebrospinal fluid [CSF]).
- No enhancement on imaging performed after administration of a contrast agent (post-contrast imaging).
- May be associated with a tethered cord.

OTHER RECOMMENDED TESTING

- Electromyography and nerve conduction velocity testing is indicated if radiculopathy is present and to rule out amyotrophic lateral sclerosis.
- Evoked potential testing is indicated to quantify spinal cord compromise.

DIFFERENTIAL DIAGNOSIS

- Normal transient dilatation of the distal spinal cord of the newborn.
- Neoplasm of the lumbar spinal cord.
- Syrinx.
- Myelomalacia.

TREATMENT

- Avoid:
  - Activities that increase risk of lumbar spine trauma, such as contact sports.
  - Extreme lumbar spine positioning during anesthesia.
  - Therapeutic manipulation of the lumbar spine.
- Conservative treatment consisting of local heat, cold, simple analgesics, and nonsteroidal anti-inflammatory agents will improve symptoms in many cases.
- Caudal epidural blocks will provide symptomatic relief if conservative therapy fails or the pain is limiting activities of daily living.
- Surgical treatment is indicated if neurologic symptoms progress.

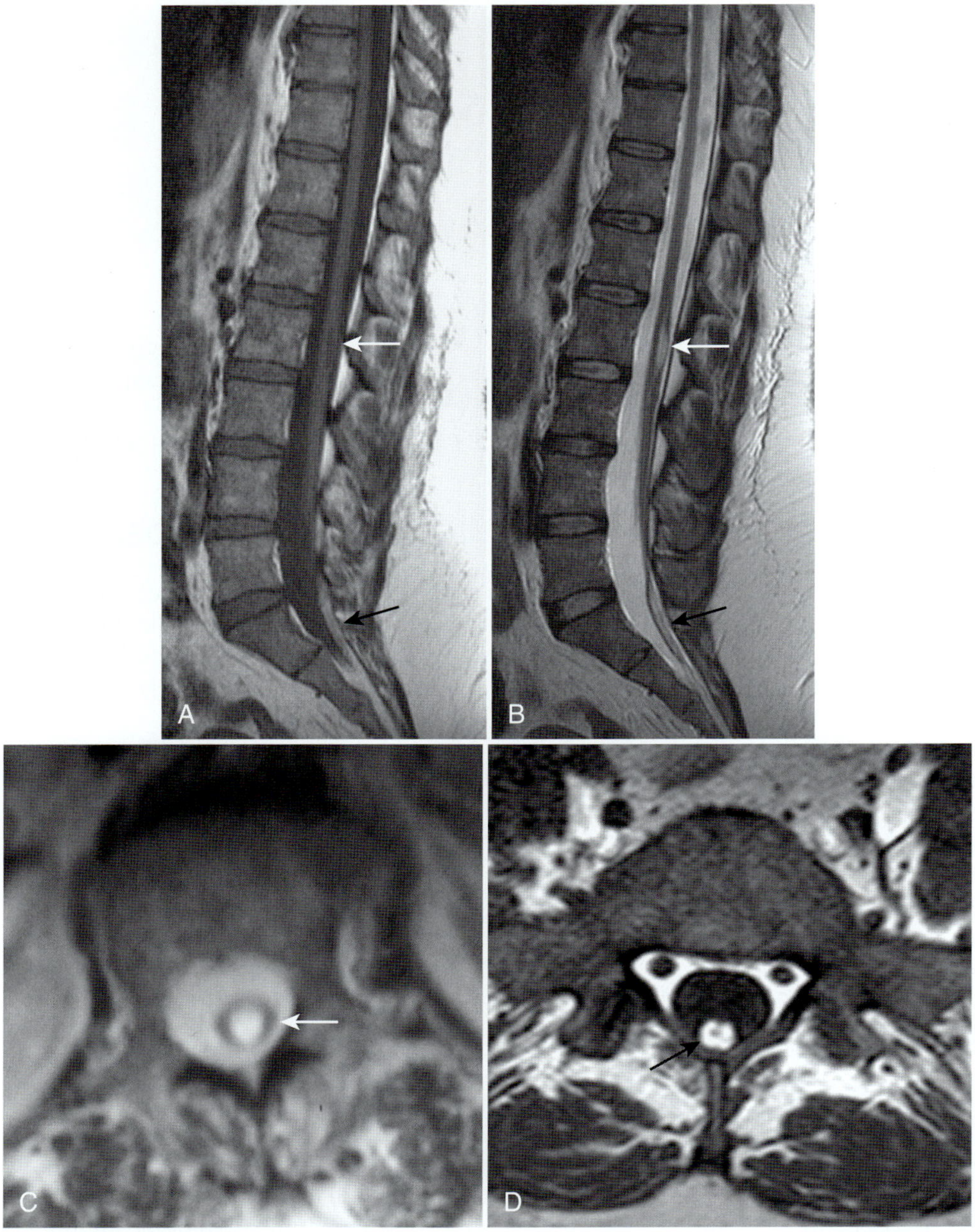

Figure 65.1 (**A**), Sagittal T1W MR image in a patient with a low-lying tethered cord and thickened filum terminale. There is a focal area of low SI within the cord at the L2 level (*white arrow*), which has high SI on the sagittal T2W MR image (**B**). (**C**), The axial T2W MR image also shows the high SI of the focal cystic lesion. No enhancement was evident on post-contrast imaging. In addition there is a small focal lipoma within the distal filum terminale at the L5-S1 level (*black arrows*), which appears as an area of high SI on both T1W and T2W MR images but which is best appreciated on the axial T1W MR image (**D**), on which it contrasts with the low SI of the CSF within the thecal sac.

CHAPTER 66

Complications of Myelography

DEFINITION

- Unexpected complications after myelography, including post–dural puncture headache, injury to neural structures, seizures, arachnoiditis, placement of contrast medium into the wrong area, reactions to contrast medium, and iatrogenic epidermoid tumor.

SIGNS AND SYMPTOMS

- Postural post–dural puncture headache, the most common complication of myelography, is characterized by postural headache, nausea, vomiting, tinnitus, cranial nerve palsies, and dizziness.
- Postural post–dural puncture headache is often associated with cranial nerve palsies, especially involving cranial nerve VI.
- The signs and symptoms of needle injury to neural structures are clinical reflections of the structure injured and the extent of injury—for example, a simple needle-stick or intraneural injection of contrast medium.
- The incidence of seizures is increased by dehydration and inadvertent placement of contrast medium into the ventricles.
- Incorrect placement of contrast medium in the subdural and/or epidural space is usually asymptomatic.
- Arachnoiditis manifests as radiculopathy and/or myelopathy.
- Reactions to contrast medium, although less common with non-ionic contrast agents, do occur; they range from life-threatening anaphylactic reactions to hives and pruritus.
- Iatrogenic epidermoid tumor is caused by the inadvertent placement of skin cells into the subarachnoid space and manifests clinically as radiculopathy and/or myelopathy, depending on which neural structures are compromised by the growing tumor.

DEMOGRAPHICS

- Incidence of post–dural puncture headache is related to the size and type of spinal needle used, with an incidence of approximately 5% if a small (25-gauge), atraumatic needle tip is used.
- Incidence of post–dural puncture headache decreases with patient age.
- Incidence of post–dural puncture headache is higher in females.
- Arachnoiditis, although rare, occurs more frequently in dehydrated patients.

IMAGING RECOMMENDATIONS

- MRI.
- CT if MRI is contraindicated:
  - NB myelography is most often used in patients in whom MRI is contraindicated.
  - Non-contrast CT may be limited in its demonstration of intrathecal abnormalities, and repeat myelography is unlikely to be recommended.

IMAGING FINDINGS

- Epidural hematoma:
  - Fluid-filled collection in the epidural space.
  - MRI signal characteristics vary according to age of the hematoma.
- Arachnoiditis:
  - Clumping of nerve roots within the thecal sac at affected level.
- Iatrogenic epidermoid:
  - Intradural mass.
  - High signal intensity (SI) on T2-weighted (T2W) MR images.
  - Intermediate SI on T1W MR images.
  - Minimal or no enhancement on imaging obtained after administration of a contrast agent.

OTHER RECOMMENDED TESTING

- Electromyography and nerve conduction velocity testing are indicated if trauma to a nerve root is suspected.
- Evoked potential testing to quantify spinal cord compromise if cord damage is suspected.

DIFFERENTIAL DIAGNOSIS

- Intracranial hypotension.
- Meningitis.
- Cerebrospinal fluid (CSF) leak unrelated to myelogram.
- Malingering.

TREATMENT

- Treat allergic reactions to contrast medium aggressively with fluids, diphenhydramine, steroids, and oxygen.
- Epidural blood patching should be performed to treat post–dural puncture headache if symptoms do not abate with 24 hours of conservative treatment.
- Surgical excision of epidermoid tumor if patient is symptomatic.

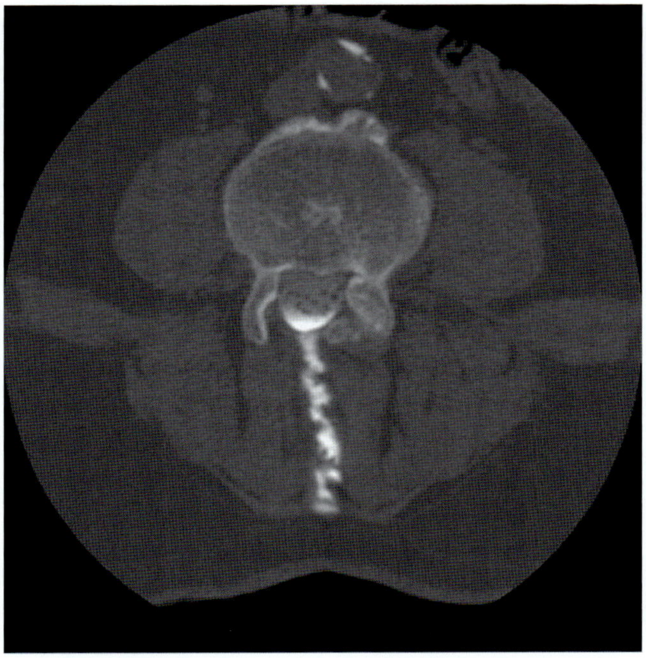

Figure 66.1 Axial CT scan acquired after removal of the spinal needle from a patient who underwent lumbar puncture for a myelogram. There was dramatic and immediate leak of CSF, and the CT scan shows the high-density contrast medium leaking posteriorly within the paraspinal soft tissues. The patient experienced a severe low-pressure headache and was observed for 24 hours. The CSF leak resolved spontaneously.

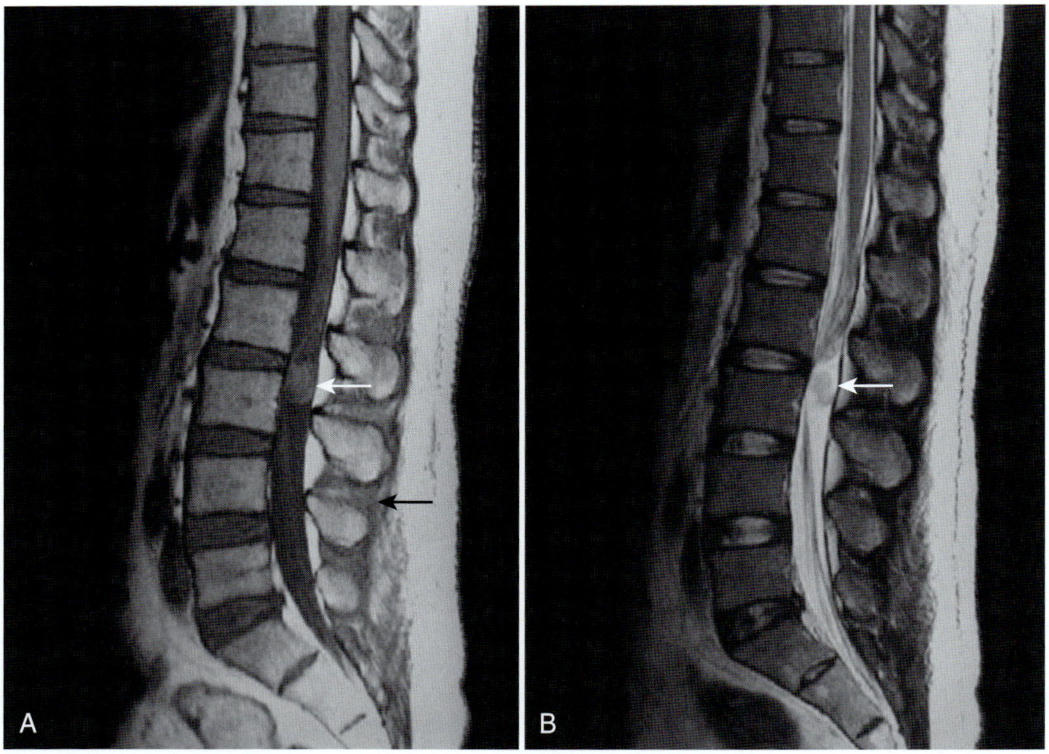

Figure 66.2 (**A**), Sagittal T1W MR image of a patient with onset of bilateral buttock and calf pain 5 years after repeated lumbar punctures. There is an intermediate-SI intradural mass (*white arrow*), which has high SI on the sagittal T2W MR image (**B**) (*white arrow*). The mass was removed, and an iatrogenic epidermoid tumor was confirmed. *(From Park JC, Chung CK, Kim HJ: Iatrogenic spinal epidermoid tumor: A complication of spinal puncture in an adult. Clin Neurol Neurosurg 2003;105:281-285.)*

CHAPTER 67

Epidural Fibrosis

DEFINITION

- Fibrosis and scarring surrounding the thecal sac and exiting nerve roots at the site of previous spine surgery.

SIGNS AND SYMPTOMS

- Usually asymptomatic.
- Onset of symptoms is insidious after what appears to be successful spine surgery.
- Gradual and subtle onset of lumbar radiculopathy and/or myelopathy.
- Back pain with radicular and nonradicular radiation of pain.
- Lower extremity numbness, weakness, and reflex changes progressing to spastic paresis.
- Loss of proprioception and vibratory sensation.
- Ataxic, spastic gait.
- Hyperreflexia.
- Pathologic reflexes (e.g., Babinski reflex) present.
- Bowel and bladder symptomatology.
- More sudden onset of symptoms following trauma to the lumbar spine.

DEMOGRAPHICS

- Adults who undergo spine surgery.
- Incidence: Male = Female.

IMAGING RECOMMENDATIONS

- MRI is the primary investigation;
  - Post-contrast (obtained after administration of a contrast agent) images may be required.
- Post-contrast CT or CT myelography if MRI is contraindicated.

IMAGING FINDINGS

- MR images obtained in first 6 months after an operation may appear very similar to preoperative images.
- Post-contrast images may be required to distinguish granulation tissue from disk material.
- Features that favor epidural fibrosis:
  - Intermediate or low signal intensity (SI) on T2-weighted (T2W) and T1W MR images.
  - No continuity with disk space.
  - Diffuse enhancement on post-contrast images.
  - In later stages, contraction and distortion of the thecal sac and nerve roots toward the area of fibrosis.
- Over 6 to 12 months, the granulation tissue usually shrinks down and the epidural fat planes return to normal.
  - Distinction between recurrent disk and postoperative fibrosis is easier in the later stages.

OTHER RECOMMENDED TESTING

- Electromyography and nerve conduction velocity testing are indicated if radiculopathy is present.
- Evoked potential testing to quantify spinal cord compromise.

DIFFERENTIAL DIAGNOSIS

- Arachnoiditis.
- Epidural abscess.
- Subacute epidural hematoma.
- Neoplasm of the lumbar spinal cord and/or surrounding structures.
- Meningioma.
- Recurrent disk herniation.
- Pseudomeningocele.

TREATMENT

- Avoid:
  - Activities that increase the risk of lumbar spine trauma, such as contact sports.
  - Extreme lumbar spine positioning during anesthesia.
  - Therapeutic manipulation of the lumbar spine.
- Modify activity to avoid overuse of lumbar spine.
- Conservative treatment consisting of local heat, cold, simple analgesics, and nonsteroidal anti-inflammatory agents will improve symptoms in many cases.
- Physical therapy, including gentle stretching and gentle range-of-motion exercises.
- Epidural blocks will provide symptomatic relief if conservative therapy fails or the pain is limiting activities of daily living.
- Lysis of epidural adhesions (Racz procedure).
- Spinal cord stimulation.
- Surgical treatment indicated if neurologic symptoms progress.

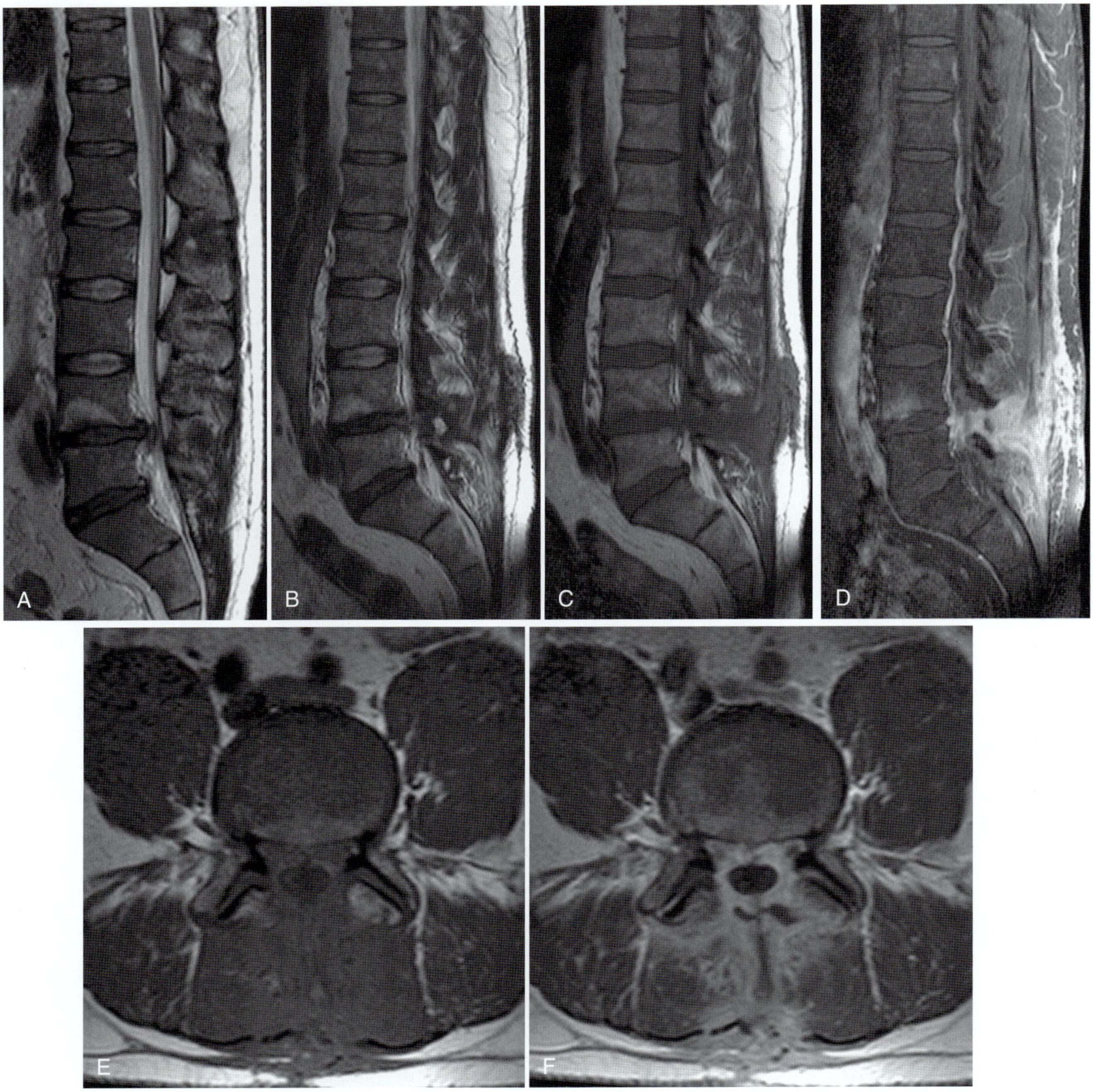

Figure 67.1 (**A**), Sagittal T2W MR image of a preoperative disk herniation at the L4-L5 level. The postoperative T2W (**B**) and T1W (**C**) MR images show no evidence of recurrent disk herniation. There is prominent postoperative low SI in the posterior structures on the T1W MR image. (**D**), The post-contrast T1W with fat suppression (FST1W) MR image demonstrates a large amount of enhancing high-SI granulation tissue in the spinal canal and the posterior soft tissues. (**E**), The axial T1W MR image demonstrates extensive low-SI granulation tissue circumferentially around the thecal sac, which enhances uniformly with high SI on the post-contrast T1W MR image (**F**). The posterior decompression is also clearly visible.

CHAPTER 68

Arachnoiditis

DEFINITION

- Inflammation of all three layers of the meninges as well as the nerve roots after myelography, spinal anesthesia, spine surgery, or infection involving these structures, that results in adhesive scarring, cerebrospinal fluid (CSF) loculation, and clumping of the nerve roots.

SIGNS AND SYMPTOMS

- Onset of symptoms is insidious following what appears to be successful myelogram, spinal anesthesia, spine surgery, or after meningeal infection.
- Gradual and subtle onset of lumbar radiculopathy and/or myelopathy.
- Back pain with radicular and nonradicular radiation of pain.
- Lower extremity numbness, weakness, and reflex changes progressing to spastic paresis.
- Loss of proprioception and vibratory sensation.
- Ataxic, spastic gait.
- Hyperreflexia.
- Pathologic reflexes (e.g., Babinski reflex) present.
- Bowel and bladder symptomatology.
- More sudden onset of symptoms following trauma to the lumbar spine.

DEMOGRAPHICS

- In adults after myelography, spinal anesthesia, spine surgery, or infection involving meninges and/or nerve roots.
- Incidence: Male = Female.
- No racial predilection.
- More common following the use of oil-based myelographic contrast medium.

IMAGING RECOMMENDATIONS

- MRI is the primary investigation.
- CT myelography is an alternative if MRI is contraindicated.

IMAGING FINDINGS

- Clumping of nerve roots within the thecal sac on axial T2-weighted (T2W) MR images.
- Adherence of the nerve roots to the dura within the thecal sac.
- In older patients, the oil-based contrast agent Myodil (no longer in use) may be seen on radiographs and as high signal intensity (SI) on T1W and T2W MR images.

OTHER RECOMMENDED TESTING

- Electromyography and nerve conduction velocity testing are indicated if radiculopathy is present.
- Evoked potential testing is used to quantify spinal cord compromise.

DIFFERENTIAL DIAGNOSIS

- Epidural fibrosis.
- Epidural abscess.
- Subacute epidural hematoma.
- Spinal stenosis.
- Neoplasm of the lumbar spinal cord, cauda equina, and/or surrounding structures.
- Meningioma.
- Carcinomatous meningitis.

TREATMENT

- Avoid:
  - Activities that increase risk of lumbar spine trauma, such as contact sports.
  - Extreme lumbar spine positioning during anesthesia.
  - Therapeutic manipulation of the lumbar spine.
- Modify activity to avoid overuse of the lumbar spine.
- Physical therapy, including gentle stretching and gentle range-of-motion exercises.
- Epidural blocks will provide symptomatic relief if conservative therapy fails or the pain is limiting activities of daily living.
- Intrathecal administration of steroids.
- Lysis of epidural adhesions (Racz procedure).
- Spinal cord stimulation.
- Surgical treatment is indicated if neurologic symptoms progress.

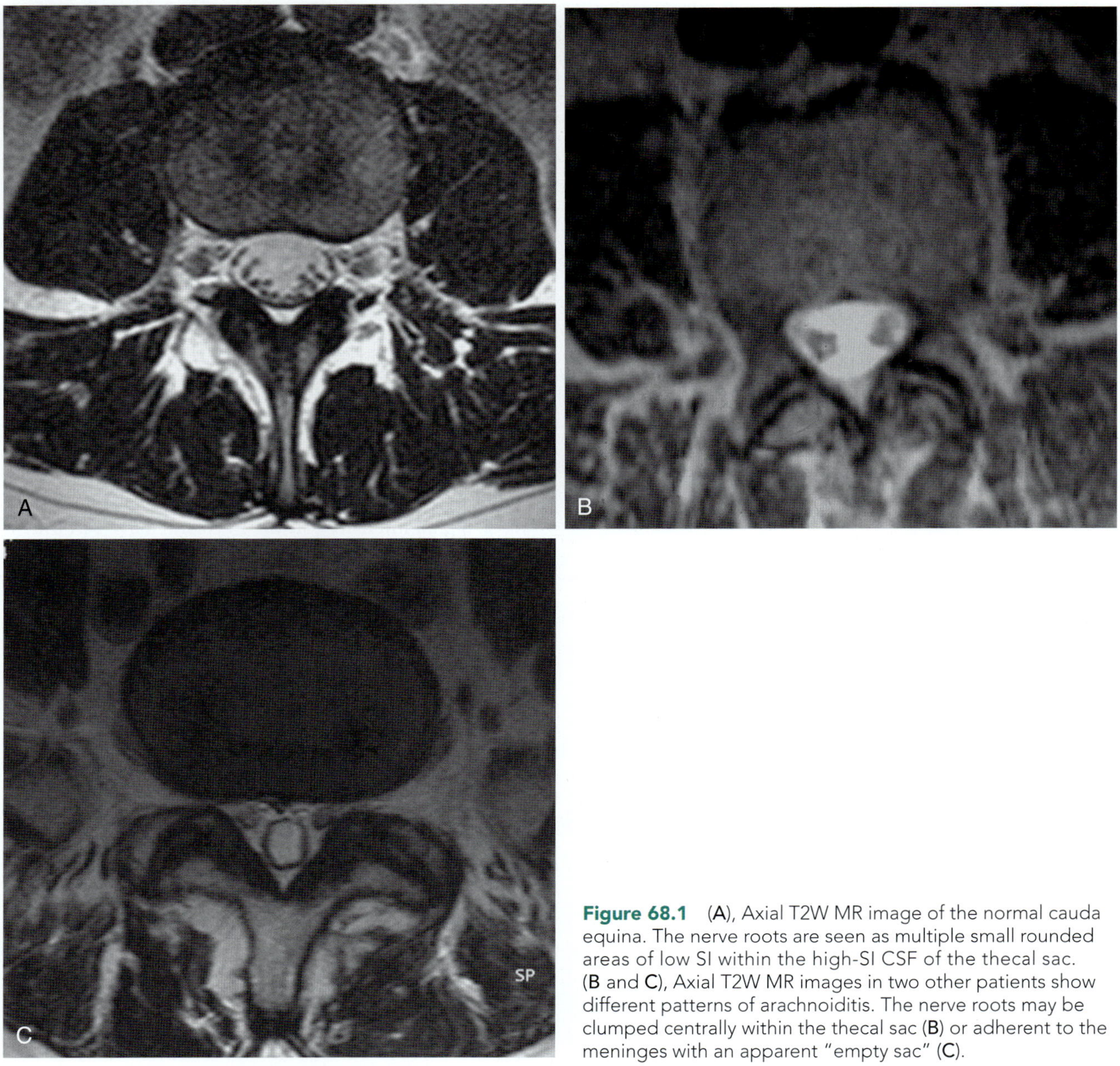

Figure 68.1 (A), Axial T2W MR image of the normal cauda equina. The nerve roots are seen as multiple small rounded areas of low SI within the high-SI CSF of the thecal sac. (B and C), Axial T2W MR images in two other patients show different patterns of arachnoiditis. The nerve roots may be clumped centrally within the thecal sac (B) or adherent to the meninges with an apparent "empty sac" (C).

CHAPTER 69

Postoperative Infections

DEFINITION

- Infection of the vertebral body and/or intervertebral disc and surrounding structures following spine surgery, most often due to a suppurative bacterial infection.

SIGNS AND SYMPTOMS

- Acute onset of localized back pain.
- Back pain may be quite focal or localized.
- Vertebral collapse with acute pain is not an uncommon sequela of infection.
- Fever that may be fulminant or subtle.
- Night sweats.
- Pain may radiate in a dermatomal or nondermatomal pattern.
- Myelopathy may be present.
- Bowel and bladder symptomatology with spinal cord compression.

DEMOGRAPHICS

- Bimodal distribution, occurring most commonly in children after scoliosis surgery and in elderly patients.
- Incidence: Male > Female.
- Increased incidence in patients with chronic diseases, such as diabetes and with immunocompromised states (e.g., human immunodeficiency virus and cancer).
- Increased incidence in intravenous drug abusers.
- *Staphylococcus aureus* is the most common pathogen.
- *Escherichia coli* is the most common gram-negative pathogen.
- *Salmonella* is the most common pathogen in patients with sickle cell disease.
- Recurrent disease is not uncommon, especially in immunocompromised patients.

IMAGING RECOMMENDATIONS

- MRI is primary investigation.
- CT may be useful:
  - With prominent MRI susceptibility artifact from orthopaedic metalwork.
  - To guide drainage procedure for deeper fluid collections if required.
- Ultrasound detects superficial soft tissue fluid collections and aids guided diagnostic aspiration and drainage procedures.

IMAGING FINDINGS

- Disc space infection:
  - High signal intensity (SI) on T2-weighted (T2W) MR images and with vertebral end-plate (VEP) erosion.
- Vertebral osteomyelitis:
  - Areas of low SI on T1W MR images and high SI on T2W or short T1 inversion recovery (STIR) MR images.
- High-SI soft tissue and epidural abscesses on T2W MR images.
- Reactive marrow edema and bony sclerosis around pedicle screws in low-grade infection.
  - Sclerosis of low-grade osteitis is well seen on CT.

OTHER RECOMMENDED TESTING

- White blood cell count, erythrocyte sedimentation rate, and serum C-reactive protein (CRP) determinations in all patients in whom postoperative infection is suspected
- Blood and urine cultures in all patients in whom postoperative infection is suspected.
- Electromyography and nerve conduction velocity testing is indicated if radiculopathy present.
- Evoked potential testing if myelopathy is present.

DIFFERENTIAL DIAGNOSIS

- Pathologic fracture due to tumor.
- Neoplasm.
- Recurrent disc herniation.
- Pott's disease.
- Degenerative VEP changes.
- Chronic hemodialysis spondyloarthropathy.
- Charcot disease of the spine.

TREATMENT

- Aggressive antibiotic therapy.
- Opioids for acute pain relief.
- Orthotic bracing.
- Emergency surgical decompression and drainage of abscess.

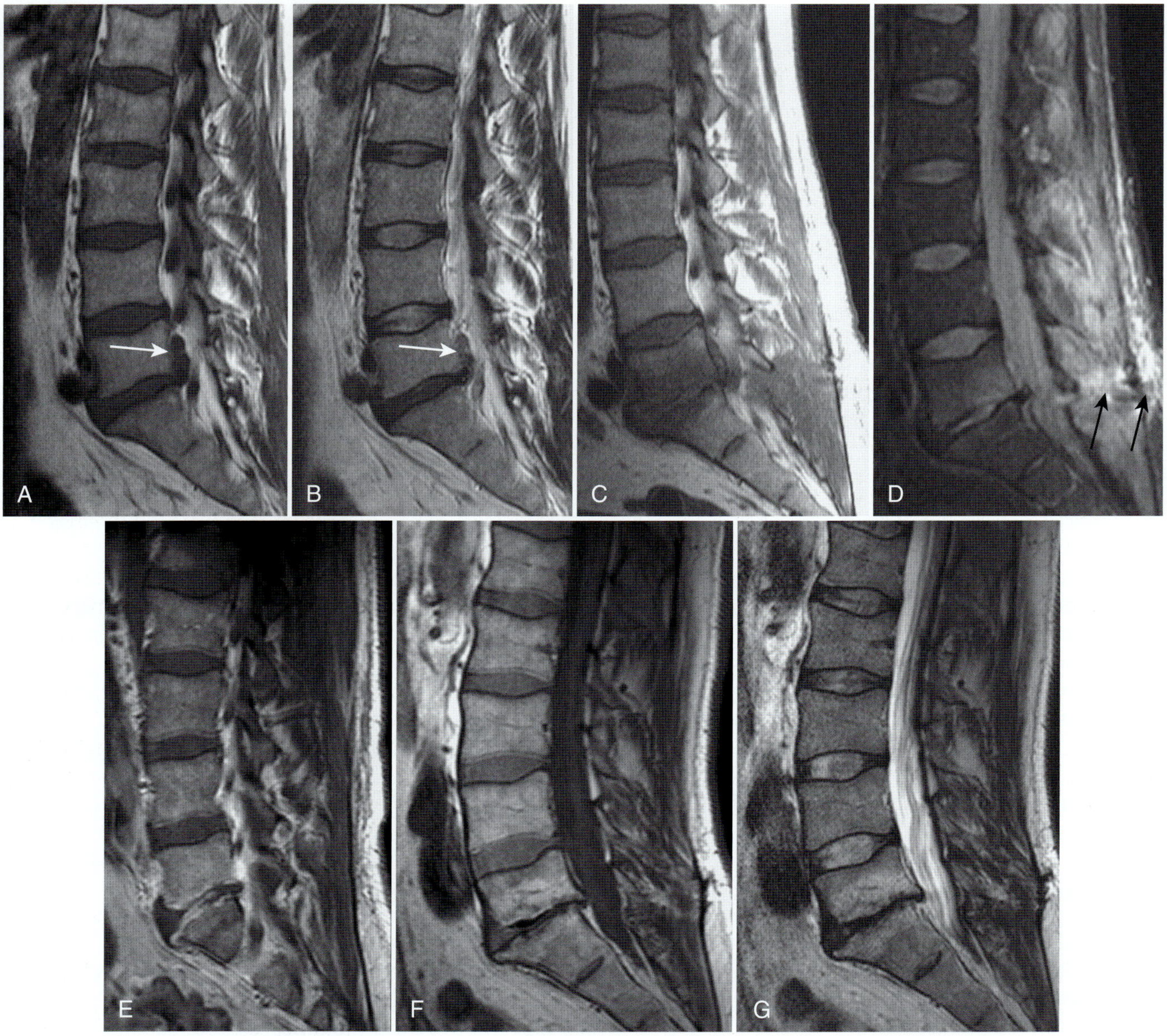

Figure 69.1 Preoperative sagittal T1W (**A**) and T2W (**B**) MR images demonstrating a degenerated L5-S1 disc with an associated disc protrusion (*white arrows*). After microdiscectomy, the patient experienced back pain and low-grade pyrexia, and an elevated CRP developed. (**C**), The sagittal T1W MR image obtained during repeat MRI demonstrates low-SI marrow edema in the L5 and S1 vertebral bodies and erosion of vertebral end plates. (**D**), On the corresponding sagittal STIR image, there is high-SI vertebral body edema and high SI within the disc, which has narrowed (compare with the preoperative image). The scar in the posterior soft tissues is clearly visible (*black arrows*). (**E**), This post-contrast sagittal T1W MR image shows high-SI enhancement within the disc and VEP. There was no paravertebral soft tissue mass or epidural abscess. The appearances are consistent with a low-grade discitis. The patient showed response to antibiotic treatment. Follow-up MRI performed a few months later shows satisfactory response. There is conversion of fatty end-plate change in the vertebral bodies, which has high SI on both the T1W (**F**) and T2W (**G**) MR images, and the disc is now low SI on the T2W MR image.

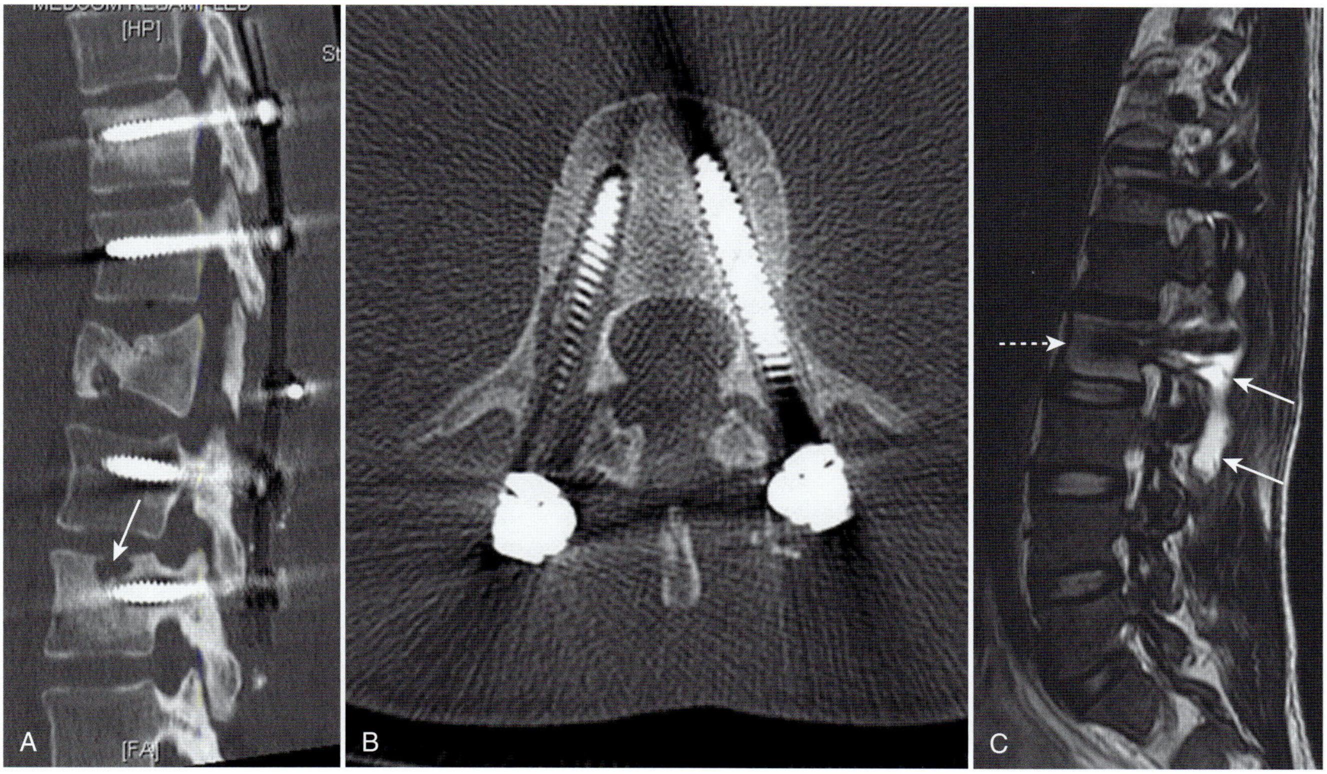

Figure 69.2 (**A** and **B**), CT scans of a patient who underwent spinal fixation for an L1 fracture complicated by a postoperative hematoma. There was a history of postoperative infected hematoma. The sagittal scan (**A**) shows sclerosis around the pedicle screws in T11 and L3 consistent with a low-grade osteitis. In addition, there is discovertebral erosion in the upper VEP of L3 due to early spread of infection into the disc space. The axial scan (**B**) demonstrates lucency around the right pedicle screw, which indicates loosening secondary to the infection. (**C**), A sagittal FST2W MR image in a different patient who underwent operative fixation demonstrates an infected high-SI fluid collection around the inferior pedicle screw (*white arrows*). In addition, there is high-SI edema in the L4 vertebral body (*broken arrow*), indicating associated infective osteitis.

CHAPTER 70

Pseudomeningocele

DEFINITION

- Cerebrospinal fluid (CSF)-containing cyst contiguous with the thecal sac that occurs following spine surgery.

SIGNS AND SYMPTOMS

- Usually asymptomatic.
- Onset of symptoms is insidious after what appears to be successful spine surgery.
- Gradual and subtle onset of lumbar radiculopathy and/or myelopathy.
- Back pain with radicular and nonradicular radiation of pain.
- Lower extremity numbness, weakness, and reflex changes progressing to spastic paresis are rare in absence of infection.
- Cyst can sometimes be palpated in the subcutaneous tissues beneath a surgical incision.

DEMOGRAPHICS

- Occurs in children or adults following spine surgery.
- Incidence: Male = Female.
- May resolve spontaneously.

IMAGING RECOMMENDATIONS

- MRI.
- CT or ultrasonography may demonstrate larger pseudomeningoceles.
- CT myelography is occasionally required to confirm communication with the CSF space.

IMAGING FINDINGS

- High-signal intensity (SI) fluid collection in soft tissues posterior to the spinal canal on T2-weighted (T2W) MR images.
- Communicates directly with the CSF space.
- Surrounding inflammatory changes are usually absent unless there is associated postoperative infection.
- Posterior bony defects following spinal decompression.

OTHER RECOMMENDED TESTING

- Electromyography and nerve conduction velocity testing are indicated if radiculopathy is present.
- Evoked potential testing is used to quantify spinal cord compromise.

DIFFERENTIAL DIAGNOSIS

- Arachnoiditis.
- Epidural abscess.
- Postoperative epidural hematoma.
- Neoplasm of the lumbar spinal cord and/or surrounding structures.
- Neurofibroma.
- Recurrent disc herniation.
- True meningocele.

TREATMENT

- Avoid:
  - Activities that increase risk of lumbar spine trauma, such as contact sports.
  - Extreme lumbar spine positioning during anesthesia.
  - Therapeutic manipulation of the lumbar spine.
- Modify activity to avoid overuse of the lumbar spine.
- Conservative treatment consisting of local heat, cold, simple analgesics, and nonsteroidal anti-inflammatory agents will improve symptoms in many cases.
- Physical therapy, including gentle stretching and gentle range-of-motion exercises.
- Epidural blocks will provide symptomatic relief if conservative therapy fails or the pain is limiting activities of daily living.
- Surgical treatment is indicated if neurologic symptoms progress.

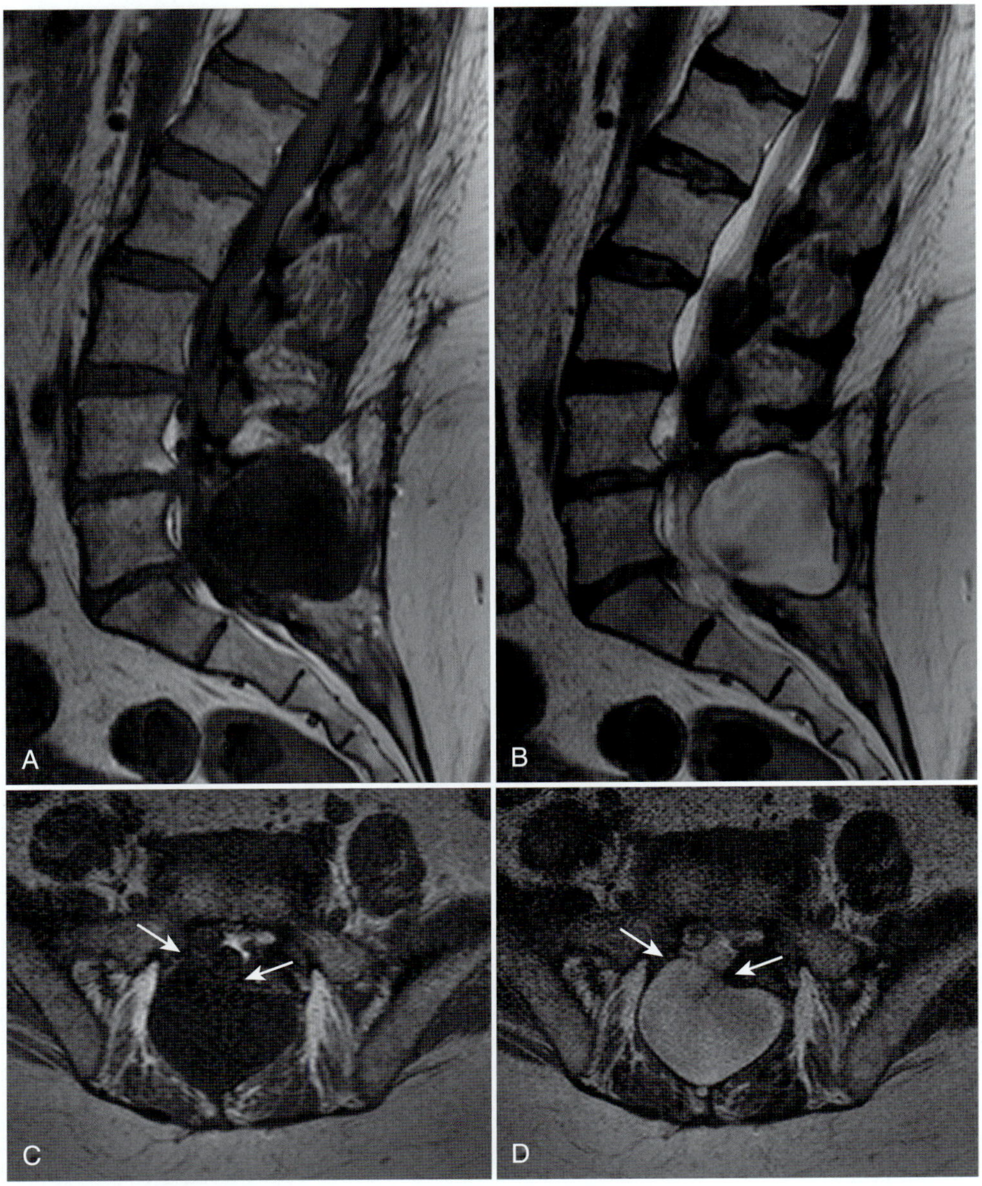

Figure 70.1 Sagittal T1W (**A**) and T2W (**B**) MR images of a patient with a pseudomeningocele that developed after a laminectomy for spinal stenosis. There is a large, rounded, fluid-filled mass posterior to the L5 vertebral level that is low-SI on the T1W MR image and high-SI on the T2W MR image. The axial T1W (**C**) and T2W (**D**) MR images also show the cysts and their relationship to the thecal sac via the laminectomy (*white arrows*).

CHAPTER 71

Accelerated Postoperative Degeneration of the Spine

DEFINITION

- Pathologic acceleration of the disc spaces and synovial lined zygapophyseal joints:
  - At levels adjacent to previous spinal fusion because of altered biomechanics at those levels.
  - After discectomy at the same level.

SIGNS AND SYMPTOMS

- May be asymptomatic.
- Onset may occur following seemingly minor trauma.
- Back pain made worse with movement of the lumbar spine.
- Worse after rest.
- Pain typically radiates into the low back and buttocks in a nondermatomal pattern.
- Pain can be made worse with axial loading combined with range of motion of the lumbar spine.

DEMOGRAPHICS

- Increased incidence with age.
- Incidence: Male = Female.
- Onset in months following spinal fusion.

IMAGING RECOMMENDATIONS

- MRI is the primary investigation:
  - Orthopaedic metalwork often does not obscure spine levels above the fusion.
- CT is alternative imaging modality if:
  - MR susceptibility artifact obscures relevant disc levels.
  - MRI is contraindicated.
- Radiography:
  - Flexion/extension views may be required to assess for instability.

IMAGING FINDINGS

- Progressive, rapid disc degeneration on serial MRI or radiographic examinations.
- Modic changes at vertebral end plate may be pronounced.
- Features of instability may be present with listhesis.
- Facet joint osteoarthritis and joint effusions.

OTHER RECOMMENDED TESTING

- Intra-articular facet injection to ascertain whether a specific facet joint is the nidus of the pain.
- Provocative discography to ascertain whether a specific disc is the nidus of the pain.

DIFFERENTIAL DIAGNOSIS

- Inflammatory arthritides, especially rheumatoid arthritis.
- Septic facet joint.
- Discitis.
- Healing facet joint fracture.
- Neoplasm.
- Spondylolysis with spondylolisthesis.
- Pseudarthrosis.

TREATMENT

- Conservative treatment consisting of local heat, cold, simple analgesics, and nonsteroidal anti-inflammatory agents will improve symptoms in many cases.
- Physical therapy, including gentle stretching, range-of-motion exercises deep heat modalities, and stretch and spray, may be beneficial in selected patients.
- Epidural and facet blocks with local anesthetic and steroid will provide symptomatic relief if conservative therapy fails or the pain is limiting activities of daily living.
- Orthotic bracing.
- Surgery including fusion of adjacent levels may be required for persistent pain or progressive neurologic symptoms.

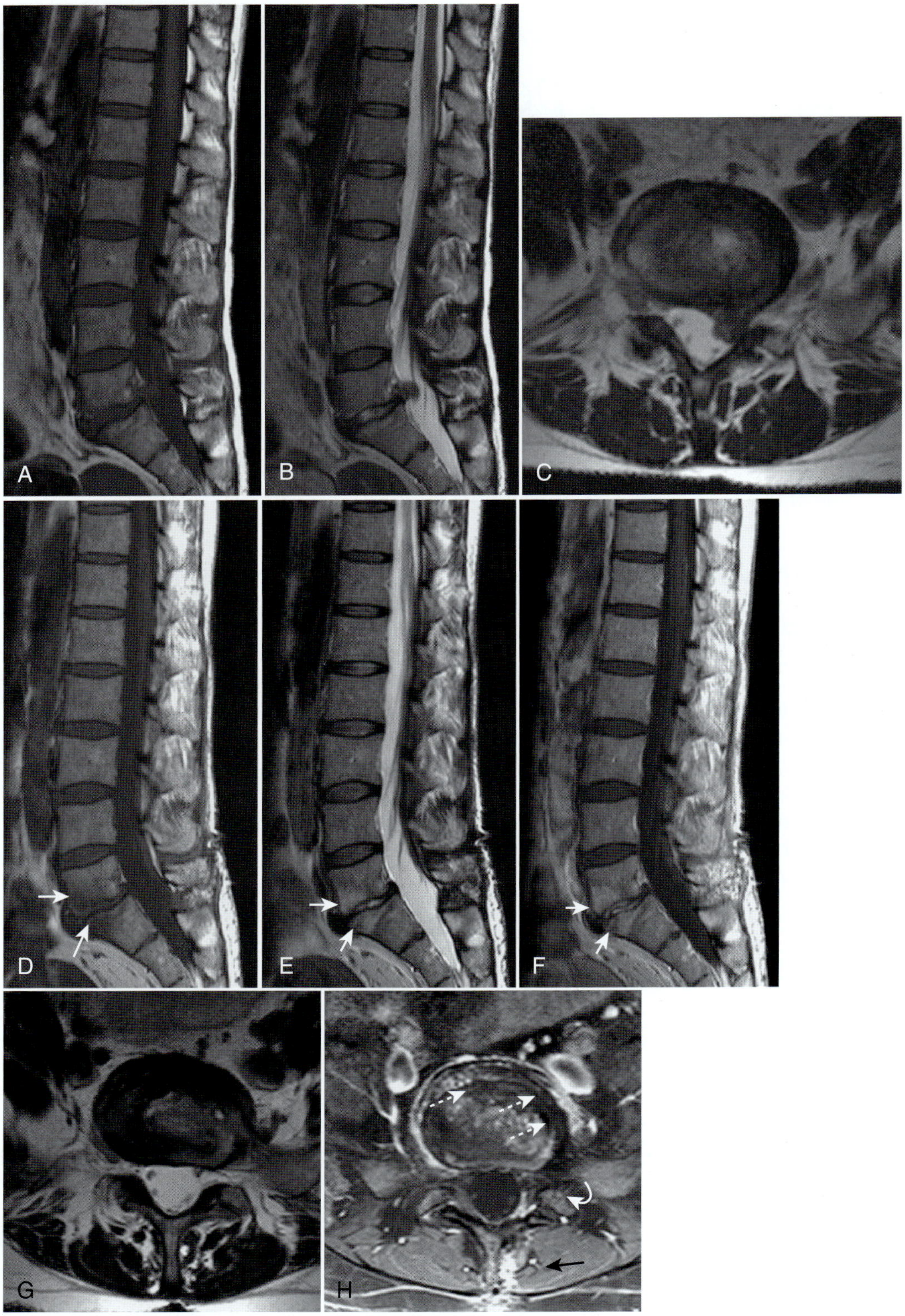

Figure 71.1 Sagittal T1-weighted (T1W) (**A**), sagittal T2W (**B**), and axial T2W (**C**) MR images demonstrate a left paracentral disc extrusion at the L5-S1 level that is compressing the S1 nerve root. There is early disc space narrowing, but discal hydration is relatively preserved, and there are no Modic changes in the vertebral end plates. The patient underwent microdiscectomy, but a few months later presented again with progressive low back pain. The sagittal T1W (**D**) and T2W (**E**) MR images obtained at this time show progressive disc space narrowing, and there are now Modic type I vertebral end-plate changes with marrow edema that has low signal intensity (SI) on the T1W MR image and high SI on the T2W MR image (*white arrows*). These areas show enhancement on the sagittal post-contrast (obtained after administration of a contrast agent) T1W MR image (**F**), and there is also discal enhancement. (**G**), The axial T2W MR image shows no evidence of recurrent disc protrusion. (**H**), The axial post-contrast T1W MR image shows patchy discal enhancement (*broken white arrows*), minor enhancing epidural fibrosis (*curved white arrow*), and enhancement along the surgical excision (*black arrow*).

CHAPTER 72

Recurrent Intervertebral Disk Herniation of the Lumbar Spine

DEFINITION

- Focal extension of the intervertebral disk of less than 50% of the disk circumference beyond the margins of the vertebra after lumbar spine surgery.

SIGNS AND SYMPTOMS

- Level, size and location (posterior, anterior, lateral, etc.) of disk herniation determines the clinical presentation.
- Back and lumbar radicular pain the most common symptoms.
- Decreased range of motion of the lumbar spine with associated muscle spasm also common.
- Pain may radiate in a dermatomal or nondermatomal pattern.
- Motor, sensory, and reflex changes may occur.
- Central disk herniation may cause compression of the lumbar spinal cord with resultant lumbar myelopathy.

DEMOGRAPHICS

- May occur following acute trauma.
- Incidence increases with age
- Repeated microtrauma to disk by repetitive activities may also increase incidence.
- Incidence: Male = Female.

IMAGING RECOMMENDATIONS

- MRI is the primary investigation.
  - Post-contrast (obtained after administration of a contrast agent) images may be required.
- Post-contrast CT or CT myelography if MRI is contraindicated.

IMAGING FINDINGS

- MR images obtained in first 6 months after operation, may appear very similar to preoperative images.
- Post-contrast images may be required to distinguish granulation tissue from disk material.
- Features that favor recurrent disk protrusion:
  - High-signal intensity (SI) disk material on T2-weighted (T2W) MR images.
  - Continuity with disk space.
  - Nonenhancement of disk material with peripheral enhancement.
  - Displacement of nerve roots and thecal sac away from disk material.
- Over 6 to 12 months, the granulation tissue usually shrinks down and the epidural fat planes return to normal.
  - Distinction between recurrent disk and postoperative fibrosis is easier in later stages.

OTHER RECOMMENDED TESTING

- Electromyography and nerve conduction velocity testing are indicated if radiculopathy is present.
- Provocative discography may serve as a useful diagnostic tool to determine whether a specific disk is serving as a nidus for the pain.

DIFFERENTIAL DIAGNOSIS

- Epidural fibrosis.
- Epidural abscess.
- Osteophyte of vertebral end plate.
- Epidural hematoma.
- Neoplasm.
- Schwannoma.

TREATMENT

- Conservative treatment consisting of local heat, cold, simple analgesics, and nonsteroidal anti-inflammatory agents will improve symptoms in many cases.
- Physical therapy, including gentle stretching, range-of-motion exercises, deep heat modalities, and stretch and spray, may be beneficial in selected patients.
- Epidural blocks will provide symptomatic relief if conservative therapy fails or the pain is limiting activities of daily living.
- Osteopathic or chiropractic manipulation may provide symptomatic relief in selected patients.
- Lysis of epidural adhesions (Racz procedure).
- Spinal cord stimulation, especially for significant epidural fibrosis and/or arachnoiditis.
- Surgery may be required for persistent pain or progressive neurologic symptoms.

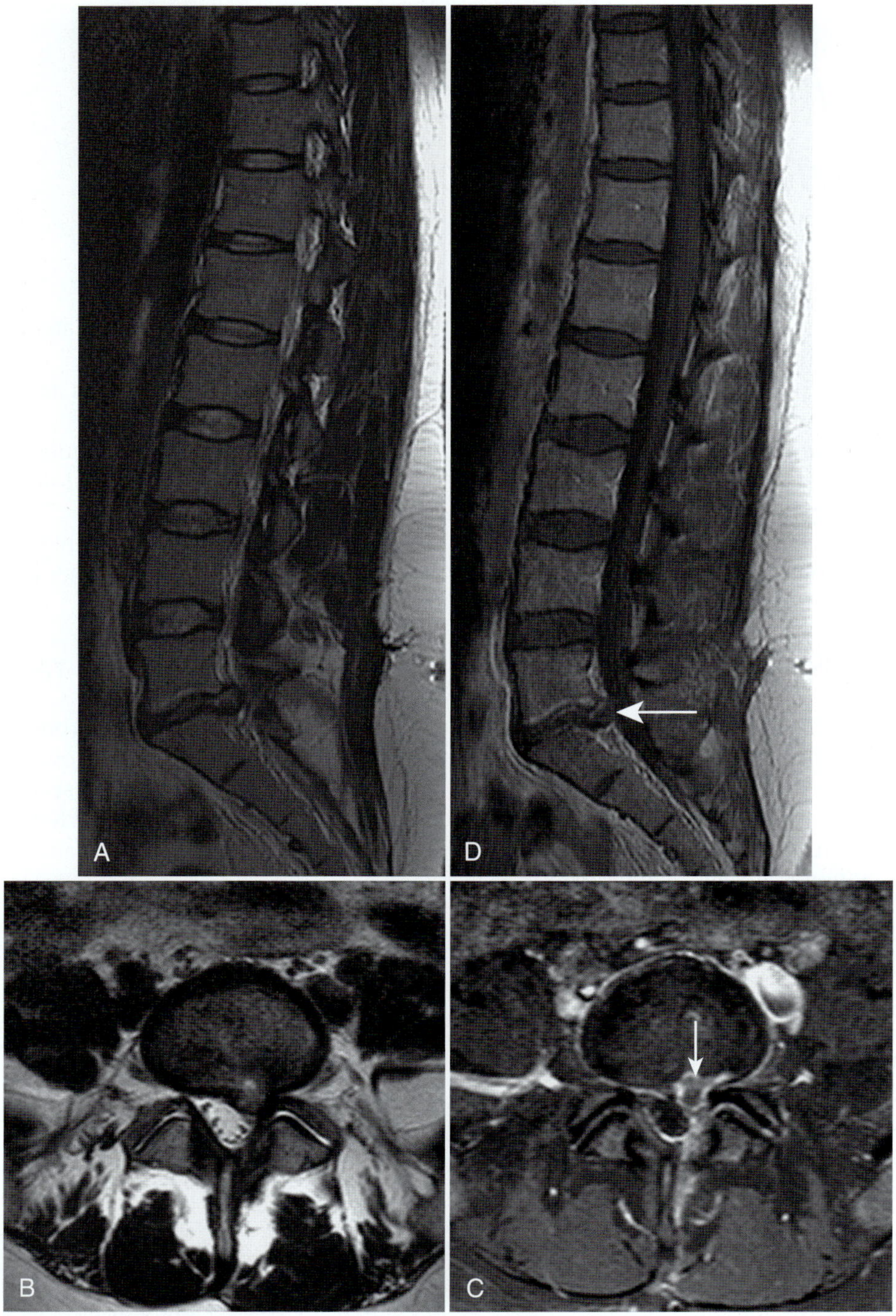

Figure 72.1 Sagittal T2W (**A**) and axial T2W (**B**) MR images demonstrating a recurrent right paracentral disk protrusion at L5-S1 that is high SI with a low-SI peripheral rim. The post-contrast sagittal T1W with fat suppression (FST1W) axial (**C**) and sagittal T1W (**D**) images show nonenhancement of the disk material (*white arrows*) with enhancement confined to the periphery of the disk.

CHAPTER 73

Hardware Failure Following Lumbar Spine Surgery

DEFINITION

- Failure of implanted hardware due to breakage or mechanical malfunction following lumbar spine surgery.

SIGNS AND SYMPTOMS

- Clinical presentation is determined by the type of hardware failure and its effect on the biomechanics of the area in which it was implanted:
  - Impingement of hardware on neural structures tends to cause significant radicular and/or myelopathic signs and symptoms.
  - Loosening or fracturing of hardware that allows movement of a segment that was intended to be fused will cause both mechanical low back pain and radicular and/or myelopathic signs and symptoms.
- Back and lumbar radicular pain is the most common symptom.
- Decreased range of motion of the lumbar spine with associated muscle spasm are also common.
- Pain may radiate in a dermatomal or nondermatomal pattern.
- Motor, sensory, and reflex changes may occur.

DEMOGRAPHICS

- Occurs primarily in adults.
- Incidence: Male = Female.
- May occur following acute trauma.
- Incidence increases with time after lumbar spine surgery, especially if osseous fusion does not occur.

IMAGING RECOMMENDATIONS

- Radiography is the primary investigation:
  - Comparison of previous radiographs is essential.
- CT is a useful adjunct for:
  - Identifying hardware failure.
  - Assessing bony fusion.
- MRI is restricted mainly to neurologic complications, infection, and so on.
- CT or CT myelography is used for neurologic complications when MRI is contraindicated or is nondiagnostic because of MRI susceptibility artifact.

IMAGING FINDINGS

- Postoperative hematomas.
- Backing-out or fracture of screws.
- Bending or fracture of rods.
- CT is more accurate for:
  - Malposition of pedicle screws.
  - Loosening of screws with surrounding bony lysis.
- Neural compression or impingement due to badly placed pedicle screws or recurrent disc protrusions.
- Bony sclerosis, erosion, and destruction in cases of infected metalwork.

OTHER RECOMMENDED TESTING

- Electromyography and nerve conduction velocity testing are indicated if radiculopathy is present.
- Provocative discography may serve as a useful diagnostic tool to determine whether a specific disc is serving as a nidus for the pain.

DIFFERENTIAL DIAGNOSIS

- Other causes of failed back surgery that may be causing symptomatology in the presence of failed hardware.

TREATMENT

- Conservative treatment consisting of local heat, cold, simple analgesics, and nonsteroidal anti-inflammatory agents will improve symptoms in many cases.
- Epidural blocks may provide symptomatic relief if conservative therapy fails or the pain is limiting activities of daily living.
- Surgery to remove, repair, or replace the failed hardware may be required for persistent pain, functional disability, or progressive neurologic symptoms.

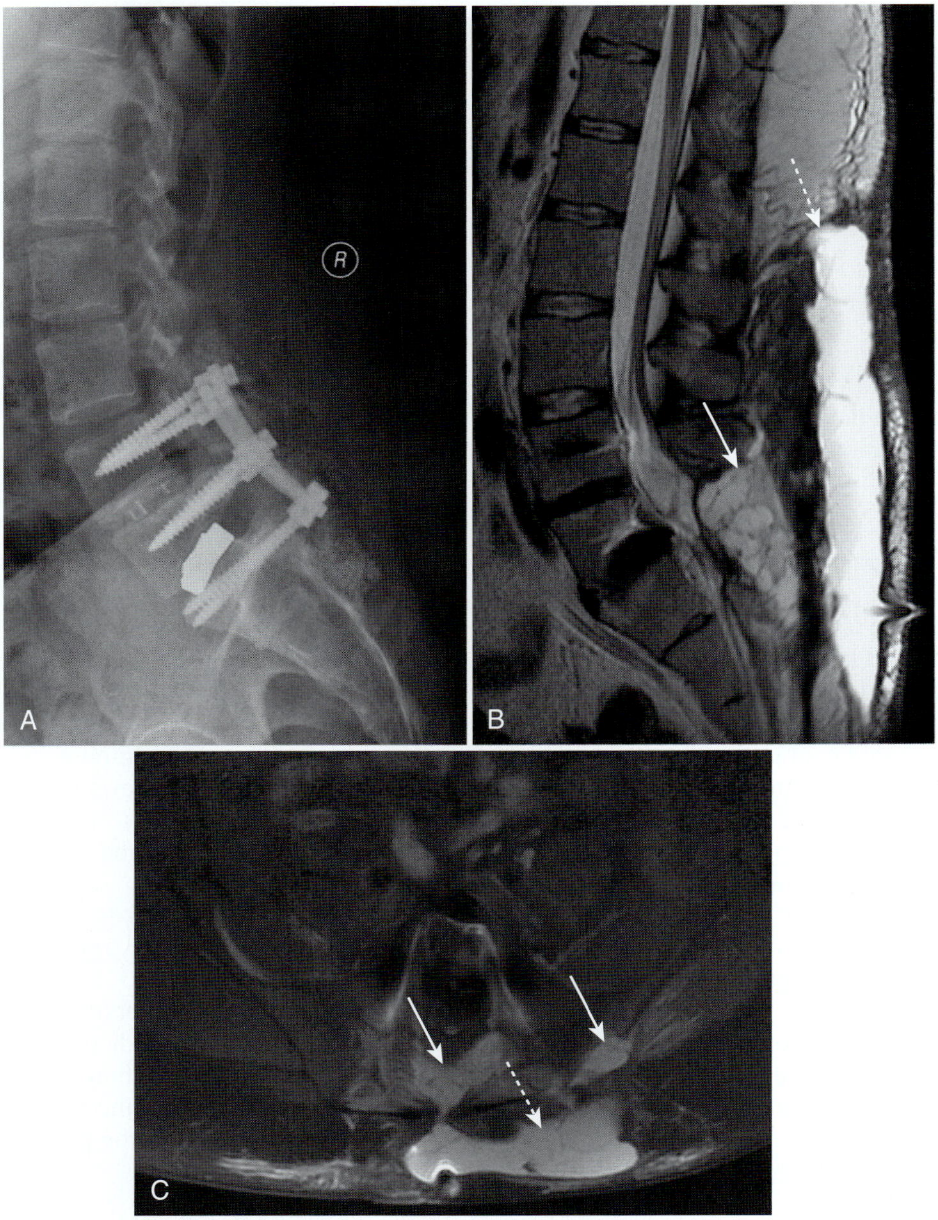

Figure 73.1 (**A**), Postoperative lateral radiograph of an anterior spinal fusion from L5 through S1, with posterior fusion from L4 through S1 and bone grafting. The patient had pain and swelling, but the radiographic findings are normal. The sagittal (**B**) and axial (**C**) T2-weighted (T2W) MR images, however, show both deep (*solid arrows*) and superficial (*broken arrow*) hematoma with high signal intensity. Aspiration and drainage revealed no evidence of infection.

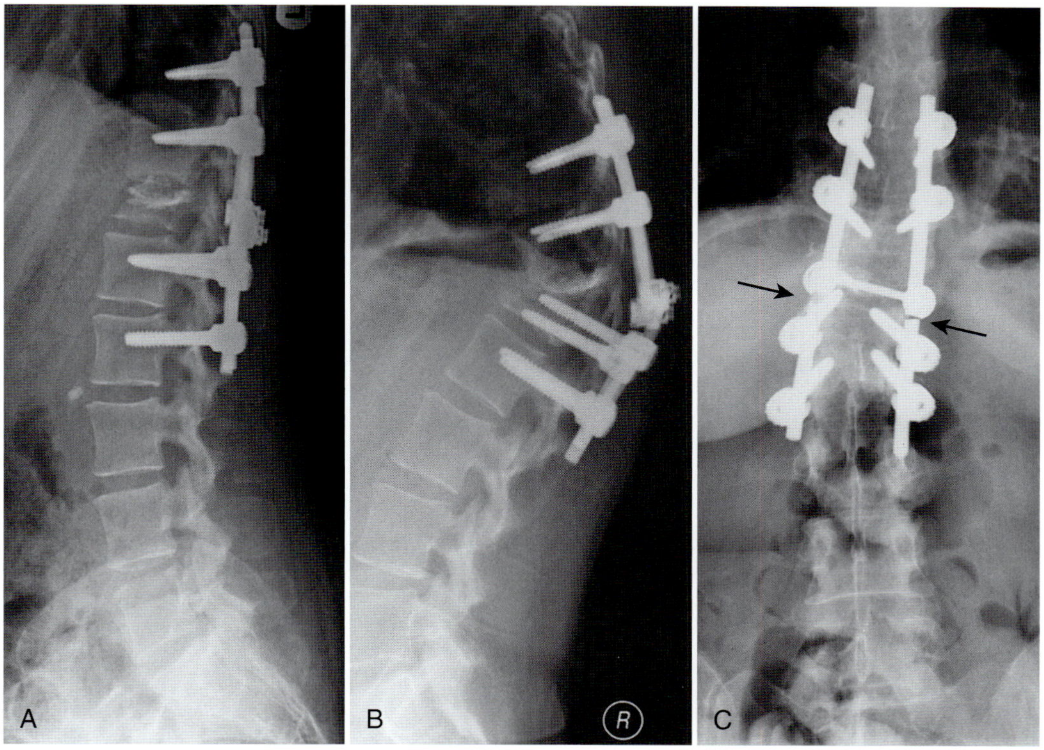

Figure 73.2 (**A**), Lateral radiograph of a patient who underwent instrumented posterior spinal fusion from T10 through L2 for a fractured L2, with calcium phosphate cement augmentation. There is good alignment of the spine and orthopedic hardware. The patient presented a few months later with increasing kyphosis and spine pain. (**B**), The lateral radiograph obtained at that time demonstrates the kyphotic angulation and increasing vertebral collapse. (**C**), Fracturing of both the spinal rods (*black arrows*) is apparent on the AP radiograph.

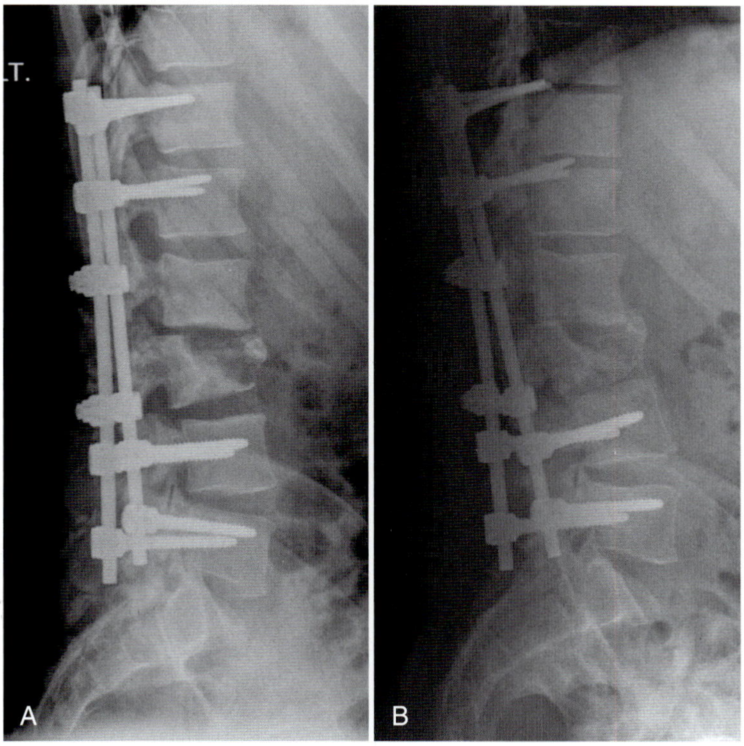

Figure 73.3 (**A**), Lateral radiograph of a patient with posterior fusion from T12 through L5 for fractured L3 with good alignment of fracture and orthopedic metalware. (**B**), However, a radiograph obtained a few months later shows backing-out of the pedicle screws at D12 and L1.

CHAPTER 74

Charcot Arthropathy of the Lumbar Spine

DEFINITION

- A destructive arthropathy that occurs in joints with normal mobility that have lost normal sensation and proprioception as a result of impairment of these protective neurologic functions by diabetes, spinal cord injury, or other neurologic diseases, such as neurosyphilis.

SIGNS AND SYMPTOMS

- May initially be asymptomatic owing to impaired nociception.
- Patient may complain of sensation of spine instability.
- Onset may occur following seemingly minor trauma.
- Back pain made worse with movement of lumbar spine.
- Pain typically radiates into the low back and buttocks in a nondermatomal pattern.
- Pain can be made worse with axial loading combined with range of motion of the lumbar spine.

DEMOGRAPHICS

- Incidence: Male = Female.
- Onset of symptoms may be delayed because of impaired nociception and proprioception.
- Diabetes is the most common cause.
- Often involves other joints.

IMAGING RECOMMENDATIONS

- Radiography.
- MRI.
- CT:
  - Assessment of extent of bony destruction.

IMAGING FINDINGS

- Narrowed or obliterated disc space.
- Marked bony sclerosis, fragmentation, and osteophyte formation.
- Progressive scoliosis and subluxation.
- Typically, no paravertebral mass.
- Changes may also occur around a fracture site.
- MRI may also show:
  - Previous cord injury.
  - Progressive syrinx formation.
- Cord atrophy.

OTHER RECOMMENDED TESTING

- Electromyography and nerve conduction velocity testing are used to determine presence or absence of neuropathy.
- Laboratory testing, including cerebrospinal fluid analysis for *Treponema pallidum* if neurosyphilis is suspected.

DIFFERENTIAL DIAGNOSIS

- Inflammatory arthritides, especially rheumatoid arthritis.
- Septic facet joint.
- Osteomyelitis of vertebral body.
- Healing facet joint fracture.
- Neoplasm.
- Degenerative disc disease with instability.

TREATMENT

- Conservative treatment consisting of local heat, cold, simple analgesics, and nonsteroidal anti-inflammatory agents will improve symptoms in many cases.
- Epidural or facet blocks with local anesthetic and a steroid will provide symptomatic relief if conservative therapy fails or the pain is limiting activities of daily living.
- Orthotic bracing.
- Surgery may be required for persistent pain or progressive neurologic symptoms.

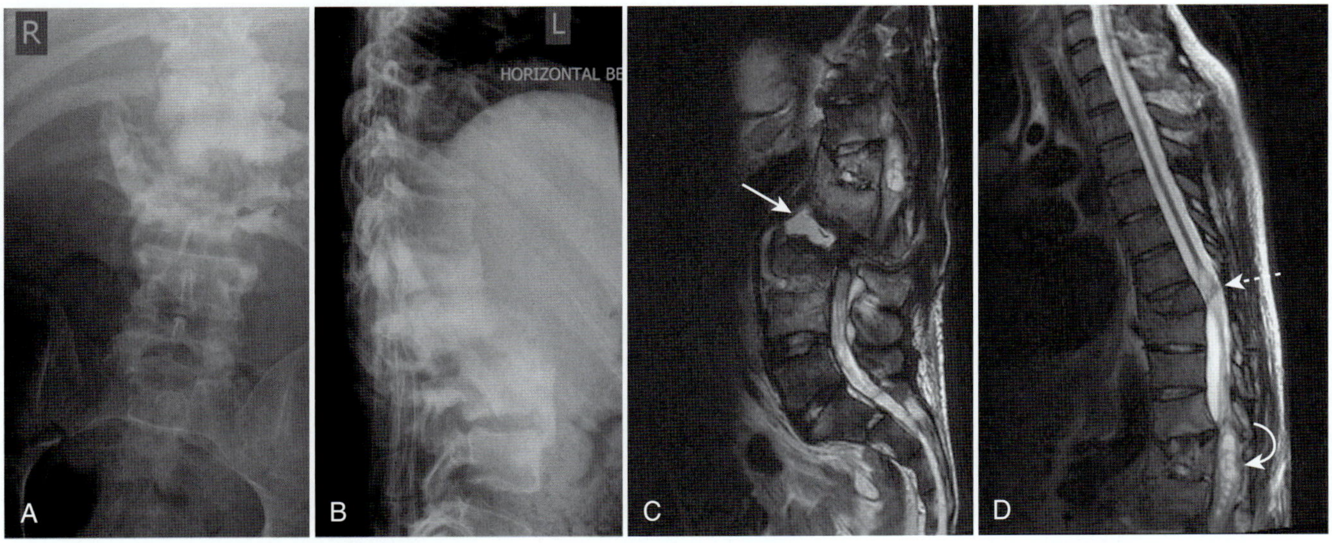

Figure 74.1 Patient with a complete cord injury at the midthoracic level. The AP (**A**) and lateral (**B**) radiographs of the lumbar spine show extensive bony destruction with prominent new bone formation and osteophytosis at the L1-L3 level with severe subluxation and scoliosis due to Charcot arthropathy. (**C**), The sagittal T2-weighted MR image with fat suppression (FST2W) of the lumbar spine demonstrates high–signal intensity (SI) fluid within the pseudarthrosis (*white arrow*), and there is reactive high-SI marrow edema in the adjacent vertebral bodies. (**D**), The sagittal FST2W MR image image of the dorsal spine demonstrates the original cord injury at the T7 level (*broken white arrow*) with an associated vertebral fracture. The distal cord is atrophic, and there are focal areas of cystic dilatation within the conus (*curved white arrow*).

CHAPTER 75

Paget Disease

DEFINITION

- Chronic metabolic disorder of bone metabolism caused by overactive osteoclasts and osteoblasts resulting in a characteristic disordered abnormal bone remodeling that produces classic ivory and picture frame vertebrae.

SIGNS AND SYMPTOMS

- May be asymptomatic initially because of impaired nociception.
- Patient may complain of sensation of dull, deep aching of the spine.
- Onset may occur after seemingly minor trauma.
- Palpable swelling may be present because of abnormal bone remodeling.
- Back pain made worse with movement of the lumbar spine.
- Pain typically radiates into the low back and buttocks in a nondermatomal pattern.
- Radiculopathy and myelopathy may occur.

DEMOGRAPHICS

- Onset of symptoms from middle fifth to eighth decade of life.
- Incidence: Female > Male.
- More common in white persons and those of Northern European descent.
- Rare in Asian and African American persons.
- Any bone in the skeleton may be affected.

IMAGING RECOMMENDATIONS

- Radiography is usually diagnostic.
- Isotope bone scanning:
  - Assess the entire skeleton.
  - Assess response to treatment.
- MRI or CT may provide additional diagnostic information in indeterminate cases.

IMAGING FINDINGS

- Spinal involvement is most common in:
  - Vertebral body.
  - Sacrum.
- Disease may be limited to a single vertebra or to multiple levels.
- Radiography/CT demonstrates:
  - Bony sclerosis.
  - Bony expansion.
  - Cortical thickening.
  - Trabecular coarsening.
- Mixed areas of low signal intensity (SI) and high SI on both T1-weighted (T1W) and T2W MR images.
- New areas of bony lysis or soft tissue mass suggest possible sarcomatous transformation.

OTHER RECOMMENDED TESTING

- Electromyography and nerve conduction velocity testing to identify presence of neuropathy.
- Laboratory testing to identify increases in serum alkaline phosphatase and urine hydroxyproline levels.

DIFFERENTIAL DIAGNOSIS

- Osteoblastic metastatic disease of the vertebral body.
- Vertebral hemangioma.

TREATMENT

- Drugs that inhibit osteoclastic bone resorption, including the bisphosphonates, calcitonin, and mithramycin.
- Conservative treatment consisting of local heat, cold, simple analgesics, and nonsteroidal anti-inflammatory agents will improve symptoms in many cases.

- Epidural or facet blocks with local anesthetic and steroid will provide symptomatic relief if conservative therapy fails or the pain is limiting activities of daily living.
- Surgery may be required for persistent pain or progressive neurologic symptoms due to spinal stenosis.

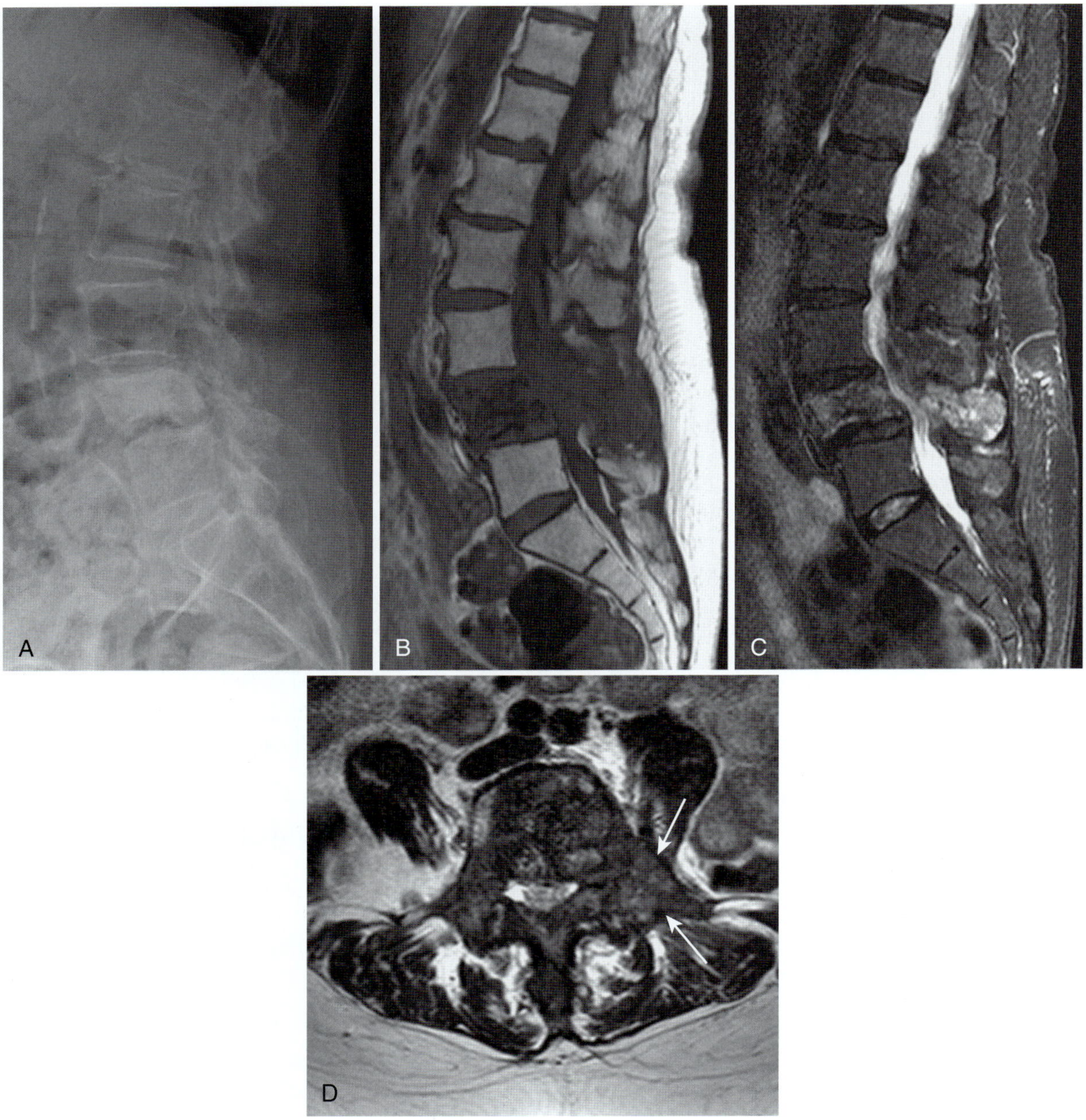

Figure 75.1 Elderly woman with low back pain. (**A**), The lateral radiograph shows a densely sclerotic and partly collapsed L4 vertebral body. (**B**) The sagittal T1W MR image shows a low-SI osteoblastic lesion involving the vertebral body and spinous process, which is mixed low and high SI on the short T1 inversion recovery (STIR) MR image (**C**). There is also bony expansion that is typical of Paget disease and is most obvious in the right transverse process on the axial T2W MR image (**D**) (*white arrows*).

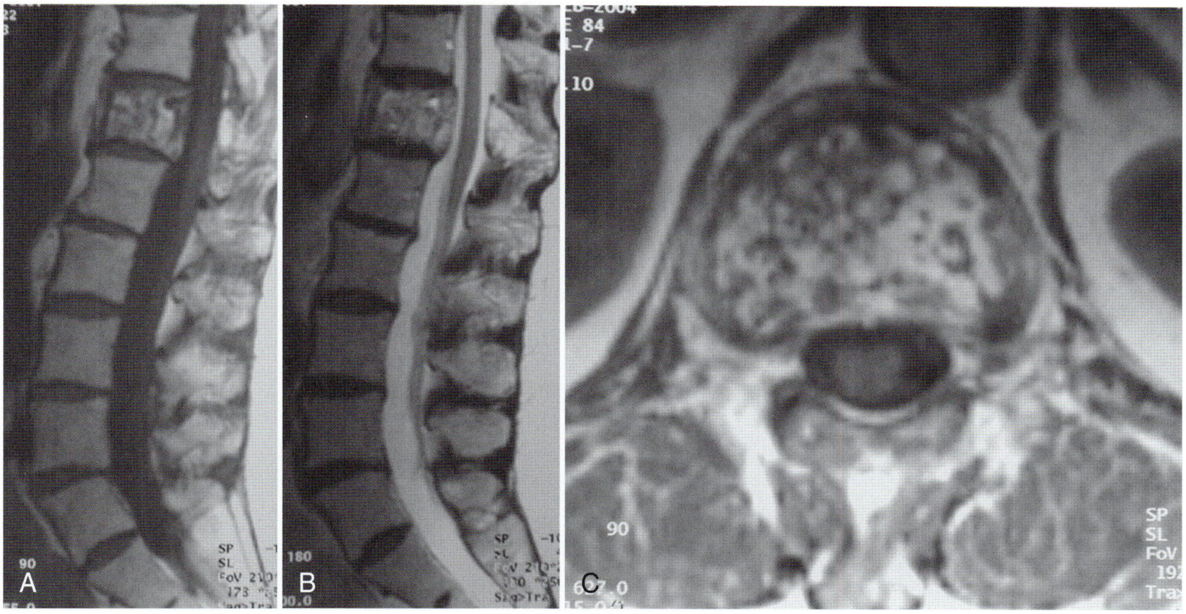

Figure 75.2 Sagittal T1W (**A**) and T2W (**B**) and axial T1W (**C**) MR images of another patient with Paget disease show more obvious bony expansion of the involved T12 vertebral body, with a greater fatty component consistent with long-standing inactive disease.

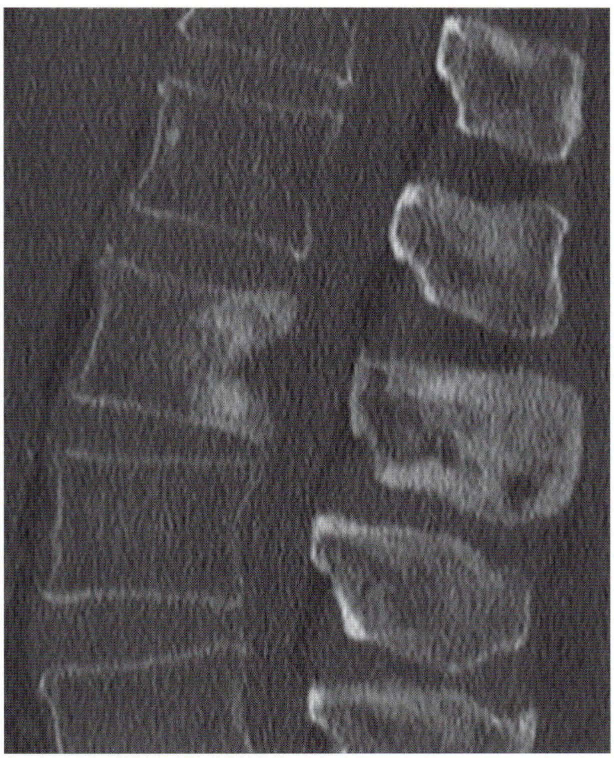

Figure 75.3 Sagittal CT scan of a patient demonstrating sclerosis of the posterior aspect of the L3 vertebral body and spinous process. The MRI examination had been misinterpreted as showing a metastasis from breast carcinoma, but the pattern of bony sclerosis and expansion is typical of Paget disease.

CHAPTER 76

Multiple Myeloma

DEFINITION

- Multifocal malignant proliferation of monoclonal plasma cells that produces characteristic skeletal abnormalities and associated anemia and renal disease.

SIGNS AND SYMPTOMS

- Usually manifests as bone pain.
- Patient may complain of sensation of dull, deep aching in the spine or other affected bone.
- Onset of symptoms may occur following seemingly minor trauma.
- Back pain made worse with movement of the lumbar spine.
- Pain typically radiates into the low back and buttocks in a nondermatomal pattern.
- Radiculopathy and myelopathy may occur.

DEMOGRAPHICS

- Onset of symptoms from middle fourth to eighth decade of life.
- Incidence: Male > Female.
- More common in African American persons.
- Less common in Asian persons.
- Anemia and renal failure often present.
- Increased incidence of amyloidosis in patients with multiple myeloma.
- Increased risk following ionizing radiation and pesticide exposures.
- Increased incidence in patients with human immunodeficiency virus.

IMAGING RECOMMENDATIONS

- Radiography:
  - Skeletal survey.
- MRI:
  - Whole-body MRI is an alternative to radiographic skeletal survey.
  - Spinal MRI for localized spinal pain or neurologic deficit.

IMAGING FINDINGS

- Focal well-defined areas of bony lysis and destruction.
- Rare occurrence of sclerotic myeloma.
- On MRI, focal deposits are typically:
  - Rounded.
  - Of low signal intensity (SI) on T1-weighted T1W MR images.
  - Of high SI on T2W or short T1 inversion recovery (STIR) MR images.
- Diffuse marrow changes may be due to red marrow reconversion or diffuse myeloma.
- Osteoporotic fractures are common and more frequent than pathologic fractures.

OTHER RECOMMENDED TESTING

- Electromyography and nerve conduction velocity testing to identify presence of neuropathy.
- Laboratory testing to identify increased serum calcium level.
- Serum protein electrophoresis to identify monoclonal gammopathy.
- Urine analysis for Bence Jones proteinuria.

DIFFERENTIAL DIAGNOSIS

- Osteoblastic metastatic disease of the vertebral body.
- Vertebral hemangioma.

TREATMENT

- Drugs that inhibit osteoclastic bone resorption, including the bisphosphonates, calcitonin, and mithramycin.
- Erythropoietin for anemia.
- Chemotherapy.
- Thalidomide.
- Bone marrow transplantation.
- Conservative treatment consisting of local heat, cold, simple analgesics, and nonsteroidal anti-inflammatory agents will improve symptoms in many cases.

- Epidural or facet blocks with local anesthetic and steroid will provide symptomatic relief if conservative therapy fails or the pain is limiting activities of daily living.
- Vertebroplasty for vertebral fracture and collapse.
- Surgery may be required for persistent pain or progressive neurologic symptoms due to spinal stenosis.

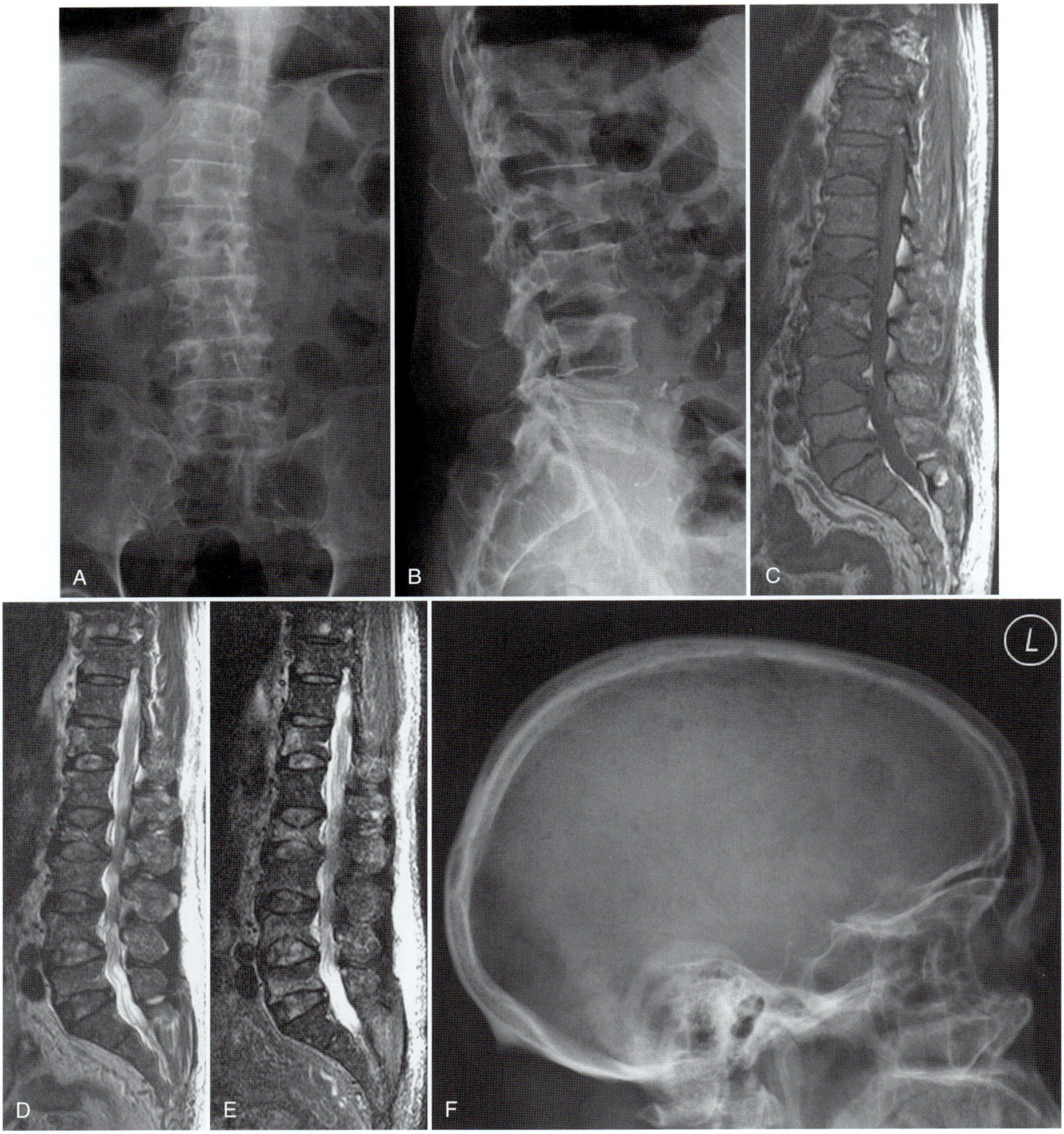

Figure 76.1 Elderly patient presenting with low back pain. AP (**A**) and lateral (**B**) radiographs show a presumed insufficiency fracture of L2 with minor end-plate collapse of L3. The sagittal T1W (**C**), T2W (**D**), and STIR (**E**) MR images acquired a few months later show multilevel vertebral fractures. There are also diffuse abnormality of the bone marrow with a generally patchy appearance and some rounded areas of high SI on the T2W and STIR images. The appearances are strongly suspicious for disorders such as plasma cell dyscrasias and other reticuloendothelial disorders. Immunoglobulin testing yielded results positive for myeloma, and a subsequent skeletal survey showed lytic lesions in the skull (**F**) typical of multiple myeloma.

CHAPTER 77

Anatomy: Special Imaging Considerations of the Sacroiliac Joint and Bony Pelvis

OSSEOUS STRUCTURES

Sacrum. Collectively made up of four broad bony segments that become progressively narrower caudally in both the coronal and sagittal planes. Centrally, the sacral segments are separated by rudimentary fibrous discs. The sacral segments fuse laterally to form the sacral alae, lateral to which lie the articular surfaces of the sacroiliac joints. Each sacral segment possesses a pair of foramina, which are directed anterolaterally. The foramina have dorsal and ventral openings for the passage of the paired sacral nerves.

Sacroiliac Joint (SIJ). Formed by the articulation between the sacrum and iliac bones. The joint surfaces are twisted craniocaudally, with the dorsal edge projecting more laterally than the ventral edge at S1, and vice versa at S3. This varying anatomy must be considered during SIJ injection. There is no true joint capsule, because the joint is bordered anteriorly and posteriorly by sacroiliac ligaments. The superior two thirds of the SIJ is bridged posteriorly by the fibrous interosseous ligament. The inferior one third is a synovial compartment, which is thus targeted during joint injection.

Iliac Bone. Each iliac bone articulates with the sacrum via a flattened inferior synovial part that has an upper fibrous part. The broad and concave iliac crests extend from the upper margins of the SIJs and arch anterolaterally before ending at the anterosuperior iliac spines, which bear the origin of the sartorius muscles. The anteroinferior iliac spines lie below and bear the attachments of the rectus femoris muscles. The lateral surface of the iliac bone curves inferiorly to form the roof and lateral rim of the acetabulum.

Pubic Bone. The bodies of the paired bones meet anteriorly in the midline, forming the pubic symphysis. The curved superior pubic ramus projects laterally from the body to form both the anterior column of the acetabulum and the anterior one third of the acetabular fossa. The body of the pubis gives rise to the adductor tubercle on its inferior aspect, lateral to which the inferior pubic ramus curves inferiorly and posteriorly. The adductor tubercle bears the insertion of the adductor longus and gracilis muscles. The inferior ramus continues posteriorly, where it then merges with the ischium just anterior to the ischial tuberosity.

Ischium. The anterior aspect of this bone blends with the inferior pubic ramus before broadening to form the ischial tuberosity, which bears the attachment of the hamstring muscles. It then curves posterosuperiorly, widening as it does so to form the posterior column of the acetabulum as well as deepening to form the posterior one third of the acetabular fossa.

PELVIC MUSCULATURE

Iliacus. This strong broad muscle arises from the inner surface of the iliac bone. It narrows distally, forming a tendon that blends with the psoas tendon to form the strong iliopsoas tendon, which is a powerful hip flexor.

Psoas Major. A long thick muscle that arises from the lumbar transverse processes and descends in a paraspinal location to enter the pelvis before narrowing and forming a strong tendon a few centimeters proximal to the hip joint. The tendon joins with that of the iliacus to form the iliopsoas tendon, which inserts on the lesser trochanter of the femur to produce hip flexion.

Obturator Internus. Arises from the inner surface of the medial acetabular wall and extends posteriorly, arching around the ischium almost at right angles to then project laterally. It inserts on the posterior facet of the greater trochanter to perform external rotation of the hip.

Obturator Externus. Arises from the ischium and pubis at the outer margin of the obturator foramen before narrowing as it extends laterally to insert on the posterior facet of the greater trochanter just below the obturator internus tendon to produce external rotation of the hip.

Piriformis. A triangular muscle that arises from its broad base on the lateral border of the sacrum, projecting and tapering laterally to insert on the internal surface of the greater trochanter. It covers the sciatic nerve as it exits the pelvis through the greater sciatic notch.

Pelvic Floor Musculature. The major component of the pelvic floor muscle group is the levator ani, which is a broad, inferiorly curved, diaphragm-like muscle. The levator ani arises from the posterior surfaces of the pubic rami, the ischia, and the obturator fascia of the lateral pelvic wall. Along with the puborectalis muscle, the levator ani supports the pelvic viscera.

NEURAL STRUCTURES

Lumbar Plexus. Formed from the L1 to L3 and part of the L4 ventral rami, the lumbar plexus lies within the psoas major muscle, anterior to the lumbar transverse processes. The lumbar plexus branches into the muscular, iliohypogastric, ilioinguinal, genitofemoral, lateral femoral cutaneous, femoral, obturator, and accessory obturator nerves. Some of these nerves are described in further detail.

Ilioinguinal Nerve. Arises from the L1 ventral ramus and traverses the quadratus lumborum to enter the inguinal canal and supply the skin of the proximal medial thigh and the root of the penis in the male and labium majus in the female.

Femoral Nerve. Descends between the psoas and iliacus, posterior to the inguinal ligament, giving off branches to the iliacus and pectineus.

Obturator Nerve. Descends within the psoas, emerging at the level of the pelvic brim to course over the obturator internus muscle to enter the obturator foramen and then into the thigh. There are no branches in the pelvis.

Sacral Plexus. This is formed by the ventral and dorsal divisions of the L5, S1 to S4, and part of the L4 nerves. After exiting the sacral foramina, the sacral nerves give off various contributing branches within the presacral space. The branches of the sacral plexus are: the nerves to the superior and inferior gemelli, quadratus femoris, and piriformis muscles; the superior and inferior gluteal, posterior femoral cutaneous, tibial (sciatic) and common peroneal (sciatic), and pudendal nerves; and the nerves to the pelvic floor musculature.

Sciatic Nerve. Formed by branches of L4, L5, and S1 to S3 nerves, which make up the divisions that distally divide into the tibial and common peroneal nerves. The sciatic nerve is the largest nerve in the body, and it leaves the pelvis through the greater sciatic foramen, passing deep to the piriformis. It then runs between the greater trochanter and ischial tuberosity.

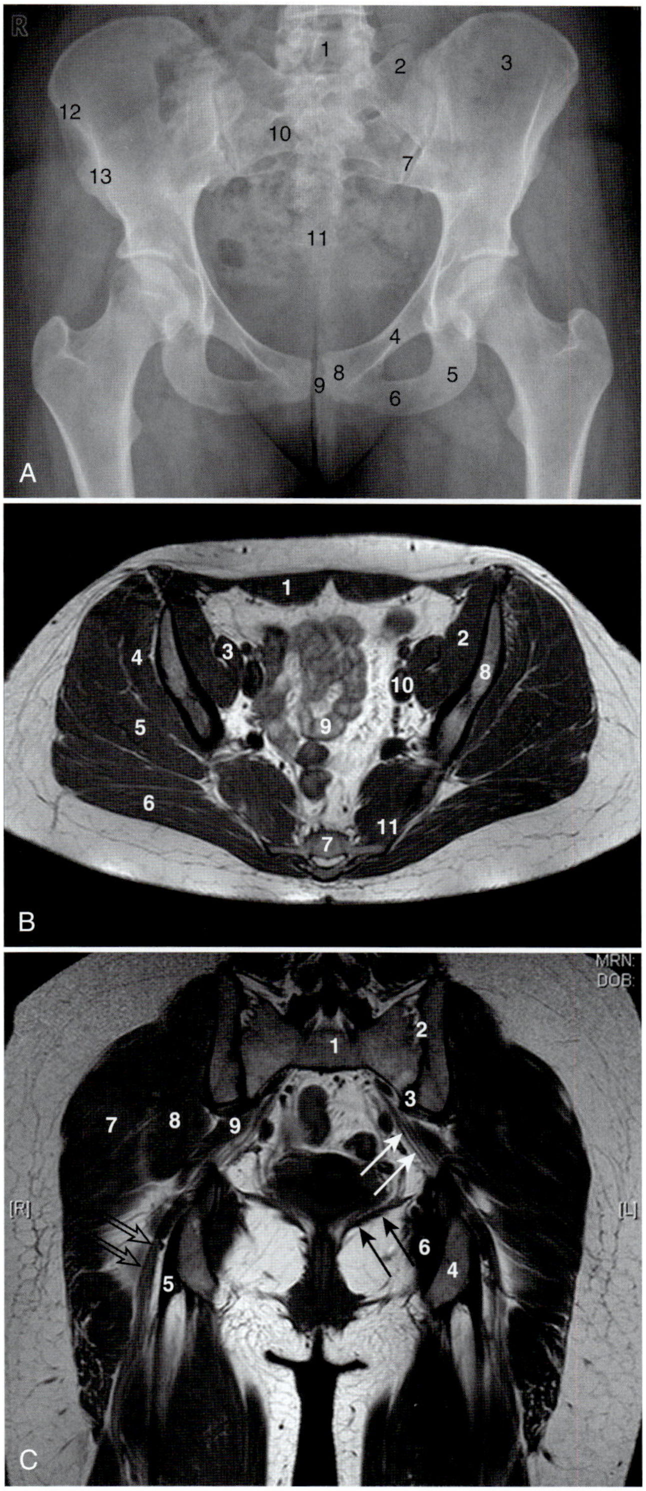

Figure 77-1 (**A**), Anteroposterior radiograph of the pelvis: 1, fifth lumbar vertebra; 2, left sacral ala; 3, iliac bone; 4, superior pubic ramus; 5, ischium; 6, inferior pubic ramus; 7, sacroiliac joint (synovial part); 8, body of the pubic bone; 9, pubic symphysis; 10, first sacral foramen; 11, sacrococcygeal junction; 12, anterosuperior iliac spine; 13, anteroinferior iliac spine. (**B**), Axial T1-weighted MR image of the pelvis: 1, rectus abdominis; 2, iliacus; 3, psoas major; 4, gluteus minimus; 5, gluteus medius; 6, gluteus maximus; 7, sacrum; 8, iliac bone; 9, small bowel; 10, common iliac vein; 11, piriformis (upper border). (**C**), Coronal T1-weighted MR image of the pelvis: 1, first sacral segment; 2, upper fibrous part of sacroiliac joint; 3, lower synovial part of sacroiliac joint; 4, ischial tuberosity; 5, hamstring tendon origin; 6, obturator internus; 7, gluteus maximus; 8, gluteus medius; 9, piriformis; *white arrows,* sacral plexus; *black arrows,* levator ani muscle; *open black arrows,* sciatic nerve.

CHAPTER 78

Sacroiliac Joint Disorders

DEFINITION

- Arthropathy of the sacroiliac joint (SIJ) from a variety of etiologies not included in the category "inflammatory seronegative spondyloarthropathies." This term includes SIJ dysfunction in young adults, stress-related disorders such as osteitis condensans ilii, osteoarthritis, diffuse idiopathic skeletal hyperostosis (DISH syndrome), gout, infection, and hyperparathyroidism.

SIGNS AND SYMPTOMS

- The most common presentation is pain localized around the SIJ and upper leg.
- The pain may radiate into the posterior buttocks and the backs of the legs.
- The pain does not radiate below the knees.
- Activity makes the pain worse.
- Rest and heat provide some relief.
- The pain is constant and characterized as aching.
- The pain may interfere with sleep.
- Tenderness to palpation of the affected SIJ.
- Patient often favors the affected leg and exhibits a list to the unaffected side.
- Spasm of the lumbar paraspinal musculature is often present.
- Limitation of range of motion of the lumbar spine in the erect position that improves in the sitting position because of relaxation of the hamstring muscles.
- Positive result of pelvic rock test.

DEMOGRAPHICS

- Incidence: Male > Female.
- Often occurs after seemingly minor trauma to SIJ.
- In absence of infection involving the SIJ, erythrocyte sedimentation rate and white blood cell count are not elevated.

IMAGING RECOMMENDATIONS

- Radiographs of the pelvis.
- CT or MRI of SIJs.
  - Disease characterization for indeterminate cases.

IMAGING FINDINGS

- SIJ dysfunction:
  - Imaging findings are usually normal.
- Osteitis condensans ilii:
  - Sclerosis confined to the iliac side of the SIJ.
- Osteoarthritis:
  - Joint space narrowing, sclerosis, and osteophyte formation.
  - In older patients, the anterior aspect of the joint may be fused.
- Gout:
  - Large unilateral punched-out erosions.
  - High-density masses around erosions on CT due to the presence of crystals.
- Infection:
  - Unilateral SIJ involvement.
  - Joint widening, erosion of subchondral bone plate, soft tissue thickening, and abscess formation.
  - Prominent marrow edema on short T1 inversion recovery (STIR) MR images.
  - Ankylosis in late stages.

OTHER RECOMMENDED TESTING

- HLA-B27 testing in all patients with sacroiliac pain to rule out seronegative spondyloarthropathy.
- Erythrocyte sedimentation rate measurement in all patients with sacroiliac pain to rule out infection.
- White blood cell count in all patients with sacroiliac pain to rule out infection.
- Serum uric acid measurement in all patients with sacroiliac pain to rule out gout.
- Serum calcium measurement to rule out hyperparathyroidism.

DIFFERENTIAL DIAGNOSIS

- Seronegative spondyloarthropathy.
- Inflammatory bowel disease.
- Septic SIJ.
- Healing SIJ fracture.
- DISH syndrome.
- Chronic juvenile arthritis.
- Retinoid therapy.
- Neoplasm.

TREATMENT

- Conservative treatment consisting of local heat, cold, simple analgesics, and nonsteroidal anti-inflammatory agents will improve symptoms in many cases.
- Physical therapy, including gentle stretching, range-of-motion exercises, deep heat modalities, and stretch and spray, may be beneficial in selected patients.
- Injections with local anesthetic and steroid to symptomatic joints will provide symptomatic relief if conservative therapy fails or the pain is limiting activities of daily living.
- Disease-modifying drugs such as methotrexate and sulfasalazine.
- Surgery may be required for persistent pain or progressive neurologic symptoms.
- Biopsy and appropriate antibiotic therapy for infective sacroiliitis.

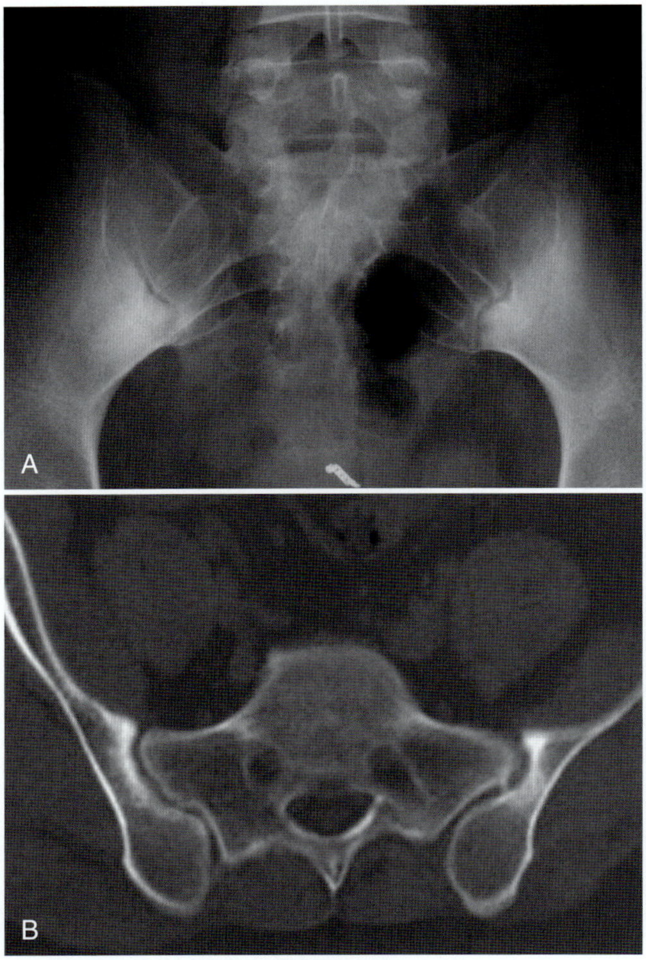

Figure 78.1 (**A**), AP radiograph of a young postpartum woman with SIJ pain. Sclerosis confined to the iliac aspect of both SIJs is due to osteitis condensans ilii. (**B**), An axial CT scan in a different patient with stress-induced changes due to athletic activity shows the same features of sclerosis of the iliac aspect of the SIJ. Note that in both cases, the joint space is preserved and there is no loss of clarity of the subchondral bone plate and no erosive change.

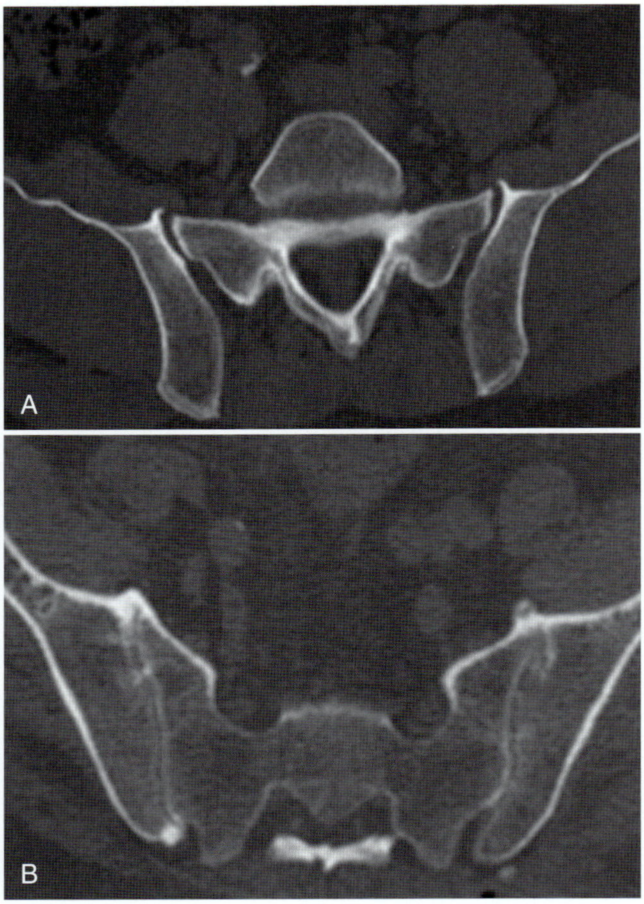

Figure 78.2 (**A**), Axial CT scan in a patient with early osteoarthritis (OA) of the SIJs. Osteophyte formation is affecting the anterior aspect of the synovial compartment of the joints. (**B**), More advanced OA is present on the axial CT scan in an elderly patient, in whom the osteophytes have fused across the anterior aspects of the joints. This appearance should not be confused with the more extensive ankylosis that occurs with ankylosing spondylitis.

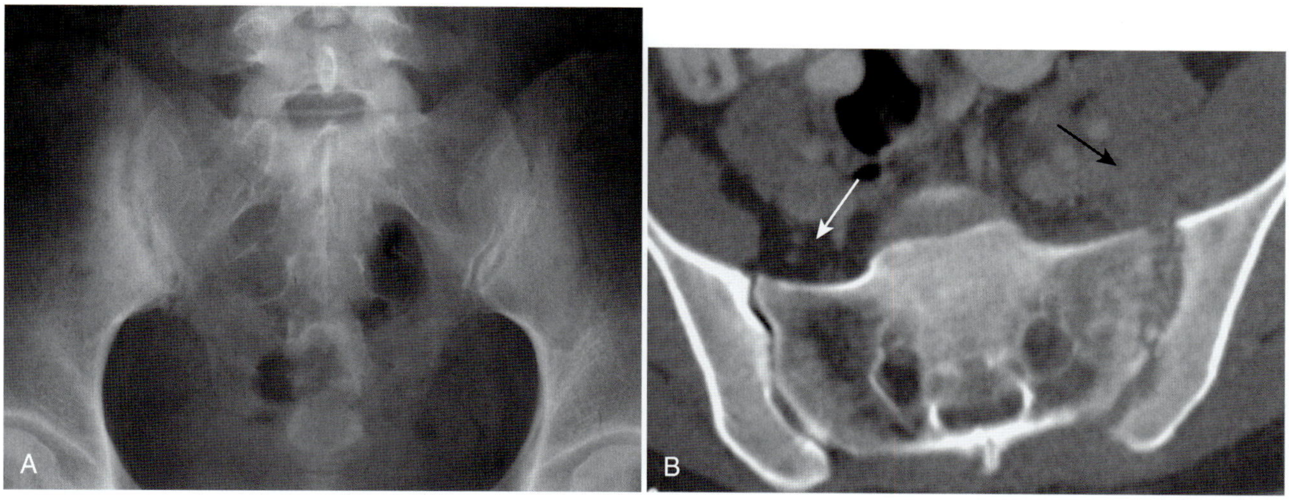

Figure 78.3 (A), AP radiograph of a patient with right-sided unilateral infective sacroiliitis. There is widening of the joint with loss of the crisp margin of the subchondral bone plate and ill-defined sclerosis. (B), The axial CT scan of a different patient with SIJ infection shows the same features in the left SIJ. Compare the anterior soft tissue inflammatory mass (*black arrow*) with the normal low-attenuation retroperitoneal fat on the opposite side (*white arrow*).

CHAPTER 79

Sacral Insufficiency Fracture

DEFINITION

- Fracture of the sacrum due to weakened osteoporotic bone under normal physiologic stress.

SIGNS AND SYMPTOMS

- Acute onset of low back, groin, buttock, or hip pain.
- Pain may radiate in a radicular or nondermatomal pattern.
- Tenderness over the sacrum may be present.
- Exacerbation of pain with weight bearing.
- Exacerbation of pain with activity.

DEMOGRAPHICS

- Onset in the sixth to eight decade in patients with osteoporosis.
- Incidence in patients with osteoporosis: Female > Male.
- No racial predilection.

IMAGING RECOMMENDATIONS

- Radiographic findings are often normal.
- MRI is the primary investigation for patients with suspected sacral insufficiency fractures.
- Isotope bone scanning and CT are alternative investigations.

IMAGING FINDINGS

- Insufficiency fractures typically have three components:
  - Tranverse fracture of the mid-sacrum.
  - Vertical fractures through the sacral ala.
- Classic "Honda sign" on isotope bone scan.
- Low-signal intensity (SI) fracture lines on all MRI pulse sequences with surrounding bone marrow edema pattern.
- Combination of low-density fractures with areas of diffuse sclerosis on CT.
- Stress fractures in athletes are typically unilateral vertical fractures.

OTHER RECOMMENDED TESTING

- In patients with osteoporosis, testing for hyperparathyroidism, panhypopituitarism, and sex hormone deficits.
- Electromyography and nerve conduction velocity testing are indicated if radiculopathy is present.

DIFFERENTIAL DIAGNOSIS

- Pathologic fracture due to tumor.
- Sacroiliitis.
- Muscle strain.
- Osteomyelitis.
- Insufficiency fractures of pelvis.

TREATMENT

- Opioids for acute pain relief.
- Caudal epidural injections of local anesthetics, opioids, and/or corticosteroids for pain not relieved by opioids.
- Decreased activity if fracture is due to overtraining.
- Bisphosphonates and calcitonin for osteoporosis.

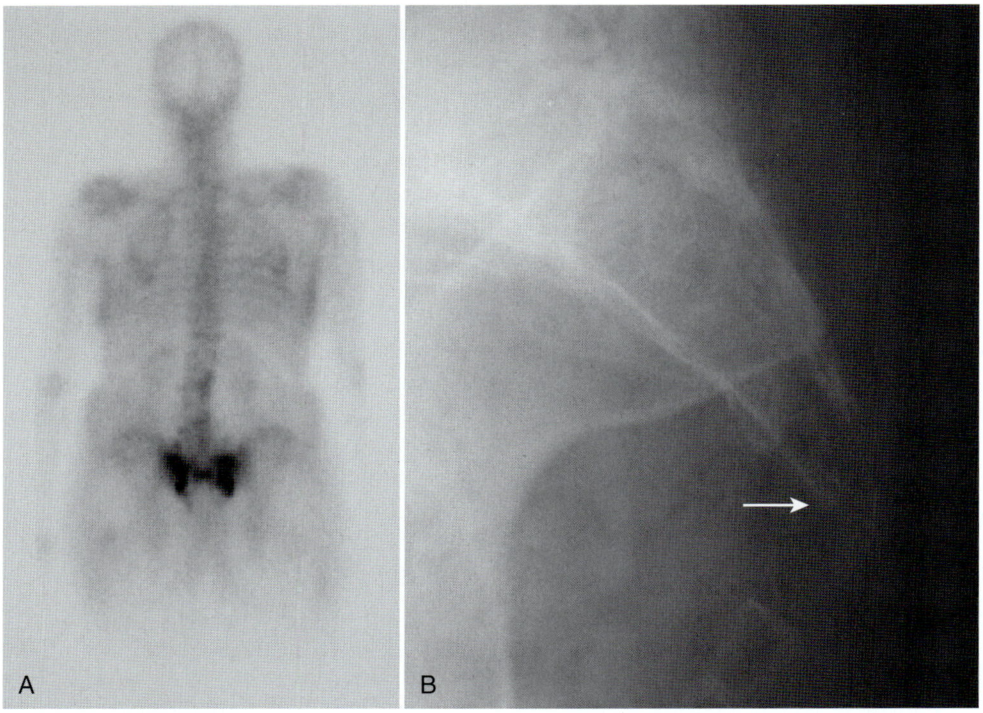

Figure 79.1 (A), Isotope bone scan of an elderly woman with sacral pain. There is an H-shaped area of increased uptake ("Honda sign") in the sacrum that is typical of a sacral insufficiency fracture. (B), The lateral radiograph demonstrates the transverse component of the fracture (*white arrow*).

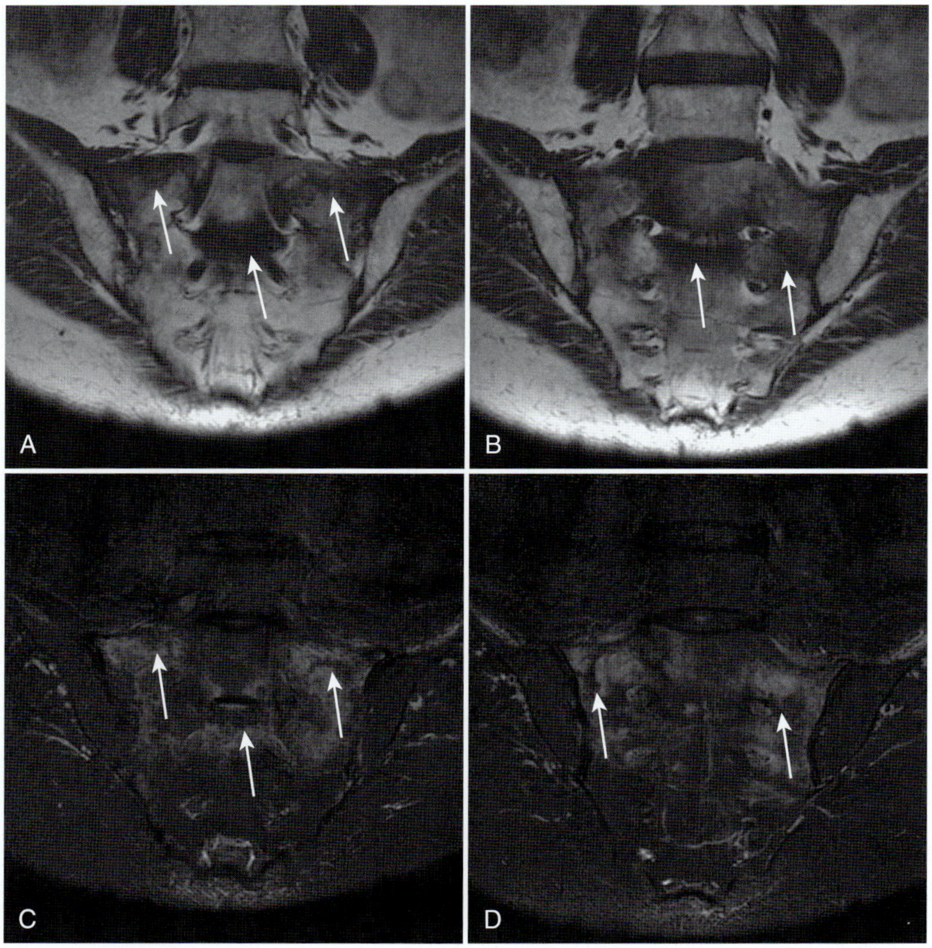

Figure 79.2 Coronal T1-weighted (T1W) (A and B) and coronal short T1 inversion recovery (STIR) (C and D) MR images of a patient with an insufficiency fracture of the sacrum. There are multiple areas of low-SI fracture lines on both the T1W and STIR images (*white arrows*). The associated marrow edema is best appreciated on the STIR images as areas of diffuse surrounding high SI.

CHAPTER 80

Insufficiency Fractures of the Pubic Rami

DEFINITION

- Fracture of the pubic rami secondary to normal physiologic stresses placed on an osteoporotic bone.
  - Stress fractures of normal bone under abnormal load may occur in athletes.

SIGNS AND SYMPTOMS

- Acute onset of groin, buttocks, and thigh pain.
- Pain may radiate in a radicular or nondermatomal pattern.
- Point tenderness over fracture may be present.
- Painful external hip rotation.
- Painful active resisted adduction.
- Antalgic gait.
- Presence of stork sign (patient unable to stand unassisted on the affected lower extremity).
- Previous dorsal kyphotic deformity may be clinically apparent, suggesting preexisting osteoporosis.

DEMOGRAPHICS

- Peak incidence in the sixth to eight decade if due to osteoporosis.
- Also seen in young athletes secondary to overtraining.
- Incidence in patients with osteoporosis: Female > Male.
- No racial predilection.

IMAGING RECOMMENDATIONS

- Radiography is the primary investigation.
- MRI or CT may be helpful for occult fractures.
- Isotope bone scanning is useful to assess the entire skeleton for multiple insufficiency fractures.

IMAGING FINDINGS

- Generalized osteopenia.
- Specific features of osteomalacia may be present.
- Fracture through pubis or pubic rami.
- Hypertrophic callus formation fractures may be prominent and may simulate a pathologic fracture.
- MRI demonstrates marrow edema on short T1 inversion recovery (STIR) images and a low-signal intensity (SI) fracture line on T1-weighted (T1W) MR images.

OTHER RECOMMENDED TESTING

- In patients with osteoporosis, testing for hyperparathyroidism, panhypopituitarism, and sex hormone deficits.
- Electromyography and nerve conduction velocity testing are indicated if radiculopathy is present.
- Evoked potential testing if myelopathy present.

DIFFERENTIAL DIAGNOSIS

- Pathologic fracture due to tumor.
- Avulsion fracture of pubic ramus.
- Insufficiency fracture of the hip.
- Osteomyelitis.
- Muscle strain.

TREATMENT

- Opioids for acute pain relief.
- Caudal epidural injections of local anesthetics, opioids, and/or corticosteroids for pain not relieved by opioids.
- Surgical treatment for non-union.
- Bisphosphonates and calcitonin for osteoporosis.

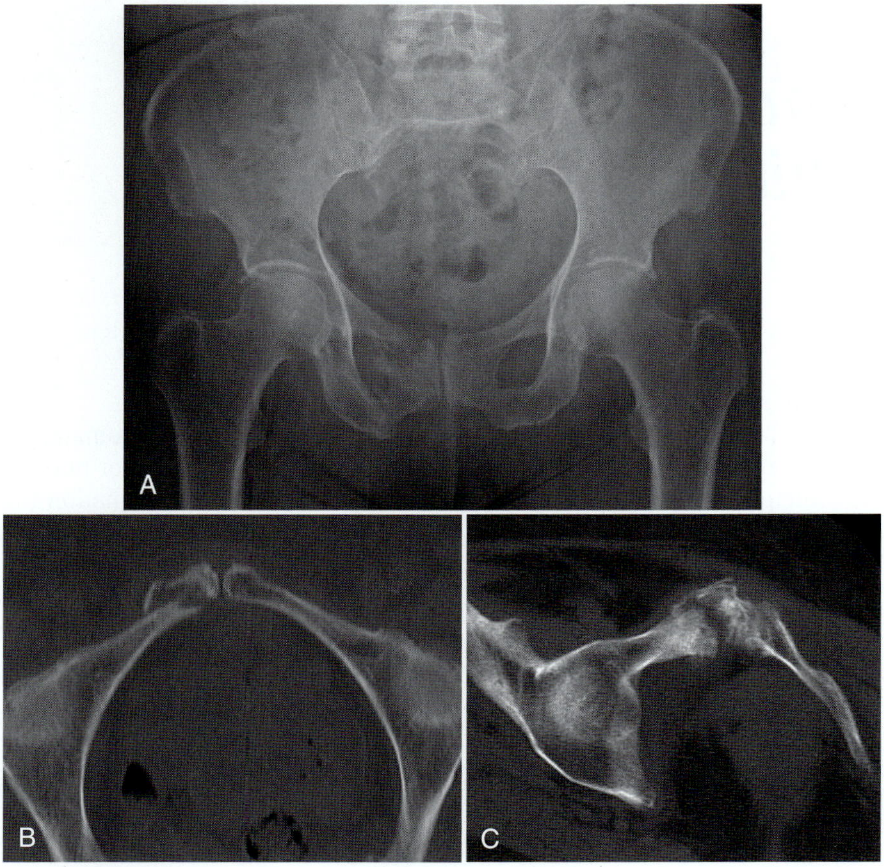

Figure 80.1 (A), Radiograph of an elderly woman with right hip pain. The hip joint is normal, but there are fractures of the pubic rami on the right side. (B and C), The CT scans demonstrate the wide fracture lines with prominent callus formation but no bony union and no soft tissue mass or lytic bony destruction. Insufficiency fractures of the sacrum were also present (*not shown*).

CHAPTER 81

Avulsion Fracture of the Ischial Tuberosity

DEFINITION

- Disruption of the cartilage or bone a resulting in a fracture due to abnormal forces placed on the musculotendinous unit of the hamstring tendon.

SIGNS AND SYMPTOMS

- Acute onset of groin, gluteal, or hip pain.
- Pain may radiate in a radicular or nondermatomal pattern.
- Tenderness over the ischial tuberosity may be present.

DEMOGRAPHICS

- Bimodal incidence, with fractures seen in younger patients after extreme passive stretching, repetitive stress, or forced contraction of the hamstring as well as in patients with osteoporosis in the sixth to eight decade of life.
- Incidence in patients with osteoporosis: Female > Male.
- Seen in ballet dancers, hurdlers, and gymnasts.
- No racial predilection.

IMAGING RECOMMENDATIONS

- Radiography.
- MRI:
  - Normal or equivocal radiographic findings.
  - Assessment of associated soft tissue injury.

IMAGING FINDINGS

- Bony avulsion of the ischial tuberosity.
- Exuberant callus formation may develop in untreated cases.
  - A rare cause of sciatica.
- Hamstring origin usually remains attached to the avulsed fragment.
- In acute injuries, MRI may demonstrate associated muscle tears around the hip.

OTHER RECOMMENDED TESTING

- In patients with osteoporosis, testing for hyperparathyroidism, panhypopituitarism, and sex hormone deficits.
- Electromyography and nerve conduction velocity testing are indicated if radiculopathy is present.

DIFFERENTIAL DIAGNOSIS

- Pathologic fracture due to tumor.
- Muscle strain.
- Piriformis syndrome.
- Tendinitis.
- Osteomyelitis.
- Insufficiency fractures.

TREATMENT

- Opioids for acute pain relief.
- Caudal epidural injections of local anesthetics, opioids, and/or corticosteroids for pain not relieved by opioids.
- Decreased activity if fracture is due to overtraining.
- Bisphosphonates and calcitonin for osteoporosis.

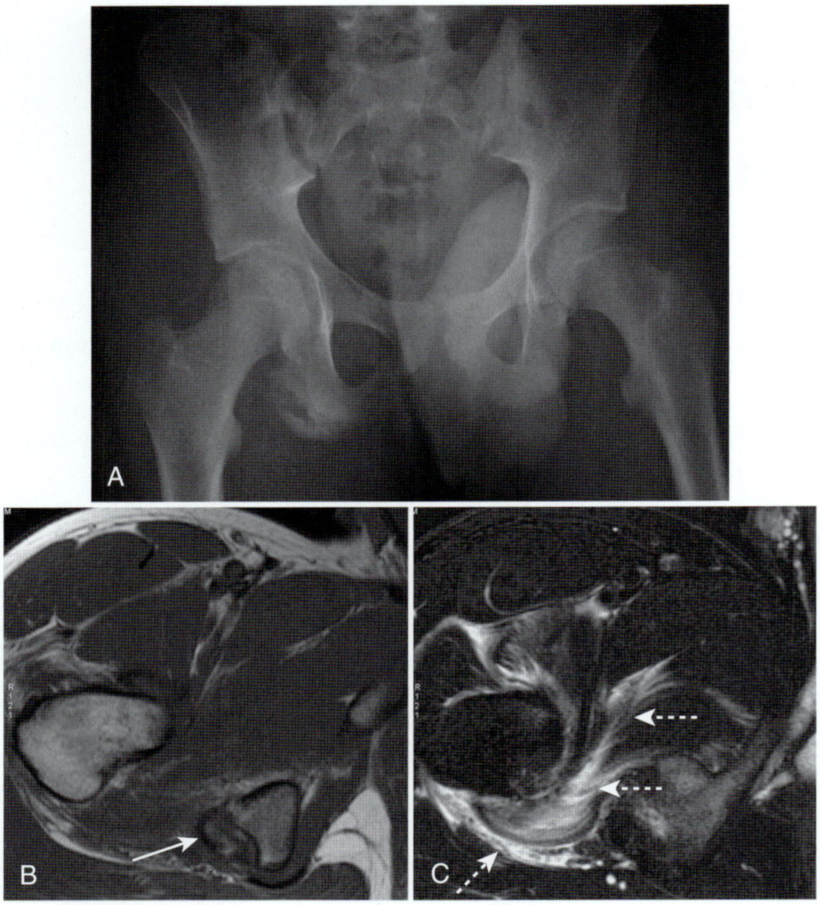

Figure 81.1 (**A**), Pelvic radiograph of a young male gymnast with avulsion of the right ischial tuberosity. (**B**), The axial T1-weighted (T1W) MR image shows the bony avulsion *(white arrow)*. (**C**), The extensive associated muscle injury is clearly evident on the axial T2W with fat suppression (FST2W) MR image, with areas of high signal intensity due to hemorrhage and soft tissue edema (*broken white arrows*).

CHAPTER 82

Osteitis Pubis

DEFINITION

- Noninfectious inflammation of the pubic synthesis that produces characteristic bony sclerosis.

SIGNS AND SYMPTOMS

- Onset may be acute or insidious.
- Moderate to severe groin pain.
- Pain may radiate to the hip or medial thigh.
- Tenderness over the pubic symphysis is often present.
- Characteristic waddling gait.
- Pain made worse with lying on one side.
- Patient may complain of clicking sensation when walking on uneven surfaces or turning over in bed.
- Exacerbation of pain with jogging, kicking, or rolling over in bed.

DEMOGRAPHICS

- Most commonly seen in third decade of life in women and fourth or fifth decade in men.
- Incidence: Female > Male.
- More common in patients with active lifestyles.
- Seen following pelvic and urologic operations and pregnancy.
- Higher rate in Europe, where playing soccer is more common.
- No racial predilection.

IMAGING RECOMMENDATIONS

- Radiography.
- MRI to assess bone and soft tissue structures.

IMAGING FINDINGS

- Bony sclerosis and irregularity of the pubic symphysis.
- MRI findings include:
  - Marrow edema on short T1 inversion recovery (STIR) MR images.
  - Adjacent soft tissue edema on STIR MR images.
  - Abnormal clefts in the symphyseal disc.
  - Chronic tendinopathy or tears of the adductor origin.

OTHER RECOMMENDED TESTING

- In patients with osteoporosis, testing for hyperparathyroidism, panhypopituitarism, and sex hormone deficits.
- Electromyography and nerve conduction velocity testing are indicated if radiculopathy is present.

DIFFERENTIAL DIAGNOSIS

- Pathologic fracture due to tumor.
- Muscle strain.
- Piriformis syndrome.
- Tendinitis of the groin.
- Osteomyelitis.
- Insufficiency fractures.

TREATMENT

- Opioids for acute pain relief.
- Injection of the pubic symphysis with local anesthetics and corticosteroids.
- Decreased activity if osteitis due to overtraining.
- Local ice application.

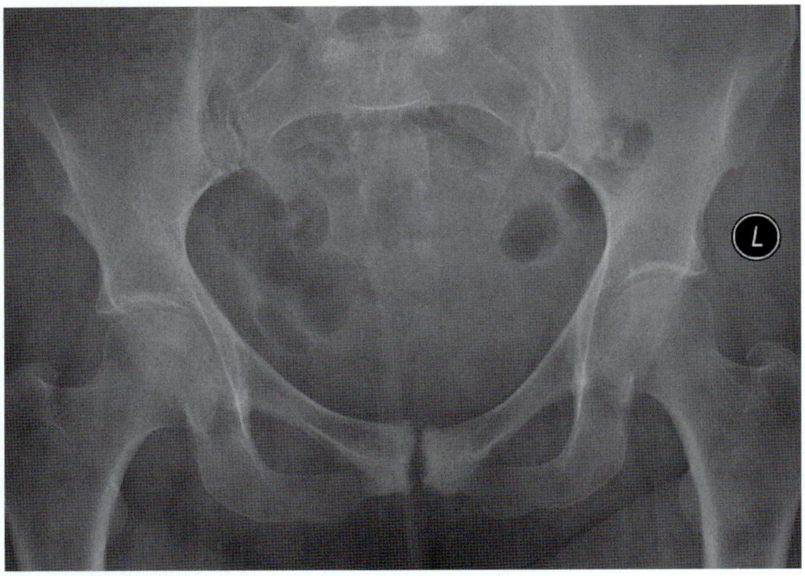

Figure 82.1 AP radiograph of the pelvis demonstrating chronic stress-related noninfective changes around the symphysis pubis with bony sclerosis and erosion of the bony margins.

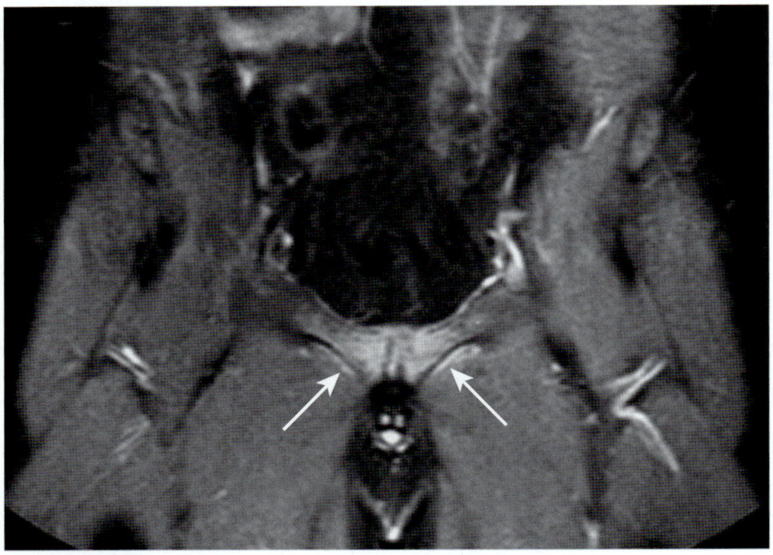

Figure 82.2 Coronal STIR MR image of osteitis pubis with high–signal intensity (SI) marrow edema in both pubic bones (*white arrows*). There is also minor periosteal edema.

CHAPTER 83

Intrasacral Meningocele

DEFINITION

- Cysts within the sacrum that typically do not transgress the margins of the sacrum.
- A variety of intrasacral "cysts" occur, and classification depends partly on the presence of nerve root fibers within the wall of the cyst. These include:
  - Tarlov perineural cysts.
  - Intradural arachnoid cysts.
  - Extradural arachnoid cysts.

SIGNS AND SYMPTOMS

- Often an incidental finding on imaging.
- Insidious onset of low back pain.
- Pain may radiate in a radicular or nondermatomal pattern.
- Bladder dysfunction may be present.

DEMOGRAPHICS

- All ages.
- Incidence: Female > Male.
- No racial predilection.

IMAGING RECOMMENDATIONS

- MRI.
- CT myelography:
  - Alternative to MRI.

IMAGING FINDINGS

- Rounded "cystic" dilatation within the sacral canal.
- Pressure erosion of sacral bodies or neural foramen.
- Rarely transgresses anterior margin of anterior wall.
- Delayed filling with contrast agent on myelography.
- Important to differentiate intrasacral cysts from:
  - Solid masses with bone destruction.
  - Meningoceles.

OTHER RECOMMENDED TESTING

- Electromyography and nerve conduction velocity testing are indicated if radiculopathy is present.
- Evoked potential testing is indicated if myelopathy is present.

DIFFERENTIAL DIAGNOSIS

- Pathologic fracture due to tumor.
- Tarlov cyst.
- Dural dysplasia.
- Sacral dysgenesis with true sacral meningocele or myelomeningocele.
- Sacral chordoma.

TREATMENT

- Opioids for acute pain relief.
- Caudal epidural injections of local anesthetics, opioids, and/or corticosteroids for pain not relieved by opioids.
- Surgery for persistent pain and/or neural dysfunction.

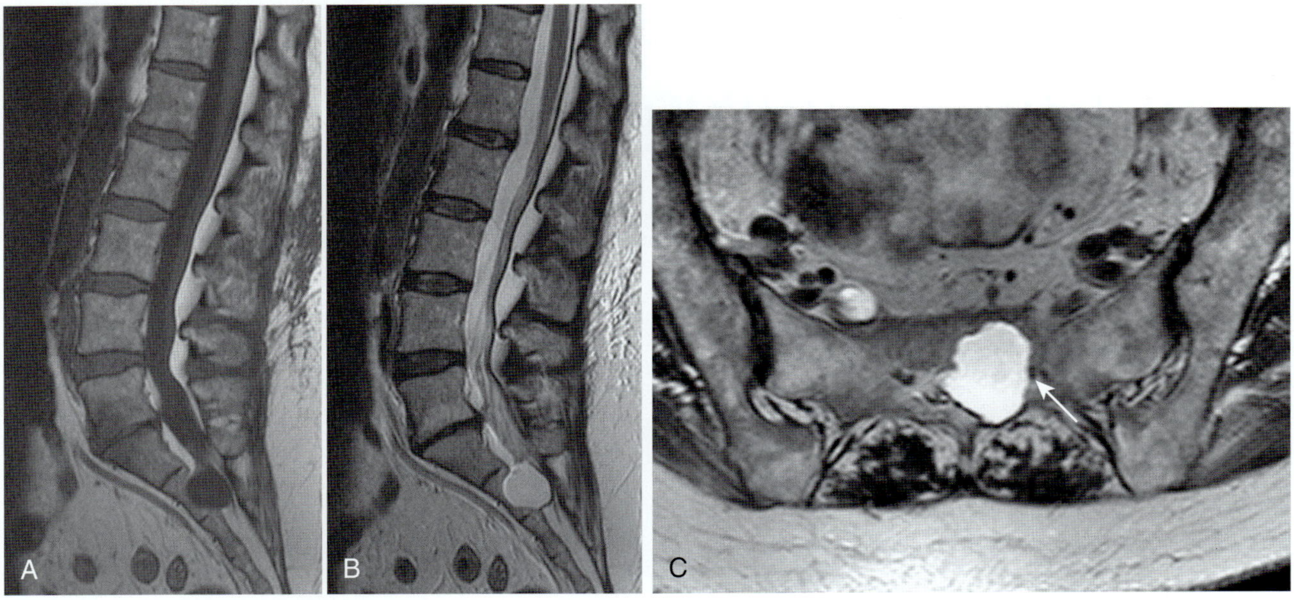

Figure 83.1 (**A**), Sagittal T1-weighted (T1W) MR image with an intermediate–signal intensity (SI) rounded lesion within the sacral canal that is causing pressure erosion of the posterior wall of the S2 segment. (**B**),The lesion has the same SI as cerebrospinal fluid on the T2W MR image, confirming its cystic nature, and the appearances are consistent with a small arachnoid cyst. (**C**), The axial T2W MR image shows the traversing nerve root fibers within the lateral wall of the cyst (*white arrow*). The patient has disc degeneration at the L5-S1 level with Modic type I (marrow edema) vertebral end-plate changes. This is more likely than the intrasacral cyst to be the cause of the back pain.

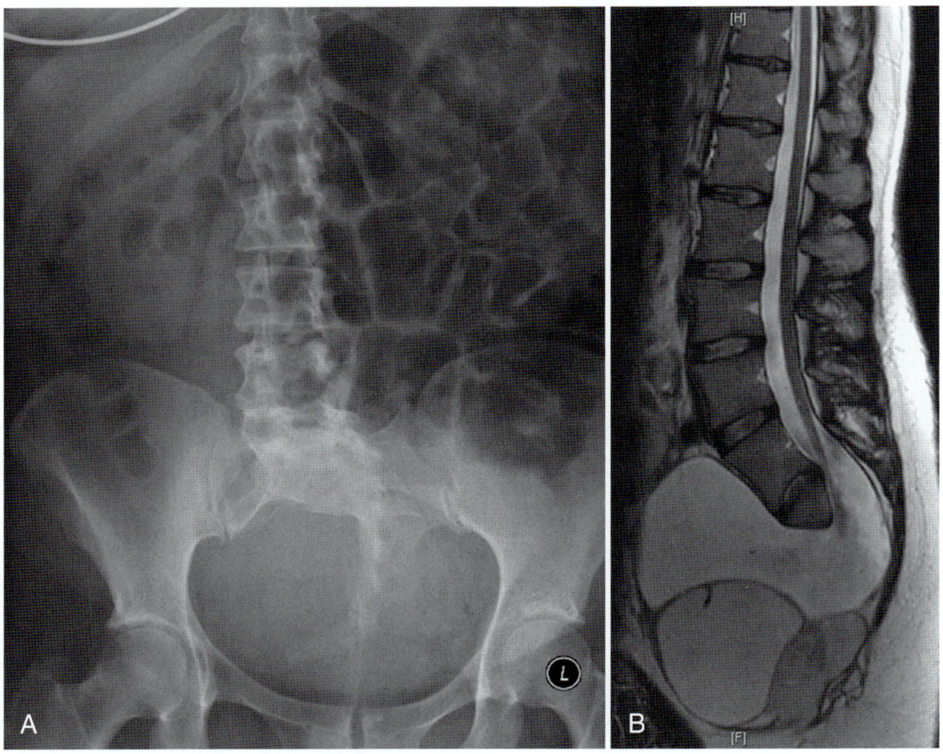

Figure 83.2 (**A**), AP radiograph of a patient with congenital partial sacral dysgenesis. The right half of the sacrum is absent, and there is a rotational deformity of the lower lumbar spine. (**B**), The sagittal T2W MR image shows the sacral dysgenesis associated with a large sacral and intrapelvic cyst. There is also a low-lying tethered cord with neural elements entering the cyst, confirming the diagnosis of a myelomeningocele.

PART 3 • THE EXTREMITIES

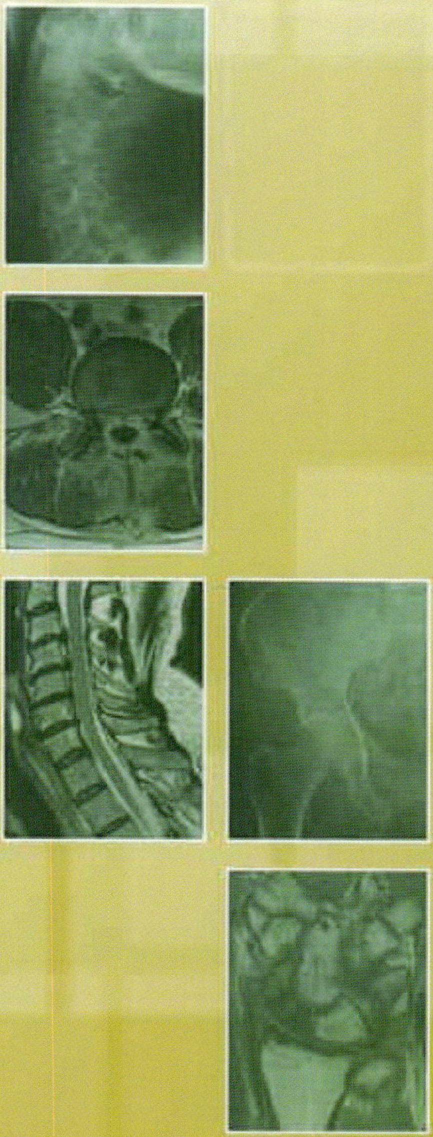

CHAPTER 84

General Principles of Joint Imaging

General Principles

Synovial joints are affected by a variety of pathologic processes, which include the following:

- Physical trauma:
  - Acute or chronic due to repetitive trauma.
- Arthritis:
  - Osteoarthritis.
  - Inflammatory arthritides.
  - Crystal arthropathies.
  - Connective tissue disorders.
- Infection.
- Avascular necrosis.
- Proliferative synovial disorders:
  - Pigmented villonodular synovitis (PVNS).
  - Synovial osteochondromatosis.
  - Amyloid.
  - Lipoma arborescens.

IMAGING SUPPLEMENTS

- Clinical history and physical examination.
- Laboratory tests.
- Joint aspiration.
- Synovial biopsy.

IMAGING RECOMMENDATIONS

The clinical diagnosis helps define standard radiologic investigative pathways.

Physical Trauma

- Radiography.
- CT:
  - Acute injuries to define fracture anatomy prior to surgery.
  - Loose bodies.
- MRI:
  - Occult osteochondral injury.
  - Ligamentous and fibrocartilage injury.
  - Tendon and other juxta-articular soft tissue injuries.
- MR/CT arthrography:
  - Preferred for articular and fibrocartilage injuries in some joints.

Arthritis

- Radiography:
  - Joint space narrowing.
  - Soft tissue swelling.
  - Bone loss:
    Osteopenia.
    Erosions.
    Subchondral cysts.
  - Reactive bone formation:
    Subchondral sclerosis.
    Osteophyte formation.
    Entheseal bone formation.
    Periostitis.
  - Soft tissue calcification.
  - Joint alignment.
- US:
  - Screening for synovitis and erosions.
  - To guide joint aspirations and injections.
- MRI:
  - Problem-solving tool for monoarthropathy:
    Differentiation from other synovial proliferative disorders.
  - Early osteoarthritis of the large joints.

Septic Arthritis

- Radiography.
- US:
  - Identification of joint effusions.
  - To guide joint aspiration.
- MRI:
  - Suspected complication of osteomyelitis.

Avascular Necrosis

- Radiography.
- MRI:
  - Staging of avascular necrosis and detection of occult disease.

Proliferative Synovial Disorders

- Radiography:
  - Soft issue swelling.
  - Erosions.
  - Soft tissue calcification.

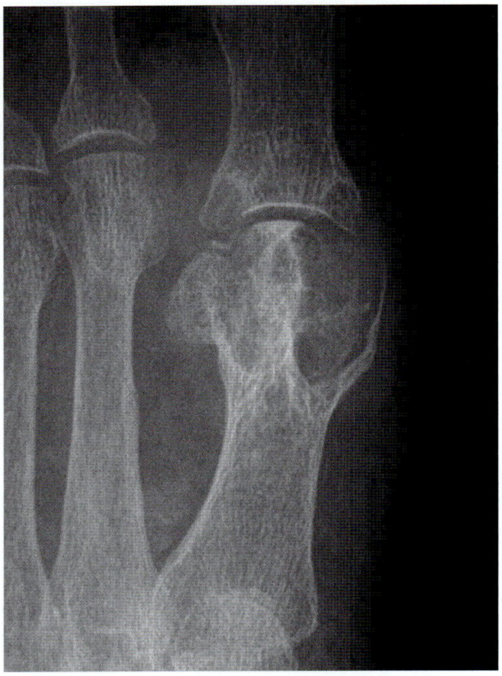

Figure 84.1 AP radiograph of the large toe in a patient with gout. There are generalized osteopenia and a large punched-out bone erosion of the first metacarpal, with smaller erosions in the proximal phalanx.

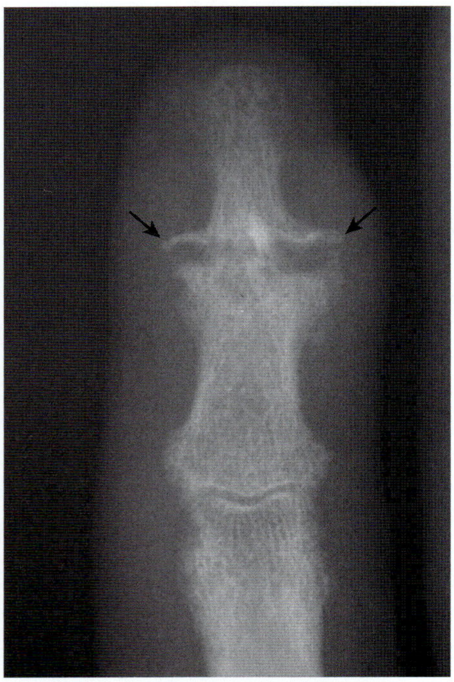

Figure 84.2 AP radiograph of the index finger, showing erosion around the distal interphalangeal joint and prominent entheseal bone formation (*black arrows*). These features are typical of psoriatic arthropathy.

- MRI:
  - Specific MRI features:
    Hemosiderin deposition (PVNS/hemophilic arthropathy).
    Cartilaginous metaplasia (osteochondromatosis).
    Fat (lipoma arborescens).

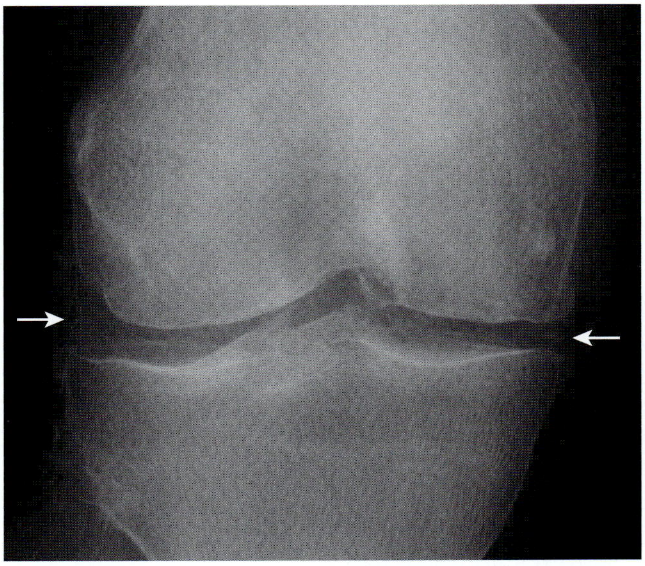

Figure 84.3 AP radiograph of a knee with chondrocalcinosis in the fibrocartilaginous menisci (*white arrows*) due to calcium pyrophosphate dihydrate (CPPD) deposition disease.

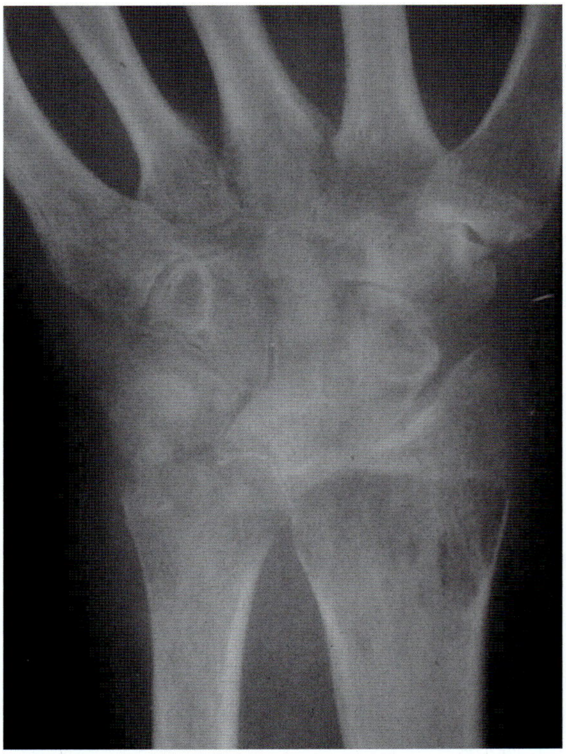

Figure 84.4 AP radiograph of the wrist of a patient with an acute monoarthropathy. There are profound osteopenia and joint space narrowing due to septic arthritis. The diagnosis was confirmed by US and joint aspiration.

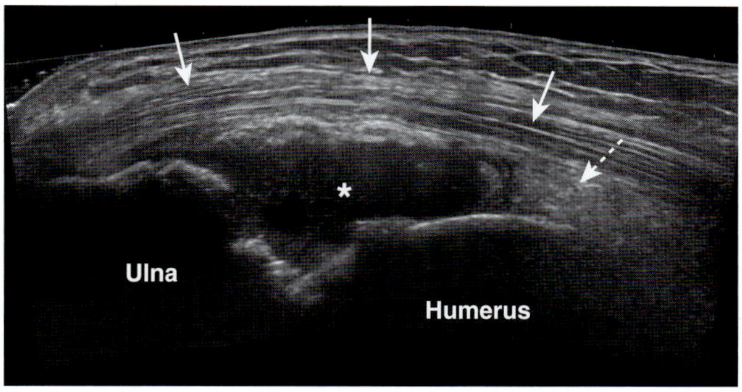

Figure 84.5 Longitudinal US image of the elbow of a patient with rheumatoid arthritis. A prominent low-reflective joint effusion (*asterisk*) deep to the triceps tendon (*white arrows*) is displacing the hyper-reflective posterior fat pad (*broken white arrow*).

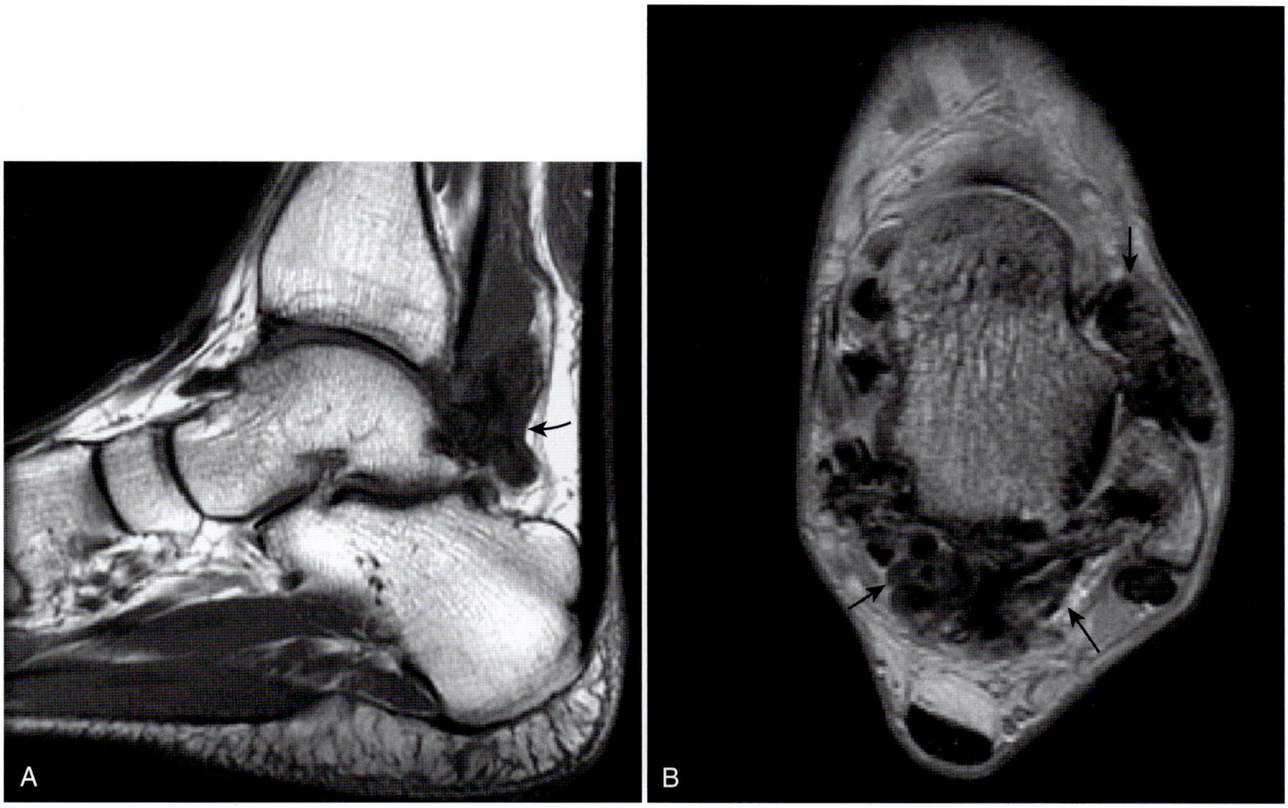

Figure 84.6 Sagittal T1-weighted (T1W) (**A**) and axial T2W (**B**) MR images demonstrating low–signal intensity (SI) synovial thickening around the ankle joint (*black arrows*) on both pulse sequences. These features are due to hemosiderin deposition in a patient with PVNS. Similar low-SI changes within a joint may be seen with calcification, amyloid deposition, or gas.

CHAPTER 85

Anatomy: Special Imaging Considerations of the Shoulder

- The shoulder comprises the glenohumeral joint, acromioclavicular joint, rotator cuff muscles, and associated tendons and ligaments.
- These structures interact to provide multiaxial movement of the upper limb, but at the cost of inherent instability.
- The shoulder can be imaged by various modalities, depending on the specific clinical question and on the specific anatomic structure forming the focus of the examination.

OSSEOUS STRUCTURES

Humeral Head (HH). Incomplete sphere covered by articular cartilage.

Greater Tuberosity. Superolateral aspect of HH anteriorly and centrally that bears the insertion or footprint of the supraspinatus tendon (SST). The infraspinatus tendon (IST) and teres minor tendon insert posteriorly.

Lesser Tuberosity. Vertically oriented ridge on the anterior aspect of the HH bearing the insertion of the subscapularis tendon (SCT).

Bicipital Groove. Osseous groove between the lesser and greater tuberosities within which runs the long head of the biceps tendon (LHB).

Glenoid. Concave ovoid surface covered by hyaline cartilage arising from the scapula neck, which articulates with the humeral head.

Acromion. Anteriorly projecting process arising from the lateral end of the scapula spine that bears the insertion of the deltoid muscle on the lateral and posterior aspects and of the coracoacromial ligament anteriorly. The acromion forms a synovial joint with the lateral end of the clavicle.

Coracoid Process. Arises from the anterosuperior aspect of the scapula head and projects anteriorly, bearing attachments of the coracoacromial ligament, coracoclavicular ligament, coracobrachialis muscle, and short head of the biceps muscle.

Clavicle. S-shaped bone articulating medially with the manubrium to form the sternoclavicular joint (SCJ), and the acromion laterally, to form the acromioclavicular joint (ACJ).

JOINTS

Glenohumeral Joint (GHJ). A synovial ball-and-socket joint formed by articulation of the humeral head with the glenoid and capable of a multiaxial range of motion. GHJ stability is increased by the glenoid labrum, a fibrocartilaginous ring attached to the glenoid rim that increases contact surface area. The GHJ possesses a synovial capsule that is lax anteriorly and inferiorly, facilitating abduction and external rotation.

Acromioclavicular Joint. A synovial joint formed between the lateral end of the clavicle and the acromion, often containing an articular disc. The ACJ is stabilized by the joint capsule and the coracoclavicular ligament.

SOFT TISSUES

Rotator Cuff Muscles

Subscapularis. A broad, vertically oriented muscle arising from the anterior surface of the scapula, forming a tendon (SCT) insertion on the lesser tuberosity, and acting to perform internal shoulder rotation.

Supraspinatus. Arises within the supraspinous fossa of the scapula, forming a broad tendon insertion (footprint) on the greater tuberosity and acting to perform shoulder abduction.

Infraspinatus. Arises from the posterior scapula, inferior to the scapula spine, and inserts laterally, forming a broad, obliquely orientated tendon (IST) insertion immediately behind the SST on the greater tuberosity.

Teres Minor. Arises from the scapula along the inferior border of the infraspinatus and projects laterally to form a tendon insertion on the posterolateral humeral neck below the IST insertion.

Other Soft Tissue Structures

Long Head of Biceps Tendon. Runs vertically within the bicipital groove to enter the GHJ, then courses medially between the anterior border of the SST and upper border of the SCT in a space called the *rotator interval*. The LHB inserts into the superior labrum and supraglenoid tubercle, forming the biceps anchor.

Subacromial Bursa. A synovium-lined space covering the IST and SST footprints, extending medially beneath the ACJ. It is continuous with the subdeltoid bursa laterally and posteriorly and with the subscapularis bursa anteriorly.

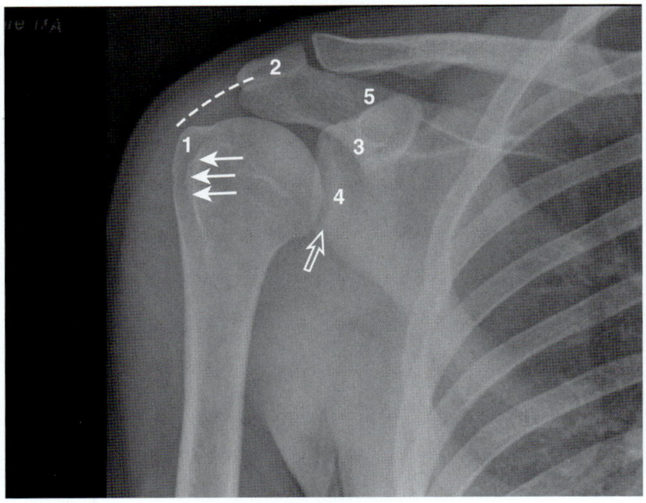

Figure 85.1 AP radiograph of the shoulder: 1, greater tuberosity; 2, acromion; 3, coracoid process; 4, glenoid (anterior rim); 5, scapula spine; *white solid arrows,* lesser tuberosity; *black solid arrow,* acromioclavicular joint; *white open arrow,* glenohumeral joint; *dashed line,* subdeltoid fat plane (outline of subacromial bursa).

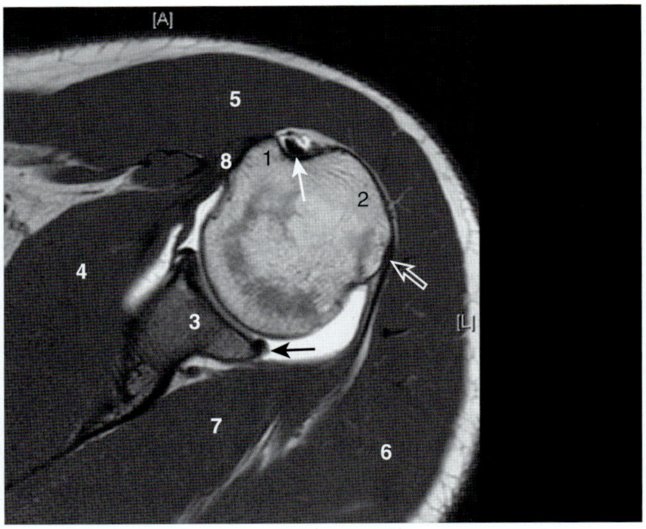

Figure 85.3 Axial T1-weighted MR arthrogram image of the shoulder: 1, lesser tuberosity; 2, greater tuberosity; 3, glenoid; 4, subscapularis muscle; 5, anterior deltoid muscle; 6, posterior deltoid muscle; 7, teres minor muscle; 8, subscapularis tendon; *white arrow,* long head of biceps (LHB) tendon; *open white arrow,* teres minor tendon; *black arrow,* glenoid labrum.

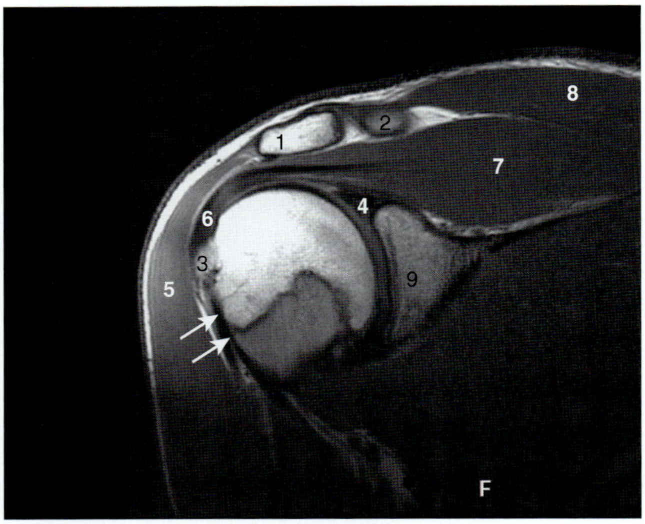

Figure 85.2 Coronal proton density–weighted MR image of the shoulder: 1, acromion; 2, lateral end of clavicle; 3, greater tuberosity; 4, glenoid labrum; 5, deltoid muscle; 6, supraspinatus tendon insertion (footprint); 7, supraspinatus muscle; 8, trapezius; 9, glenoid; *white arrows,* long head of biceps (LHB) tendon.

CHAPTER 86

Osteoarthritis of the Glenohumeral Joint

DEFINITION

- Degenerative arthritis characterized by destruction of the chondral surfaces, subchondral cysts, synovitis, and osteophyte formation.

SIGNS AND SYMPTOMS

- Gradual onset of pain with range of motion of the shoulder joint.
- Effusion may be present.
- Crepitus may be present.
- Gradual decrease in range of motion.

DEMOGRAPHICS

- Incidence: Male > Female.
- Most common in elderly patients; also seen in younger patients after shoulder joint trauma and/or surgery.
- Universal finding after fifth decade of life.
- Often a history of joint trauma.
- May be a genetic predisposition.

IMAGING RECOMMENDATIONS

- Radiography is the first-line investigation of arthropathy.
- MRI:
  - Assess intra-articular structures and status of rotator cuff.
  - Assess cartilage loss.
- MR/CT arthrography:
  - Specialist investigation for associated abnormalities such as instability, to assess labrum, ligaments, and articular cartilage.
- US:
  - Assessment of rotator cuff.
  - Identification of effusions and synovitis.
  - Guidance for joint aspiration and injection.

IMAGING FINDINGS

- Joint space narrowing, subchondral sclerosis, subchondral cysts, and osteophyte formation.
- Narrowing of subacromial space on radiographs indicates rotator cuff failure.
- Frequent association with osteoarthritis (OA) in the acromioclavicular (AC) joint.

OTHER RECOMMENDED TESTING

- Laboratory testing to rule out inflammatory arthritis.
- Joint aspiration to rule out crystal arthropathies.
- Joint aspiration to rule out infection.

DIFFERENTIAL DIAGNOSIS

- Inflammatory arthritides, especially rheumatoid arthritis.
- Septic shoulder joint.
- Healing shoulder joint fracture, especially of the glenoid rim.
- Rotator cuff tear.
- Crystal arthropathy of shoulder.
- Avascular osteonecrosis.

TREATMENT

- Conservative treatment consisting of local heat, cold, simple analgesics, and nonsteroidal anti-inflammatory agents will improve symptoms in many cases.
- Physical therapy, including gentle stretching, range-of-motion exercises, and deep heat modalities, may be beneficial in selected patients.
- Intra-articular injection with local anesthetic and steroid will provide symptomatic relief if conservative therapy fails or the pain is limiting activities of daily living.
- Surgery may be required for persistent pain or progressive functional disability.

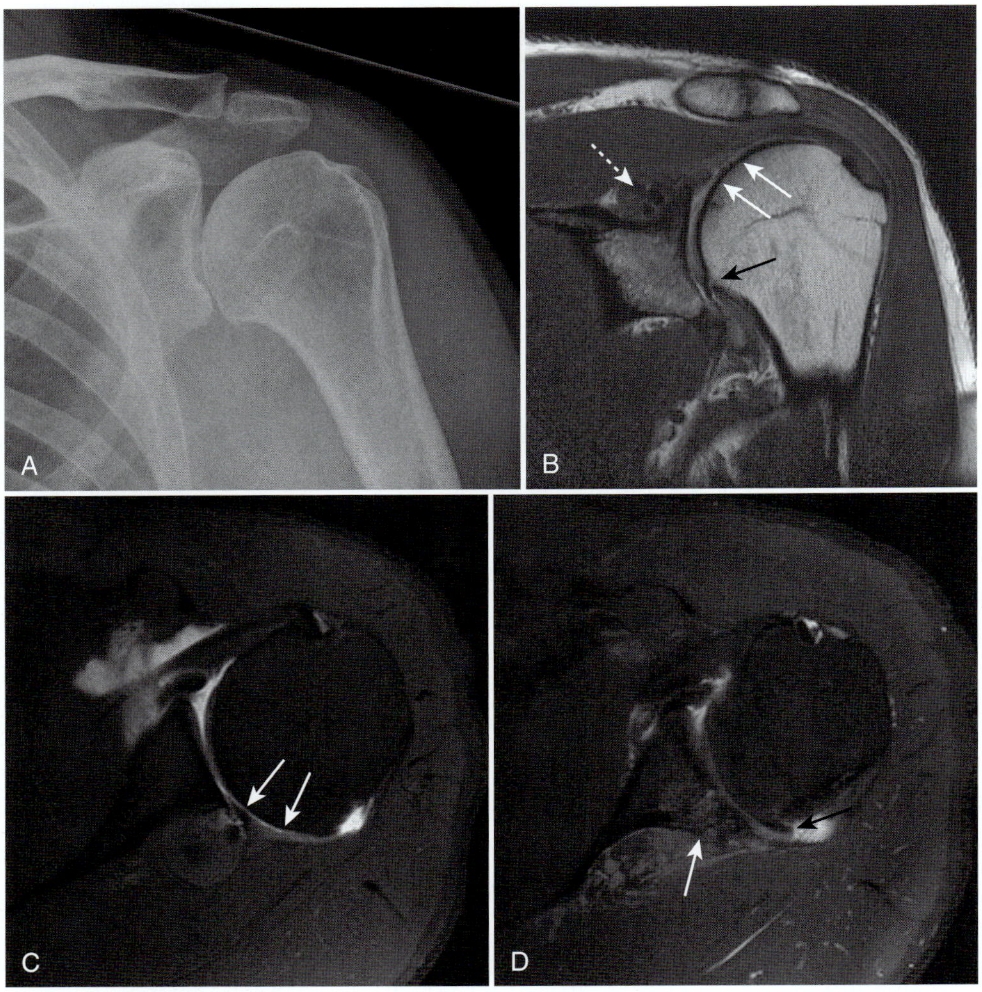

Figure 86.1 (**A**), AP radiograph of a patient with early OA of the glenohumeral joint. There is asymmetrical joint space narrowing and minor inferior osteophyte formation. The AC joint is normal, and the subacromial space is preserved. (**B**), The coronal T1-weighted (T1W) MR arthrogram image demonstrates chondral thinning (*white arrows*), the inferior osteophyte (*black arrow*), and low–signal intensity (SI) loose bodies within the spinoglenoid notch (*broken arrow*). (**C**), The chondral thinning is also seen on an axial T1W with fat suppression (FST1W) MR image (*white arrows*). (**D**), On a more inferior axial FST1W MR image, the osteophytes (*black arrow*) are visualized in association with bony eburnation of the posterior glenoid (*thick white arrow*).

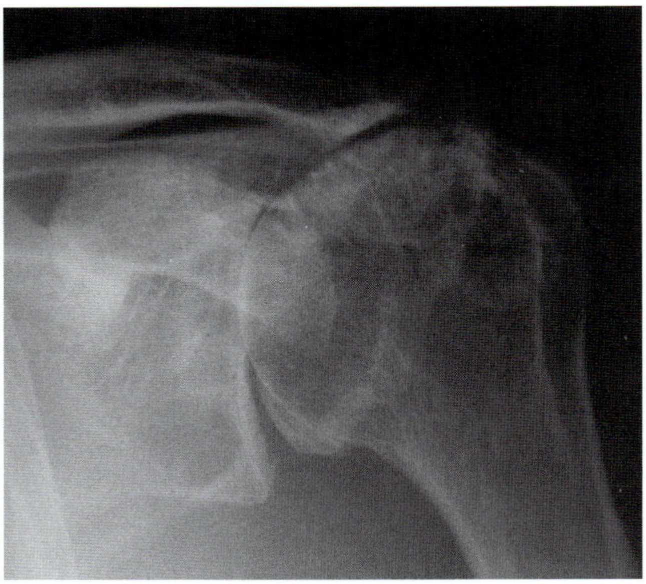

Figure 86.2 AP radiograph of a patient with severe glenohumeral joint OA secondary to rotator cuff failure (cuff arthropathy). Note the superior migration of the humeral head with complete loss of the subacromial space and bony eburnation of the acromion.

CHAPTER 87

Osteonecrosis of the Glenohumeral Joint

DEFINITION

- The death of cellular components of bone due to interruption of the blood supply with resultant pain, collapse and destruction of bone, and loss of function.

SIGNS AND SYMPTOMS

- Gradual onset of pain with decreasing range of motion of the shoulder joint.
- Crepitus may be present.
- Functional disability may be severe.

DEMOGRAPHICS

- Incidence: Male > Female.
- Age at onset related to date of trauma or onset of underlying disease, with sickle cell disease being the most common inciting factor in younger patients.
- Most common following shoulder joint trauma that disrupts the vascular supply.
- Common site of involvement by dysbaric osteonecrosis in deep sea divers.
- More common in patients with sickle cell disease, Gaucher disease, Fabry disease, systemic lupus erythematosus (SLE), and gout.
- Associated with exogenous steroid therapy and heavy alcohol intake.

IMAGING RECOMMENDATIONS

- Radiography.
- MRI:
  - Normal or equivocal radiographic findings.
  - Preoperative planning.

IMAGING FINDINGS

- Radiography:
  - Sclerosis in the subarticular humeral head.
  - In later stages, subchondral lucency and collapse eventually leading to fragmentation and destruction of the articular surface.
  - Serpiginous lines of sclerosis in intramedullary infarcts.
- MRI:
  - High-signal intensity (SI) edema in the humeral head on short T1 inversion recovery (STIR) images.
  - Low-SI subchondral sclerosis on T1-weighted (T1W) and T2W MR images.
  - Subchondral crescent sign.
  - Eventual subchondral collapse and fragmentation.
  - Double-line sign of intramedullary infarcts on T2W MR images.

OTHER RECOMMENDED TESTING

- Laboratory testing to rule out SLE.
- Laboratory testing to rule out gout.
- Joint aspiration to rule out crystal arthropathies.
- Joint aspiration to rule out infection.

DIFFERENTIAL DIAGNOSIS

- Inflammatory arthritides, especially SLE.
- Osteoarthritis.
- Bone marrow tumors.
- Primary bone tumors.
- Metastatic tumors.
- Osteochondral injuries.

TREATMENT

- Conservative treatment consisting of local heat, cold, simple analgesics, and nonsteroidal anti-inflammatory agents will improve symptoms in many cases.
- Physical therapy, including gentle stretching, range-of-motion exercises, and deep heat modalities, may be beneficial in selected patients.
- Intra-articular injection with local anesthetic and steroid will provide symptomatic relief if conservative therapy fails or the pain is limiting activities of daily living.
- Surgery may ultimately be required for persistent pain or progressive functional disability.

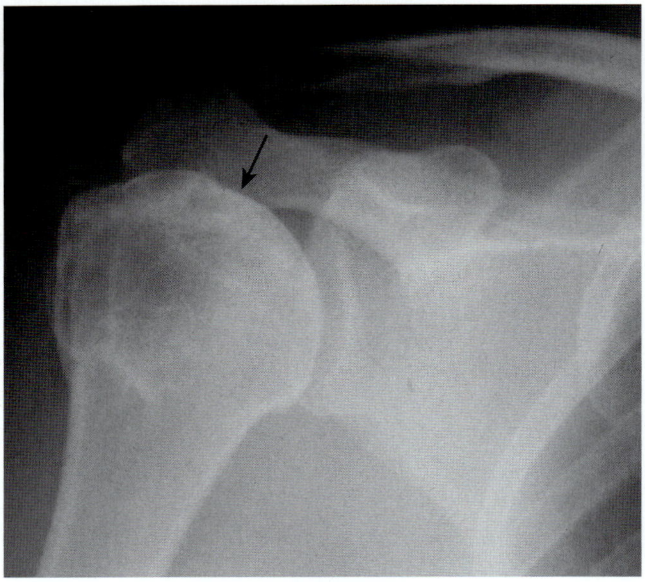

Figure 87.1 AP radiograph of a patient with dysbaric osteonecrosis. There is ill-defined subchondral sclerosis in the humeral head as well as early subchondral collapse and flattening of the articular surface (*black arrow*).

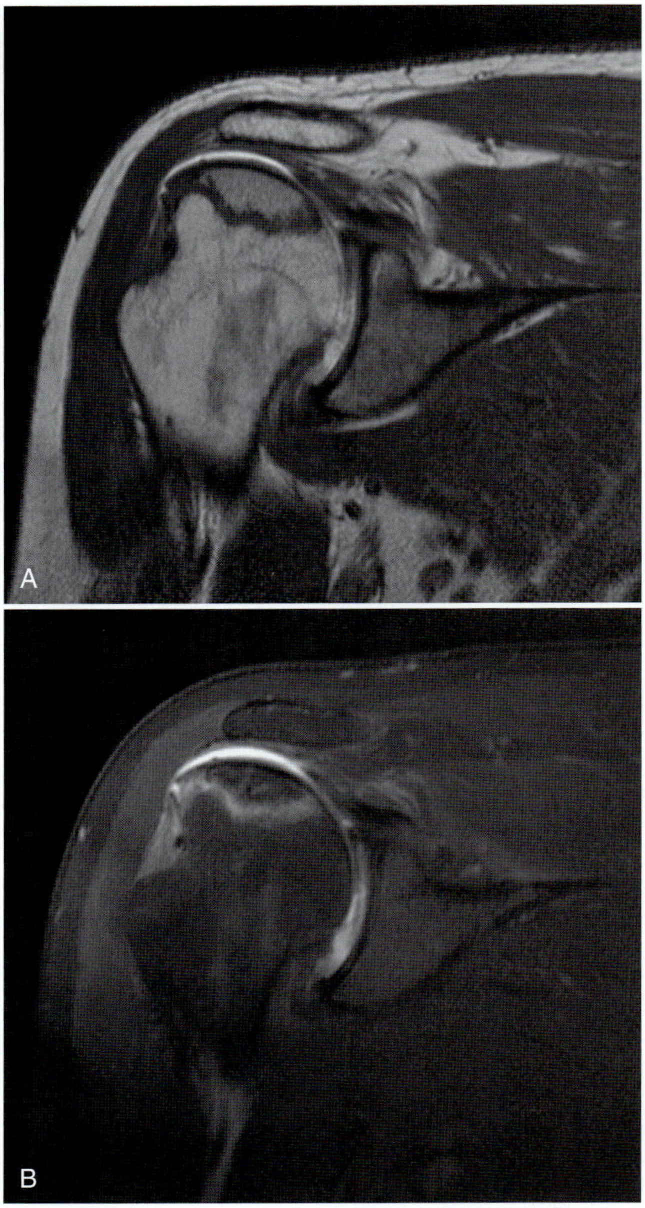

Figure 87.2 Coronal T1W (**A**) and T2W with fat suppression (FST2W) (**B**) MR images of a patient with previous dislocation of the shoulder show a large bony defect of the lateral aspect of the proximal humerus. In addition, there is early secondary avascular necrosis (AVN) of the superior aspect of the humeral head. A subchondral crescent marks the boundary of the area of AVN, which has low SI on the T1W MR image and high SI on the FST2W MR image.

CHAPTER 88

Rheumatoid Arthritis of the Glenohumeral Joint

DEFINITION

- Symmetrical inflammatory arthritis characterized by synovitis, joint space narrowing, effusions, erosions, and elevation of serum rheumatoid factor combined with a constellation of other clinical signs and symptoms.

SIGNS AND SYMPTOMS

- Pain with range of motion of the shoulder joint.
- Synovitis.
- Effusion often present.
- Warmth often present.
- Crepitus may be present.
- Morning stiffness.
- Gelling phenomenon.
- Gradual decrease in range of motion.
- Fatigue, lassitude, and mild fever.
- Symmetrical polyarthritis involving three or more joints invariably present on careful inspection.

DEMOGRAPHICS

- Incidence: Female > Male.
- Adult form most common, although juvenile form should be considered in any child with polyarthritis.
- Peak onset between the fourth and sixth decade of life.

IMAGING RECOMMENDATIONS

- Radiography is the primary investigation for arthropathy.
- MRI:
  - Assess synovitis, early erosions.
  - Assess cartilage loss.
- US:
  - Identify synovitis, effusions, and early erosions.
  - Guide joint aspiration and injection.

IMAGING FINDINGS

- Joint space narrowing, erosions, osteopenia.
- Reactive bone formation with osteophytes and sclerosis occurs only with secondary osteoarthritis (OA).
- Commonly, erosive disease in the acromioclavicular joint.
- Subacromial narrowing associated with rotator cuff failure.

OTHER RECOMMENDED TESTING

- Laboratory testing, including complete blood count, blood chemistry profile, and erythrocyte sedimentation rate measurement, to rule out extra-articular manifestations of the disease.
- Antinuclear antibody testing and systemic lupus erythematosus preparation test if diagnosis is in doubt.
- Joint aspiration to rule out crystal arthropathies.
- Joint aspiration to rule out infection.

DIFFERENTIAL DIAGNOSIS

- Other inflammatory arthritides, especially systemic lupus erythematosus arthritis.
- Charcot shoulder joint.
- Osteoarthritis.
- Psoriatic arthritis.
- Crystal arthropathy of the shoulder.
- Avascular osteonecrosis.

TREATMENT

- Disease-modifying agents, including gold salts, penicillamine, azathioprine, and cyclosporine A, can dramatically slow the progression of the disease, albeit not without side effects.
- Cytotoxic drugs, including methotrexate.
- Biologic agents, including interleukin and tumor necrosis factor-alpha (TNF-α).
- Salicylates, nonsteroidal anti-inflammatory agents, and corticosteroids.
- Physical and occupational therapies.
- Intra-articular injection of local anesthetic and corticosteroid for symptomatic relief and to aid in physical therapy.
- Surgery may be required for persistent pain or progressive functional disability.

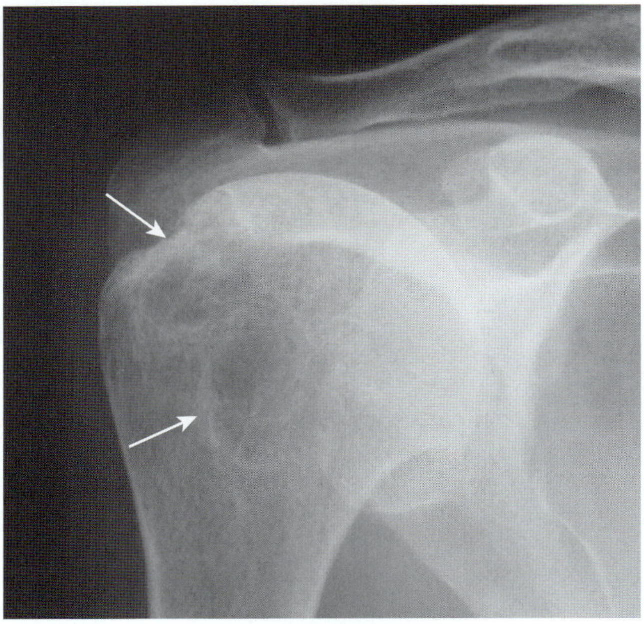

Figure 88.1 AP radiograph of the shoulder of a patient with rheumatoid arthritis. There are large erosions on the humeral head (*white arrows*), and the subacromial space is narrowed because of secondary cuff failure.

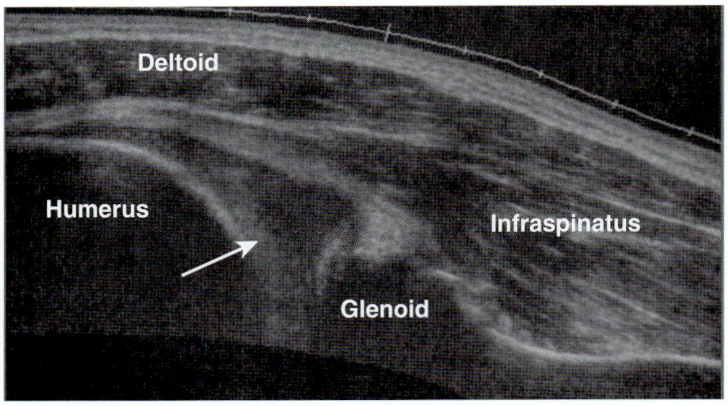

Figure 88.3 Transverse US image of the posterior aspect of the glenohumeral joint in a patient with rheumatoid arthritis. There is an effusion with echogenic debris (*white arrow*) due to the presence of fibrinous exudates.

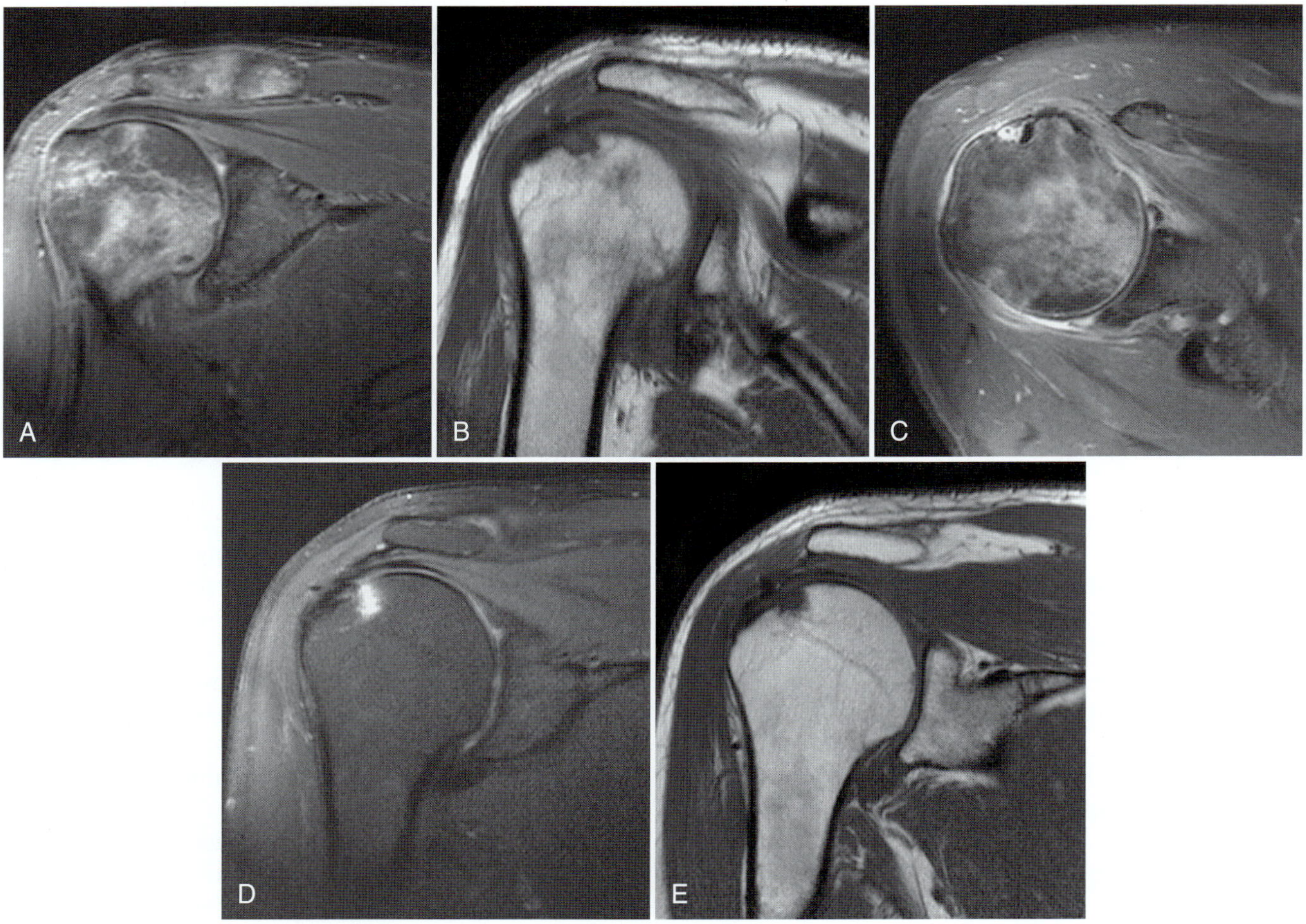

Figure 88.2 (**A**), Coronal T2-weighted MR image with fat suppression (FST2W) of a patient with an acute flare-up of rheumatoid arthritis. Radiographs showed only joint space narrowing. There is diffuse marrow edema in the humeral head as well as joint space narrowing with cartilage loss. (**B**), The coronal T1W MR image demonstrates a small erosion on the posterior humeral head. (**C**), There is diffuse high–signal intensity (SI) synovial enhancement on this axial FST1W MR image, which was acquired after intravenous administration of a contrast medium. Coronal FST2W (**D**) and T1W (**E**) MR images obtained a few weeks later, after anti–TNF-α therapy, show resolution of the marrow edema and synovitis. There is persistent joint space narrowing due to cartilage loss, but the bony erosion has not progressed.

CHAPTER 89

Osteoarthritis of the Acromioclavicular Joint

DEFINITION

- Degenerative arthritis characterized by destruction of the chondral surfaces, subchondral cysts, synovitis, and osteophyte formation.

SIGNS AND SYMPTOMS

- Gradual onset of anterosuperior pain with abnormal range of motion of the acromioclavicular (AC) joint.
- Effusion may be present.
- Crepitus may be present.
- Clicking or catching sensation may be present.
- Provocation of AC pain (positive result) with cross-body adduction test.
- Gradual decrease in range of motion.

DEMOGRAPHICS

- Incidence: Male > Female.
- Most common in elderly patients and seen in younger patients following shoulder joint trauma and/or surgery.
- Universal finding after the fifth decade of life.
- Often a history of joint trauma.

IMAGING RECOMMENDATIONS

- Radiography:
  - Lordotic and oblique views.
- MRI:
  - Part of assessment of rotator cuff in patients with impingement.
- US:
  - Demonstrates only the superior aspect of the joint.
  - May be used to identify dynamic instability.
  - Guides therapeutic injections.

IMAGING FINDINGS

- Osteophytes, sclerosis, and subchondral cysts.
- MRI also demonstrates:
  - Marrow edema.
  - Capsular thickening.
  - Pericapsular edema.
  - Associated subacromial bursitis and osteophyte impingement on the rotator cuff.
- AC joint synovial cysts in association with rotator cuff tears:
  - "Geyser" phenomenon.

OTHER RECOMMENDED TESTING

- Intra-articular injection of contrast agent and local anesthetic.
- Laboratory testing to rule out inflammatory arthritis.
- Joint aspiration to rule out crystal arthropathies.
- Joint aspiration to rule out infection.

DIFFERENTIAL DIAGNOSIS

- AC joint separation.
- Os acromiale.
- Post-traumatic arthritides.
- Inflammatory arthritides, especially rheumatoid arthritis.

TREATMENT

- Conservative treatment consisting of local heat, cold, simple analgesics, and nonsteroidal anti-inflammatory agents will improve symptoms in many cases.
- Physical therapy, including gentle stretching, range-of-motion exercises, and deep heat modalities, may be beneficial in selected patients.
- Intra-articular injection with local anesthetic and steroid will provide symptomatic relief if conservative therapy fails or the pain is limiting activities of daily living.
- Surgery may be required for persistent pain or progressive functional disability.

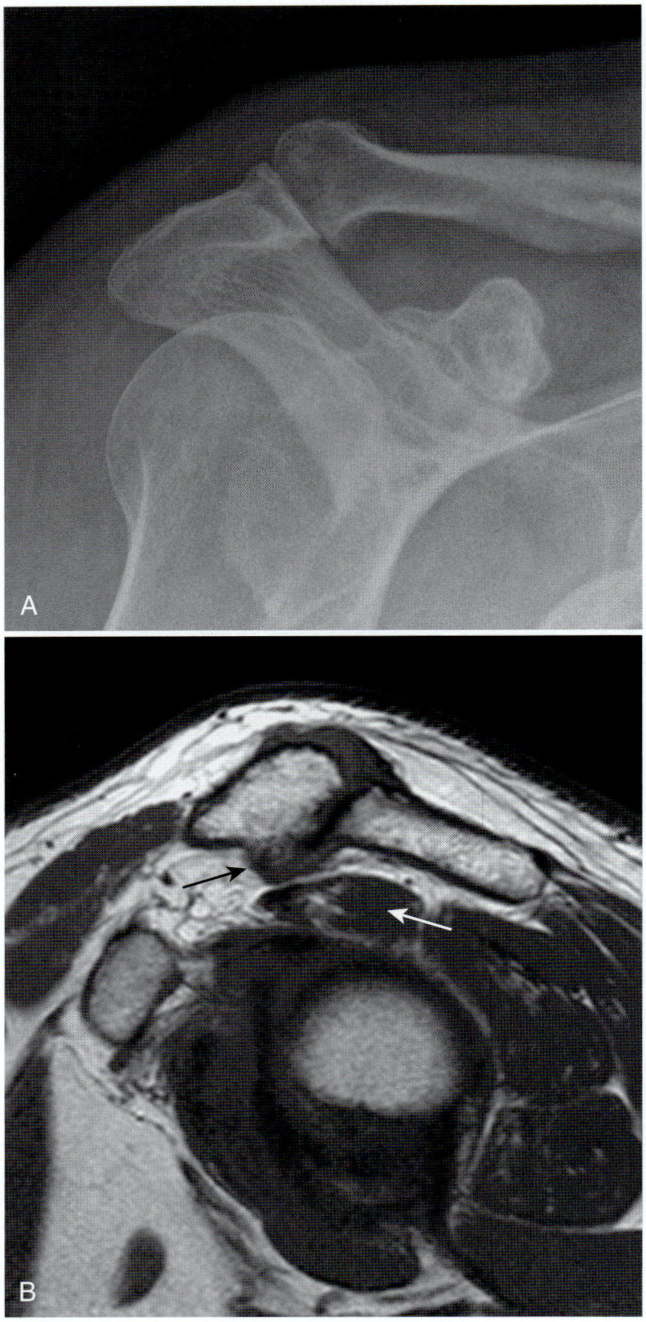

Figure 89.1 (**A**), Oblique radiograph demonstrating typical features of osteoarthritis (OA) changes with osteophytes and sclerosis. (**B**), The sagittal oblique T1-weighted (T1W) MR image shows the inferior osteophyte formation (*black arrow*), which does not impinge on the supraspinatus tendon (*white arrow*).

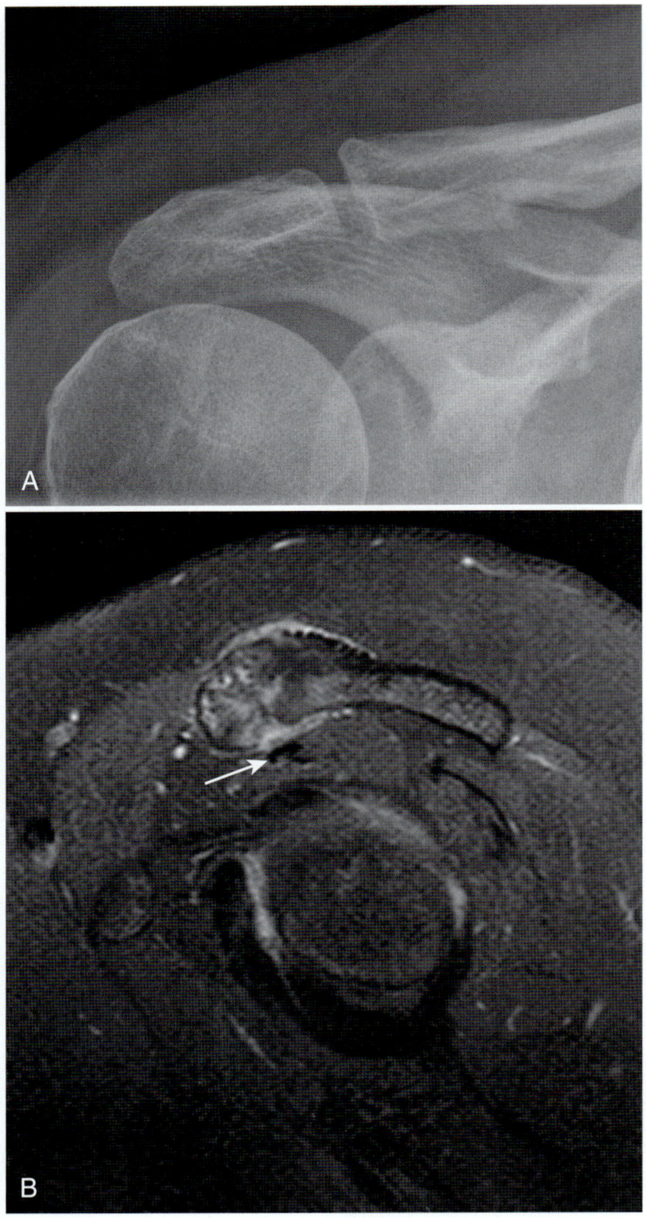

Figure 89.2 (**A**), AP radiograph of a patient with AC joint pain. There are no features of OA on the radiograph. (**B**), The oblique sagittal T2W MR image with fat suppression (FST2W), however, shows capsular thickening with high–signal intensity (SI) marrow edema and pericapsular edema in close relation to the supraspinatus muscle and tendon (*white arrow*).

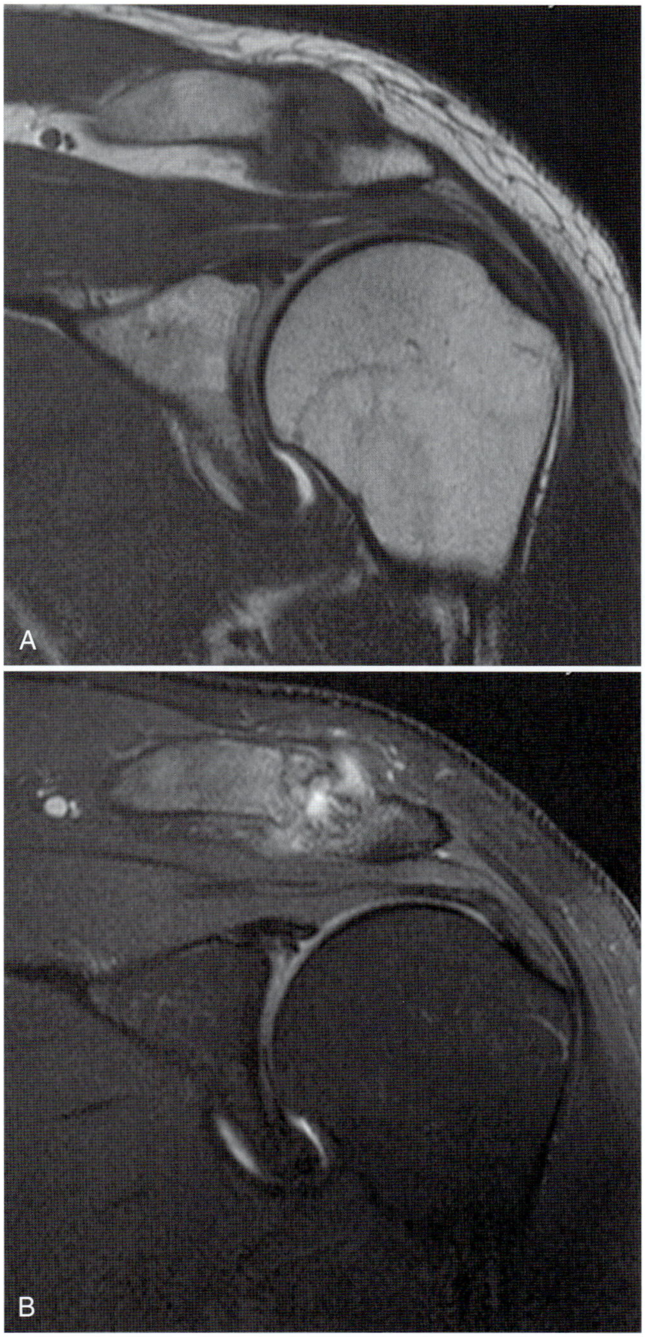

Figure 89.3 Coronal oblique T1W (**A**) and FST2W (**B**) MR images of a patient with OA of the AC joint with marrow edema and subchondral cyst formation. In addition, there is subluxation of the joint, indicating joint instability, which may contribute to subacromial impingement.

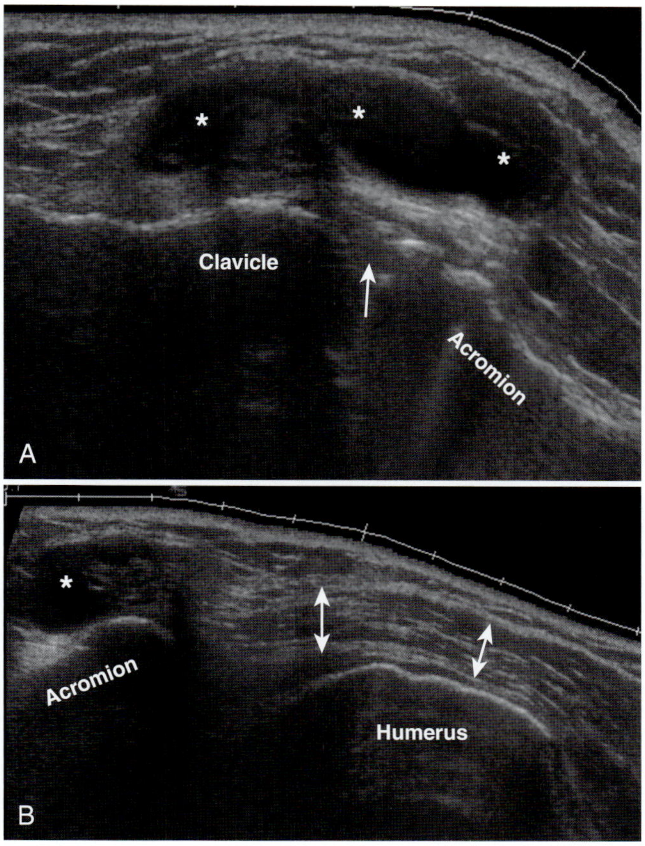

Figure 89.4 (**A**), Coronal US image of the AC joint (*white arrow*) with an overlying loculated anechoic cystic structure (*asterisks*). (**B**), The coronal image of the rotator cuff shows the deltoid muscle (*double-headed arrows*) lying directly on the humeral head with absence of the supraspinatus as a result of a massive cuff tear. The cyst occurs as a result of glenohumeral joint fluid communicating through the AC joint in association with the cuff tear, a finding referred to as the "geyser" phenomenon. A portion of the cyst is also visible on this image (*asterisk*).

CHAPTER 90

Os Acromiale

DEFINITION

- Failure of normal fusion of one or more of the distal ossification centers, resulting in separate distal ossicles. May contribute to external impingement.

SIGNS AND SYMPTOMS

- Gradual onset of anterosuperior shoulder pain.
- Exacerbation of pain with abduction of the shoulder.
- Exacerbation of pain with forward flexion of the shoulder.
- Clicking or catching sensation may be present.

DEMOGRAPHICS

- Incidence: Male > Female.
- Most common early in the third decade of life.
- Commonly associated with impingement syndrome.
- Commonly associated with rotator cuff tendinopathy.

IMAGING RECOMMENDATIONS

- Radiography:
  - Best visualized on subaxial view.
- MRI.

IMAGING FINDINGS

- Non-united ossification center.
- Reactive sclerosis in the pseudoarticulation is unusual, although there may be associated enthesopathy of the acromion owing due to impingement.
- Reactive edema may be seen in adjacent bone ends on short T1 inversion recovery (STIR) MR images.

OTHER RECOMMENDED TESTING

- Intra-articular injection of contrast medium and local anesthetic.
- If diagnosis is in question:
  - Laboratory testing to rule out inflammatory arthritis.
  - Joint aspiration to rule out crystal arthropathies and infection.

DIFFERENTIAL DIAGNOSIS

- Acromioclavicular joint separation.
- Distal clavicular fracture.
- Post-traumatic arthritides.
- Inflammatory arthritides, especially rheumatoid arthritis.
- Large subacromial vessel.

TREATMENT

- Conservative treatment consisting of local heat, cold, simple analgesics, and nonsteroidal anti-inflammatory agents will improve symptoms in many cases.
- Physical therapy, including gentle stretching, range-of-motion exercises, and deep heat modalities, may be beneficial in selected patients.
- Intra-articular injection with local anesthetic and steroid will provide symptomatic relief if conservative therapy fails or the pain is limiting activities of daily living.
- Surgery may be required for persistent pain or progressive functional disability.

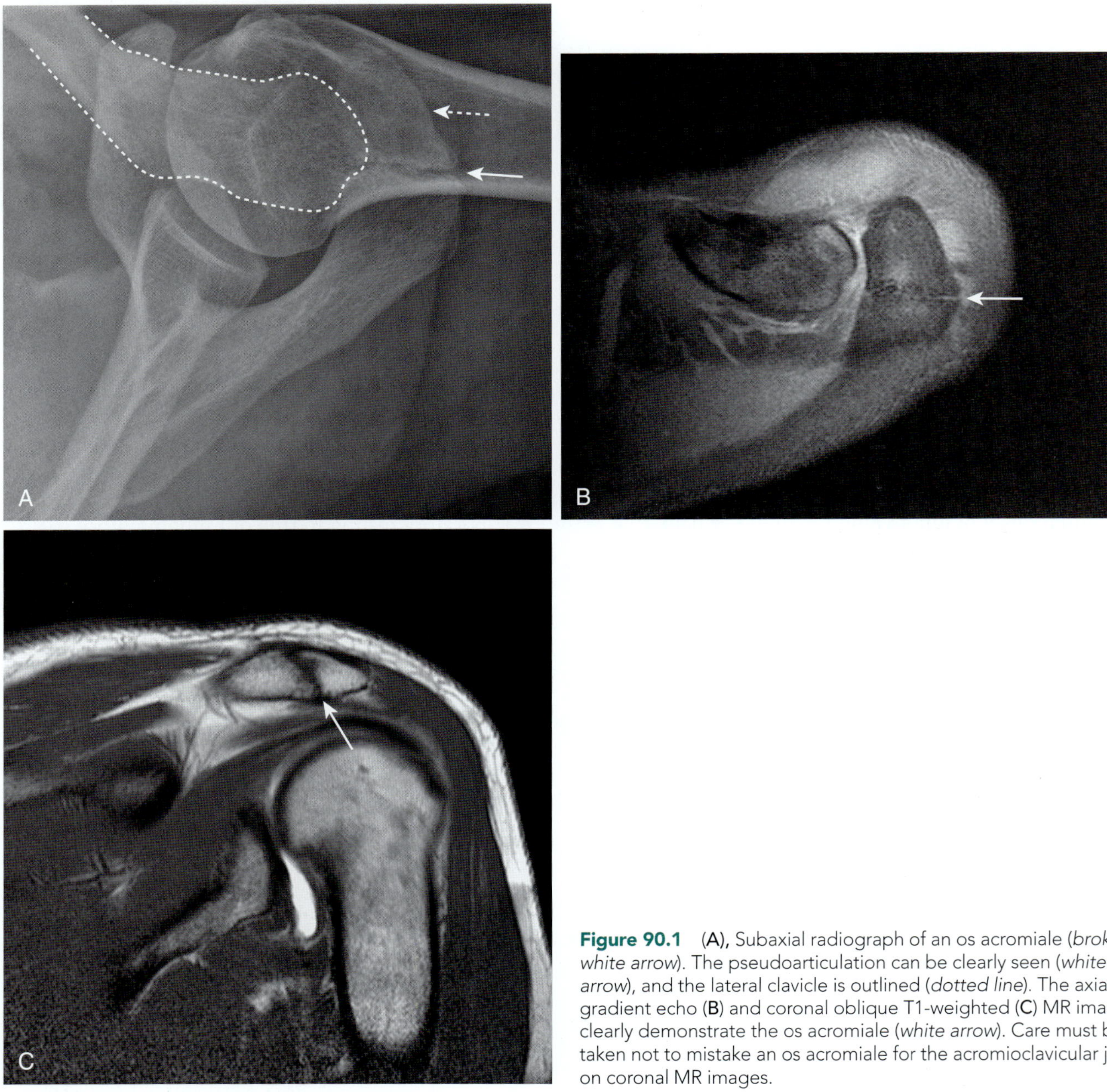

Figure 90.1 (A), Subaxial radiograph of an os acromiale (*broken white arrow*). The pseudoarticulation can be clearly seen (*white arrow*), and the lateral clavicle is outlined (*dotted line*). The axial gradient echo (B) and coronal oblique T1-weighted (C) MR images clearly demonstrate the os acromiale (*white arrow*). Care must be taken not to mistake an os acromiale for the acromioclavicular joint on coronal MR images.

CHAPTER 91

Rotator Cuff Tendinopathy

DEFINITION

- Degeneration of the collagenous elements of the tendons that make up the rotator cuff.

SIGNS AND SYMPTOMS

- Gradual onset of anterolateral pain with decreased range of motion of the shoulder joint.
- Weakness.
- Crepitus may be present.
- Exacerbation of pain with overhead activities.
- Pain often worse at night.
- Patient unable to sleep on affected shoulder.
- Gradual decrease in range of motion.

DEMOGRAPHICS

- Slight female preponderance.
- Young athletes often affected.
- 40- to 50-year-old persons most commonly affected.
- Supraspinatus tendon most commonly affected.
- More common after trauma, including repetitive stress injuries.

IMAGING RECOMMENDATIONS

- MRI or US.
- Radiography:
  - To exclude calcific tendinitis.
  - To exclude associated glenohumeral arthropathy in older patients.
- Imaging mainly required to:
  - Exclude rotator cuff tear.
  - Identify associated features of external impingement.

IMAGING FINDINGS

- Tendon thickening.
- High signal intensity (SI) within tendon on T2-weighted (T2W) MR images or T2W MR images with fat saturation.
  - Short TE MR images are subject to magic angle effects: (artifact creating increased SI within tendons)
- Low-echo change and loss of fibrillar pattern on US.
- Features of external impingement:
  - Subacromial bursitis.
  - Enthesopathy of acromion and tuberosity.
  - Osteoarthritis in the acromioclavicular joint.
  - Abnormality of acromial morphology.

OTHER RECOMMENDED TESTING

- Laboratory testing to rule out inflammatory arthritis.
- Joint aspiration to rule out crystal arthropathies.
- Joint aspiration to rule out infection if diagnosis is in question.

DIFFERENTIAL DIAGNOSIS

- Calcific tendinitis.
- Partial-thickness rotator cuff tear.
- Complete rotator cuff tear.
- Cyst involving one of the tendons of the rotator cuff.
- Posterosuperior glenoid impingement syndrome.

TREATMENT

- Conservative treatment consisting of local heat, cold, simple analgesics, and nonsteroidal anti-inflammatory agents will improve symptoms in many cases.
- Physical therapy, including gentle stretching, range-of-motion exercises, and deep heat modalities, may be beneficial in selected patients.
- Injection with local anesthetic and steroid will provide symptomatic relief if conservative therapy fails or if the pain is limiting activities of daily living.
- Surgery may be required for persistent pain or progressive functional disability.

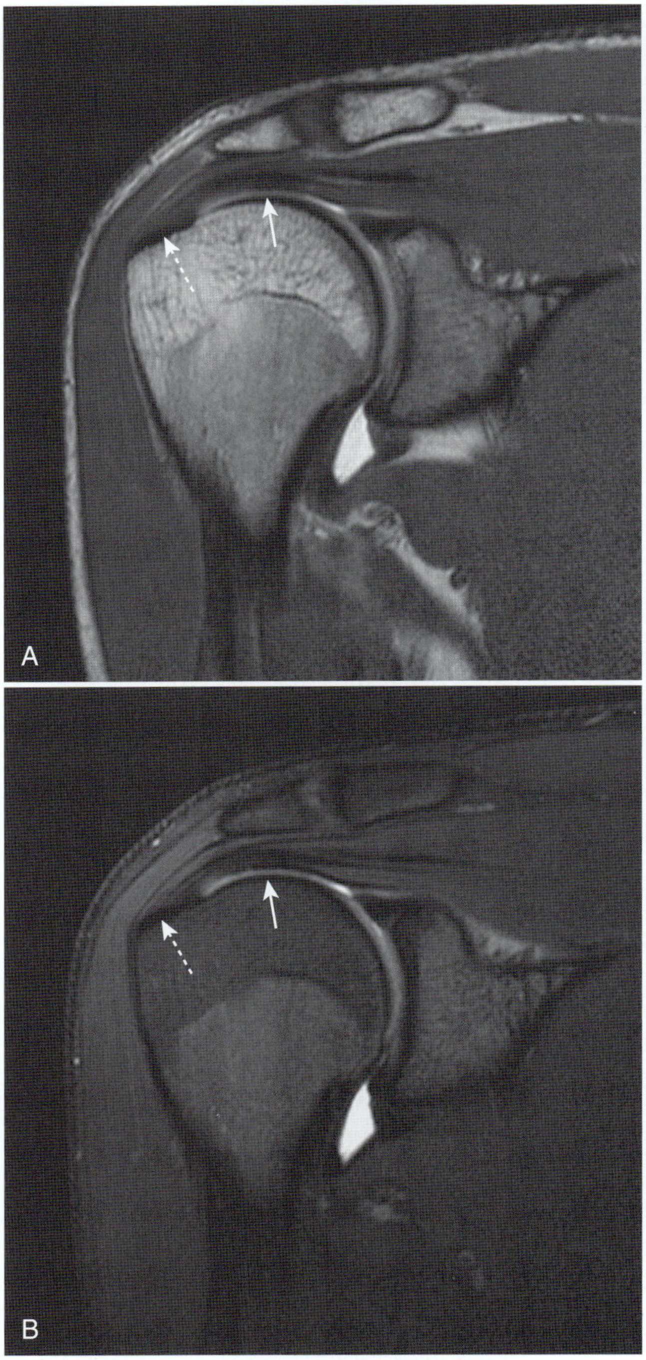

Figure 91.1 Coronal oblique T1W (**A**) and T2W MR images with fat suppression (FST2W) and (**B**) MR images of a normal supraspinatus tendon (*white arrows*), which inserts on the greater tuberosity (*broken white arrows*). The tendon has low SI on both pulse sequences.

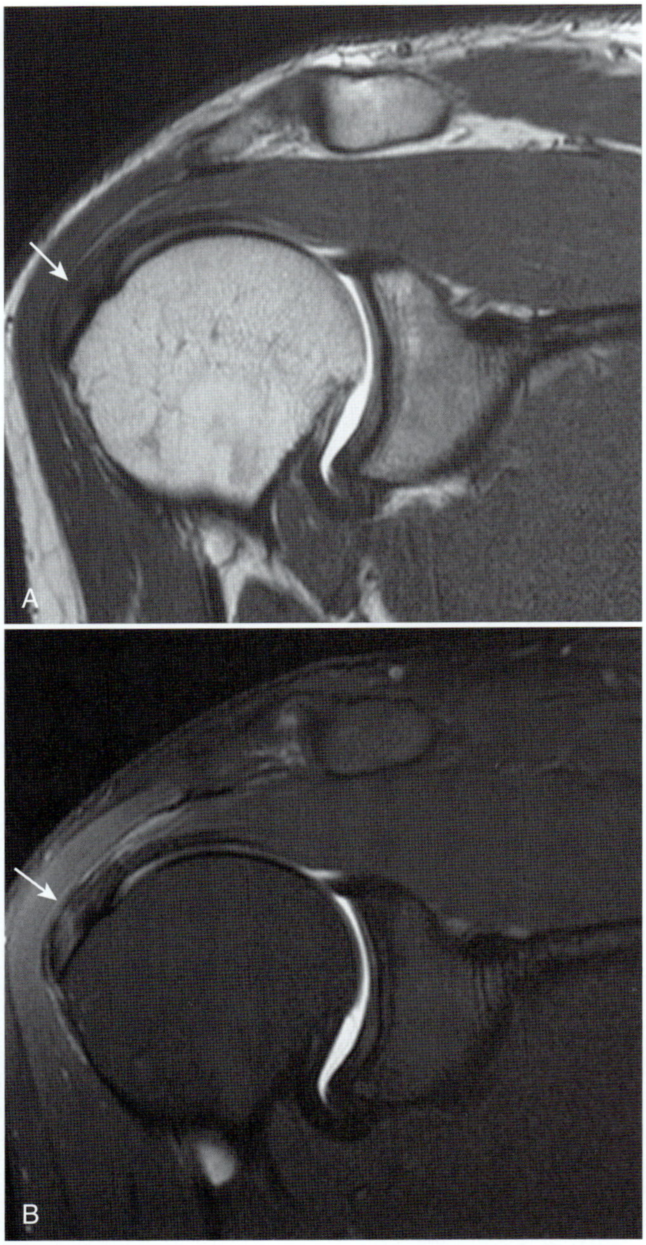

Figure 91.2 Coronal oblique T1W (**A**) and FST2W (**B**) MR images of a patient with supraspinatus tendinopathy. The distal tendon is thickened with increased SI on both pulse sequences (*white arrows*). There is no evidence of tendon tear.

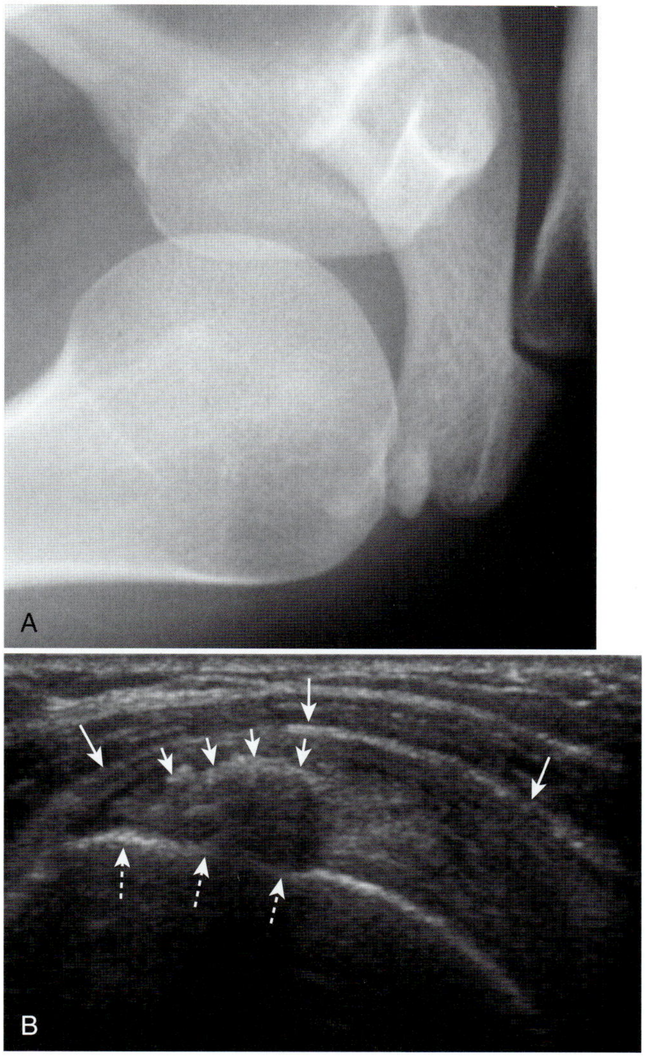

Figure 91.3 (A), AP radiograph of a patient with calcific tendinitis affecting the supraspinatus tendon. (B), The corresponding longitudinal US image shows the area of calcification within the tendon substance (*small white arrows*) with posterior acoustic shadowing. The subdeltoid fat plane superficial to the tendon (*large white arrows*) and the tendon insertion on the greater tuberosity (*broken white arrows*) can both be clearly seen.

CHAPTER 92

Partial Thickness Tear of the Rotator Cuff

DEFINITION

- Degeneration of the collagenous elements of the tendons of the rotator cuff, resulting in a partial tear.

SIGNS AND SYMPTOMS

- Gradual onset of anterolateral shoulder pain that is made worse with muscle contraction.
- Sudden onset of anterolateral shoulder pain following trauma.
- Weakness.
- Crepitus may be present.
- Exacerbation of pain with overhead activities.
- Pain often worse at night.
- Patient unable to sleep on the affected shoulder.
- Gradual decrease in range of motion.
- Clinical differentiation from SLAP (superior labral tear from anterior to posterior) lesions can be difficult.

DEMOGRAPHICS

- Incidence: Male = Female.
- Throwing athletes and workers doing heavy labor are often affected.
- Forty to 50-year-old persons most commonly affected, but affected patients are generally younger than those with complete cuff tears.
- Supraspinatus tendon most commonly affected.
- More common after trauma, including repetitive stress injuries.

IMAGING RECOMMENDATIONS

- Radiography not routinely required in younger patients.
- MR arthrography is the gold standard investigation.
  - Also useful to exclude associated SLAP lesions.
- Conventional MRI and US are less accurate for diagnosis of partial tears, with variability in reported sensitivity and specificity rates.

IMAGING FINDINGS

- Graded according to thickness of tendon involved:
  - Grade 1: <25%.
  - Grade 2: 25%-50%.
  - Grade 3: >50%.
- High-signal intensity (SI) clefts in the tendon at the margin of the tuberosity footprint on T2-weighted (T2W) MR images or T2W with fat suppression (FST2W) MR images.
- Focal areas of tendon attenuation or roughening.
- Low-reflection clefts on US.
- Focal defects of tendon outlined by contrast medium on MR arthrography.
- ABER (abduction and external rotation) imaging may improve visualization of partial tears.
- Bursal surface tears are less common.
- Distinguishing partial tears from tendinopathy can be difficult.
- Imbibing of contrast agent in areas of tendinopathy may occur, so that arthrographic appearance mimics that of a partial tear.

OTHER RECOMMENDED TESTING

- Laboratory testing to rule out inflammatory arthritis.
- Joint aspiration to rule out crystal arthropathies if diagnosis is in question.
- Joint aspiration to rule out infection if diagnosis is in question.

DIFFERENTIAL DIAGNOSIS

- Calcific tendinitis.
- Rotator cuff tendinopathy.
- Complete rotator cuff tear.
- Cyst involving one of the tendons of the rotator cuff.
- Adhesive capsulitis of the glenohumeral joint.

TREATMENT

- Conservative treatment consisting of local heat, cold, simple analgesics, and nonsteroidal anti-inflammatory agents will improve symptoms in many cases.
- Physical therapy, including gentle stretching, range-of-motion exercises, and deep heat modalities, may be beneficial in selected patients.

- Injection with local anesthetic and steroid will provide symptomatic relief if conservative therapy fails or if the pain is limiting activities of daily living.
- Surgery may be required for persistent pain or progressive functional disability.

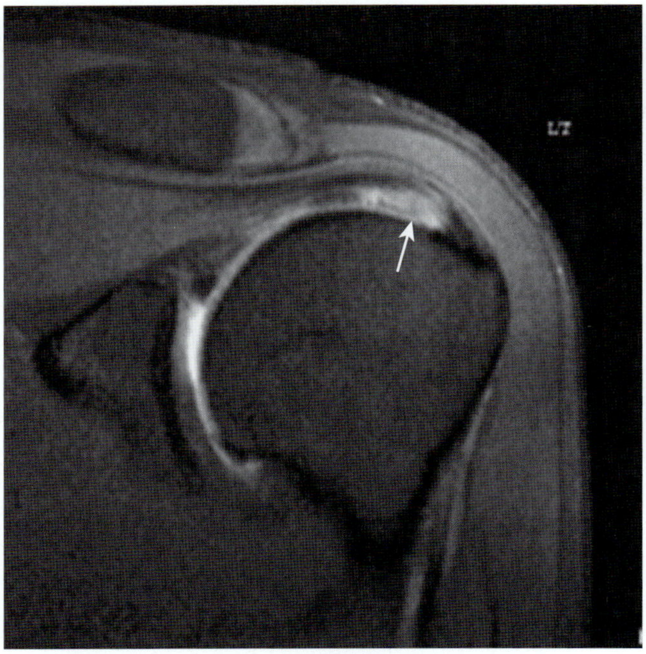

Figure 92.1 Coronal oblique MR arthrogram image demonstrating a partial articular surface tear of the supraspinatus tendon filled by high-SI contrast medium (*white arrow*). The tear involves >50% of the tendon thickness but does not communicate with the bursal surface of the tendon. *(Reproduced with permission from Campbell RSD & Dunn A. External impingement of the shoulder. Seminars In Musculoskeletal Radiology. 2008:12(2); 107-126.)*

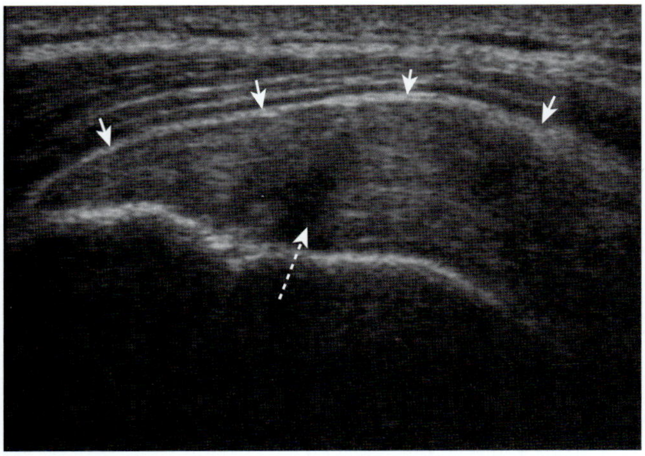

Figure 92.3 Longitudinal US image of a partial–articular surface supraspinatus tear with a well-demarcated, focal low-echo area within the tendon substance (*broken white arrow*) at the margin of the tuberosity. The tear does not extend through to the bursal surface of the tendon (*white arrows*). *(Reproduced with permission from Campbell RSD & Dunn A. External impingement of the shoulder. Seminars In Musculoskeletal Radiology. 2008:12(2); 107-126.)*

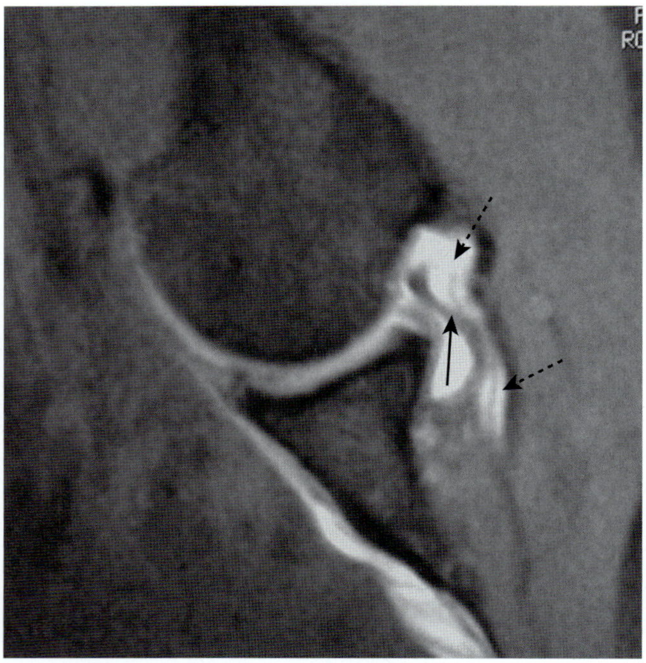

Figure 92.2 FST1W MR arthrogram image obtained in the ABER position. There is a partial supraspinatus tear with tendon delamination. The frayed articular component of the tendon (*black arrow*) is detached from its origin on the tuberosity, and high-SI contrast medium extends along the tendon delamination (*broken black arrows*). *(Reproduced with permission from Campbell RSD & Aniq H Protocols for orthopaedic shoulder imaging. Radiology Update 2008:7(1); 44-57.)*

CHAPTER 93

Full Thickness Tear of the Rotator Cuff

DEFINITION

- Complete tear of one or more of the tendons of the rotator cuff.

SIGNS AND SYMPTOMS

- Gradual onset of anterolateral shoulder pain that is made worse with muscle contraction.
- Sudden onset of anterolateral shoulder pain following trauma.
- Weakness with positive drop test result.
- Crepitus may be present.
- Exacerbation of pain with overhead activities.
- Pain often worse at night.
- Patient unable to sleep on the affected shoulder.
- Gradual decrease in range of motion.

DEMOGRAPHICS

- Incidence: Male > Female.
- Throwing athletes often affected.
- Persons older than 40 through 50 years of age most commonly affected.
- Supraspinatus tendon most commonly affected.
- More common after trauma, including repetitive stress injuries.

IMAGING RECOMMENDATIONS

- Radiography in older patients to exclude associated glenohumeral arthropathy.
- MR arthrography is the gold standard investigation, but conventional MRI and US are sufficiently accurate in most cases (approaching 100% accuracy for full-thickness tears).

IMAGING FINDINGS

- Primary signs:
  - Focal defect of tendon.
  - Tendon retraction in complete massive tears.
- Secondary signs:
  - Combined effusion in subacromial bursa and glenohumeral joint.
  - Herniation of deltoid into tendon defect.
  - Subacromial narrowing.
  - Superior migration of the humeral head with secondary eburnation of the acromion.
- Superior migration of the humeral head and narrowing of the subacromial space in chronic cuff tears.
- Secondary osteoarthritis in the glenohumeral joint (cuff arthropathy) occurs with massive cuff failure.
- Muscle atrophy can be assessed by both MRI and US.

OTHER RECOMMENDED TESTING

- Laboratory testing to rule out inflammatory arthritis.
- Joint aspiration to rule out crystal arthropathies if diagnosis is in question.
- Joint aspiration to rule out infection if diagnosis is in question.

DIFFERENTIAL DIAGNOSIS

- Calcific tendinitis.
- Rotator cuff tendinopathy.
- Partial rotator cuff tear.
- Cyst involving one of the tendons of the rotator cuff.
- Rheumatoid arthritis.
- Adhesive capsulitis of the glenohumeral joint.

TREATMENT

- Conservative treatment consisting of local heat, cold, simple analgesics, and nonsteroidal anti-inflammatory agents will improve symptoms in many cases.
- Physical therapy, including gentle stretching, range-of-motion exercises, and deep heat modalities, may be beneficial in selected patients.
- Injection with local anesthetic and steroid will provide symptomatic relief if conservative therapy fails or the pain is limiting activities of daily living.
- Surgery may be required for persistent pain or progressive functional disability.

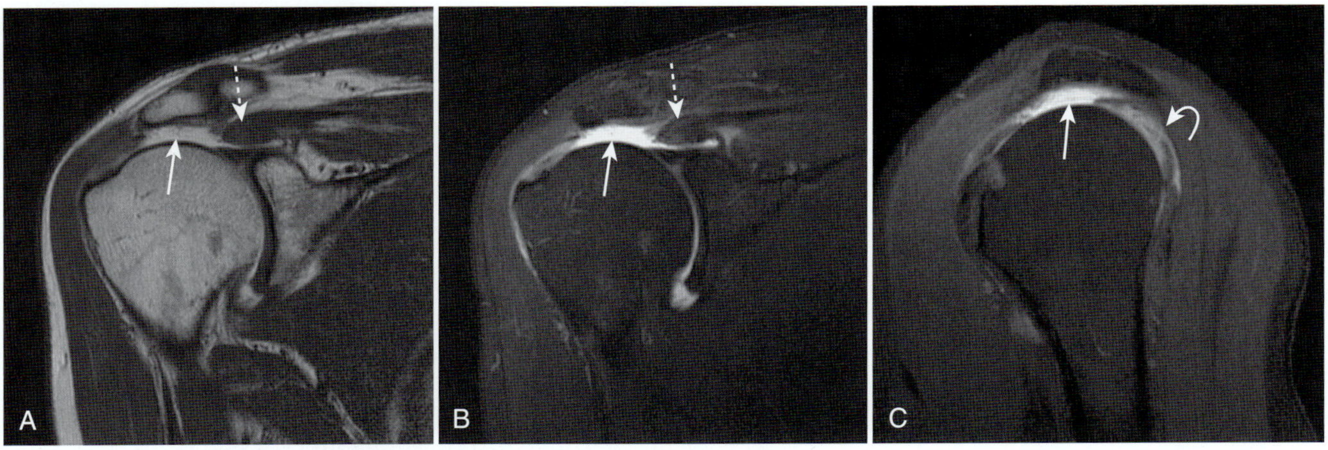

Figure 93.1 Coronal oblique T1-weighted (T1W) (**A**) and T2W with fat suppression (FST2W) (**B**) MR arthrogram images of a patient with a full-thickness tear of the supraspinatus tendon. The tendon defect is outlined by the high-SI contrast medium (*white arrows*), and the torn tendon end is visible medially (*broken white arrows*). (**C**), The sagittal oblique FST2W MR image also demonstrates the tendon tear (*white arrow*), and the infraspinatus tendon posteriorly (*curved arrow*) is thickened and has high-SI because of associated tendinopathy.

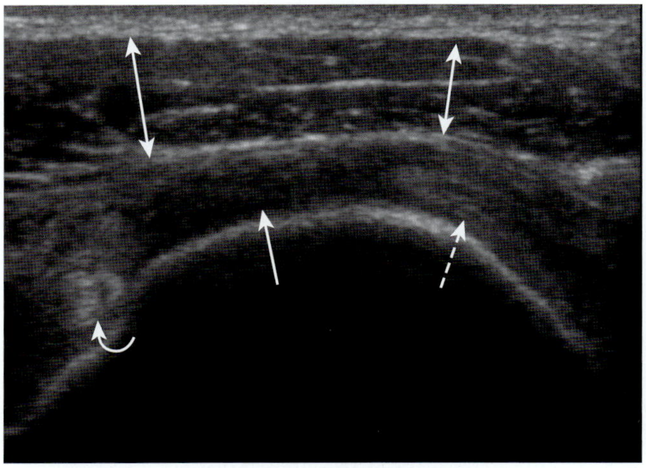

Figure 93.2 Transverse US image of a torn supraspinatus tendon. The image is comparable with Figure 103.1C. The tendon defect is filled by low-echo fluid (*white arrow*); it lies between the biceps tendon anteriorly (*curved arrow*) and the infraspinatus posteriorly (*broken white arrow*) and is deep to the deltoid muscle (*double-headed white arrows*).

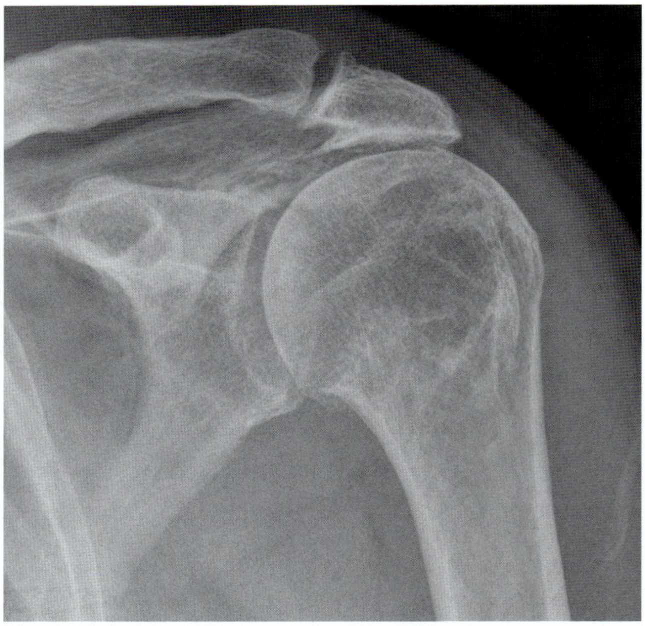

Figure 93.3 AP radiograph of the shoulder in a patient with a chronic rotator cuff tear. There is marked narrowing of the subacromial space secondary to proximal humeral head migration.

CHAPTER 94

Adhesive Capsulitis of the Shoulder

DEFINITION

- A progressive restriction of shoulder range of motion associated with pain and contracture of the joint.

SIGNS AND SYMPTOMS

- Gradual onset of painful movement of the shoulder with associated limited range of motion.
- Elevation and rotation of shoulder especially painful.
- Crepitus may be present.
- Pain often worse at night.
- Patient unable to sleep on the affected shoulder.
- Gradual decrease in range of motion.

DEMOGRAPHICS

- Incidence: Female > Male.
- Often associated with rotator cuff pathology.
- Forty to 70-year-old persons most commonly affected.
- Increased incidence:
  - In patients with diabetes mellitus, especially if insulin dependent.
  - In patients with HLA-B27.
- After shoulder trauma, including fractures of the humerus.

IMAGING RECOMMENDATIONS

- Clinical diagnosis for which imaging usually is not required.
- MRI or US:
  - To exclude other shoulder pathology
- Arthrography:
  - As a part of distention arthrography for treatment of capsulitis.

IMAGING FINDINGS

- MRI:
  - Joint effusion.
  - Thickening and high-signal intensity (SI) of inferior glenohumeral ligament (IGHL) and axillary pouch (becomes low-SI with chronic adhesive capsulitis).
  - Effacement of normal fat planes within the rotator interval.
- Arthrogram:
  - Restriction of joint capsule with pain on injection.
- US:
  - Doppler signal within rotator interval (although may be seen with any cause of synovitis).

OTHER RECOMMENDED TESTING

- Laboratory testing to rule out inflammatory arthritis.
- Laboratory testing to rule out diabetes mellitus.
- Joint aspiration to rule out crystal arthropathies if diagnosis in question.
- Joint aspiration to rule out infection if diagnosis in question.

DIFFERENTIAL DIAGNOSIS

- Osteoarthritis of shoulder.
- Rotator cuff tendinopathy.
- Complete rotator cuff tear.
- Impingement syndromes.

TREATMENT

- Conservative treatment consisting of local heat, cold, simple analgesics, and nonsteroidal anti-inflammatory agents and opioids will provide some symptomatic relief.
- Physical therapy, including gentle stretching, range-of-motion exercises, and deep heat modalities may be beneficial in selected patients.
- Injection with local anesthetic and steroid will provide symptomatic relief if conservative therapy fails or the pain is limiting activities of daily living.
- Manipulation under anesthesia may be required for more advanced cases.
- Surgery may be required for persistent pain or progressive functional disability.

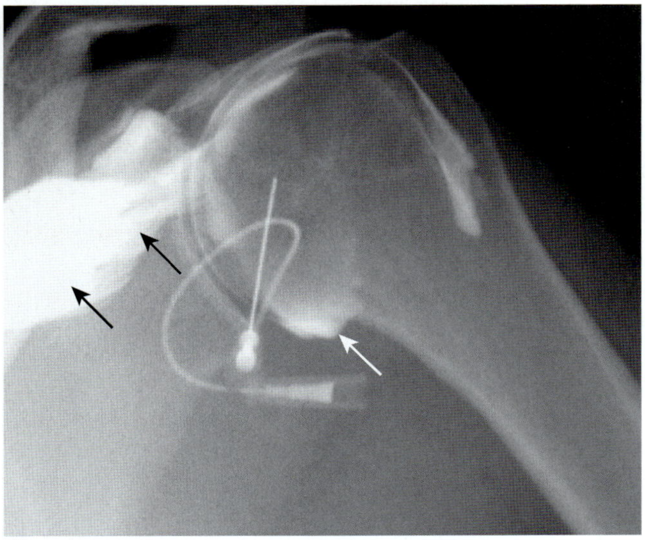

Figure 94.1 Fluoroscopic image obtained during a distention arthrogram procedure in a patient with adhesive capsulitis. The axillary pouch is underdistended (*white arrow*) because of contraction of the joint capsule, and there is early extravasation of contrast medium from the joint (*black arrows*).

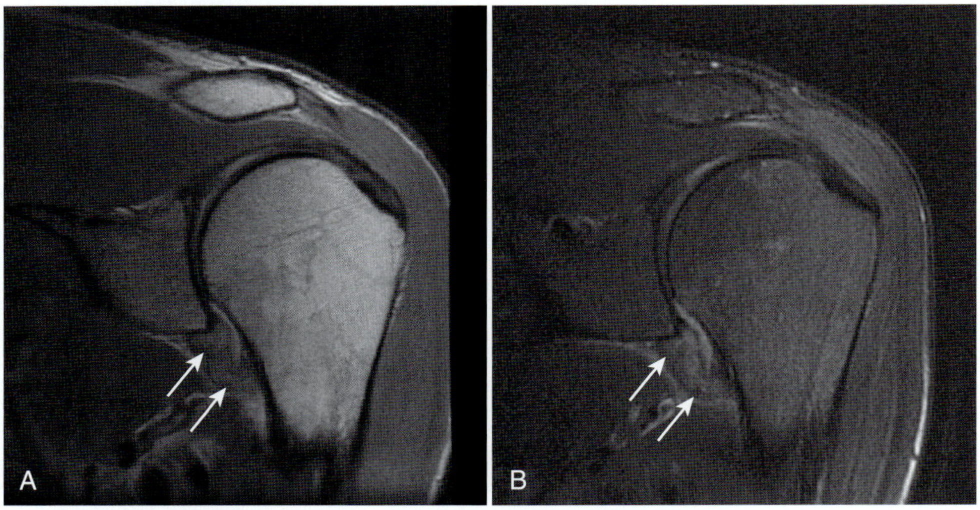

Figure 94.2 Coronal proton density (**A**) and T2-weighted with fat suppression (FST2W) (**B**) MR images in a different patient with adhesive capsulitis. There are thickening and high SI within the Inferior glenohumeral ligament and the capsule of the axillary pouch (*white arrows*). Only a small joint effusion is present.

CHAPTER 95

Labral Tear of the Shoulder

DEFINITION

- Tear of the cartilaginous labrum of the shoulder due to trauma, including traumatic instability secondary to dislocation, repetitive overhead stress with internal impingement, and direct trauma.

SIGNS AND SYMPTOMS

- Sudden onset of shoulder pain following trauma.
- Subluxation may be present.
- Exacerbation of pain with flexion, adduction, and internal rotation.
- Pain often worse at night.
- Patient unable to sleep on the affected shoulder.
- Gradual decrease in range of motion.

DEMOGRAPHICS

- Incidence: Male > Female.
- Throwing and swimming athletes often affected.
- Younger patients most commonly affected.
- Increased incidence in patients with major motor seizures.
- More common after trauma, including repetitive stress injuries.

IMAGING RECOMMENDATIONS

- MR arthrography is usually regarded as the gold standard investigation.
- CT arthrography is an alternative if MRI is contraindicated.
- Conventional MRI has lower sensitivity and specificity than arthrography for labral tears.
- Conventional CT may be useful to assess the size and extent of bony glenoid rim defects.

IMAGING FINDINGS

- Two common patterns of involvement: traumatic instability and superior labral tear from anterior to posterior (SLAP) lesions:
  - Overlap of these two patterns may occur.
- Traumatic instability:
  - Anteroinferior instability more common.
  - Variable patterns of labral tears and detachments (Bankart lesion).
  - Bony glenoid rim defects are common (bony Bankart lesion).
  - Associated bony defects on humeral head (Hill-Sachs lesion).
  - Associated injury to glenohumeral ligaments (inferior glenohumeral ligament is the most important stabilizer).
- SLAP lesion:
  - Tear of the superior labrum that may involve the biceps tendon anchor.
  - Grades 1 to 4 are the most common (although up to 12 grades have been described).
  - Extent of tear is more important than grading.

OTHER RECOMMENDED TESTING

- Laboratory testing to rule out inflammatory arthritis if diagnosis is in question.
- Joint aspiration to rule out crystal arthropathies if diagnosis is in question.
- Joint aspiration to rule out infection if diagnosis is in question.

DIFFERENTIAL DIAGNOSIS

- Humeral fractures.
- Rotator cuff tendinopathy.
- Partial rotator cuff tears.
- Complete rotator cuff tear.
- Cyst involving one of the tendons of the rotator cuff.
- Teres minor avulsion.

TREATMENT

- Conservative treatment consisting of local heat, cold, simple analgesics, and nonsteroidal anti-inflammatory agents will improve symptoms in many cases.
- Physical therapy, including gentle stretching, range-of-motion exercises, and deep heat modalities, may be beneficial in selected patients.
- Injection with local anesthetic and steroid will provide symptomatic relief if conservative therapy fails or the pain is limiting activities of daily living.
- Surgery often required for persistent pain or progressive functional disability.

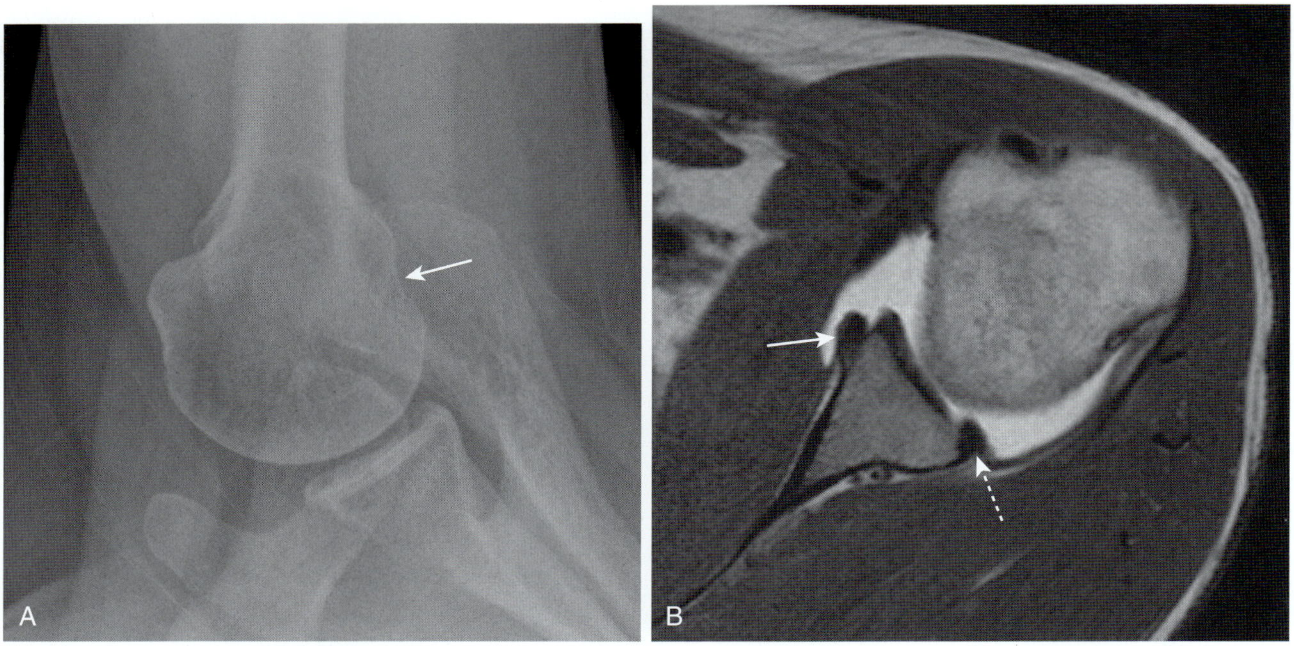

Figure 95.1 (**A**), Subaxial radiograph of the shoulder in a patient with traumatic instability. There is a shallow posterior Hill-Sachs lesion due to impaction fracture (*white arrow*). (**B**), The axial T1-weighted (T1W) MR arthrogram image shows a tear of the fibrocartilaginous labrum, which is displaced medially along the glenoid neck (*white arrow*). Compare with the normal position of the posterior labrum (*broken white arrow*).

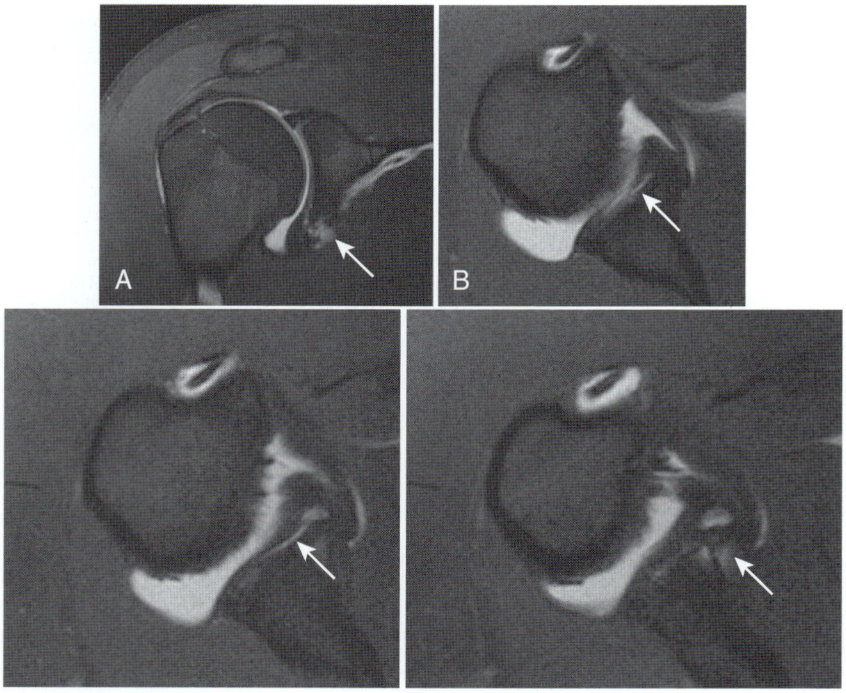

Figure 95.2 (**A**), Coronal T2W with fat suppression (FST2W) MR arthrogram image demonstrating a high–signal intensity (SI) paralabral cyst at the anteroinferior margin of the glenoid in a patient with previous dislocation. (**B**), Three consecutive axial FST1W MR arthrogram images show the high-SI contrast medium (*white arrows*) extending through a labral tear and communicating with the cyst.

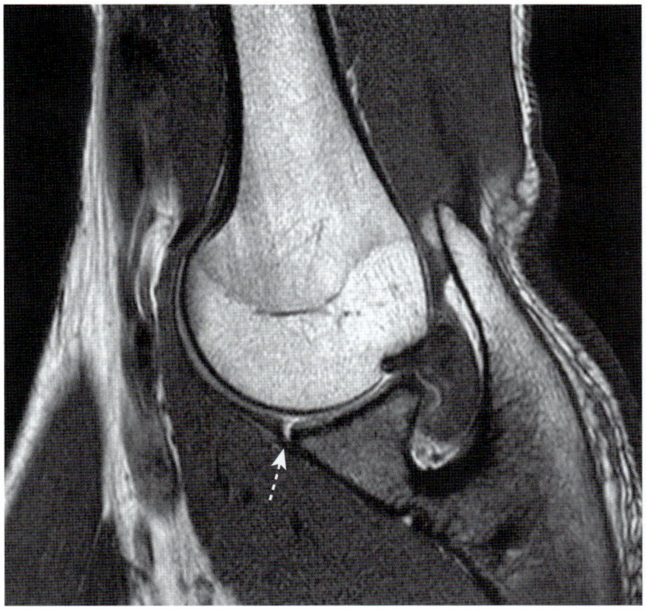

Figure 95.3 T1W MR arthrogram image in the abduction and external rotation (ABER) position of a patient with instability. There is partial detachment of the anteroinferior labrum (*broken white arrow*), demonstrated with the inferior glenohumeral ligament under tension, which was not visible on the routine axial images.

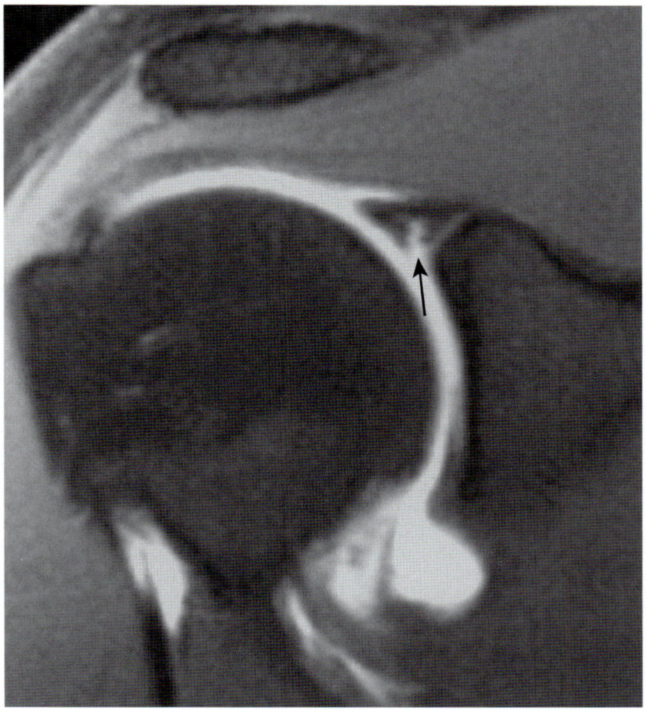

Figure 95.4 Coronal FST2W MR arthrogram image in a swimmer with shoulder pain. There is a tear of the superior labrum (SLAP lesion) with high-SI contrast medium undercutting the base of the low-SI labrum (*black arrow*). The biceps anchor was intact.

CHAPTER 96

Biceps Tendinopathy

DEFINITION

- Degeneration of the long head of the biceps (LHB) due to repetitive microtrauma to the musculotendinous unit.

SIGNS AND SYMPTOMS

- Gradual onset of dull, ill-defined anterior shoulder pain.
- Pain often radiates into the upper arm.
- Positive results of:
  - Speed test.
  - Yergason test.
  - O'Brien test.
- Crepitus may be present.
- Exacerbation of pain with overhead activities, pulling, and/or lifting.
- Patient unable to sleep on the affected shoulder.

DEMOGRAPHICS

- Incidence: Male = Female.
- Young athletes participating in throwing and overhead sports are often affected.
- Forty to 50-year-old persons most commonly affected.
- Subacromial impingement often present.
- More common after trauma, including repetitive stress injuries.

IMAGING RECOMMENDATIONS

- Imaging indicated primarily to exclude associated rotator cuff disease.
- MRI or US can be used to assess the LHB tendon.
- Radiography is of limited value for isolated biceps tendon abnormalities.

IMAGING FINDINGS

- Primary signs:
  - Tendon thickening.
  - Increased signal intensity (SI) on T1-weighted (T1W) and T2W MR imaging.
  - Hyporeflective tendon on US.
  - Tendon splitting may occur with partial tearing.
- Secondary signs:
  - Localized effusions within the tendon sheath in the bicipital groove.
  - Enthesophytes impinging on the tendon within the bicipital groove.
  - Associated rotator cuff tear.

OTHER RECOMMENDED TESTING

- Laboratory testing to rule out inflammatory arthritis.
- Joint aspiration to rule out crystal arthropathies.
- Joint aspiration to rule out infection if diagnosis is in question.

DIFFERENTIAL DIAGNOSIS

- Calcific tendinitis.
- Partial-thickness rotator cuff tear.
- Complete rotator cuff tear.
- Cyst involving one of the tendons of the rotator cuff.
- SLAP (superior labral tear from anterior to posterior) lesions.
- Labral tear of the shoulder.

TREATMENT

- Conservative treatment consisting of local heat, cold, simple analgesics, and nonsteroidal anti-inflammatory agents will improve symptoms in many cases.
- Physical therapy, including gentle stretching, range-of-motion exercises, and deep heat modalities, may be beneficial in selected patients.
- Injection with local anesthetic and steroid will provide symptomatic relief if conservative therapy fails or the pain is limiting activities of daily living.
- Surgery may be required for persistent pain or progressive functional disability.

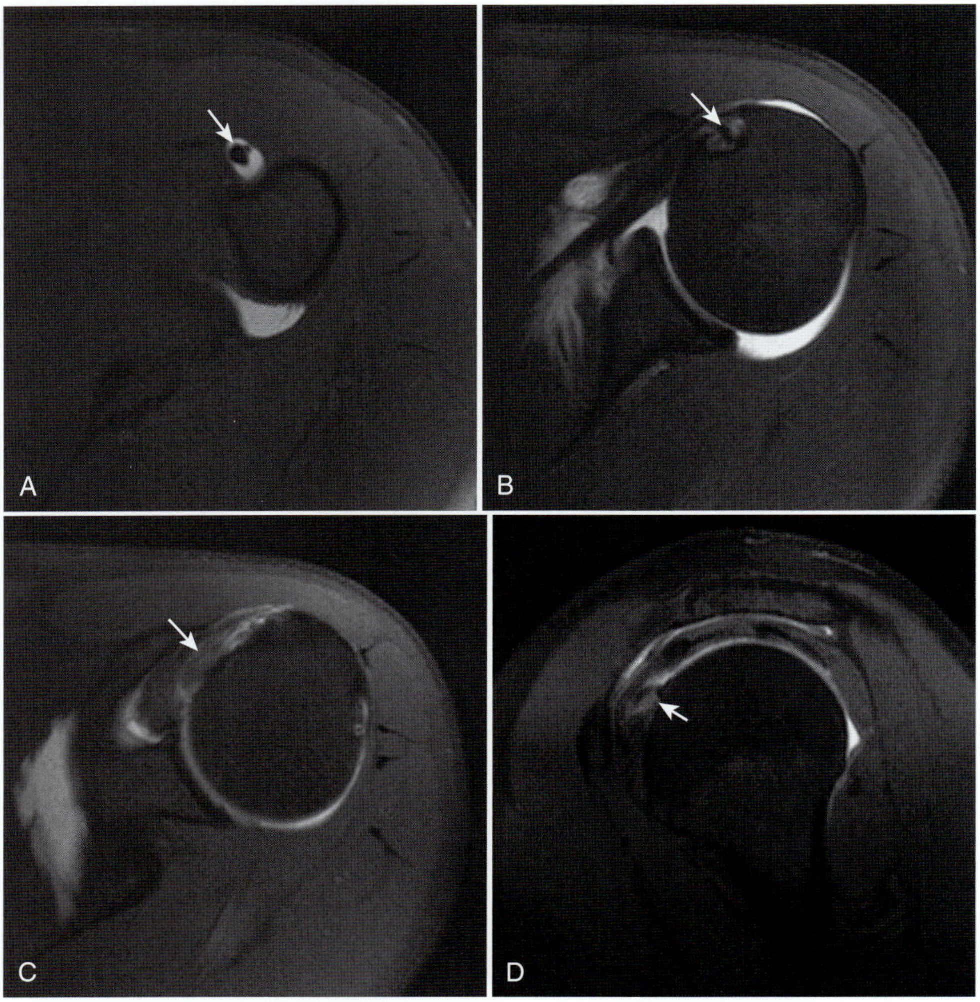

Figure 96.1 Axial (**A** to **C**) and sagittal oblique (**D**) T1W with fat suppression (FST1W) MR arthrogram images of the LHB tendon (*white arrows)* in a patient with pain over the biceps. (**A**), The LHB tendon in the distal tendon sheath is normal. (**B**), More proximally, the tendon is attenuated and is surrounded by intermediate-SI soft tissue thickening, with osteophytes arising from the lesser tuberosity in the medial aspect of the bicipital groove. (**C**), and (**D**), In the rotator interval, the tendon is thickened and demonstrates areas of increased SI due to tendinopathy.

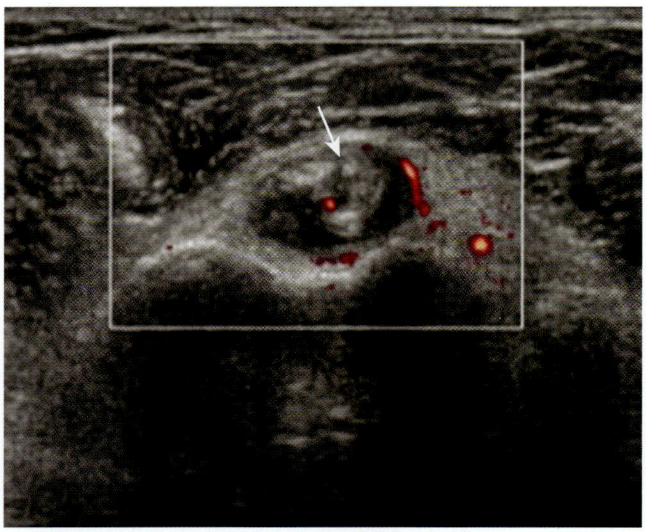

Figure 96.2 Transverse power Doppler US image of the biceps tendon within the bicipital groove (*white arrow*). There is anechoic fluid within the tendon sheath, which in isolation is not a significant finding. However, the tendon is heterogeneous in echo texture with an area of low-echo change, and there is abnormal vascularity within the tendon and the synovial tendon sheath, indicating biceps tendinopathy.

CHAPTER 97

Biceps Tendon Disruption

DEFINITION

- Rupture of the long head of the biceps (LHB).

SIGNS AND SYMPTOMS

- Sudden onset of dull, ill-defined anterior shoulder pain after seemingly minor trauma.
- Pain often radiates into the upper arm.
- Positive results of:
  - Ludington ("Popeye") test because of muscle belly retraction.
  - Speed test.
  - Yergason test.
  - O'Brien test.
- Crepitus may be present.
- Exacerbation of pain with overhead activities, pulling, and/or lifting.
- Patient unable to sleep on the affected shoulder.

DEMOGRAPHICS

- Incidence: Male > Female.
- Young athletes participating in throwing and overhead sports are often affected.
- Subacromial impingement often present.
- More common after trauma, including repetitive stress injuries.

IMAGING RECOMMENDATIONS

- Usually a clinical diagnosis.
- Imaging indicated primarily to exclude associated rotator cuff disease.
- MRI or US can be used to assess the LHB tendon.
- Radiography is of limited value for isolated biceps tendon abnormalities.

IMAGING FINDINGS

- Loss of visualization of the tendon within the bicipital groove.
- Retracted musculotendinous junction in upper arm, with "Popeye" sign giving a pseudomass.
- Associated rotator cuff tears are common.
- Important to differentiate biceps tendon dislocation associated with subscapularis tear from biceps tendon rupture.

OTHER RECOMMENDED TESTING

- Laboratory testing to rule out inflammatory arthritis.
- Joint aspiration to rule out crystal arthropathies.
- Joint aspiration to rule out infection if diagnosis is in question.

DIFFERENTIAL DIAGNOSIS

- Calcific biceps tendinitis.
- Partial-thickness rotator cuff tear.
- Complete rotator cuff tear.
- Cyst involving one of the tendons of the rotator cuff.
- SLAP (superior labral tear from anterior to posterior) lesions.
- Labral tear of the shoulder.
- Fractures of the greater tuberosity of the humerus.

TREATMENT

- Conservative treatment consisting of local heat, cold, simple analgesics, and nonsteroidal anti-inflammatory agents will improve symptoms in many cases.
- Physical therapy, including gentle stretching, range-of-motion exercises, and deep heat modalities, may be beneficial in selected patients.
- Injection with local anesthetic and steroid will provide symptomatic relief if conservative therapy fails or the pain is limiting activities of daily living.
- Surgery may be required for persistent pain or progressive functional disability.

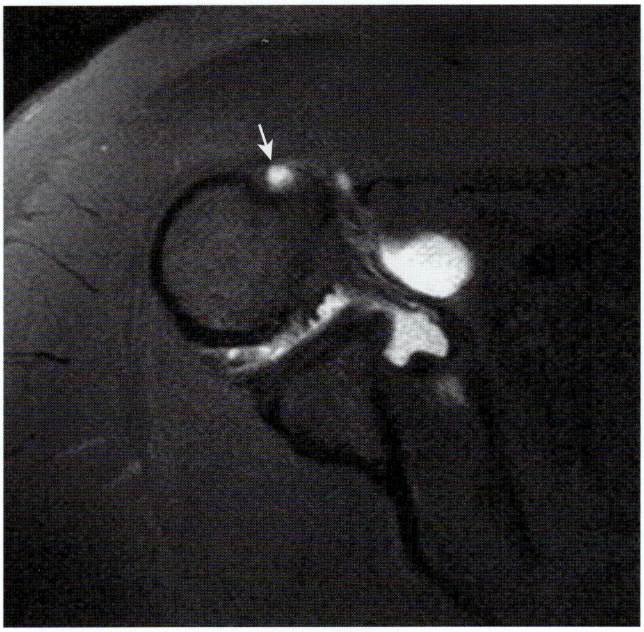

Figure 97.1 Axial T1-weighted with fat suppression (FST1W) MR arthrogram image of a patient with an extensive rotator cuff tear and rupture of the LHB tendon. The tendon sheath within the bicipital groove is filled by high–signal intensity (SI) contrast, and no tendon is visible (*white arrow*).

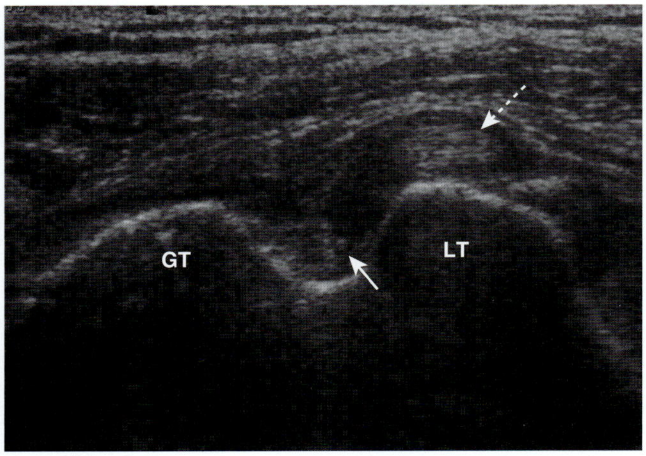

Figure 97.2 Transverse US image of the proximal humerus demonstrating an empty bicipital groove (*white arrow*). However, the LHB tendon is subluxated medially and is clearly visible lying on the lesser tuberosity (*broken white arrow*). When the tendon is dislocated more medially, it can be difficult to identify and can be mistaken for a tendon rupture. GT, greater tuberosity; LT, lesser tuberosity.

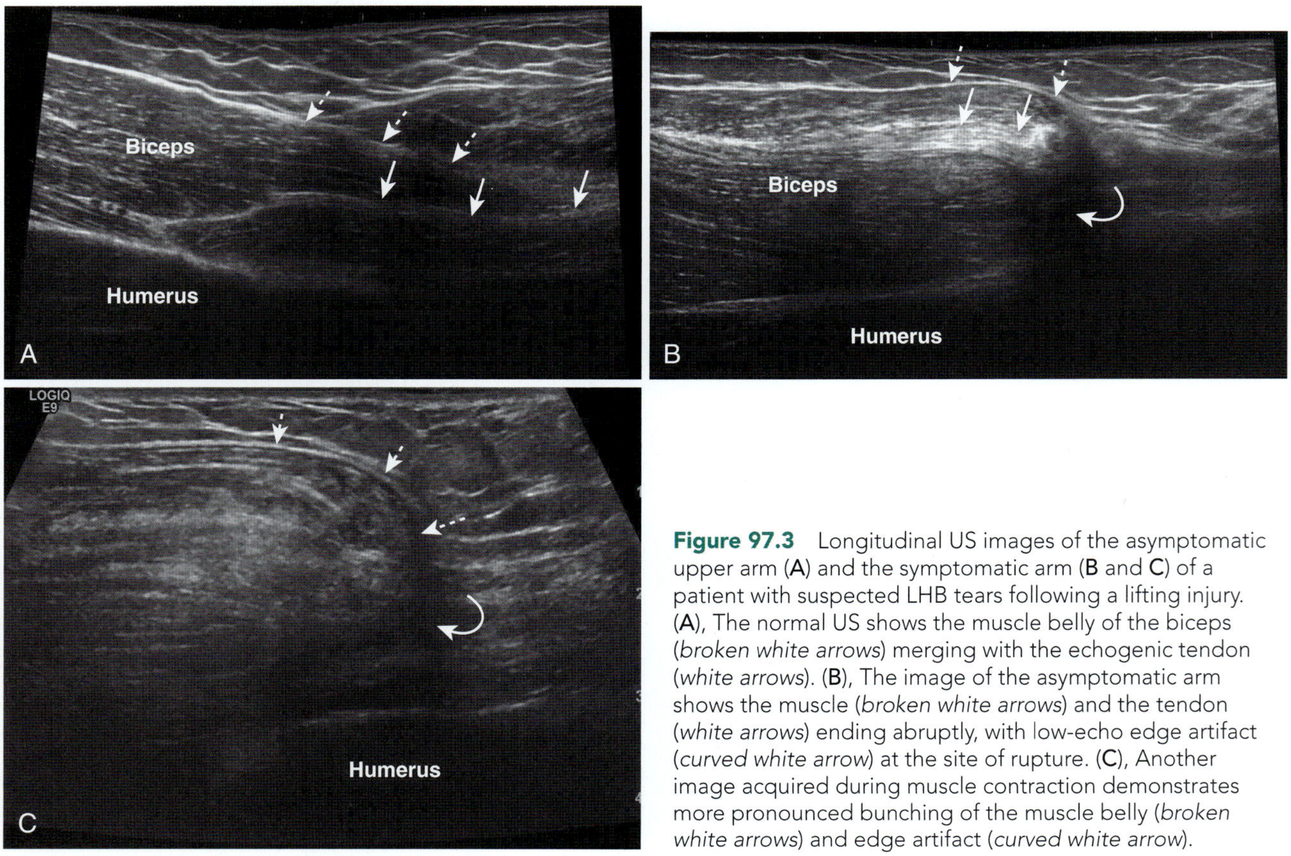

Figure 97.3 Longitudinal US images of the asymptomatic upper arm (**A**) and the symptomatic arm (**B** and **C**) of a patient with suspected LHB tears following a lifting injury. (**A**), The normal US shows the muscle belly of the biceps (*broken white arrows*) merging with the echogenic tendon (*white arrows*). (**B**), The image of the asymptomatic arm shows the muscle (*broken white arrows*) and the tendon (*white arrows*) ending abruptly, with low-echo edge artifact (*curved white arrow*) at the site of rupture. (**C**), Another image acquired during muscle contraction demonstrates more pronounced bunching of the muscle belly (*broken white arrows*) and edge artifact (*curved white arrow*).

CHAPTER 98

Subacromial Impingement

DEFINITION

- Painful impingement of the supraspinatus tendon and subacromial bursa between the head of the humerus and the coracoacromial arch.

SIGNS AND SYMPTOMS

- Gradual onset of shoulder pain with abduction and forward flexion.
- Range of motion preserved, but painful.
- Weakness of supraspinatus muscle.
- Positive Neer test result.
- Positive Hawkins test result.
- Patient unable to sleep on the affected shoulder.

DEMOGRAPHICS

- Incidence: Male > Female.
- Young athletes involved in overhead activities often affected.
- Forty to 50-year-old persons most commonly affected.
- More common after trauma, including repetitive stress injuries.

IMAGING RECOMMENDATIONS

- MRI or US:
  - Primarily indicated to exclude rotator cuff tear.
- Imaging can identify abnormalities associated with external impingement, but such abnormalities have limited correlation with symptoms of impingement.
- Diagnosis of impingement is usually based on either:
  - Clinical findings.
  - Diagnostic injection of anesthetic in subacromial bursa.

IMAGING FINDINGS

- Subacromial bursitis.
- Enthesopathy of acromion and tuberosity:
  - Bony sclerosis, cortical roughening, and bone spur formation.
- Osteoarthritic changes in the acromioclavicular (AC) joint.
- Morphologic abnormalities of acromion:
  - Os acromiale.
  - Lateral downsloping.
  - Hooked acromion.
- Impingement of the bursa may be seen on dynamic US examination.

OTHER RECOMMENDED TESTING

- If diagnosis is in question:
  - Laboratory testing to rule out inflammatory arthritis.
  - Joint aspiration to rule out crystal arthropathies.
  - Joint aspiration to rule out infection.

DIFFERENTIAL DIAGNOSIS

- Calcific tendinitis.
- Partial-thickness rotator cuff tear.
- Rotator cuff pathology.
- Cyst involving the tendon of the supraspinatus muscle.
- Posterosuperior glenoid impingement syndrome.
- Os acromiale.

TREATMENT

- Conservative treatment consisting of local heat, cold, simple analgesics, and nonsteroidal anti-inflammatory agents will improve symptoms in many cases.
- Physical therapy, including gentle stretching, range-of-motion exercises, and deep heat modalities, may be beneficial in selected patients.
- Injection with local anesthetic and steroid will provide symptomatic relief if conservative therapy fails or the pain is limiting activities of daily living.
- Surgery may be required for persistent pain or progressive functional disability.

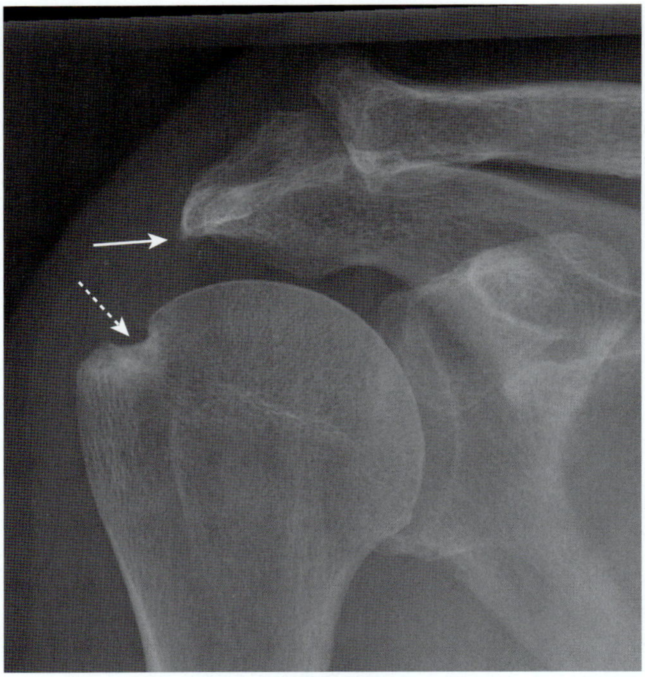

Figure 98.1 AP radiograph of the shoulder with osteoarthritic change in the AC joint, but there is also enthesopathy with bone formation on the acromion (*white arrow*) and sclerosis and notching of the greater tuberosity (*broken white arrow*).

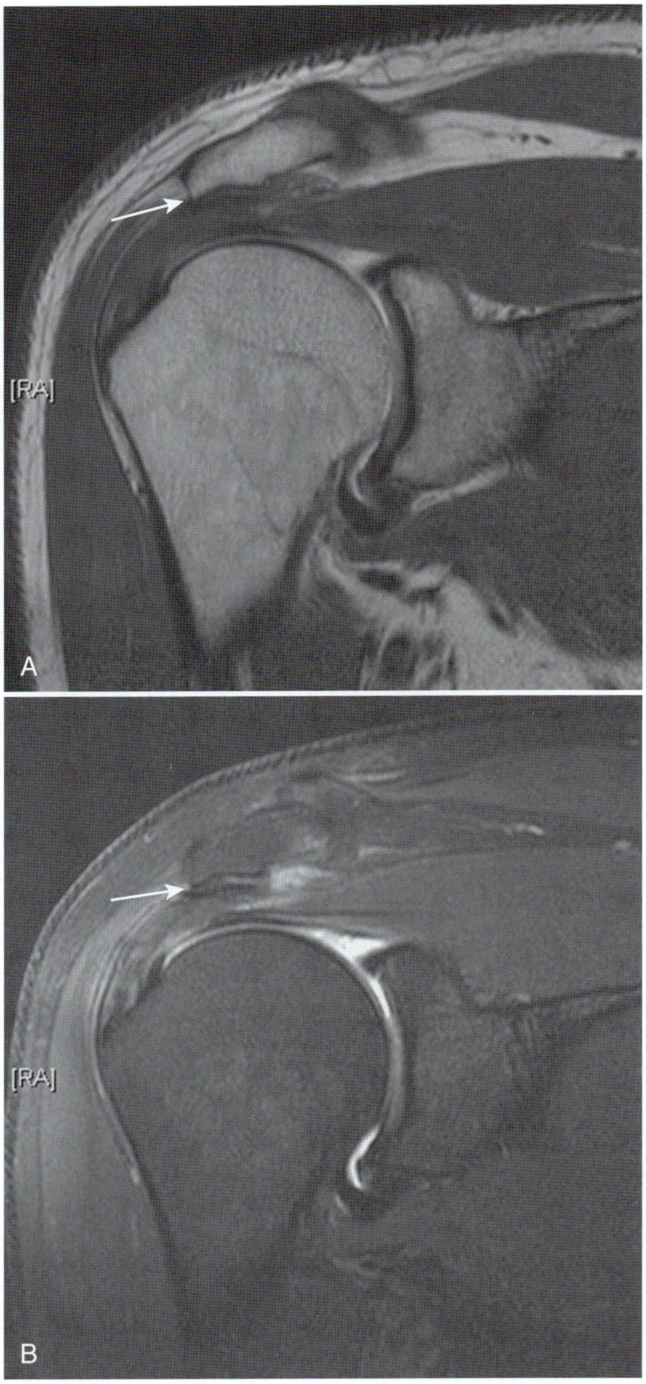

Figure 98.2 Coronal T1-weighted (T1W) (**A**) and T2W with fat suppression (FST2W) (**B**) MR arthrogram images demonstrating enthesopathy of the acromion (*white arrows*) with impingement of the supraspinatus tendon, which is thickened and tendinopathic. There is early subacromial bursitis.

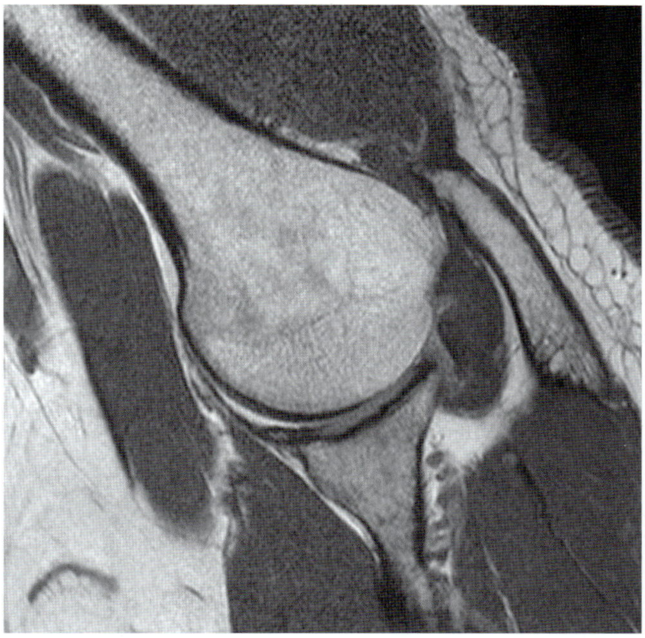

Figure 98.3 T1W MR image acquired in the abduction and external rotation (ABER) position, with direct contact apparent between the greater tuberosity of the humerus and the acromion, both of which show enthesopathic bone formation.

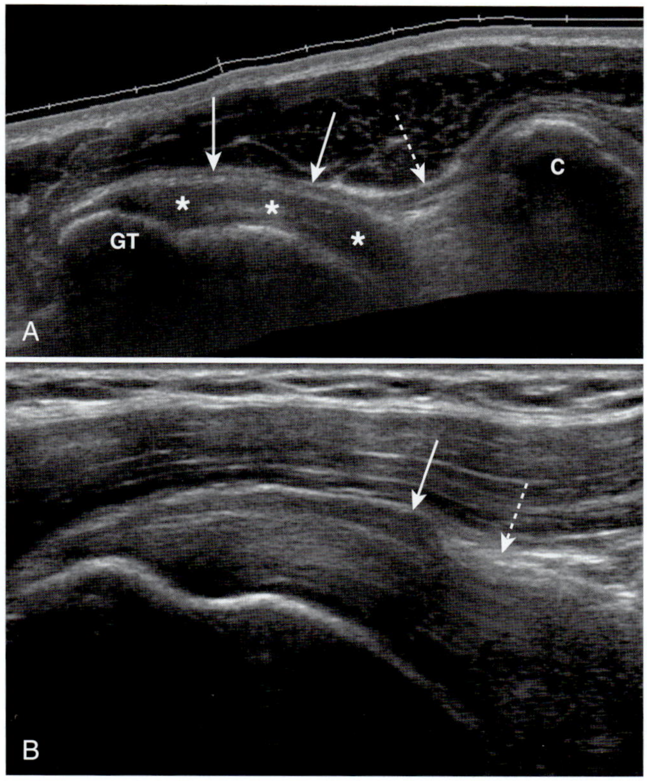

Figure 98.5 (**A**), US image of the normal relationship between the rotator cuff *(asterisks)*, the subacromial bursa (*white arrows*), and the coracohumeral ligament (CAL) (*broken white arrow*). The bursa normally glides smoothly beneath the CAL during abduction. (**B**), A US image acquired during dynamic evaluation in a patient with impingement syndrome demonstrates bunching of the bursa (*white arrow*) just proximal to the CAL (*broken white arrow*), which is referred to as the "step" sign. (**C**), coracoid; GT, greater tuberosity.

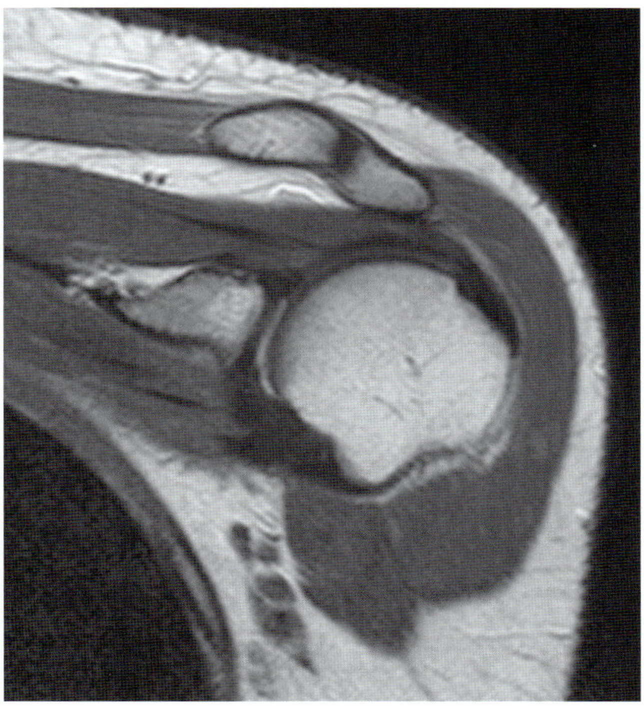

Figure 98.4 Coronal T1W MR image demonstrating lateral downsloping of the acromion, a pattern of acromial morphology thought to be associated with impingement.

CHAPTER 99

Subdeltoid Bursitis

DEFINITION

- Inflammation of the bursa that lies under the acromion between the deltoid muscle and the joint capsule.

SIGNS AND SYMPTOMS

- Pain localized underneath the deltoid muscle that is made worse with any shoulder movement.
- Pain may radiate to proximal humerus.
- Tenderness to palpation of the subdeltoid bursa.
- Warmth may be present.
- Shoulder may feel boggy or edematous.
- Crepitus or catching sensation may be present.
- Exacerbation of pain with resisted abduction.
- Pain often worse at night.
- Patient unable to sleep on the affected shoulder.
- Gradual decrease in range of motion.
- May progress to frozen shoulder if left untreated.

DEMOGRAPHICS

- Incidence: Male = Female.
- Young athletes often affected.
- Forty to 50-year-old persons most commonly affected.
- More common after trauma, including repetitive stress injuries.
- Increased incidence with jobs that require working with the arm across the body.
- May be associated with inflammatory or crystal arthropathies.

IMAGING RECOMMENDATIONS

- MRI or US.
- Imaging primarily used to identify associated rotator cuff disease.

IMAGING FINDINGS

- Fluid within the subdeltoid bursa:
  - Usually small effusions when secondary to impingement.
- Associated features of external impingement and rotator cuff disease.
- Inflammatory or crystal arthropathy:
  - Effusions may be prominent.
  - Synovial thickening:
    - Enhancement on post–contrast (obtained after administration of contrast agent) MR images.
    - Increased vascularity on Doppler imaging.
- Fibrinous exudates with "rice bodies" in rheumatoid arthritis.
- Echogenic effusions with crystals on US.

OTHER RECOMMENDED TESTING

- Laboratory testing to rule out inflammatory arthritis.
- Bursal aspiration with Gram staining and culture and sensitivity testing if infection is in question or to rule out crystal arthropathy.

DIFFERENTIAL DIAGNOSIS

- Calcific tendinitis.
- Partial-thickness rotator cuff tear.
- Complete rotator cuff tear.
- Frozen shoulder.
- Septic arthritis of the shoulder.

TREATMENT

- Conservative treatment consisting of local heat, cold, simple analgesics, and nonsteroidal anti-inflammatory agents will improve symptoms in mild cases.
- Physical therapy, including gentle stretching, range-of-motion exercises, and deep heat modalities, may be beneficial in selected patients.
- Injection with local anesthetic and steroid will provide symptomatic relief if conservative therapy fails or if the pain is limiting activities of daily living.
- Surgery may be required for persistent pain or progressive functional disability.

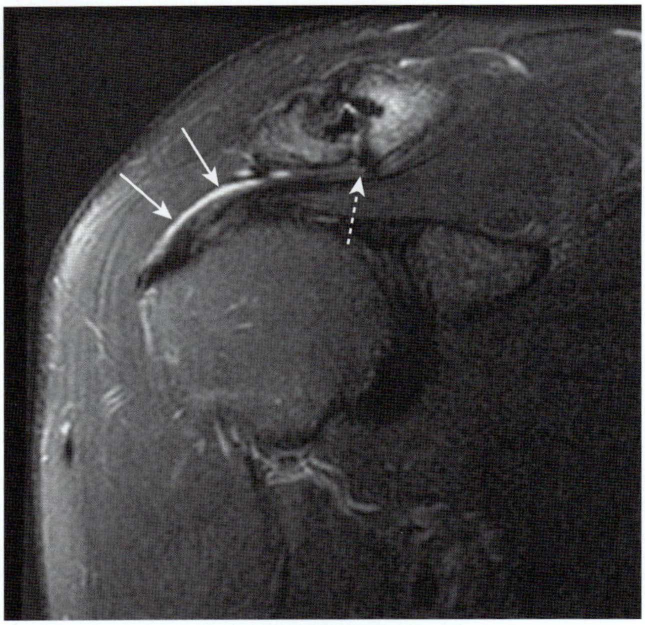

Figure 99.1 Coronal T2-weighted with fat suppression (FST2W) MR image of a patient with subacromial impingement. A small bursal effusion is present, which appears as a thin rim of high signal intensity (SI) (*white arrows*) superficial to the rotator cuff. There are also osteoarthritic changes in the acromioclavicular joint with inferior osteophytes impinging on the supraspinatus musculotendinous junction (*broken white arrow*). *(Reproduced with permission from Campbell RSD & Dunn A. External Impingement of the Shoulder. Seminars In Musculoskeletal Radiology. 2008:12(2);107-126.)*

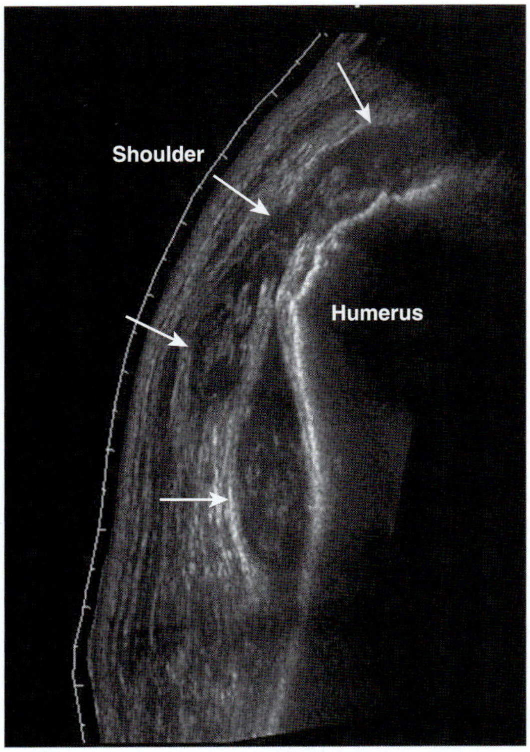

Figure 99.3 Coronal panoramic US image of an infected subacromial bursa that is distended by low-echo fluid (*white arrows*) but contains areas of echogenic exudate. Rheumatoid arthritis might give a similar appearance, and infection was proved by aspiration.

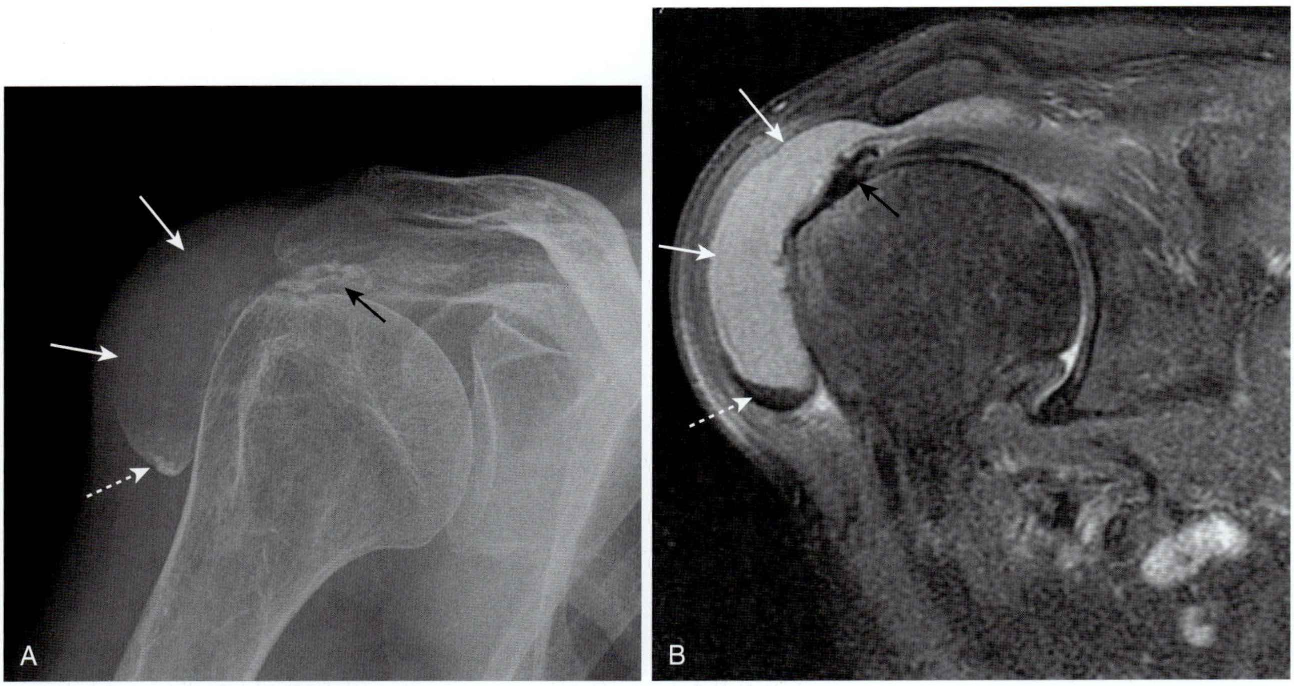

Figure 99.2 (**A**), AP radiograph of a patient with an acute inflammatory subacromial bursitis. There is soft tissue thickening (*white arrows*) due to bursal distention, with crystals collecting in the dependent portion of the bursa (*broken white arrow*), originating from a focus of calcific tendinitis within the rotator cuff (*black arrow*). (**B**), The corresponding coronal FST2W MR image shows the same features with a high-SI fluid-filled bursa (*white arrows*), low-SI crystals within the bursa (*broken white arrow*), and the supraspinatus tendon (*black arrow*).

CHAPTER 100

Quadrilateral Space Syndrome

DEFINITION

- Entrapment of the axillary nerve within the quadrilateral space by mass, tumor, aberrant fibrous band, or fracture.

SIGNS AND SYMPTOMS

- Paresthesias radiating into the lateral shoulder and upper posterior upper extremity.
- Passive range of motion preserved.
- Weakness of teres minor and deltoid muscles.
- Tenderness to palpation of the quadrilateral space.
- Neurapraxia often present.

DEMOGRAPHICS

- Incidence: Male > Female.
- Young athletes often affected.
- Can occur acutely following trauma.
- Twenty to 30-year-old persons most commonly affected.
- More common after trauma, including repetitive stress injuries.

IMAGING RECOMMENDATIONS

- MRI or US:
  - To exclude compressive soft tissue mass or bony abnormality.
- MRI:
  - Most sensitive technique to identify muscle denervation edema, although US will document fatty atrophy.

IMAGING FINDINGS

- Soft tissue mass or underlying bony abnormality adjacent to or within quadrilateral space.
- Identification of the axillary nerve may not be possible.
- High–signal intensity (SI) muscle edema within deltoid and/or teres minor muscle on short T1 inversion recovery (STIR) MR images.
- High-SI fatty replacement and atrophy of muscles on T1-weighted (T1W) MR images in later stages:
  - Echogenic muscle tissue on US.

OTHER RECOMMENDED TESTING

- Electromyography and nerve conduction velocity testing of the cervical nerve roots, brachial plexus, and axillary nerve.

DIFFERENTIAL DIAGNOSIS

- Parsonage-Turner syndrome.
- Hematoma.
- Benign neoplasm.
- Malignant neoplasm.
- Humeral fracture.
- Anterior shoulder dislocation.

TREATMENT

- Conservative treatment consisting of local heat, cold, simple analgesics, and nonsteroidal anti-inflammatory agents will improve symptoms in mild self-limited cases.
- Physical therapy, including gentle stretching, range-of-motion exercises, and local heat modalities, may be beneficial in selected patients to maintain function.
- Injection of the axillary nerve with local anesthetic and steroid may provide symptomatic relief if conservative therapy fails or the pain is limiting activities of daily living.
- Surgery may be required to relieve entrapment of the axillary nerve.

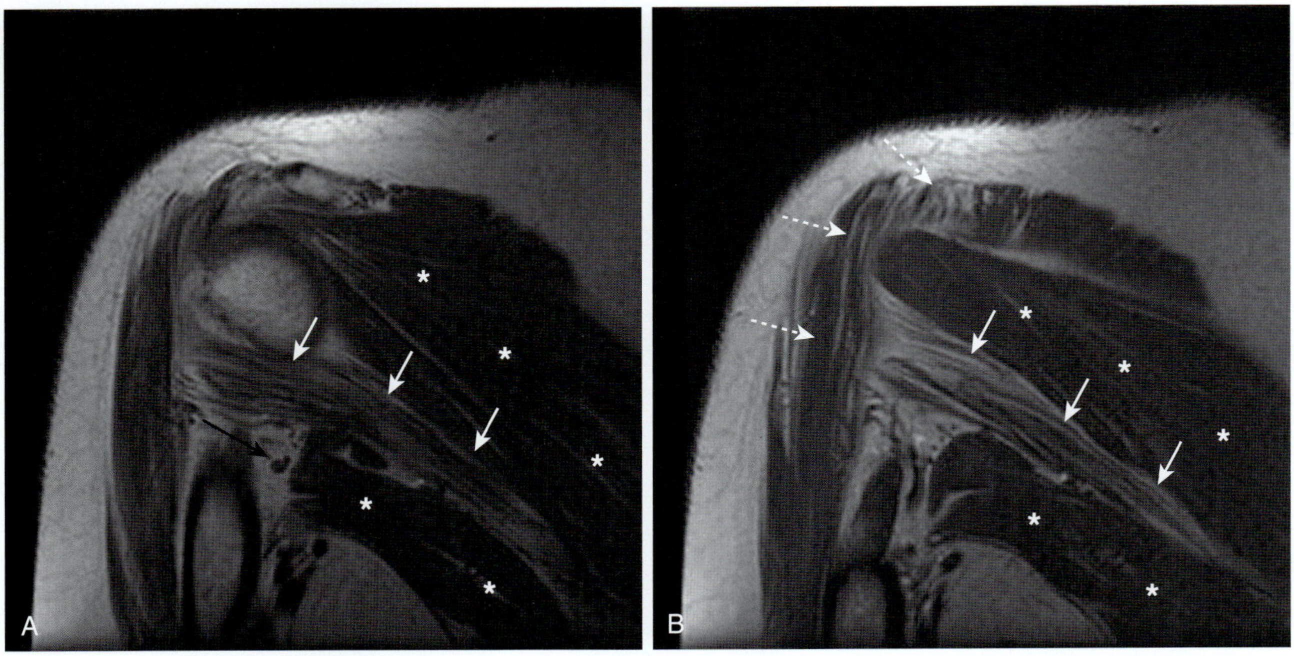

Figure 100.1 (A and B), Consecutive coronal T1W MR images in a patient with chronic quadrilateral space syndrome. The axillary nerve is clearly demonstrated (*black arrow*). There are pronounced atrophy and fat infiltration within the teres minor (*white arrows*) and also within the posterior deltoid (*broken white arrows*). Compare with the normal appearance of the infraspinatus, triceps, teres major, and latissimus dorsi muscles (*asterisks*). No abnormal muscle edema was present on T2W with fat suppression MR images in this chronic case, and no compressive lesion was identified. The axillary nerve is visible within the fat-filled quadrilateral space (*broken black arrow*).

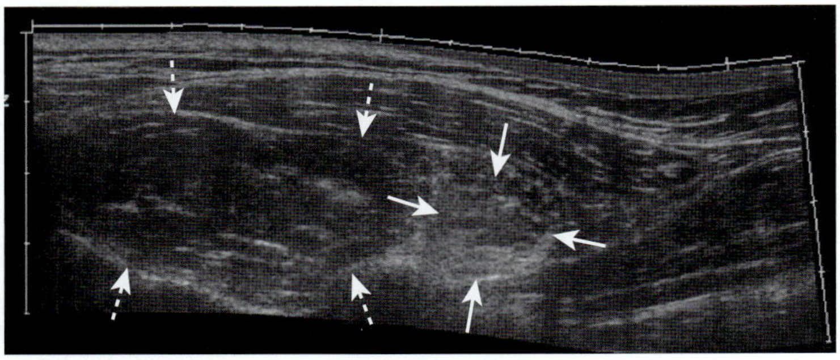

Figure 100.2 US image of another case of quadrilateral space syndrome. The teres minor muscle (*white arrows*) is small and echogenic, in comparison with the infraspinatus muscle (*broken white arrows*), because of fat infiltration and atrophy.

CHAPTER 101

Suprascapular Nerve Entrapment

DEFINITION

- Entrapment of the suprascapular nerve, as it passes through the suprascapular notch, by the transverse scapular ligament or a mass, tumor, aberrant fibrous band, scapular fracture, or paralabral cyst.

SIGNS AND SYMPTOMS

- Paresthesias radiating into the shoulder and upper posterior upper extremity.
- Passive range of motion preserved.
- Weakness of supraspinatus and infraspinatus muscles.
- Tenderness to palpation of the suprascapular nerve as it exits the suprascapular notch.
- Neurapraxia often present.

DEMOGRAPHICS

- Incidence: Male > Female.
- Young athletes involved in overhead sports such as tennis and volleyball often affected.
- Can occur acutely following trauma.
- Twenty to 30-year-old persons most commonly affected.
- More common after trauma, including repetitive stress injuries.
- Can result from wearing a backpack that is too heavy.

IMAGING RECOMMENDATIONS

- Radiography:
  - To exclude bony abnormality.
- MRI or US:
  - To exclude compressive soft tissue mass.
  - MRI is a more sensitive technique to identify muscle denervation edema, although US will document fatty atrophy.

IMAGING FINDINGS

- Soft tissue mass or underlying bony abnormality in the spinoglenoid notch.
- High-signal intensity (SI) muscle edema within supraspinatus and infraspinatus muscles on short T1 inversion recovery (STIR) MR images:
  - Isolated infraspinatus involvement may occur.
- In later stages, high-SI fatty replacement and atrophy of muscles on T1-weighted (T1W) MR images.
  - Echogenic muscle tissue on US.
- May be the presentation of a SLAP (superior labral tear from anterior to posterior) lesion with paralabral cyst formation.

OTHER RECOMMENDED TESTING

- Electromyography and nerve conduction velocity testing of the cervical nerve roots, brachial plexus, and suprascapular nerve.

DIFFERENTIAL DIAGNOSIS

- Parsonage-Turner syndrome.
- Hematoma.
- Benign neoplasm.
- Malignant neoplasm.
- Scapular fracture.
- Rotator cuff pathology.

TREATMENT

- Conservative treatment consisting of local heat, cold, simple analgesics, and nonsteroidal anti-inflammatory agents will improve symptoms in mild, self-limited cases.
- Physical therapy to maintain function, including gentle stretching, range-of-motion exercises, and local heat modalities may be beneficial in selected patients.
- Injection with local anesthetic and steroid of the suprascapular nerve may provide symptomatic relief if conservative therapy fails or the pain is limiting activities of daily living.
- Surgery may be required to relieve entrapment of the suprascapular nerve.

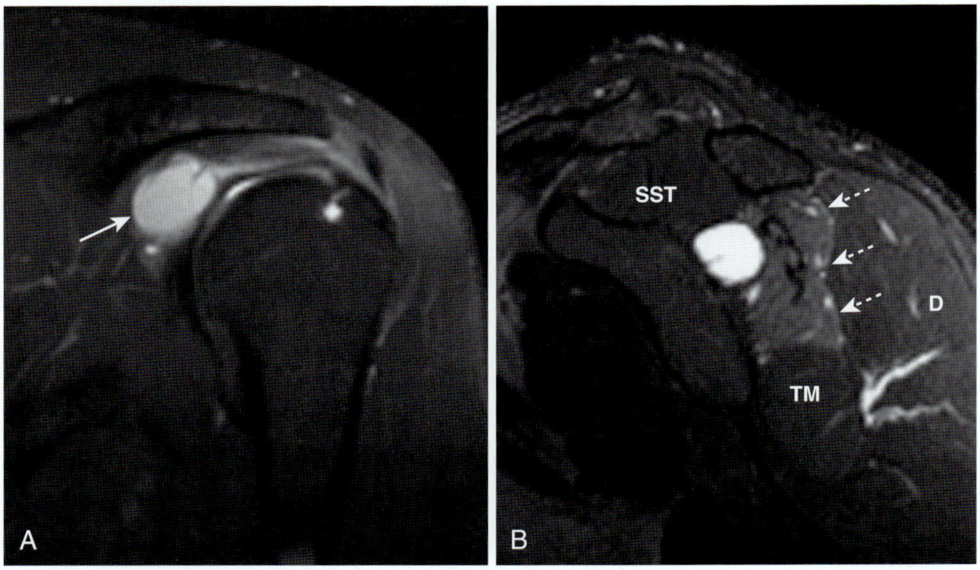

Figure 101.1 (A), Coronal oblique T2W with fat suppression (FST2W) MR image of a patient with a high-SI paralabral cyst in the spinoglenoid notch (*white arrow*). (B), A sagittal oblique FST2W MR image shows the cyst. There is also high SI within the infraspinatus muscle belly (*broken white arrows*) in comparison with the supraspinatus, teres minor, and deltoid muscle bellies. This finding indicates muscle denervation edema due to compression of the suprascapular nerve by the cyst. D, deltoid; SST, supraspinatus; TM, teres minor. *(Image courtesy of Dr. Phil Robinson, Leeds, United Kingdom.)*

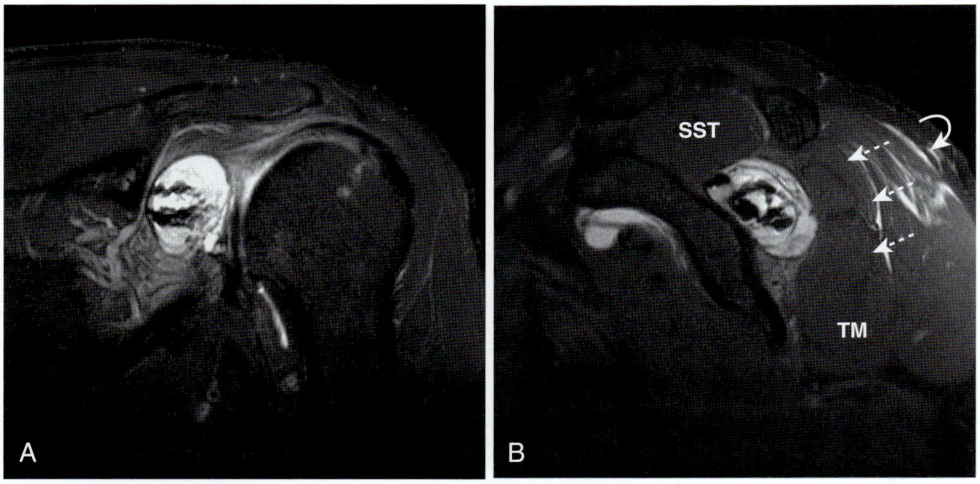

Figure 101.2 (A), Coronal oblique FST2W MR arthrogram image of a patient with symptoms of a SLAP lesion. There is a paralabral cyst similar to that shown in Figure 101.1 that contains some low-SI loose bodies. In this case, however, the sagittal oblique FST2W MR image (B) demonstrates normal SI within the infraspinatus *(broken white arrows)*, and there is no evidence of suprascapular nerve entrapment. High SI within the posterior soft tissues is due to local anesthetic used during the arthrogram procedure (*curved white arrow*). SST, supraspinatus; TM, teres minor.

CHAPTER 102

Anatomy: Special Imaging Considerations of the Elblow

OSSEOUS STRUCTURES

Humerus. The distal end of the humerus is made up of the trochlear and capitellum, which form the elbow joint, and the extra-articular medial epicondyle and lateral condyle, on which insert the common flexor and extensor muscle origins, respectively.

Radius. The proximal radius has a flattened, disc-shaped head covered in hyaline cartilage that articulates with the capitellum as well as the proximal ulna. Distal to the capsular insertion is the radial tuberosity bearing the insertion of the distal biceps tendon.

Ulna. The proximal ulna is made up of the olecranon bearing the triceps insertion, the trochlear notch, and the coronoid process further distally, which articulate with the trochlear of the humerus.

JOINTS

The elbow is a complex synovial hinge joint made up of three separate articulations:

Humeroulnar Joint. Articulation of the concave trochlear of the humerus with the trochlear notch of the ulna, also referred to as the *ulnotrochlear compartment* of the elbow.

Humeroradial Joint. Articulation between the anterior convexity of the humeral capitellum and the slightly concave, discoid radial head, also referred to as the *radiocapitellar compartment*.

Proximal Radioulnar Joint (PRUJ). Formed by the radial head and the articular groove on the lateral surface of the proximal ulna.

SOFT TISSUES

Medial Stabilizers. Ulnar collateral ligament complex composed of anterior, transverse, and posterior bundles.

Lateral Stabilizers. Radial collateral ligament and lateral ulnar collateral ligament, which also contribute to the posterior stability of the radial head.

Annular Ligament. An intra-articular bandlike ligament that wraps around the radial head, stabilizing the PRUJ.

Common Flexor Origin (CFO). A group of muscles forming the superficial flexor compartment of the forearm and taking origin from a common tendon insertion of the medial epicondyle of the humerus.

Common Extensor Origin (CEO). A group of muscles forming the superficial extensor compartment of the forearm and taking origin from a common tendon insertion of the lateral epicondyle of the humerus.

Distal Biceps Tendon. Forms proximal to the elbow by fusion of the long and short heads of the biceps, inserts onto the radial tuberosity, and is stabilized by the bicipital aponeurosis.

NERVES

Median Nerve. Descends in the upper arm medial to the brachial artery and gives off branches to the brachial artery and pronator teres. It then enters the cubital fossa lying deep to the bicipital aponeurosis, anterior to the brachialis. An anatomic variant known as the *ligament of Struthers* may be present arising from the anterior humerus proximal to the elbow, which may produce median nerve entrapment.

Ulnar Nerve. Descends in the upper arm medial to the brachial artery and does not give off any branches in the arm proximal to the elbow. It courses along the medial head of the triceps to enter the ulnar tunnel between the medial epicondyle and the olecranon. The roof of the ulnar tunnel is formed by Osborne ligament.

Radial Nerve. Descends posteriorly in the upper arm, giving off branches to triceps as it runs along the spiral groove. From the lateral border of the humerus, it then pierces the intermuscular membrane to enter the anterior compartment between the brachialis and brachioradialis. The radial nerve divides into the posterior interosseous nerve (PIN) and superficial terminal branches anterior to the lateral epicondyle. The PIN may become compressed as it passes beneath the origin of the supinator muscle in a region known as the arcade of Frohse.

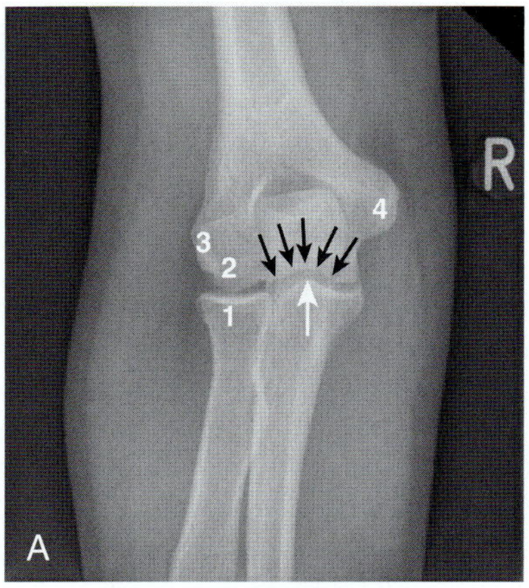

Figure 102.1 1, Radial head; 2, capitellum; 3, lateral epicondyle; 4, medial epicondyle; *black arrows,* trochlear; *white arrow,* coronoid process.

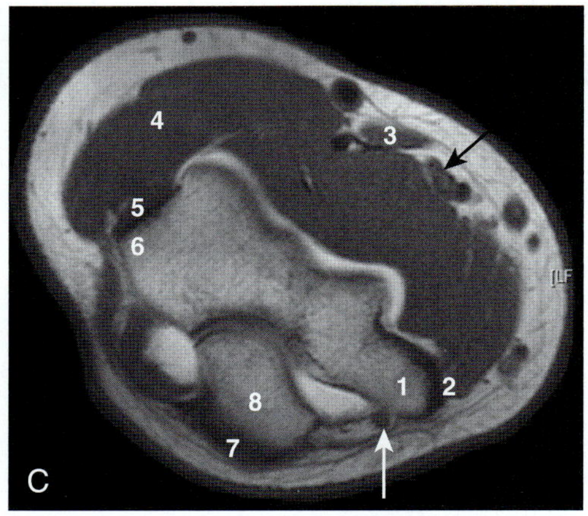

Figure 102.3 Axial T1-weighted MR arthrogram image of the elbow. 1, Medial epicondyle; 2, common flexor origin ; 3, distal biceps tendon; 4, brachioradialis muscle; 5, common extensor origin; 6, lateral epicondyle; 7, triceps tendon; 8, olecranon process; *white arrow,* ulnar nerve; *black arrow,* median nerve.

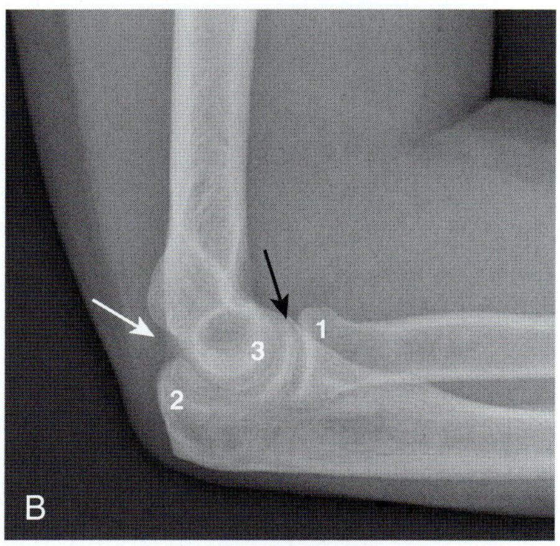

Figure 102.2 1, Radial head; 2, olecranon; 3, capitellum; *white arrow,* olecranon fossa; *black arrow,* coronoid process.

CHAPTER 103

Tennis Elbow

DEFINITION

- Degeneration of the extensor tendons due to repetitive microtrauma at the origin of the musculotendinous unit at the lateral epicondyle.

SIGNS AND SYMPTOMS

- Gradual onset of dull lateral elbow pain.
- Worse with activity.
- Pain often radiates into the upper forearm.
- Pain worse with activities such as holding a coffee cup and using a hammer.
- Point tenderness at the origin of the musculotendinous unit at the lateral epicondyle.
- Pain worse with resisted wrist extension.
- Patient experiences sleep disturbance.

DEMOGRAPHICS

- Incidence: Male = Female.
- Associated with activities that require repeated valgus stress on the elbow.
- Worse in tennis players with forward-leading backhand stroke.
- More common after trauma, including repetitive stress injuries.

IMAGING RECOMMENDATIONS

- Imaging not routinely indicated.
- MRI or US may be useful for refractory cases.

IMAGING FINDINGS

- High signal intensity (SI) and thickening of the tendon on T2-weighted with fat suppression (FST2W) MR images.
  - Focal fluid SI or tendon defect present with tendon tears.
- Low reflectivity, tendon thickening on US:
  - Neovascularization on Doppler imaging.
- Bony enthesophyte formation may be present in chronic cases.
- Occasional radial collateral ligament tears may be present in refractory cases.
  - May be associated with posterolateral instability.

OTHER RECOMMENDED TESTING

- Electromyography and nerve conduction velocity testing to rule out radial tunnel syndrome.
- Laboratory testing to rule out inflammatory arthritis.
- Joint aspiration to rule out crystal arthropathies.
- Joint aspiration to rule out infection if diagnosis in question.

DIFFERENTIAL DIAGNOSIS

- Calcific tendinitis.
- Radial tunnel syndrome.
- Gout.
- Occult elbow fracture.
- Posterior elbow instability.

TREATMENT

- Conservative treatment consisting of local heat, cold, simple analgesics, and nonsteroidal anti-inflammatory agents will improve symptoms in many cases.
- Physical therapy, including gentle stretching, range-of-motion exercises, and deep heat modalities, may be beneficial in selected patients.
- Injection with local anesthetic and steroid will provide symptomatic relief if conservative therapy fails or the pain is limiting activities of daily living.
- Surgery may be required for persistent pain or progressive functional disability.

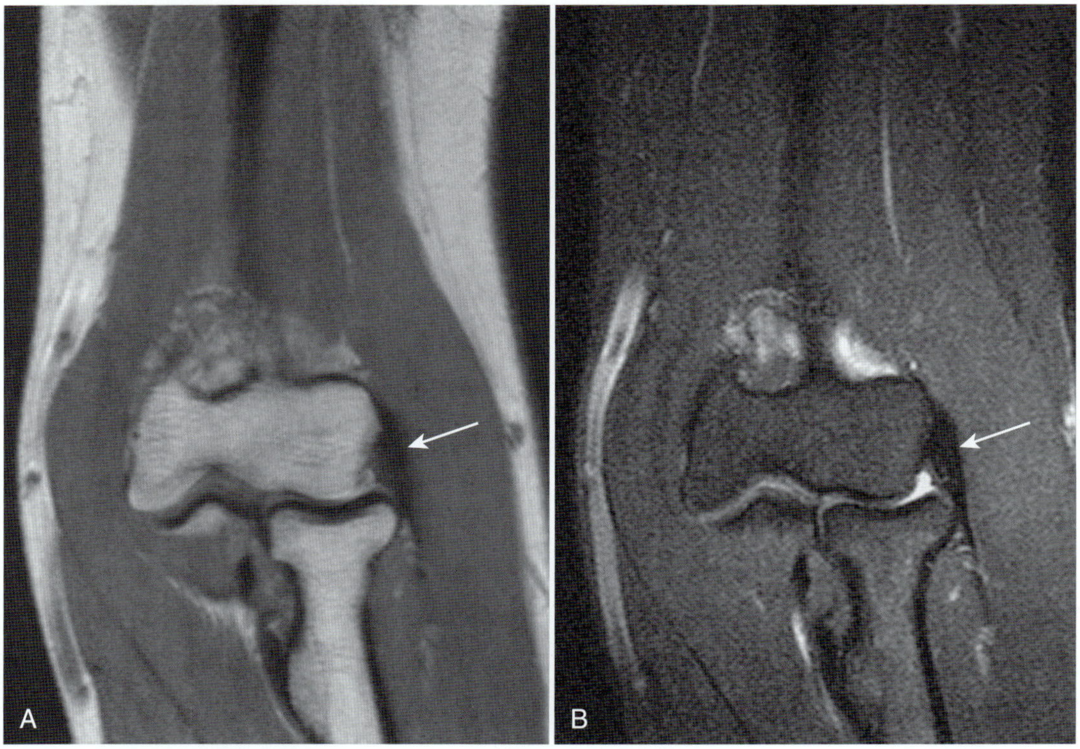

Figure 103.1 Coronal proton density (PD) (**A**) and FST2W (**B**) MR images of a normal elbow. Note the low SI of the common extensor origin tendon (*white arrows*), which arises from the lateral humeral epicondyle.

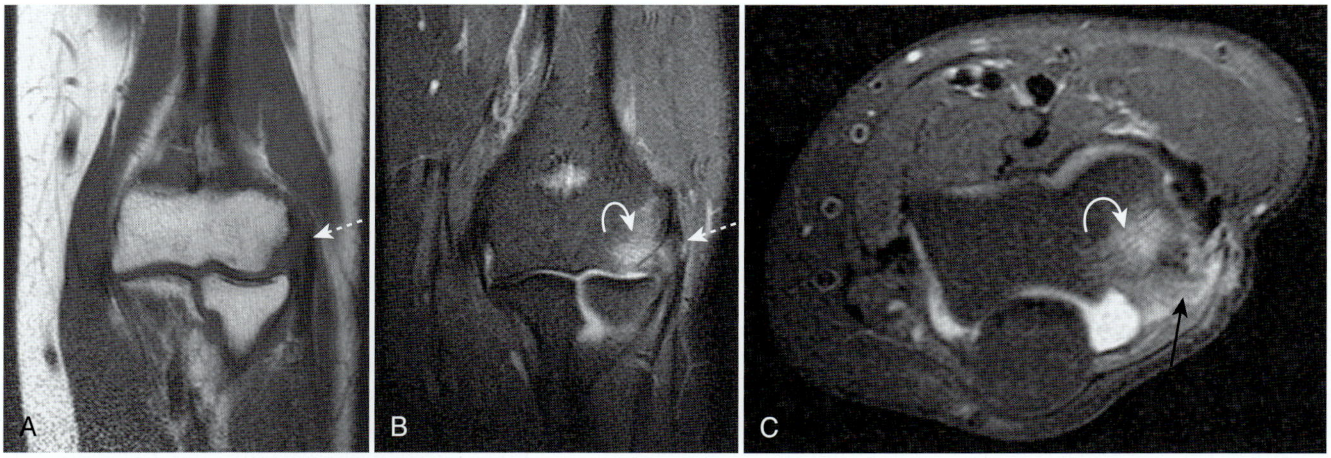

Figure 103.2 Coronal PD (**A**) and FST2W (**B**) MR images of a patient with tennis elbow. There are thickening and increased SI within the common extensor tendon (*broken white arrow*) along with associated underlying bone marrow edema (*curved arrow*). (**C**), The bone marrow is also seen on the axial FST2W MR image (*curved arrow*), and the soft tissue thickening and increased SI posterior to the extensor tendon probably reflect associated soft tissue impingement (*black arrow*).

CHAPTER 104

Golfer's Elbow

DEFINITION

- Degeneration of the flexor pronator group resulting in an overuse tendinopathy at the medial epicondyle.

SIGNS AND SYMPTOMS

- Gradual onset of dull medial elbow pain.
- Worse with activity.
- Pain often radiates into upper forearm.
- Pain worse with activity such as throwing a ball.
- Point tenderness at the origin of the musculotendinous unit at the medial epicondyle.
- Pain worse with resisted wrist flexion.
- Patient may experience sleep disturbance.

DEMOGRAPHICS

- Incidence: Male = Female.
- Most common in the third to fifth decade of life.
- Most common in the dominant hand of golfers and throwing athletes.
- Associated with activities that require repeated valgus stress on the elbow.
- More common after trauma, including repetitive stress injuries.

IMAGING RECOMMENDATIONS

- Imaging not routinely indicated.
- MRI or US may be useful for refractory cases.

IMAGING FINDINGS

- High signal intensity (SI) and thickening of tendon on T2-weighted with fat suppression (FST2W) MR images:
  - Focal fluid SI or tendon defect is present with tendon tears.
- Low reflectivity, tendon thickening on US:
  - Neovascularization on Doppler imaging.
  - Focal areas of microcalcification.
- Bony enthesophyte formation may be present in chronic cases.
- Occasional ulnar collateral ligament tears may be present in refractory cases.

OTHER RECOMMENDED TESTING

- Electromyography and nerve conduction velocity testing to rule out ulnar neuropathy.
- Laboratory testing to rule out inflammatory arthritis.
- Joint aspiration to rule out crystal arthropathies.
- Joint aspiration to rule out infection if diagnosis in question.

DIFFERENTIAL DIAGNOSIS

- Calcific tendinitis.
- Ulnar neuropathy.
- Gout.
- Occult elbow fractures.
- Posterior elbow instability.

TREATMENT

- Conservative treatment consisting of local heat, cold, simple analgesics, and nonsteroidal anti-inflammatory agents will improve symptoms in many cases.
- Physical therapy, including gentle stretching, range-of-motion exercises, and deep heat modalities, may be beneficial in selected patients.
- Injection with local anesthetic and steroid will provide symptomatic relief if conservative therapy fails or the pain is limiting activities of daily living.
- Surgery may be required for persistent pain or progressive functional disability.

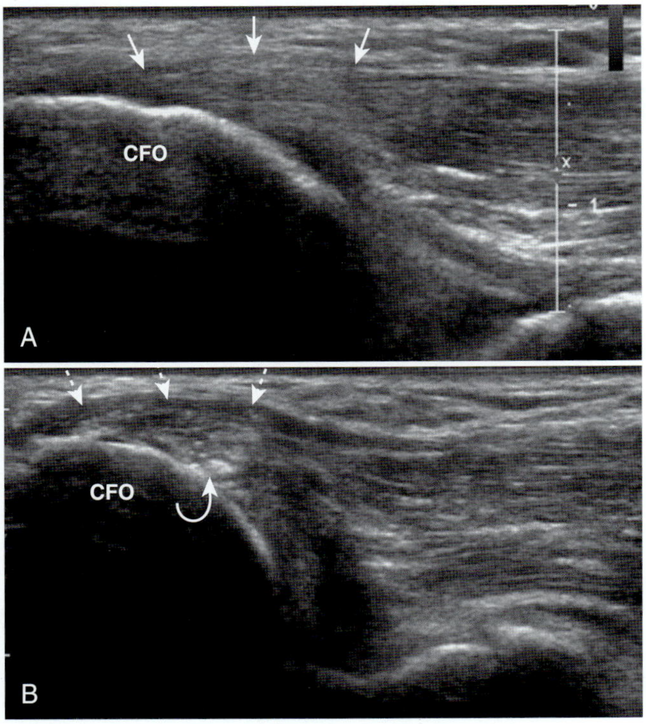

Figure 104.1 (A), Longitudinal US image of the asymptomatic elbow of a patient presenting with golfer's elbow. The common flexor origin (CFO) of the medial humeral epicondyle gives rise to a normal echogenic common flexor tendon (*white arrows*). (B), On the affected side, the tendon is thickened with heterogeneous low-echo change (*broken white arrows*), and there are small areas of echo-bright degenerative microcalcification (*curved white arrow*). These US features are typical of insertional tendinopathy associated with golfer's or tennis elbow.

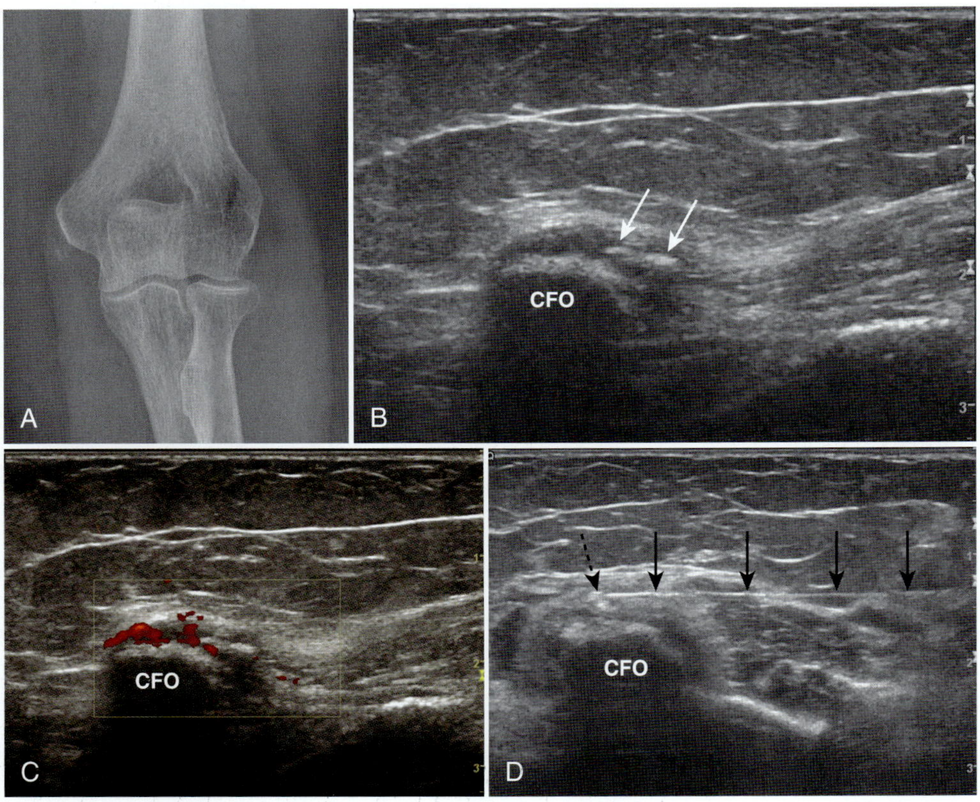

Figure 104.2 (A), Radiograph of a middle-aged woman with golfer's elbow demonstrates a few small areas of calcification in the CFO adjacent to the medial epicondyle. (B and C), The corresponding US images show an echo-poor tendon with small echogenic foci of calcification (*white arrows*) and neovascularization, as evident by increased blood flow on Doppler imaging (C) consistent with tendinopathy. (D), US-guided injection and dry needling shows the needle (*black arrows*) with the tip adjacent to the areas of calcification (*broken black arrow*).

CHAPTER 105

Little Leaguer's Elbow

DEFINITION

- Repetitive stress injury resulting in a traction apophysitis that manifests as delayed closure of the medial epicondylar epiphysis or avulsion fracture of the medial epicondyle.

SIGNS AND SYMPTOMS

- Gradual onset of dull medial elbow pain.
- Worse with activity.
- Pain often radiates into upper forearm.
- Pain worse with activity such as throwing a ball.
- Point tenderness at the origin of the musculotendinous unit at the medial epicondyle.
- Pain worse with resisted wrist flexion.
- Pain improves with reduction in valgus stress activities.
- Gradual loss of range of motion.
- Patient may experience sleep disturbance.

DEMOGRAPHICS

- Incidence: Male > Female.
- Most common in children but can occur in adults.
- Most common in the dominant hand of a throwing athlete.
- Associated with activities that require repeated valgus stress on the elbow.
- More common after trauma, including repetitive stress injuries.

IMAGING RECOMMENDATIONS

- Radiography.
- MRI or US:
  - To assess soft tissue injury.

IMAGING FINDINGS

- Radiography:
  - Avulsion or fragmentation of the medial epicondylar ossification center.
- MRI:
  - Marrow edema in ossification center with or without fragmentation.
  - High-signal intensity (SI) edema in common flexor origin tendon.
  - High-SI cleft tear within flexor tendon.
  - Thickening and high SI within ulnar collateral ligament (UCL) or ligament disruption.
- US:
  - Fragmentation of ossification center.
  - Thickening and low echogenicity within tendon tears.
  - Thickening and loss of visualization of UCL.

OTHER RECOMMENDED TESTING

- Electromyography and nerve conduction velocity testing to rule out ulnar neuropathy.
- Laboratory testing to rule out inflammatory arthritis.
- Joint aspiration to rule out crystal arthropathies.
- Joint aspiration to rule out infection if diagnosis in question.

DIFFERENTIAL DIAGNOSIS

- Calcific tendinitis.
- Golfer's elbow.
- Medial collateral ligament pathology.
- Capitellar osteochondritis.
- Ulnar neuropathy.
- Gout.
- Occult elbow fracture.
- Posterior elbow instability.

TREATMENT

- Conservative treatment consisting of local heat, cold, simple analgesics, and nonsteroidal anti-inflammatory agents will improve symptoms in many cases.
- Cessation of valgus overload activities.
- Injection with local anesthetic and steroid will provide symptomatic relief if conservative therapy fails or the pain is limiting activities of daily living.
- Surgery may be required for persistent pain or progressive functional disability and for acute bony avulsion of the epicondyle.

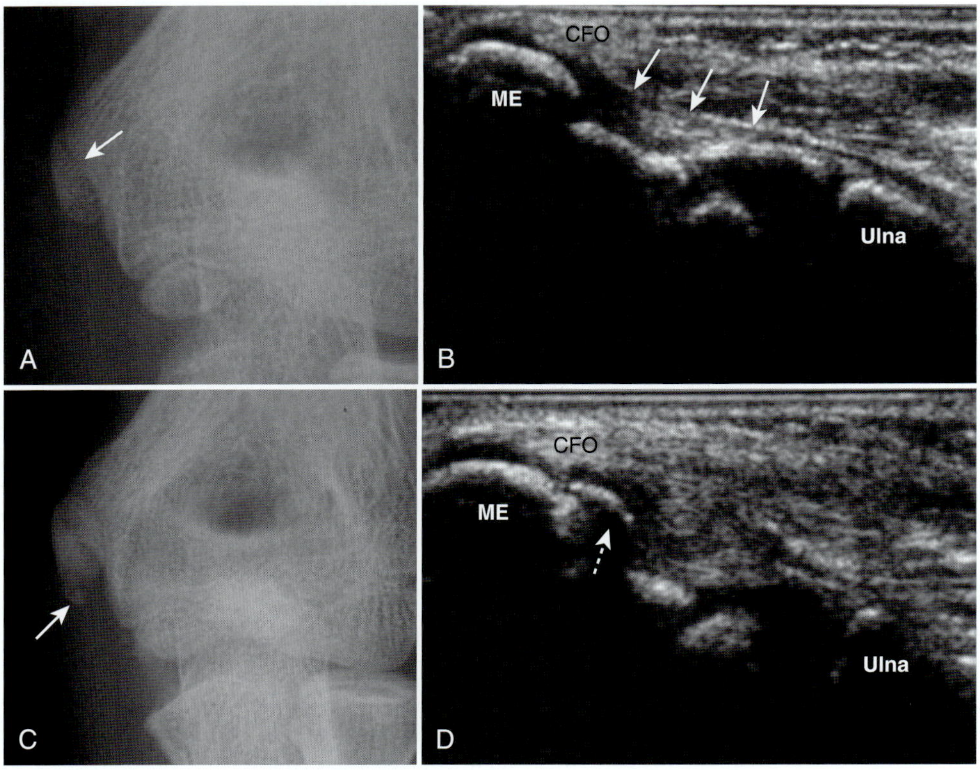

Figure 105.1 (**A**), AP radiograph of a normal medial epicondyle (*white arrow*). (**B**), The corresponding US image shows the medial epicondyle (ME) and the echogenic common flexor origin (CFO). The UCL can be seen as a thin, echo-bright structure (*white arrows*) extending from the distal humerus and attaching to the ulna. (**C**), An AP radiograph in a symptomatic child shows fragmentation of the medial epicondyle (*white arrow*). (**D**), The corresponding longitudinal US image demonstrates the fragmented epicondyle (*broken white arrow*). The UCL is not visualized because of a chronic tear.

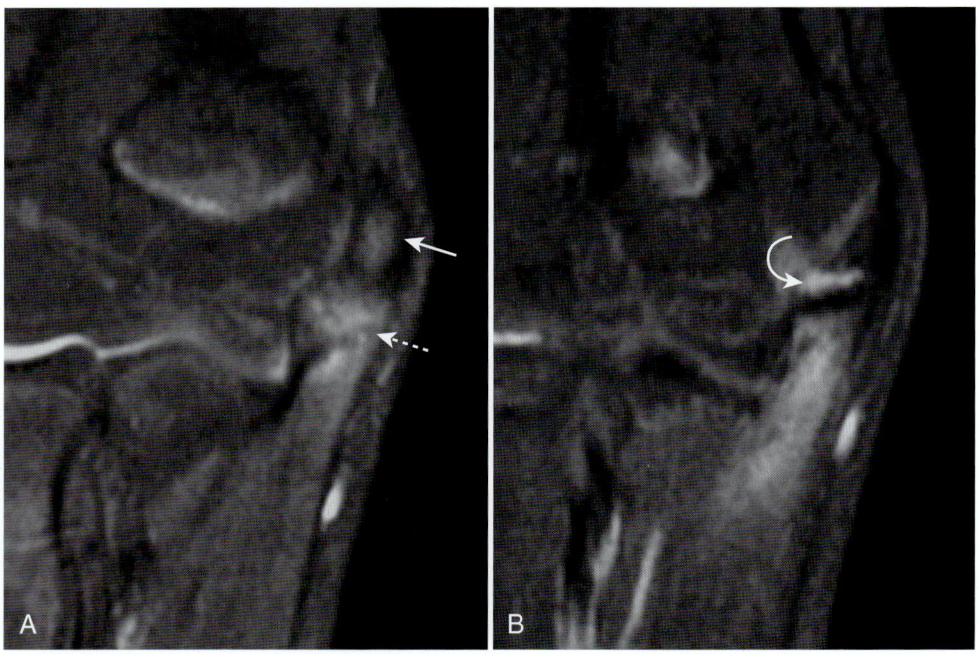

Figure 105.2 (**A** and **B**), Consecutive coronal T2-weighted with fat suppression (FST2W) MR images of the elbow in a child with recent strain injury of the medial epicondyle. The medial ossification center is not displaced (*white arrow*), but there are distal soft tissue edema (*broken white arrow*) and a high-SI cleft tear in the proximal flexor digitorum (*curved white arrow*).

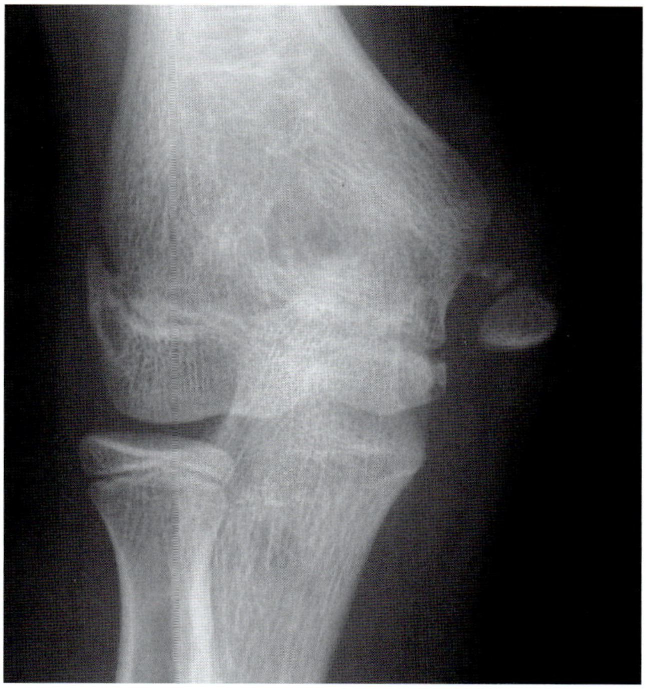

Figure 105.3 AP radiograph demonstrating an acute avulsion injury of the medial epicondylar ossification center that has been displaced and requires surgical reattachment.

CHAPTER 106

Distal Biceps Tendon Rupture

DEFINITION

- Rupture of the distal biceps tendon from the radial tuberosity.

SIGNS AND SYMPTOMS

- Sudden onset of dull, ill-defined pain after forced extension of a flexed forearm.
- Pain often radiates distally.
- Positive result of Ludington ("Popeye") test because of muscle belly retraction.
- Crepitus may be present.
- Ecchymosis in the cubital fossa.
- Exacerbation of pain with flexion of the forearm.
- Absence of the distal biceps tendon on palpation of the antecubital fossa.
- Patient unable to sleep on the affected shoulder.

DEMOGRAPHICS

- Incidence: Male > Female.
- Occurs most commonly in the fifth decade of life.
- Common in weight lifters, football players, and snowboarders.
- More common after forced extension of a flexed forearm.

IMAGING RECOMMENDATIONS

- MRI or US.

IMAGING FINDINGS

- Tears usually occur at the tendon's insertion on the radial tuberosity.
  - Less commonly, tear occurs at the musculotendinous junction.
- Tendon retraction:
  - May be limited by intact attachment to the lacertus fibrosus aponeurosis of the forearm.
- Fluid within the empty distal tendon sheath.
- Eventual atrophy of the biceps muscle belly.

OTHER RECOMMENDED TESTING

- Biopsy of undefined biceps mass to rule out neoplasm if diagnosis in question.

DIFFERENTIAL DIAGNOSIS

- Brachialis muscle rupture.
- Radial bursitis.
- Neoplasm involving the biceps muscle.

TREATMENT

- Conservative treatment consisting of local heat, cold, simple analgesics, and nonsteroidal anti-inflammatory agents will improve symptoms in many cases.
- Physical therapy to maintain range-of-motion exercises.
- Injection with local anesthetic and steroid will provide symptomatic relief if conservative therapy fails or the pain is limiting activities of daily living.
- Surgery often required for persistent pain or progressive functional disability.

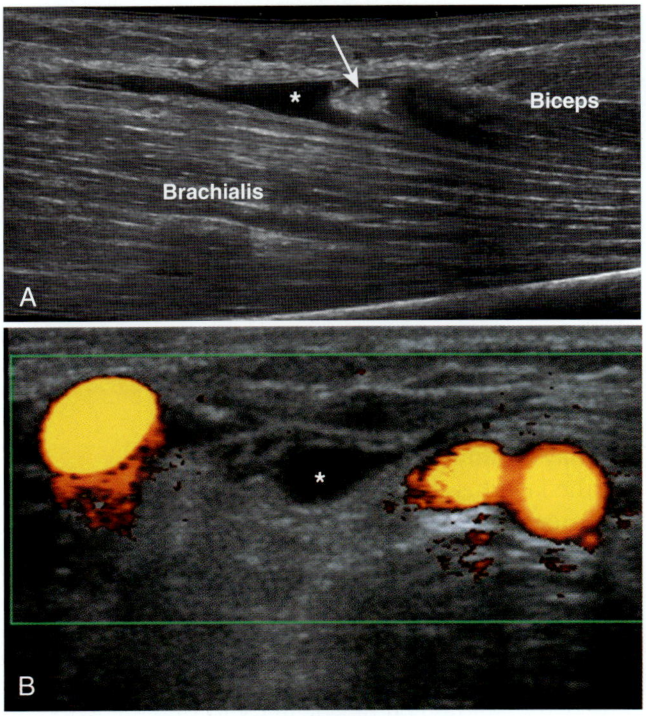

Figure 106.1 (A), Longitudinal US image of a distal biceps rupture. The torn end of the retracted tendon (*arrow*) can be seen superficial to the brachialis muscle. The empty tendon sheath (*asterisk*) is anechoic and fluid filled. (B), The axial Doppler US image differentiates the empty tendon sheath (*asterisk*) from the superficial veins.

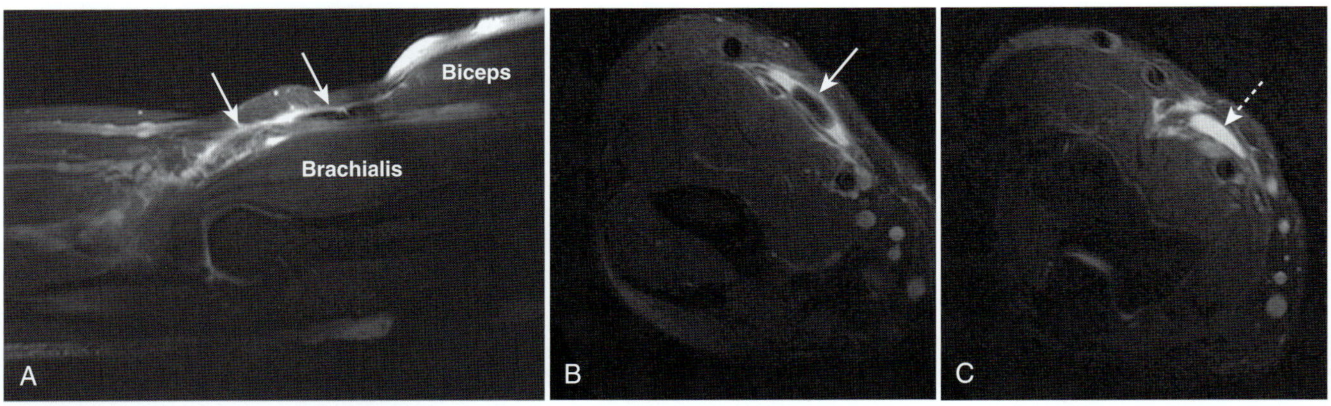

Figure 106.2 (A), Sagittal T2-weighted with fat suppression (FST2W) MR image demonstrates a torn biceps tendon (*arrows*), which is thickened and irregular, and high–signal intensity (SI) fluid within the tendon sheath. (B), The axial FST2W MR image shows the tendon in the proximal tendon sheath (*arrow*). (C), The distal tendon sheath is empty (*broken arrow*).

CHAPTER 107

Bicipital Radial Bursitis

DEFINITION

Inflammation of the bursa that lies between the biceps tendon and the anterior aspect of the radial tuberosity.

SIGNS AND SYMPTOMS

- Onset may be acute or insidious.
- Pain localized underneath the biceps tendon that is made worse with supination of the elbow.
- Pain may radiate to the proximal forearm.
- Tenderness to palpation of the antecubital fossa.
- Warmth may be present.
- Antecubital fossa may feel boggy or edematous.
- Mass may be present.
- Crepitus or catching sensation may be present.
- Exacerbation of pain with resisted supination.
- Pain often worse at night.
- Gradual decrease in range of motion.

DEMOGRAPHICS

- Incidence: Male > Female.
- Young athletes often affected.
- Forty to 50-year-old persons most commonly affected.
- More common after trauma, including repetitive stress injuries.
- Increased incidence in patients with distal biceps pathology.
- Common in rheumatoid arthritis.

IMAGING RECOMMENDATIONS

- MRI or US.

IMAGING FINDINGS

- Fluid in biceps tendon sheath with intact tendon.
- May be associated with biceps tendinopathy and tendon thickening:
  - Increased signal intensity (SI) on T1-weighted (T1W) and T2W MR images.
  - Low reflectivity on US.
- Rheumatoid arthritis:
  - Often, large bursal effusions.
  - May be echogenic because of fibrinous exudates or synovial thickening.
  - Frequently associated with inflammatory arthritis in the elbow joint.

OTHER RECOMMENDED TESTING

- Laboratory testing to rule out inflammatory arthritis.
- Bursa aspiration with gram staining and culture and sensitivity testing if infection in question.
- Joint aspiration to rule out crystal arthropathies.
- Joint aspiration to rule out infection if diagnosis in question.

DIFFERENTIAL DIAGNOSIS

- Calcific tendinitis.
- Partial distal biceps tendon tear.
- Complete distal biceps tendon tear.
- Gout.
- Occult radial head fractures.
- Capitellum osteochondritis dissecans.
- Antecubital fossa mass.
- Septic arthritis of the elbow.

TREATMENT

- Conservative treatment consisting of local heat, cold, simple analgesics, and nonsteroidal anti-inflammatory agents will improve symptoms in mild cases.
- Physical therapy, including gentle stretching, range-of-motion exercises, and deep heat modalities, may be beneficial in selected patients.
- Injection with local anesthetic and steroid will provide symptomatic relief if conservative therapy fails or the pain is limiting activities of daily living.
- Surgery may be required for persistent pain or progressive functional disability.

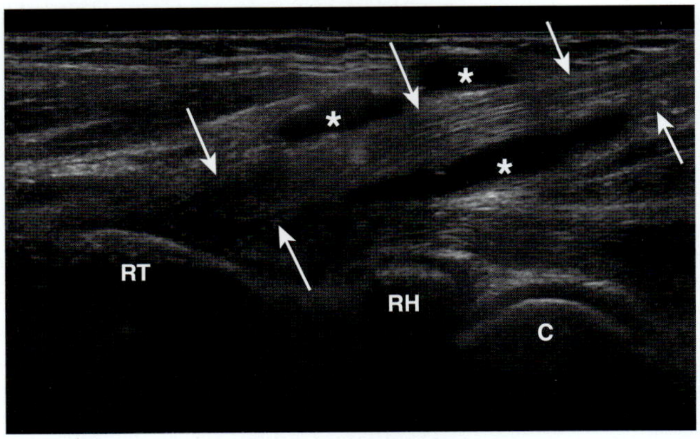

Figure 107.1 US image of a patient with bicipital radial bursitis. Anechoic fluid (*asterisks*) outlines the normal distal biceps tendon (*white arrows*), which inserts on the radial tuberosity (RT). The radiocapitellar joint is normal. C, capitellum; RH, radial head.

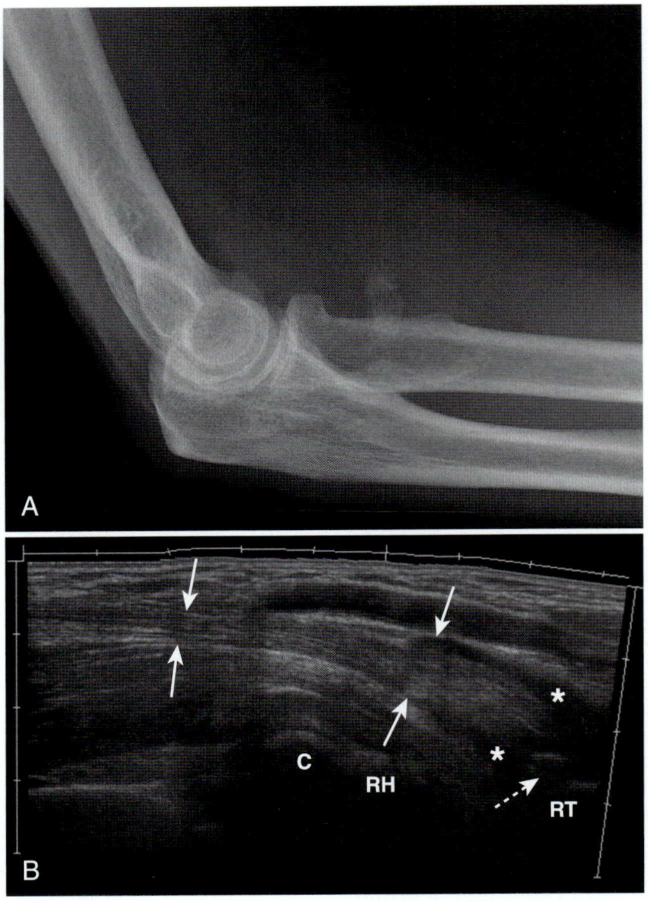

Figure 107.2 (A), Radiograph of a patient with chronic insertional tendinopathy of the distal biceps tendon with new bone formation at the radial tuberosity. (B), The corresponding US image demonstrates a thickened distal biceps tendon (*white arrows*) with associated bicipital radial bursitis and fluid in the tendon sheath (*asterisks*). New bone formation (*broken arrow*) can be seen on the radial tuberosity (RT). The radiocapitellar joint is normal. (C), capitellum; RH, radial head.

CHAPTER 108

Olecranon Bursitis

DEFINITION

- Inflammation of the bursa that lies between the triceps tendon and the tip of the olecranon.

SIGNS AND SYMPTOMS

- Onset may be acute or insidious.
- Pain is localized to posterior elbow.
- Pain is made worse with movement of the elbow.
- Large fluid collections sometimes present.
- Tenderness to palpation of the antecubital fossa.
- Warmth may be present.
- Posterior elbow may feel boggy or edematous.
- Crepitus or catching sensation may be present.
- Exacerbation of pain with resisted extension.
- Pain often worse at night.
- Gradual decrease in range of motion.

DEMOGRAPHICS

- Incidence: Male = Female.
- Often seen in students and draftspersons.
- All ages affected.
- More common after trauma, including repetitive stress injuries.
- Increased incidence in patients with calcific tendinitis of the distal triceps.
- Common finding in gout.

IMAGING RECOMMENDATIONS

- Imaging not routinely required:
  - MRI or US if there are atypical features.
  - Radiography to assess associated joint disease.

IMAGING FINDINGS

- Soft tissue thickening over olecranon on radiography.
- Fluid-filled bursa on MRI or US.
- Synovial thickening and effusions may be prominent with crystal arthropathy:
  - Enhancement on MR images obtained after administration of contrast medium.
  - Increased reflectivity and vascularity on US.

OTHER RECOMMENDED TESTING

- Laboratory testing to rule out inflammatory arthritis.
- Bursa aspiration with Gram staining and culture and sensitivity testing if infection or crystal disease in question.
- Joint aspiration to rule out crystal arthropathies.
- Joint aspiration to rule out infection if diagnosis in question.

DIFFERENTIAL DIAGNOSIS

- Calcific tendinitis.
- Partial distal triceps tendon tear.
- Complete distal triceps tendon tear.
- Gout.
- Occult olecranon fracture.
- Posterior elbow mass.
- Septic arthritis of the elbow.

TREATMENT

- Conservative treatment consisting of local heat, cold, simple analgesics, and nonsteroidal anti-inflammatory agents will improve symptoms in mild cases.
- Physical therapy, including gentle stretching, range-of-motion exercises, and deep heat modalities, may be beneficial in selected patients.
- Injection with local anesthetic and steroid will provide symptomatic relief if conservative therapy fails or the pain is limiting activities of daily living.
- Surgery may be required for persistent pain or progressive functional disability.

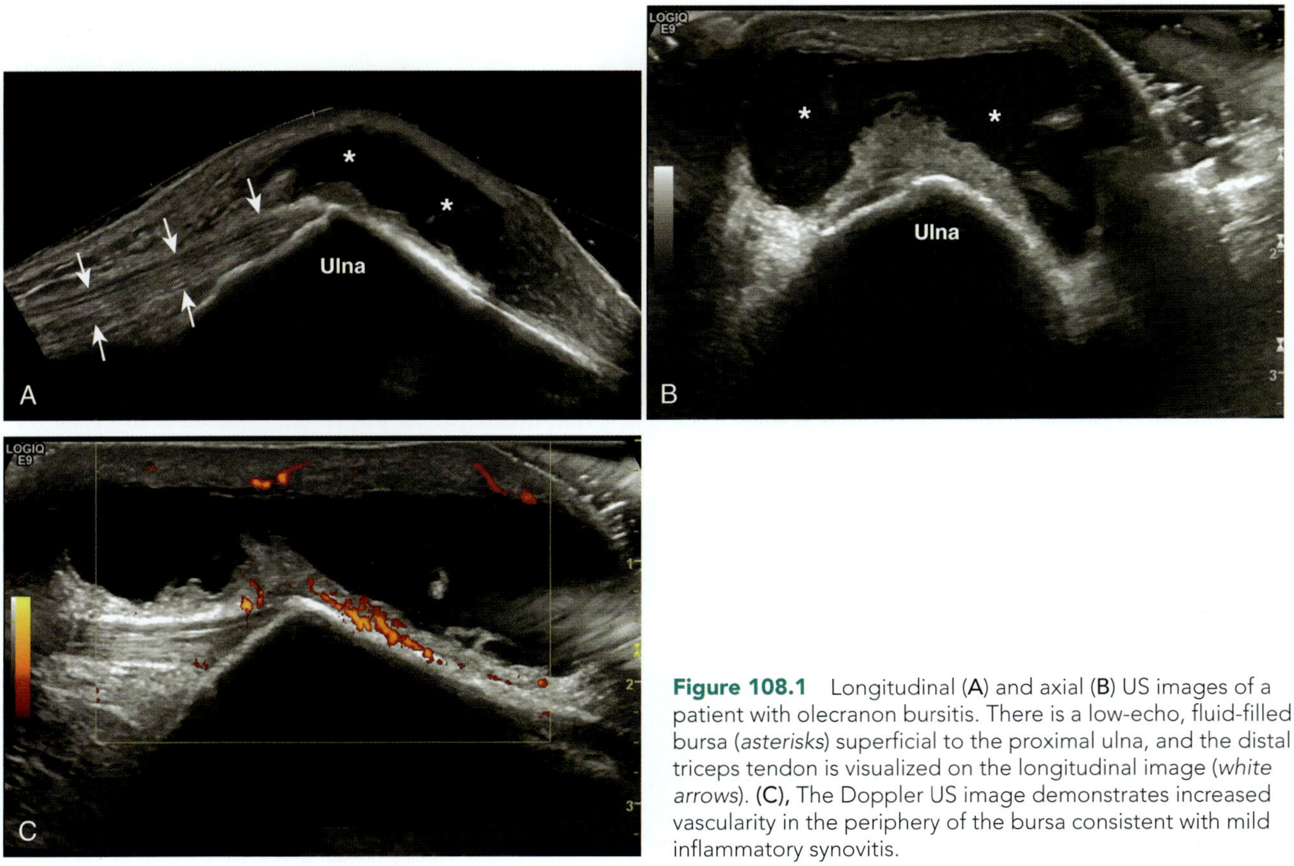

Figure 108.1 Longitudinal (**A**) and axial (**B**) US images of a patient with olecranon bursitis. There is a low-echo, fluid-filled bursa (*asterisks*) superficial to the proximal ulna, and the distal triceps tendon is visualized on the longitudinal image (*white arrows*). **(C),** The Doppler US image demonstrates increased vascularity in the periphery of the bursa consistent with mild inflammatory synovitis.

CHAPTER 109

Osteoarthritis of the Elbow

DEFINITION

- Degenerative arthritis characterized by destruction of the chondral surfaces, subchondral cysts, synovitis, and osteophyte formation.

SIGNS AND SYMPTOMS

- Gradual onset of pain with range of motion of the elbow joint.
- Effusion may be present.
- Crepitus may be present.
- Gradual decrease in range of motion.

DEMOGRAPHICS

- Incidence: Male > Female.
- Most common in elderly patients; also seen in younger patients following elbow joint trauma and/or surgery.
- Universal finding after fifth decade of life.
- A history of joint trauma common.
- Genetic predisposition possible.

IMAGING RECOMMENDATIONS

- Radiography is the primary investigation for arthropathy.
- CT/MR arthrography may be used as an adjunct to radiography for:
  - Localizing osteophytes prior to surgical excision.
  - Loose bodies.
  - Articular cartilage abnormalities.

IMAGING FINDINGS

- Joint space narrowing, subchondral cysts, sclerosis and osteophytes.
- Asymmetrical involvement is typical, but all three joint compartments may be involved:
  - Unlotrochlear.
  - Radiocapitellar.
  - Proximal radioulnar.
- Loose bodies frequently lie in the posterior olecranon fossa or the anterior coronoid fossa of the humerus.

OTHER RECOMMENDED TESTING

- Laboratory testing to rule out inflammatory arthritis.
- Joint aspiration to rule out crystal arthropathies.
- Joint aspiration to rule out infection.

DIFFERENTIAL DIAGNOSIS

- Inflammatory arthritides, especially rheumatoid arthritis.
- Septic elbow joint.
- Healing elbow joint fracture, especially of the olecranon.
- Crystal arthropathy of elbow.
- Avascular osteonecrosis.

TREATMENT

- Conservative treatment consisting of local heat, cold, simple analgesics, and nonsteroidal anti-inflammatory agents will improve symptoms in many cases.
- Physical therapy, including gentle stretching, range-of-motion exercises, and deep heat modalities, may be beneficial in selected patients.
- Intra-articular injection with local anesthetic and steroid will provide symptomatic relief if conservative therapy fails or the pain is limiting activities of daily living.
- Surgery may be required for persistent pain or progressive functional disability.

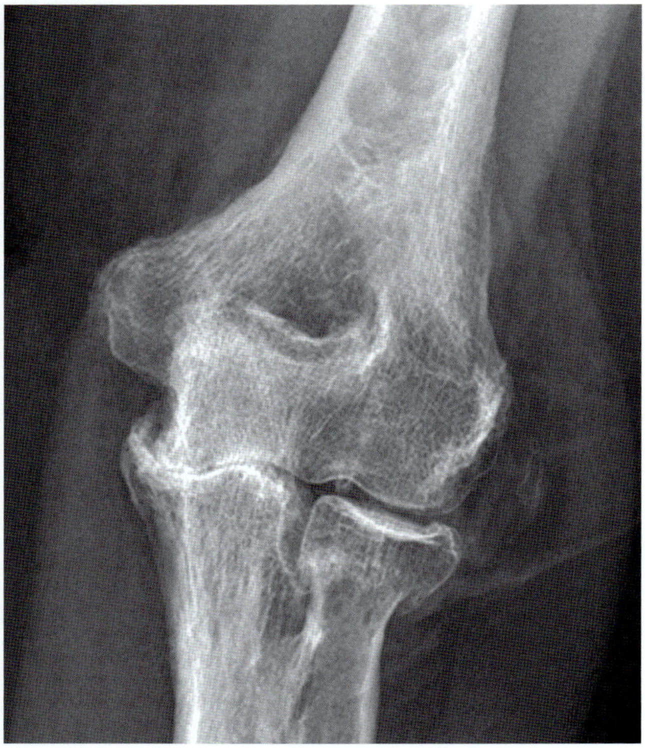

Figure 109.1 AP radiograph of an elderly patient with typical features of elbow osteoarthritis (OA). There is asymmetrical joint space narrowing, which most severely affects the ulnotrochlear joint, with osteophyte formation and subchondral sclerosis.

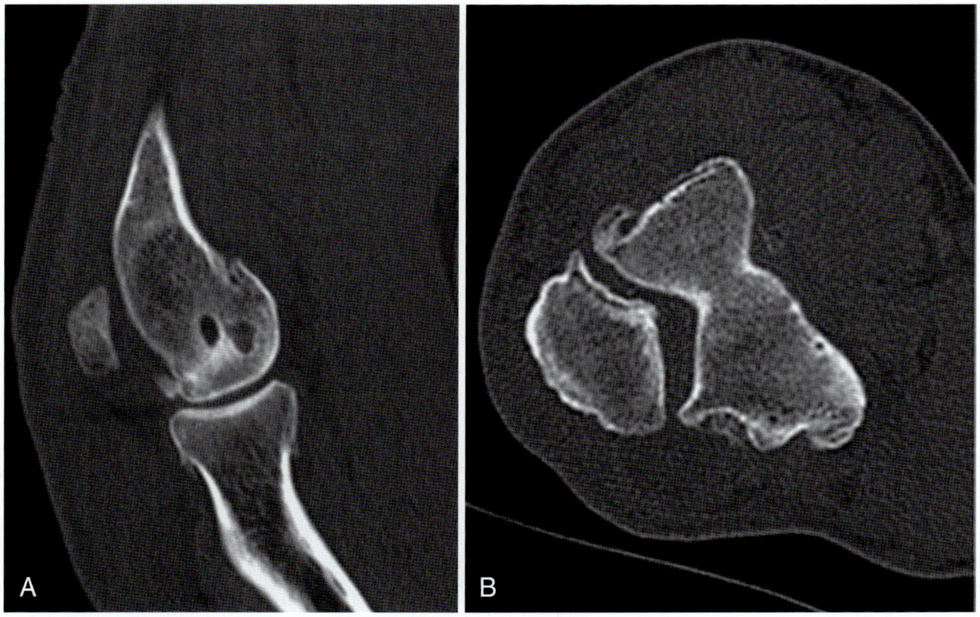

Figure 109.2 Sagittal (**A**) and axial (**B**) CT scans of elbow OA obtained prior to surgery for trimming of osteophytes. Anterior and posterior osteophytes are present in the radiocapitellar joint, with subchondral cyst formation. There are also medial and lateral osteophytes in the ulnotrochlear joint.

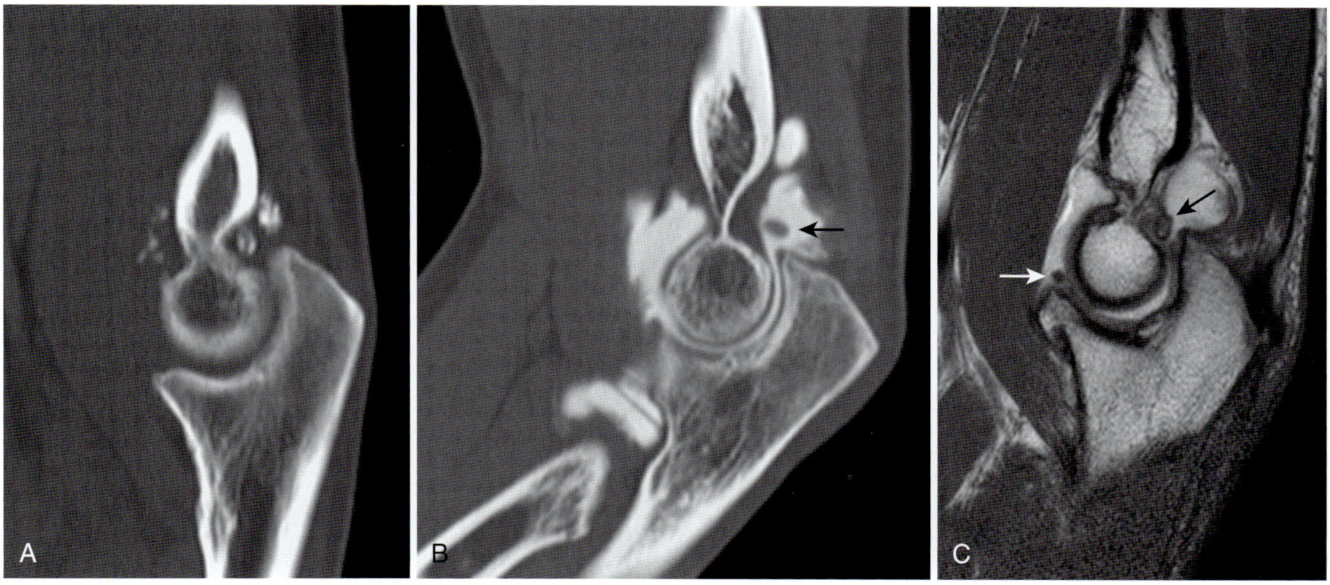

Figure 109.3 (A), Sagittal CT scan demonstrating radiopaque loose bodies in both the posterior olecranon fossa and the anterior coronoid fossa of the distal humerus. (B), A sagittal CT arthrogram in a different patient demonstrates a non-radiopaque cartilaginous loose body (*black arrow*) that was not visible on the CT scan without contrast agent. (C), A sagittal T1-weighted (T1W) MR arthrogram image from a third patient with an ossific loose body posteriorly (*black arrow*) and a second cartilaginous loose body anteriorly (*white arrow*). There are established OA changes.

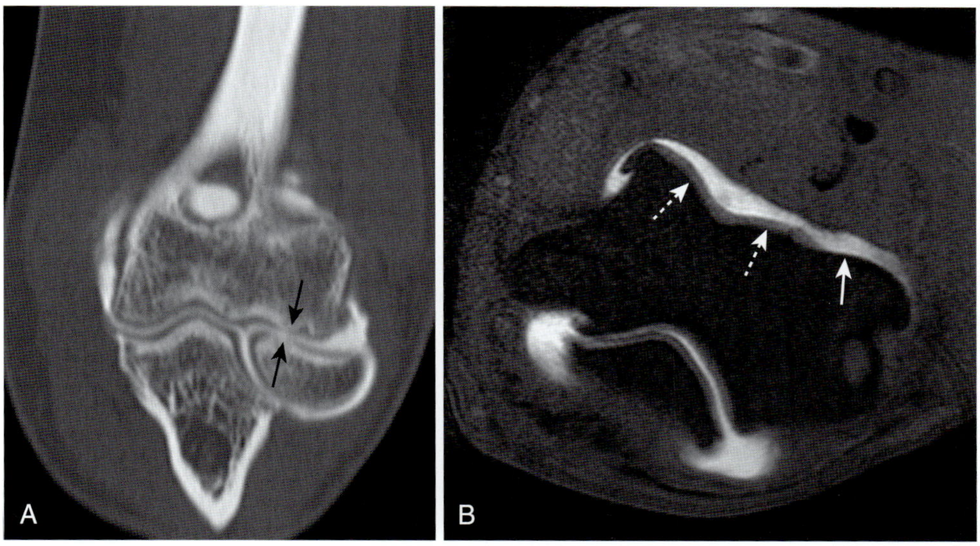

Figure 109.4 (A), Coronal CT arthrogram showing focal areas of cartilage ulceration on the capitellum and radius (*black arrows*). Radiographic findings were normal. (B), An axial T2W with fat suppresion (FST2W) MR arthrogram image of a different patient shows a focal area of full-thickness cartilage loss (*white arrow*). Compare it with the normal articular cartilage, which has intermediate signal intensity, on the remainder of the distal humerus (*broken white arrows*).

CHAPTER 110

Rheumatoid Arthritis of the Elbow

DEFINITION

- Symmetrical inflammatory arthritis characterized by synovitis, joint space narrowing, effusions and erosions, and elevation of serum rheumatoid factor combined with a constellation of other clinical signs and symptoms.

SIGNS AND SYMPTOMS

- Pain with range of motion of the elbow joint.
- Synovitis.
- Effusion often present.
- Warmth often present.
- Crepitus may be present.
- Morning stiffness.
- Gelling phenomenon.
- Gradual decrease in range of motion.
- Fatigue, lassitude, and mild fever.
- Symmetrical polyarthritis involving three or more joints invariably present upon careful inspection.

DEMOGRAPHICS

- Incidence: Female > Male.
- Adult form more common, although juvenile form should be considered in any child with polyarthritis.
- Peak onset in the fourth to sixth decade of life.

IMAGING RECOMMENDATIONS

- Radiography is the primary investigation for arthropathy.
- MRI or US:
  - Synovitis.
  - Radiographically occult erosions.
  - US to guide joint aspiration or injection.

IMAGING FINDINGS

- Joint space narrowing, erosions, and osteopenia.
- Uniform joint involvement.
- Absence of osteophytes and reactive bone formation except with secondary osteoarthritis change.
- Effusion:
  - Presence of fat pad sign on radiographs.
- Synovitis:
  - Increased signal intensity (SI) on post-contrast (obtained after administration of a contrast agent) MR images.
  - Echogenic synovium on US: Increased vascularity on Doppler imaging.

OTHER RECOMMENDED TESTING

- Laboratory testing, including complete blood count, blood chemistry profile, and erythrocyte sedimentation rate determination, to rule out extra-articular manifestations of the disease.
- Antinuclear antibody and systemic lupus erythematosus (SLE) testing if diagnosis in doubt.
- Joint aspiration to rule out crystal arthropathies.
- Joint aspiration to rule out infection.

DIFFERENTIAL DIAGNOSIS

- Other inflammatory arthritides, especially SLE arthritis.
- Charcot elbow joint.
- Olecranon bursitis.
- Bicipital radial bursitis.
- Osteoarthritis.
- Psoriatic arthritis.
- Crystal arthropathy of elbow.
- Avascular osteonecrosis.

TREATMENT

- Disease-modifying agents, including gold salts, penicillamine, azathioprine, and cyclosporine A, can dramatically slow the progression of the disease, albeit not without side effects.
- Cytotoxic drugs, including methotrexate.
- Biologic agents, including interleukin and tumor necrosis factor-α.
- Salicylates, nonsteroidal anti-inflammatory agents, and corticosteroids.
- Physical and occupational therapy.
- Intra-articular injection of local anesthetic and corticosteroid for symptomatic relief and to aid in physical therapy.
- Surgery may be required for persistent pain or progressive functional disability.

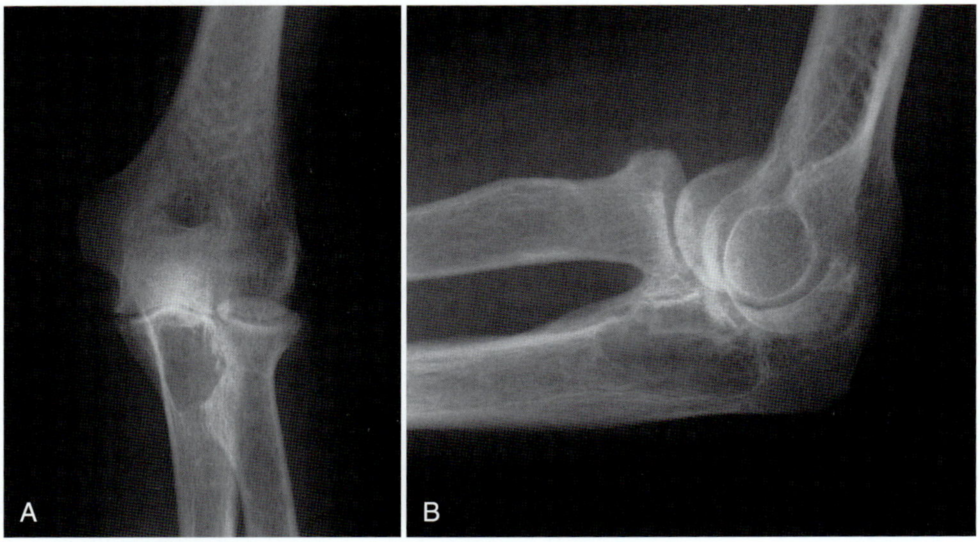

Figure 110.1 AP (**A**) and lateral (**B**) radiographs of early rheumatoid involvement of the elbow. There is global joint space narrowing and a large lucent geode is present within the proximal ulna. No erosions are present.

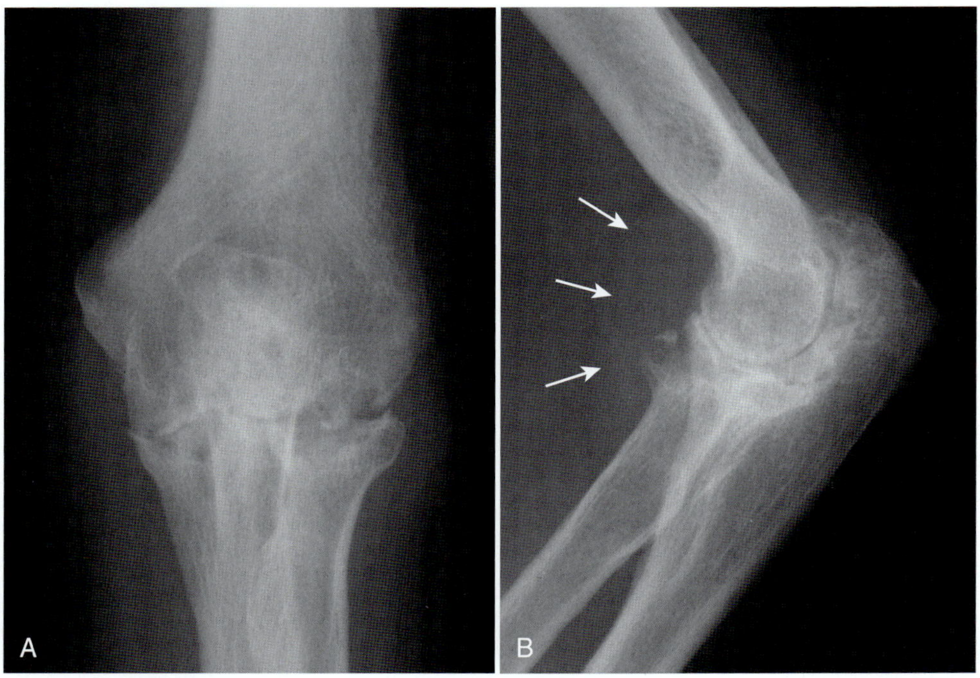

Figure 110.2 AP (**A**) and lateral (**B**) radiographs in advanced rheumatoid arthritis. Joint space narrowing and destruction with multiple joint erosions can be seen. The presence of synovitis and effusion is evident from the anterior soft tissue swelling (*white arrows*).

CHAPTER 111

Osteonecrosis of the Elbow

DEFINITION

- The death of cellular components of bone due to interruption of the blood supply, with resultant pain, collapse, and destruction of bone and loss of function.

SIGNS AND SYMPTOMS

- Gradual onset of pain with decreasing range of motion of the elbow joint.
- Crepitus may be present.
- Functional disability may be severe.

DEMOGRAPHICS

- Incidence: Male > Female.
- Age at onset is related to date of trauma or of onset of underlying disease, with sickle cell disease being the most common inciting factor in younger patients.
- Most common after elbow joint trauma that disrupts the vascular supply.
- More common in patients with sickle cell disease, Gaucher disease, Fabry disease, systemic lupus erythematosus (SLE), and gout.
- Associated with exogenous steroid administration and heavy alcohol intake.

IMAGING RECOMMENDATIONS

- Radiography.
- MRI or CT.

IMAGING FINDINGS

- Radiography:
  - Sclerosis in affected subchondral bone.
  - Later subchondral collapse and bony fragmentation.
  - Serpiginous lines of sclerosis in intramedullary infarcts.
  - Loose bodies.
- MRI:
  - High–signal intensity (SI) edema in subchondral bone.
  - Low-SI subchondral sclerosis on T1-weighted (T1W) and T2W MR images.
  - High-SI lines at base of osteochondral defects in Panner's disease indicate unstable lesions.
  - Double-line sign of intramedullary infarcts on T2W MR images.

OTHER RECOMMENDED TESTING

- Laboratory testing to rule out SLE.
- Laboratory testing to rule out gout.
- Joint aspiration to rule out crystal arthropathies.
- Joint aspiration to rule out infection.

DIFFERENTIAL DIAGNOSIS

- Inflammatory arthritides, especially SLE.
- Osteoarthritis.
- Bone marrow tumor.
- Primary bone tumor.
- Metastatic tumor.
- Osteochondral injuries.
- Panner disease (osteochondritis dissecans).
- Neuroarthropathy.

TREATMENT

- Conservative treatment consisting of local heat, cold, simple analgesics, and nonsteroidal anti-inflammatory agents will improve symptoms in many cases.
- Physical therapy, including gentle stretching, range-of-motion exercises, and deep heat modalities, may be beneficial in selected patients.
- Intra-articular injection with local anesthetic and steroid will provide symptomatic relief if conservative therapy fails or if the pain is limiting activities of daily living.
- Surgery may ultimately be required for persistent pain or progressive functional disability.

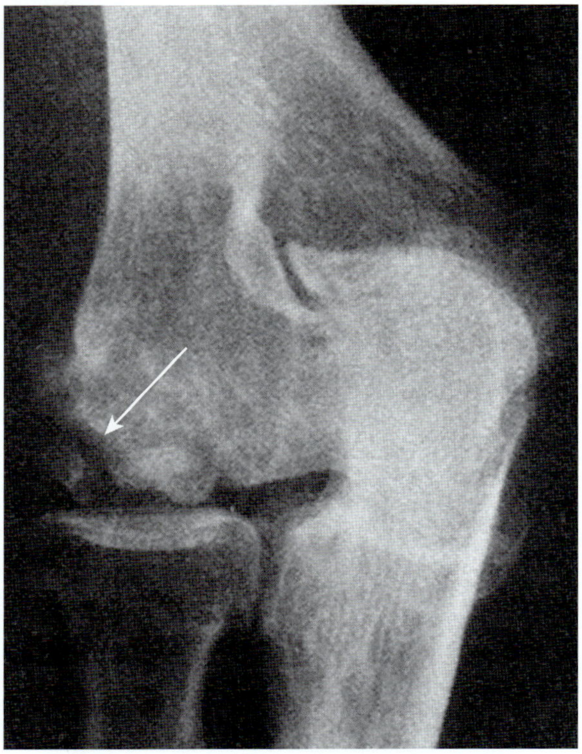

Figure 111.1 AP radiograph of a patient with SLE showing fragmentation and collapse of the capitellum (*white arrow*) due to avascular necrosis (AVN). *(From Bergstein JM, Wiens C, Fish AJ, et al: Avascular necrosis of bone in systemic lupus erythematosus. J Pediatr 1974;85:31-35.)*

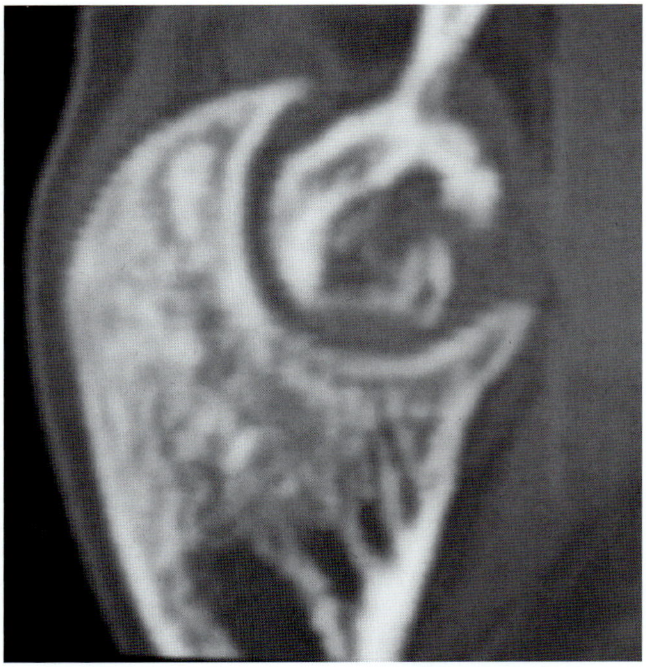

Figure 111.2 Sagittal CT scan of a patient with sickle cell anemia. There are lucency and fragmentation of the trochlea of the distal humerus due to AVN. *(From Mukisi Mukaza M, Manicom O, Fillipini P, Hernigou P: Elbow osteonecrosis in sickle cells anemia: A study of six cases. Rev Chir Orthop Traumatol 2009;95:82-84.)*

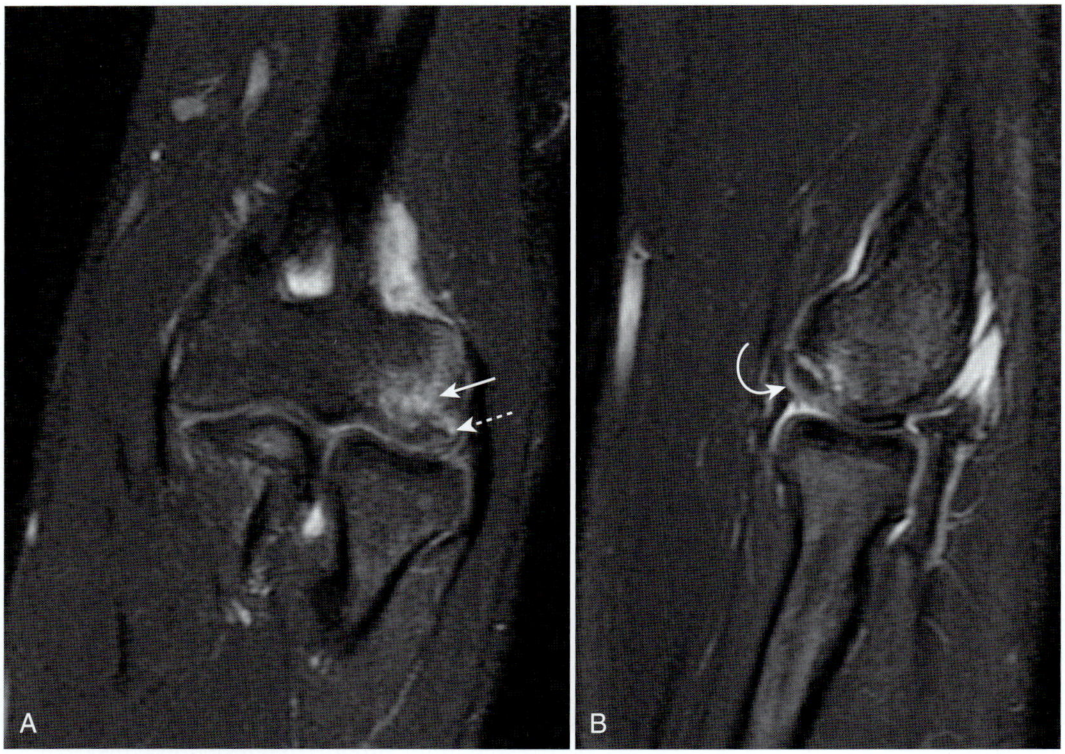

Figure 111.3 **(A),** Coronal T2W with fat suppression (FST2W) MR image demonstrating an area of high-SI marrow edema in the capitellum (*white arrow*) of an adolescent with elbow pain. There is also an area of low SI in the subchondral bone plate (*broken white arrow*), which is suggestive of an osteochondral defect. **(B),** The sagittal FST2W MR image more clearly shows the low-SI osteochondral defect (*curved white arrow*), with a linear area of high SI at its base, indicating that the lesion is likely to be unstable. These appearances are typical of Panner's disease (osteochondritis dissecans).

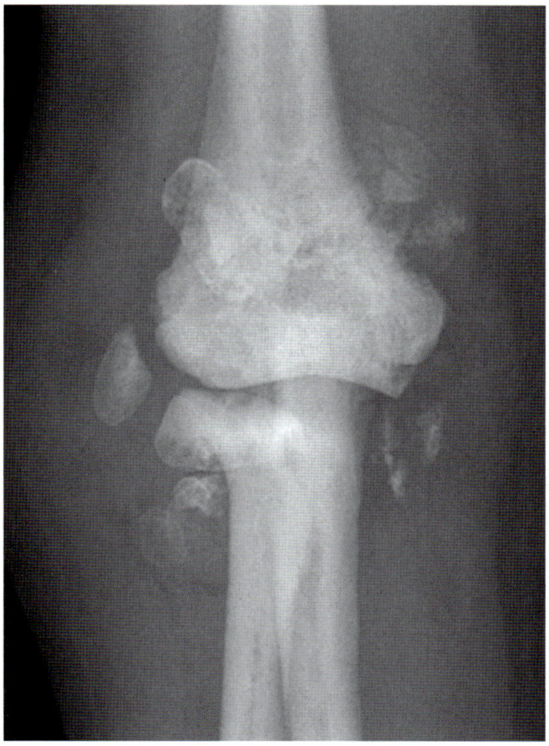

Figure 111.4 AP radiograph of the elbow of a patient with syringomyelia. There is marked bone fragmentation of the joint surfaces of the elbow with reactive sclerosis due to neuroarthropathy.

CHAPTER 112

Os Supratrochlear

DEFINITION

- Failure of normal fusion of one or more of the distal ossification centers, resulting in separate distal ossicles.

SIGNS AND SYMPTOMS

- Gradual onset of elbow pain.
- Exacerbation of pain with flexion and extension of the elbow.
- Decreased range of motion.
- Clicking, locking, grating, or catching sensation may be present.

DEMOGRAPHICS

- Incidence: Male > Female.
- Occurs in all age groups.
- Commonly associated with loose bodies.

IMAGING RECOMMENDATIONS

- Radiography.
- MRI:
  - Occasionally required to exclude other bone or soft tissue pathology.

IMAGING FINDINGS

- Well-defined bony ossicles at sites of known ossification centers after skeletal maturity has been reached:
  - Important to distinguish from areas of calcific tendinitis.
- Occasionally, larger fragments of separated ossification centers may occur as a result of trauma.
- Symptomatic lesions may demonstrate bone marrow edema and adjacent reactive soft tissue edema.

OTHER RECOMMENDED TESTING

- Intra-articular injection of contrast medium and local anesthetic.
- If diagnosis is in question:
  - Laboratory testing to rule out inflammatory arthritis.
  - Joint aspiration to rule out crystal arthropathies.
  - Joint aspiration to rule out infection.

DIFFERENTIAL DIAGNOSIS

- Panner disease.
- Occult fracture.
- Synovial chondromatosis.
- Osteochondritis dissecans.

TREATMENT

- Conservative treatment consisting of local heat, cold, simple analgesics, and nonsteroidal anti-inflammatory agents will improve symptoms in many cases.
- Physical therapy, including gentle stretching, range-of-motion exercises, and deep heat modalities, may be beneficial in selected patients.
- Intra-articular injection with local anesthetic and steroid will provide symptomatic relief if conservative therapy fails or if the pain is limiting activities of daily living.
- Surgery may be required for persistent pain or progressive functional disability.

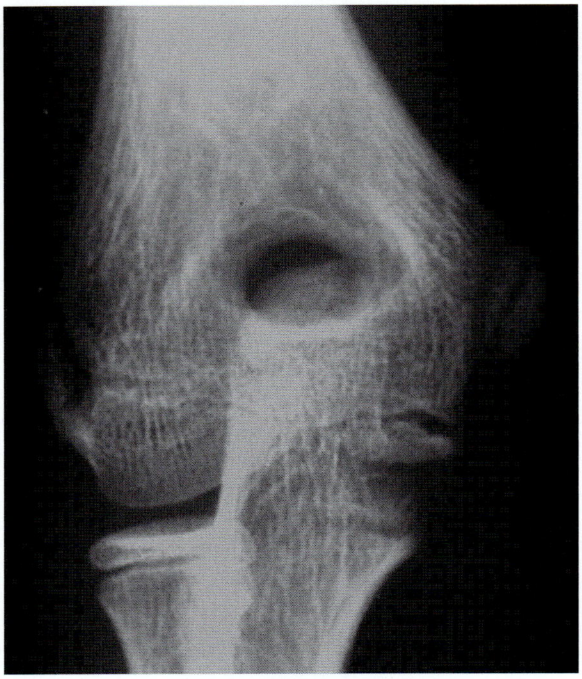

Figure 112.1 AP radiograph of a normal elbow in a child. The ossification centers for the ulna and capitel um have fused. The lateral epicondylar ossification center has partially fused. The ossification centers for the radial head, trochlea, and medial epicondyle remain unfused.

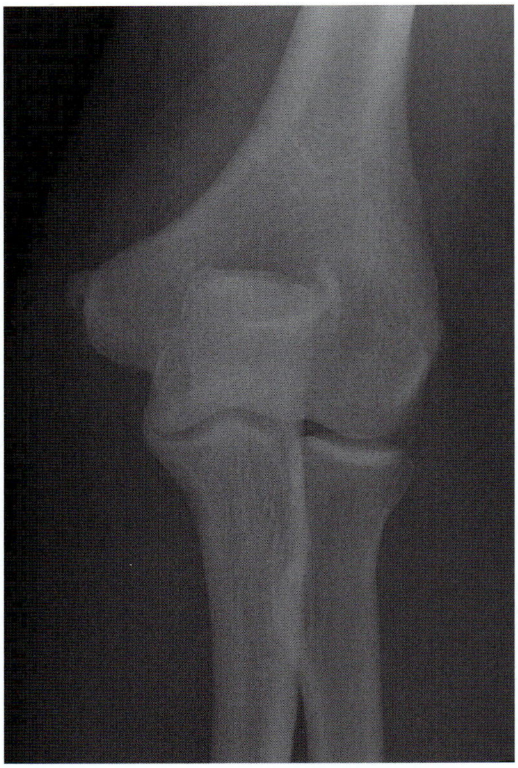

Figure 112.2 Incidental finding of an accessory ossicle adjacent to the medial epicondyle of the distal humerus on an AP radiograph.

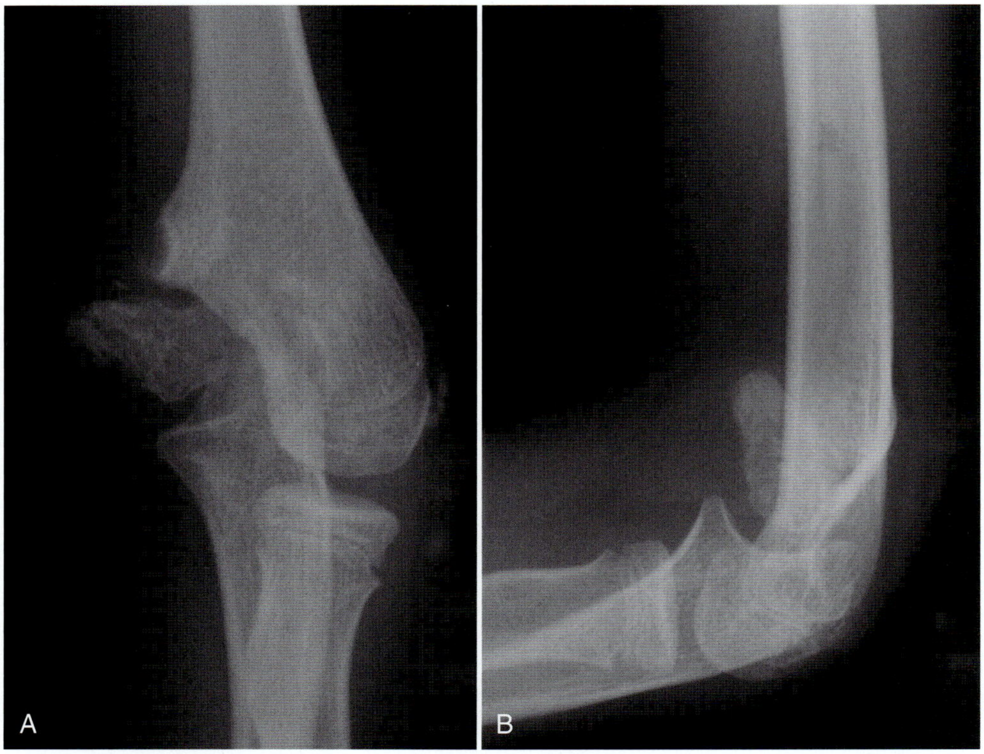

Figure 112.3 AP (**A**) and lateral (**B**) radiographs in a child with a large unfused fragment of the trochlea and medial epicondyle resulting from a non-united intercondylar fracture sustained a few years previously.

CHAPTER 113

Radial Tunnel Syndrome

DEFINITION

- Entrapment of the radial nerve at the elbow by muscle, the fibrous arch of the long head of the triceps muscle, an aberrant artery or fibrous band, or a mass, tumor, or humeral fracture.

SIGNS AND SYMPTOMS

- Exact signs and symptoms related to what portion of the radial nerve is compressed.
- Presence of Tinel sign over the entrapped nerve.
- Pain radiating into the anterolateral forearm.
- Passive range of motion preserved.
- Weakness of forearm supination and wrist extension.
- Pain over radial aspect of distal forearm with paresthesias in the radial distribution into the hand.
- Tenderness to palpation of the radial nerve at point of entrapment.
- Neurapraxia often present.

DEMOGRAPHICS

- Incidence: Male > Female.
- Young athletes involved in overhead activities such as tennis and volleyball often affected.
- Can occur acutely following trauma and fracture.
- All ages affected.
- More common after trauma, including repetitive stress injuries.

IMAGING RECOMMENDATIONS

- Radiography:
  - To exclude bony abnormality.
- MRI or US.

IMAGING FINDINGS

- Imaging findings often normal:
  - Fibrous bands at the level of arcade of Frohse are usually not visible.
- If posterior interosseous nerve is affected, edema and atrophy of affected muscles are seen:
  - Supinator.
  - Extensor carpi radialis brevis and longus.
  - Extensor digitorum and indicis.
  - Extensor carpi ulnaris.
  - Extensor pollicis longus and brevis, and abductor pollicis longus.
- Compressive soft tissue masses or neural tumors.

OTHER RECOMMENDED TESTING

- Electromyography and nerve conduction velocity testing of the cervical nerve roots, brachial plexus, and radial, ulnar, and median nerves.

DIFFERENTIAL DIAGNOSIS

- Parsonage-Turner syndrome.
- Hematoma.
- Benign neoplasm.
- Malignant neoplasm.
- Humeral fracture.
- Lateral epicondylitis.
- Median neuropathy.

TREATMENT

- Conservative treatment consisting of local heat, cold, simple analgesics, and nonsteroidal anti-inflammatory agents will improve symptoms in mild, self-limited cases.
- Physical therapy to maintain function, including gentle stretching, range-of-motion exercises, and local heat modalities, may be beneficial in selected patients.
- Splinting to preserve normal range of motion.
- Injection of the radial nerve with local anesthetic and steroid may provide symptomatic relief if conservative therapy fails or if the pain is limiting activities of daily living.
- Surgery may be required to relieve entrapment of the radial nerve.

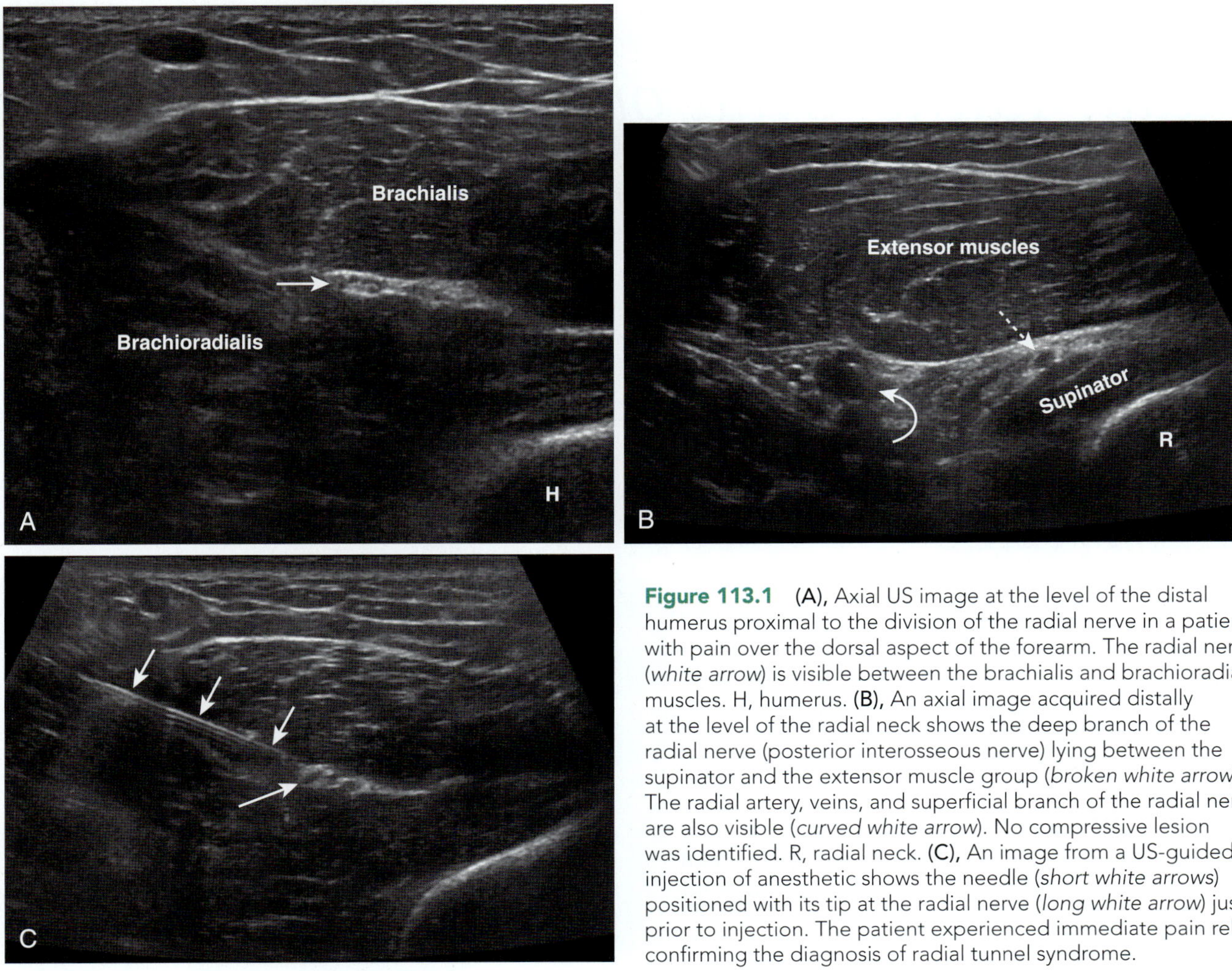

Figure 113.1 **(A)**, Axial US image at the level of the distal humerus proximal to the division of the radial nerve in a patient with pain over the dorsal aspect of the forearm. The radial nerve (*white arrow*) is visible between the brachialis and brachioradialis muscles. H, humerus. **(B)**, An axial image acquired distally at the level of the radial neck shows the deep branch of the radial nerve (posterior interosseous nerve) lying between the supinator and the extensor muscle group (*broken white arrow*). The radial artery, veins, and superficial branch of the radial nerve are also visible (*curved white arrow*). No compressive lesion was identified. R, radial neck. **(C)**, An image from a US-guided injection of anesthetic shows the needle (*short white arrows*) positioned with its tip at the radial nerve (*long white arrow*) just prior to injection. The patient experienced immediate pain relief, confirming the diagnosis of radial tunnel syndrome.

CHAPTER 114

Cubital Tunnel Syndrome

DEFINITION

- Entrapment of the ulnar nerve at the elbow as it passes through the cubital tunnel.

SIGNS AND SYMPTOMS

- Presence of Tinel sign over the entrapped nerve.
- Pain at the elbow radiating into the hand and occasionally proximally above the elbow.
- Passive range of motion preserved early on, with clawing of the fingers if left untreated.
- Weakness in ulnar nerve distribution.
- Presence of Froment sign.
- Positive results of:
  - Wartenberg test.
  - Little finger abduction test.
- Paresthesias radiating into the ring and little fingers.
- Tenderness to palpation of the ulnar nerve at the point of entrapment.
- Ulnar neurapraxia often present.

DEMOGRAPHICS

- Incidence: Female > Male.
- Second most common nerve entrapment syndrome, after carpal tunnel syndrome.
- Young athletes involved in throwing sports and adults suffering from overuse of elbow joints are primarily affected.
- Can occur acutely following trauma and fracture.
- More common after trauma, including repetitive stress injuries.

IMAGING RECOMMENDATIONS

- Radiography:
  - Exclude associated osteoarthritic change.
- MRI or US.

IMAGING FINDINGS

- Thickening of the ulnar nerve within the cubital tunnel.
- High signal intensity (SI) of nerve on T2-weighted with fat suppression (FST2W) MR images.
- Loss of fascicular pattern and low reflectivity on US.
- Compression of ulnar nerve:
  - Osteophytes or other bony abnormality.
  - Synovial disease or other soft tissue mass.
  - Accessory anconeus muscle.
- Subluxation of the tendon may be demonstrated by dynamic US.

OTHER RECOMMENDED TESTING

- Electromyography and nerve conduction velocity testing of the cervical nerve roots, brachial plexus, and ulnar, radial, and median nerves.

DIFFERENTIAL DIAGNOSIS

- Parsonage-Turner syndrome.
- Hematoma.
- Benign neoplasm.
- Malignant neoplasm.
- Elbow fracture.
- Medial epicondylitis.
- Hansen disease.

TREATMENT

- Conservative treatment consisting of local heat, cold, simple analgesics, and nonsteroidal anti-inflammatory agents will improve symptoms in mild, self-limited cases.
- Physical therapy to maintain function, including gentle stretching, range-of-motion exercises, and local heat modalities, may be beneficial in selected patients.
- Splinting to preserve normal range of motion.
- Injection of the ulnar nerve with local anesthetic and steroid may provide symptomatic relief if conservative therapy fails or the pain is limiting activities of daily living.
- Surgery may be required to relieve entrapment of the ulnar nerve.

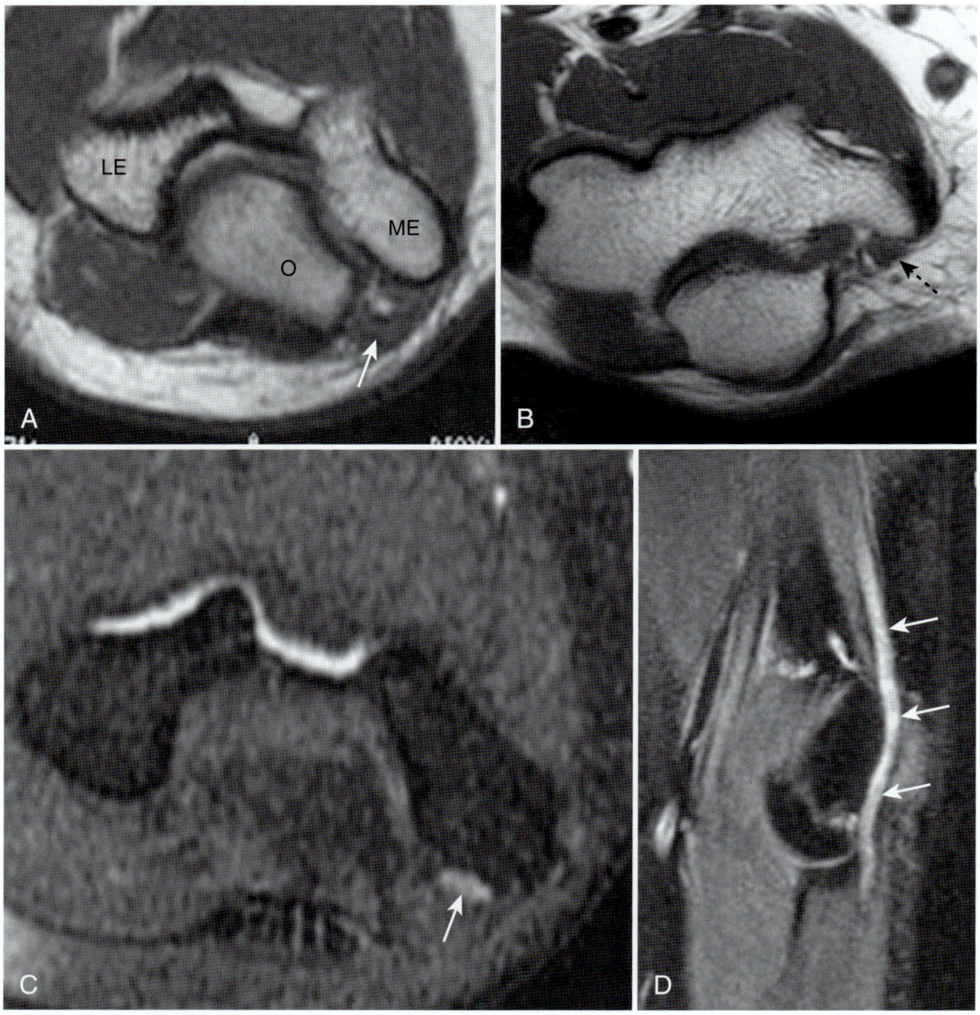

Figure 114.1 (A), Axial T1W MR image of a patient with symptoms of ulnar nerve compression. There is soft tissue within the region of the cubital tunnel (*white arrow*); it is iso-intense with normal muscle and represents an accessory anconeus muscle. The ulnar nerve is not clearly visible. LE, lateral epicondyle; ME, medial epicondyle; O, olecranon. (B), Compare this axial T1W MR image of a normal elbow with high-SI fat within the cubital tunnel around the ulnar nerve (*broken black arrow*) and no accessory muscle tissue. The axial (C) and sagittal (D) FST2W MR images demonstrate high SI within the nerve (*white arrows*) due to compression neuritis.

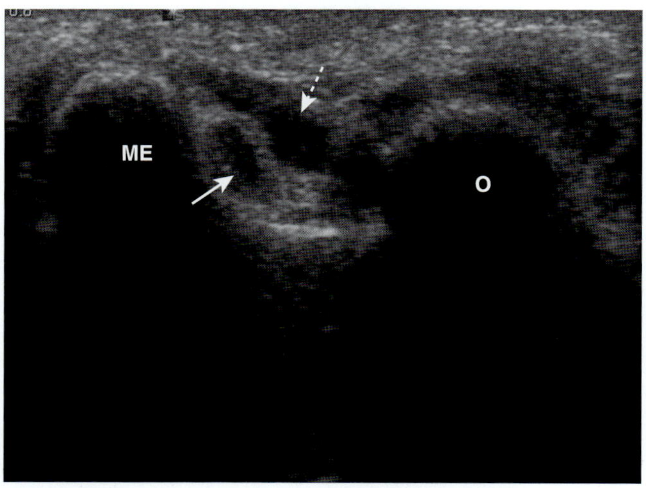

Figure 114.2 A transverse US image of a different patient with an accessory anconeus muscle (*broken white arrow*) within the cubital tunnel. The ulnar nerve (*white arrow*) is thickened and demonstrates loss of the normal fascicular pattern. ME, medial epicondyle; O, olecranon.

CHAPTER 115

Anterior Interosseous Syndrome

DEFINITION

- Entrapment of the anterior interosseous branch of the median nerve just below the elbow by an aberrant artery, a mass, bursitis, or fibrous bands.

SIGNS AND SYMPTOMS

- Presence of Tinel sign over the entrapped nerve.
- Pain over the entrapped nerve at the elbow that radiates into the hand and sometimes proximally, above the elbow.
- Passive range of motion preserved early on, with loss of function later if left untreated.
- Weakness of the flexor pollicis longus (FPL) and profundus flexors of the second and third fingers.
- No sensory deficit with pure entrapment of the anterior interosseous branch of the median nerve.
- Median neurapraxia often present.

DEMOGRAPHICS

- Incidence: Female > Male.
- Affects all ages.
- Can occur acutely following trauma and fracture.
- More common after trauma, including repetitive stress injuries.

IMAGING RECOMMENDATIONS

- MRI.
- US is an alternative to MRI but is less sensitive for early muscle denervation.

IMAGING FINDINGS

- Muscle denervation:
  - High-signal intensity (SI) edema on T2-weighted with fat suppression (FST2W) MR images.
- Later fatty atrophy:
  - Flexor pollicis longus (FPL).
  - Flexor digitorum profundus (FDP) (index and middle fingers).
  - Pronator quadratus.
  - Anomalous branches of the median nerve may affect distribution.
  - Compressive soft tissue mass lesions may be present.

OTHER RECOMMENDED TESTING

- Electromyography and nerve conduction velocity testing of the cervical nerve roots, brachial plexus, and ulnar, radial, and median nerves.

DIFFERENTIAL DIAGNOSIS

- Pronator syndrome.
- Parsonage-Turner syndrome.
- C6-C7 radiculopathy.
- Hematoma.
- Benign neoplasm.
- Malignant neoplasm.
- Elbow fracture.
- Radial neuropathy.

TREATMENT

- Conservative treatment consisting of local heat, cold, simple analgesics, and nonsteroidal anti-inflammatory agents will improve symptoms in mild, self-limited cases.
- Physical therapy, including gentle stretching, range-of-motion exercises, and local heat modalities, may be beneficial in selected patients to maintain function.
- Splinting to preserve normal range of motion.
- Injection with local anesthetic and steroid of the median nerve may provide symptomatic relief if conservative therapy fails or the pain is limiting activities of daily living.
- Surgery may be required to relieve entrapment of the median nerve.

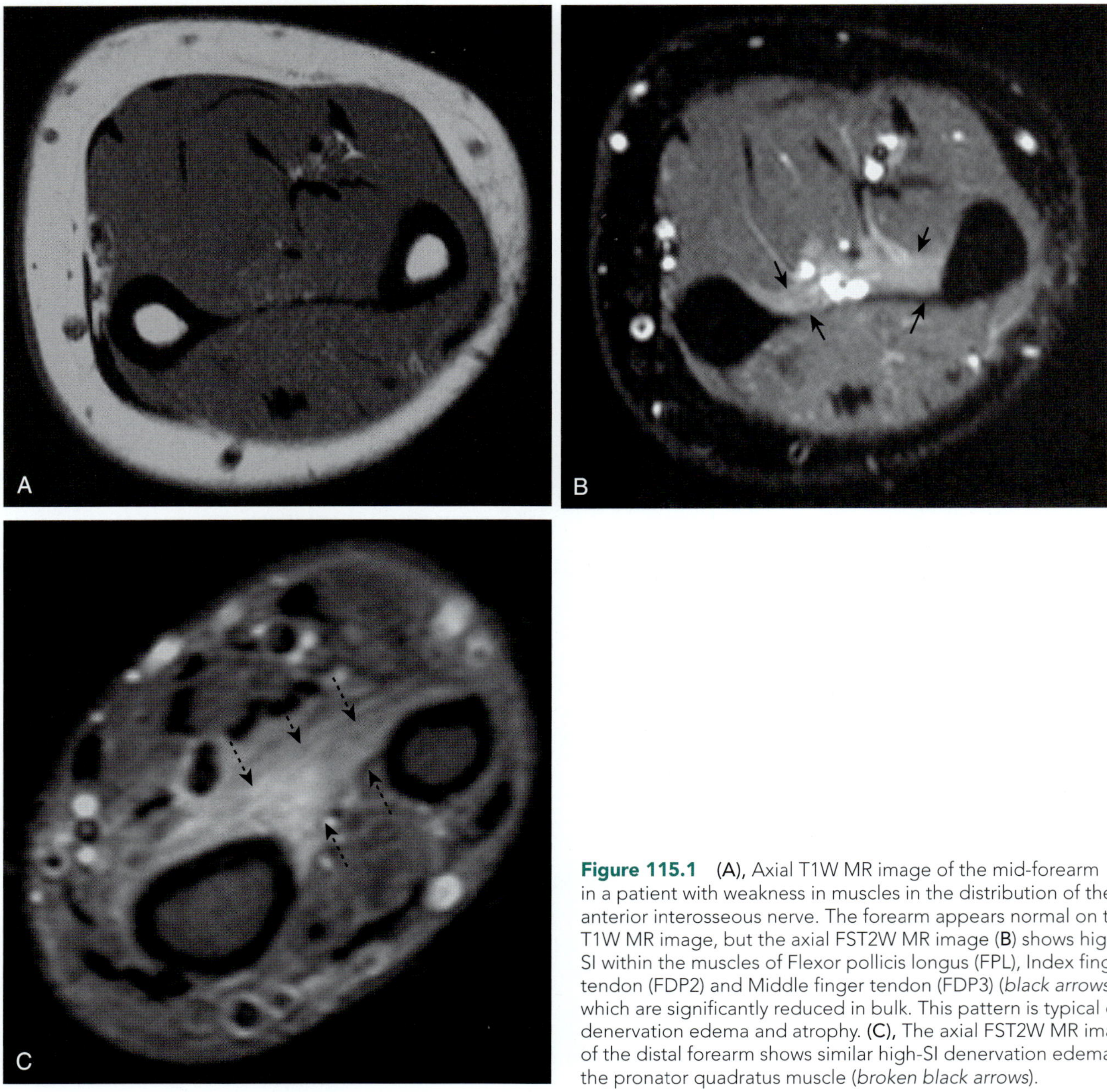

Figure 115.1 (A), Axial T1W MR image of the mid-forearm in a patient with weakness in muscles in the distribution of the anterior interosseous nerve. The forearm appears normal on the T1W MR image, but the axial FST2W MR image (B) shows high SI within the muscles of Flexor pollicis longus (FPL), Index finger tendon (FDP2) and Middle finger tendon (FDP3) (*black arrows*), which are significantly reduced in bulk. This pattern is typical of denervation edema and atrophy. (C), The axial FST2W MR image of the distal forearm shows similar high-SI denervation edema in the pronator quadratus muscle (*broken black arrows*).

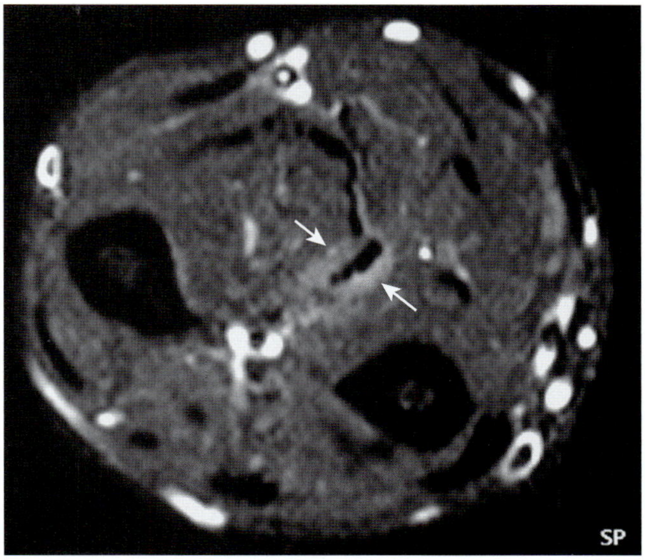

Figure 115.2 Axial FST2W MR image of the mid-forearm in a different patient, who presented with loss of flexion of the index finger alone. The initial diagnosis was rupture of the flexor tendon, but US examination demonstrated a normal tendon. There is isolated denervation edema and atrophy of the muscle of Index finger tendon (FDP2) (*white arrows*). This pattern of anterior interosseous nerve syndrome often causes clinical confusion.

CHAPTER 116

Anatomy: Special Imaging Considerations of the Forearm, Wrist, and Hand

OSSEOUS STRUCTURES

Radius. The distal radius has a broad metaphysis with a sloping distal articular surface that demonstrates medial inclination and volar tilt and has concave articular facets for the scaphoid and lunate. The medial surface of the distal radius is concave, forming the sigmoid notch of the distal radioulnar joint (DRUJ).

Ulna. The distal ulna has a convexity on the lateral surface that articulates with the radius to form the DRUJ. The distal surface of the ulna has a shallow convexity covered with hyaline cartilage, which is covered by the triangular fibrocartilage (TFC). The ulnar styloid arises from the dorsolateral aspect of the ulna and bears the ulnar attachment of the TFC.

Carpal Bones. The carpal bones are arranged into two rows of four bones. The proximal carpal row, from lateral to medial, are the scaphoid, lunate, triquetral, and pisiform. From lateral to medial, the distal carpal row consists of the trapezium, trapezoid, capitate, and hamate. The hamate possesses a hook on its volar surface on which bears the lateral attachment of the flexor retinaculum; the medial attachment is on the volar ridge of the trapezium.

JOINTS

Radiocarpal (Wrist) Joint. An ellipsoid synovial joint between the distal radius and the proximal carpal row that is capable of volar and dorsiflexion as well as ulnar and radial deviation.

Distal Radioulnar Joint. A synovial pivot joint formed by the articulation of the lateral surface of the distal ulna with the sigmoid notch of the distal radius. The distal margin of the joint is bordered by the TFC and thus normally does not communicate directly with the radiocarpal joint.

Intercarpal Joints. All the carpal bones possess articular cartilaginous surfaces, the proximal row articulating with the distal row to form synovial joints. There are distinct radiocarpal and mid-carpal compartments. The carpus is stabilized by a complex network of radiocarpal, ulnocarpal, intercarpal, and carpometacarpal ligaments. The scapholunate ligament is one of the most important; disruption of this structure can lead to instability of the proximal carpal row.

EXTRA-ARTICULAR SOFT TISSUES

Carpal Tunnel. A fibro-osseous tunnel formed by the volar surfaces of the distal carpal row and the flexor retinaculum, which forms the roof. The carpal tunnel contains the tendons of the flexor digitorum profundus and superficialis, flexor pollicis longus, and flexor carpiradialis, and the median nerve. Swelling and edema of these tendons or space-occupying lesions may produce a compressive neuropathy of the median nerve known as *carpal tunnel syndrome*.

Triangular Fibrocartilage (TFC). A fibrocartilaginous disc that forms the distal border of the DRUJ. The TFC has a thin membranous part and a thicker body; it is stabilized by dorsal and volar ligaments, each of which inserts on the radius and ulnar styloid.

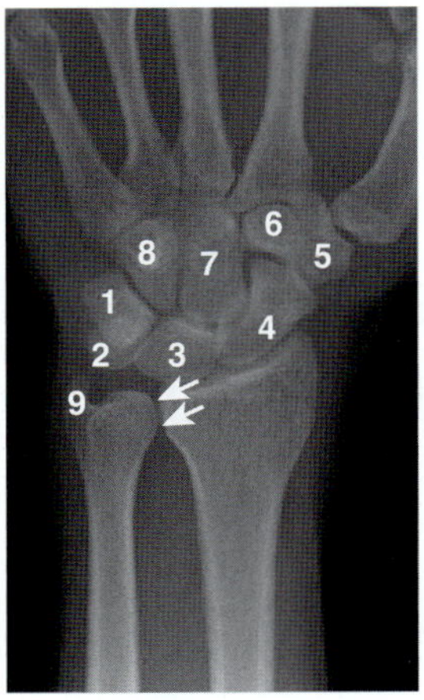

Figure 116.1 AP radiograph of the wrist: 1, triquetral; 2, pisiform; 3, lunate; 4, scaphoid; 5, trapezium; 6, trapezoid; 7, capitate; 8, hamate; 9, ulnar styloid; 10, DRUJ.

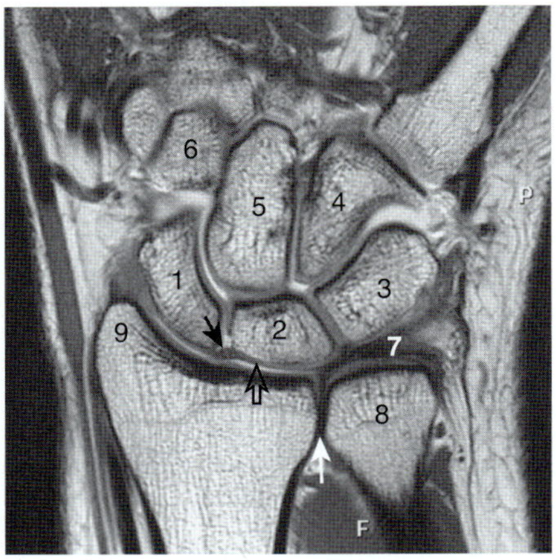

Figure 116.2 Coronal T1-weighted MR arthrogram image of the wrist: 1, scaphoid; 2, lunate; 3, triquetral; 4, hamate; 5, capitate; 6, trapezoid; 7, triangular fibrocartilage (body); 8, ulna; 9, radial styloid; *black solid arrow,* scapholunate ligament; *black open arrow,* articular cartilage; *white solid arrow,* DRUJ.

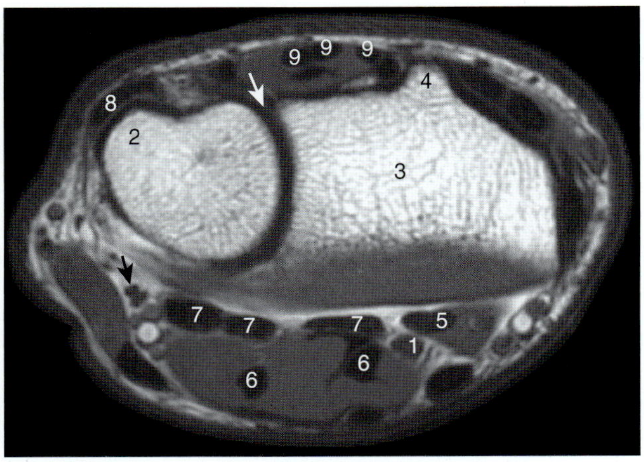

Figure 116.3 Axial T1-weighted MR image of the wrist: 1, median nerve; 2, ulnar styloid; 3, radius; 4, Lister tubercle; 5, flexor pollicis longus tendon; 6, flexor digitorum superficialis tendons; 7, flexor digitorum profundus tendons; 8, extensor carpiulnaris; 9, extensor digitorum communis tendons; *black arrow,* ulnar nerve; *white arrow,* DRUJ.

CHAPTER 117

Osteoarthritis of the Wrist

DEFINITION

- Degenerative arthritis characterized by destruction of the chondral surfaces, subchondral cysts, synovitis, and osteophyte formation.

SIGNS AND SYMPTOMS

- Gradual onset of pain with range of motion of the wrist joint.
- Effusion may be present.
- Crepitus may be present.
- Gradual decrease in range of motion.

DEMOGRAPHICS

- Incidence: Male > Female.
- Most common in elderly patients, and seen in younger patients following wrist joint trauma and/or surgery.
- Universal finding after the fifth decade of life.
- Often a history of joint trauma.

IMAGING RECOMMENDATIONS

- Radiography is primary investigation for arthropathy.
- MRI or US:
  - Identification of associated synovitis.

IMAGING FINDINGS

- Joint space narrowing, subchondral cysts, sclerosis and osteophytes.
- Primary osteoarthritis (OA) commonly affects:
  - Scaphotrapeziotrapezoid (STT) joint.
  - Carpometacarpal (CMC) joint of the thumb.
  - Interphalangeal (IP) joints of the fingers.
- Secondary OA:
  - Trauma, infection, calcium pyrophosphate dehydrate (CPPD) deposition arthropathy.
  - Radiocarpal joint.
  - Midcarpal joint and second through fifth CMC joints.

OTHER RECOMMENDED TESTING

- Laboratory testing to rule out inflammatory arthritis.
- Joint aspiration to rule out crystal arthropathies.
- Joint aspiration to rule out infection.

DIFFERENTIAL DIAGNOSIS

- Inflammatory arthritides, especially rheumatoid arthritis.
- Septic wrist joint.
- Healing wrist joint fracture, especially of the scaphoid.
- Ulnocarpal abutment syndrome.
- Kienböck disease.
- Scapulolunate instability.
- Crystal arthropathy of wrist.
- Avascular osteonecrosis.

TREATMENT

- Conservative treatment consisting of local heat, cold, simple analgesics, and nonsteroidal anti-inflammatory agents will improve symptoms in many cases.
- Physical therapy, including gentle stretching, range-of-motion exercises, and deep heat modalities, may be beneficial in selected patients.
- Intra-articular injection with local anesthetic and steroid will provide symptomatic relief if conservative therapy fails or the pain is limiting activities of daily living.
- Surgery may be required for persistent pain or progressive functional disability.

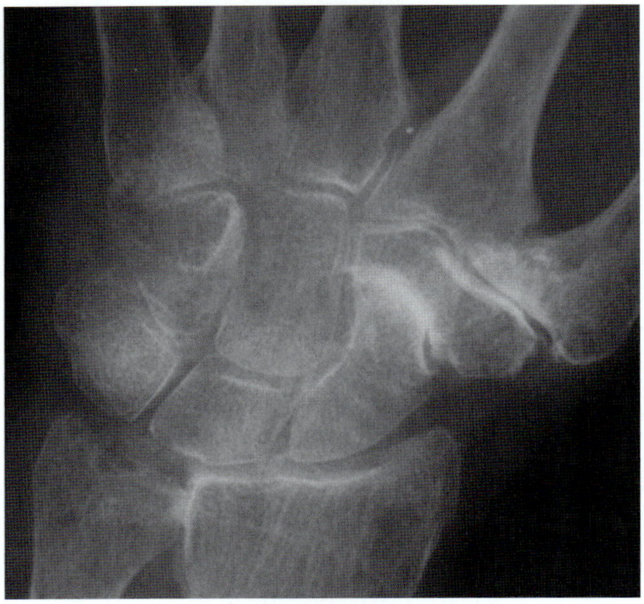

Figure 117.1 AP radiograph of an elderly patient with typical OA affecting the first CMC joint and the STT joint of the wrist with joint space narrowing, subchondral sclerosis, and early osteophyte formation. There is also OA change in the distal radioulnar joint.

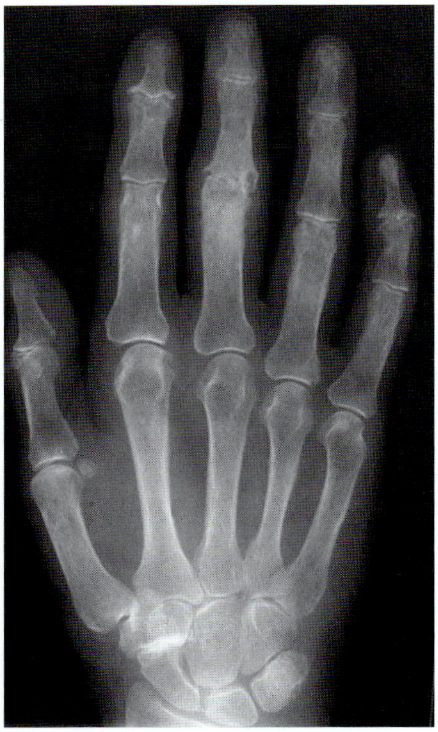

Figure 117.2 AP radiograph of a middle-aged woman with OA in the STT joint but also in several IP joints of the fingers with some erosive features. These findings are typical of inflammatory or erosive OA.

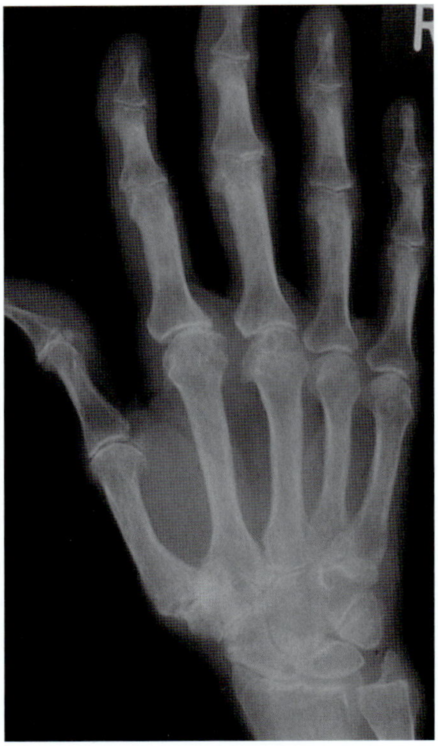

Figure 117.3 AP radiograph of a middle-aged man with OA in the first CMC and STT joints. However, there is also OA in the radiocarpal joint and in the second and third metacarpophalangeal joints with large "hook" osteophytes. These findings are consistent with secondary OA due to CPPD deposition arthropathy associated with hemachromatosis.

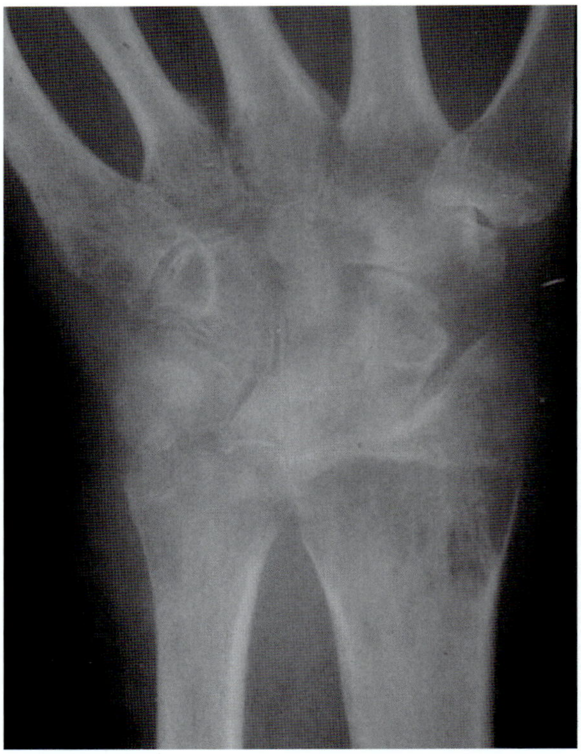

Figure 117.4 AP radiograph of an elderly man with acute monoarthritis of the wrist. Profound osteopenia can be seen, along with global joint space narrowing of the entire wrist and early bone destruction, but no features of OA change. These findings are typical of septic arthritis.

CHAPTER 118

Rheumatoid Arthritis of the Wrist

DEFINITION

- Symmetrical inflammatory arthritis characterized by synovitis, joint space narrowing, effusions and erosions, and elevation of serum rheumatoid factor combined with a constellation of other clinical signs and symptoms.

SIGNS AND SYMPTOMS

- Pain with range of motion of the wrist joint.
- Synovitis.
- Effusion often present.
- Warmth often present.
- Crepitus may be present.
- Morning stiffness.
- Gelling phenomenon.
- Gradual decrease in range of motion.
- Fatigue, lassitude, and mild fever.
- Symmetrical polyarthritis involving three or more joints invariably present on careful inspection.

DEMOGRAPHICS

- Incidence: Female > Male.
- Adult form more common, although juvenile form should be considered in any child with polyarthritis.
- Peak onset in the fourth to sixth decade of life.

IMAGING RECOMMENDATIONS

- Radiography is the primary investigation for arthropathy.
- US:
  - Identify synovitis, effusions, and early erosions.
  - Guide joint aspiration or injection.
- MRI:
  - Assess synovitis, early erosions.
  - Assess cartilage loss.

IMAGING FINDINGS

- Periarticular osteopenia.
- Joint space narrowing and erosions.
- Reactive bone formation with osteophytes and sclerosis occurs only with secondary osteoarthritis.
- Global wrist joint involvement is common, but changes may be restricted to the radiocarpal joint.
- Metacarpophalangeal (MCP) joint involvement is common, often leading to ulnar drift.
- Synovitis:
  - Enhancement of post-contrast (obtained after administration of a contrast agent) MR images.
  - Hypervascular synovial tissue on Doppler US.

OTHER RECOMMENDED TESTING

- Laboratory testing, including complete blood count, blood chemistry profile, and erythrocyte sedimentation rate determination, to rule out extra-articular manifestations of the disease.
- Antinuclear antibody and systemic lupus erythematosus (SLE) testing if diagnosis in doubt.
- Joint aspiration to rule out crystal arthropathies.
- Joint aspiration to rule out infection.

DIFFERENTIAL DIAGNOSIS

- Other inflammatory arthritides, especially SLE arthritis.
- Charcot wrist joint.
- Reflex sympathetic dystrophy.
- Infectious arthritis.
- Osteoarthritis.
- Psoriatic arthritis.
- Crystal arthropathy of wrist.
- Avascular osteonecrosis.

TREATMENT

- Disease-modifying agents, including gold salts, penicillamine, azathioprine, and cyclosporine A, can dramatically slow the progression of the disease, albeit not without side effects.
- Cytotoxic drugs, including methotrexate.
- Biologic agents, including interleukin and tumor necrosis factor-α.
- Salicylates, nonsteroidal anti-inflammatory agents, and corticosteroids.
- Physical and occupational therapy.
- Intra-articular injection of local anesthetic and corticosteroid for symptomatic relief and to aid in physical therapy.
- Surgery may be required for persistent pain or progressive functional disability.

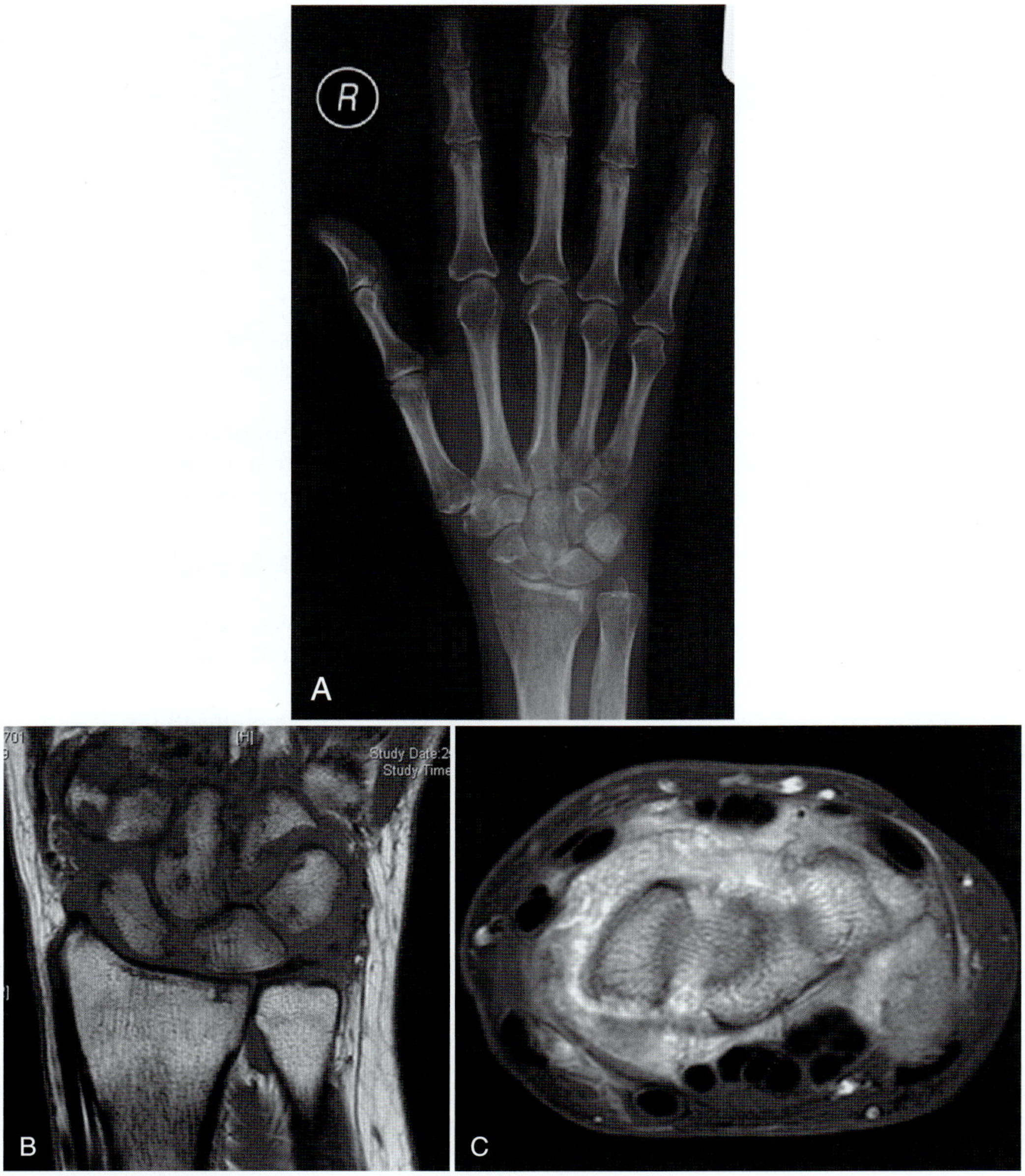

Figure 118.1 (A), Radiograph of the hand of a patient with newly diagnosed rheumatoid arthritis. There is periarticular osteopenia but no evidence of erosions. **(B),** However, a coronal T1-weighted (T1W) MR image demonstrates multiple erosions with low–signal intensity (SI) thickening of the synovium. **(C),** The axial fat sat T1W MR image acquired after administration of the contrast agent gadolinium shows the high-SI, enhancing synovitis.

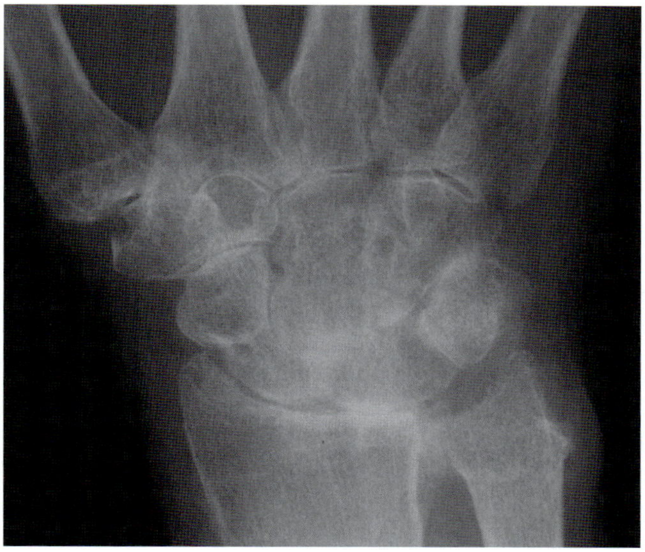

Figure 118.2 Radiograph of a patient with long-standing rheumatoid disease. There is marked joint space narrowing of the radiocarpal and mid-carpal joint with erosions of the distal ulna and the carpal bones.

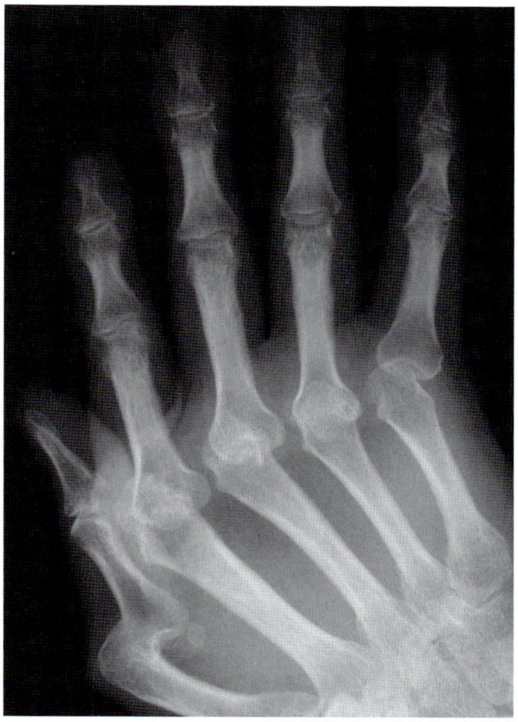

Figure 118.3 Radiograph of a patient with rheumatoid arthritis affecting the MCP joints. There are multiple metacarpal erosions associated with classic rheumatoid joint subluxation and ulnar drift.

CHAPTER 119

Scapholunate Ligament Tear Syndrome

DEFINITION

- Disruption of the intrinsic ligament between the scaphoid and lunate bones.

SIGNS AND SYMPTOMS

- Acute or gradual onset of dull, ill-defined dorsoradial wrist pain.
- Swelling over dorsoradial wrist.
- Positive result of the Watson shift ulnar deviation test.
- Crepitus may be present.
- Exacerbation of pain with ulnar deviation of wrist.
- Audible click with ulnar deviation of wrist.

DEMOGRAPHICS

- Incidence: Male = Female.
- Increased incidence in athletes involved in sports that require loading of the wrist in the presence of palmar flexion.
- Forty to 50-year-old persons most commonly affected.
- More common after trauma, including repetitive stress injuries.

IMAGING RECOMMENDATIONS

- Radiography:
  - Instability radiographs and dynamic fluoroscopy.
- Arthrography with MRI or CT is the gold standard for demonstration of intrinsic wrist ligaments.
- Conventional MRI is an alternative to MR arthrography.
- US reliably demonstrate tears of the dorsal component of the ligament.
  - This component is the strongest and functionally most important part of the ligament.

IMAGING FINDINGS

- Dorsal intercalated segmental instability (DISI) with dorsal tilt of the lunate and increased scapholunate angle on lateral radiographs.
- Scapholunate diastasis (> 3 mm) that may be apparent only on stress views.
- Abnormal communication through the scapholunate joint on arthrography.
- Deficiency of ligament on MRI or MR/CT arthrography.
- Secondary osteoarthritis (OA) changes.

OTHER RECOMMENDED TESTING

- Laboratory testing to rule out inflammatory arthritis.
- Joint aspiration to rule out crystal arthropathies.
- Joint aspiration to rule out infection if diagnosis is in question.

DIFFERENTIAL DIAGNOSIS

- Ganglion cyst.
- Calcific tendinitis.
- Scaphoid fracture.
- Scaphoid non-union.
- Distal radius fracture.
- Kienböck disease.
- De Quervain stenosing tenosynovitis.

TREATMENT

- Conservative treatment consisting of local heat, cold, simple analgesics, and nonsteroidal anti-inflammatory agents will improve symptoms in many cases.
- Physical therapy, including gentle stretching, range-of-motion exercises, and deep heat modalities, may be beneficial in selected patients.
- Injection with local anesthetic and steroid will provide symptomatic relief if conservative therapy fails or if the pain is limiting activities of daily living.
- Surgery may be required for persistent pain or progressive functional disability.

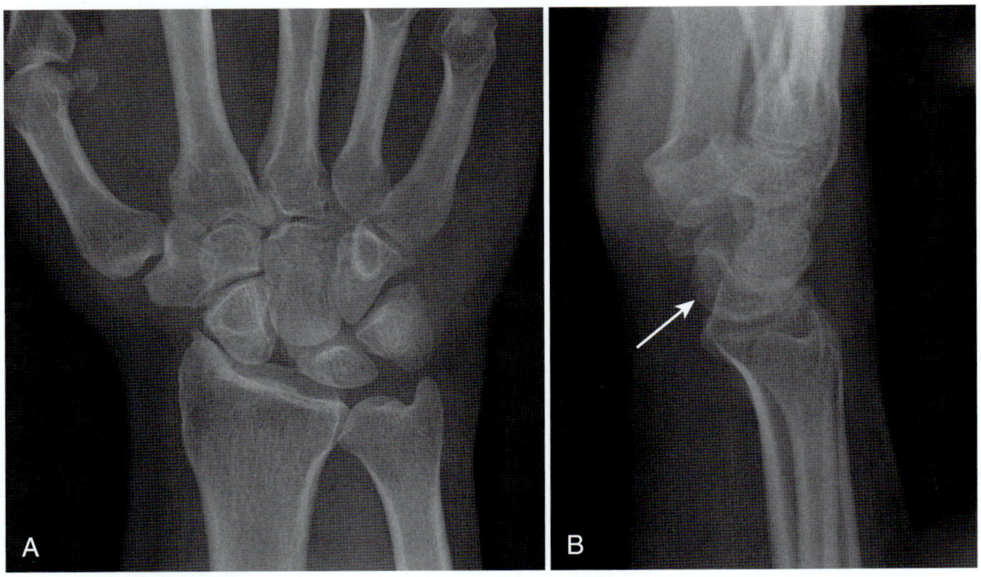

Figure 119.1 (A), AP radiograph demonstrating separation of the articulation between the scaphoid and lunate (scapholunate diastasis). There is also secondary OA change in the radiocarpal joint. (B), The lateral radiograph demonstrates dorsal tilt of the lunate (*white arrow*), indicating the presence of DISI deformity.

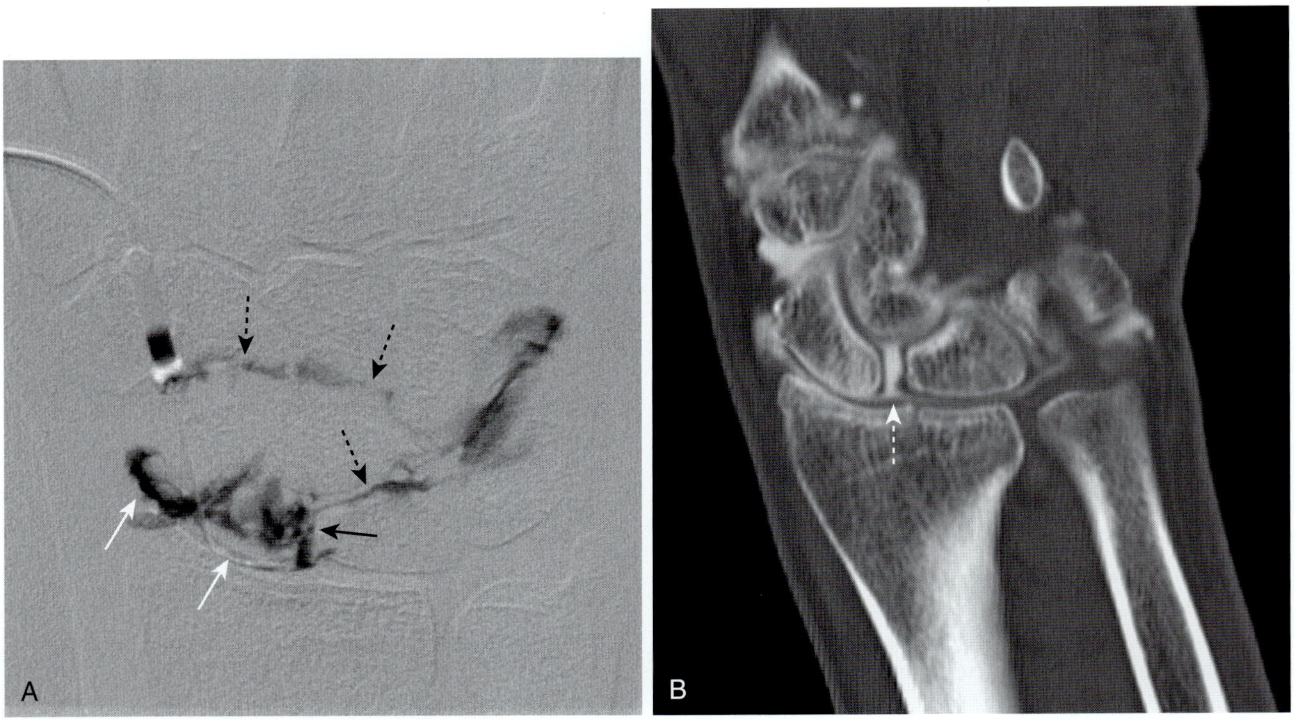

Figure 119.2 (A), A digital subtraction arthrographic image in which the outline of the carpal bones is just visible. There is contrast agent within the radiocarpal joint (*white arrows*). However, contrast agent is also shown extending through the scapholunate joint (*black arrow*) and into the midcarpal joints (*broken black arrows*), indicating a torn scapholunate ligament. (B), The comparative CT arthrographic scan clearly demonstrates absence of the scapholunate ligament and early scapholunate diastasis (broken *white arrow*).

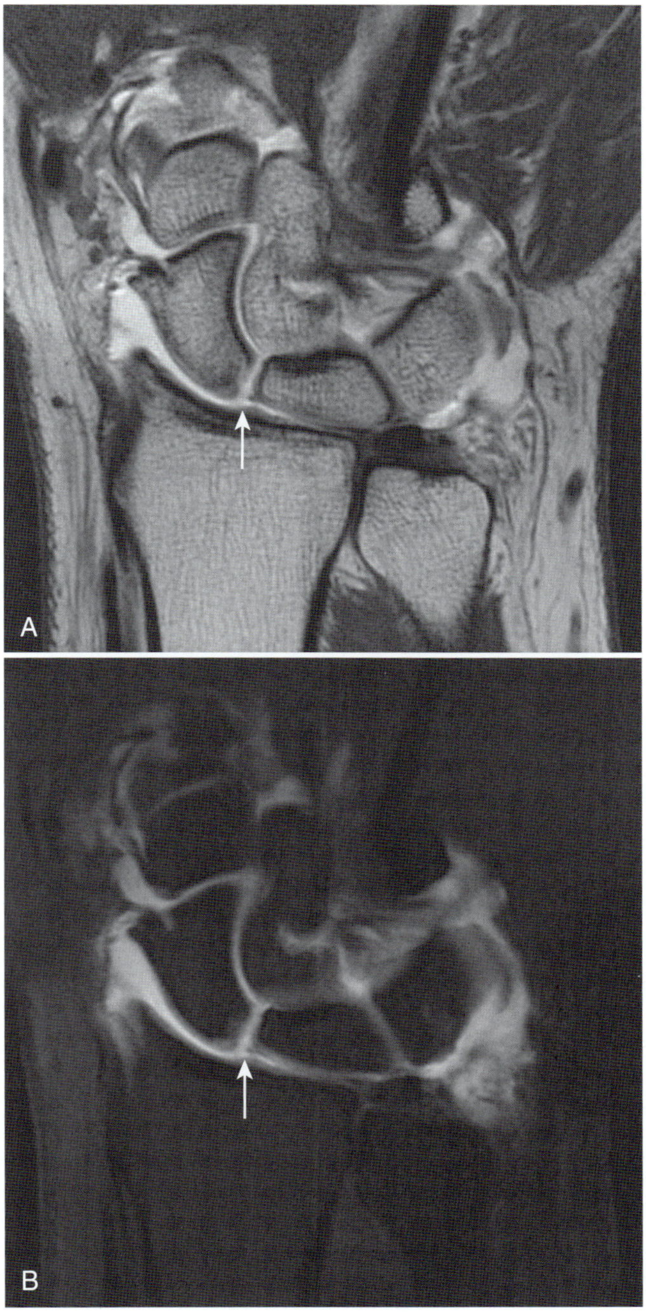

Figure 119.3 Coronal T1-weighted (T1W) (**A**) and T1W with fat suppression (FST1W) (**B**) MR arthrogram images demonstrating a tear of the scapholunate ligament (*white arrows*) without associated scapholunate diastasis. The radiographic findings were normal.

CHAPTER 120

Lunotriquetral Instability Pain Syndrome

DEFINITION

Degeneration or tear of the lunotriquetral (LT) ligament.

SIGNS AND SYMPTOMS

- Acute or gradual onset of dull, ill-defined ulnar pain.
- Swelling over ulnar aspect of wrist.
- Crepitus may be present.
- Exacerbation of pain with radial deviation of wrist.
- Audible click with radial or ulnar deviation of wrist.

DEMOGRAPHICS

- Incidence: Male = Female.
- Increased incidence following a fall on the outstretched hand or a twisting injury to the wrist.
- Forty to 50-year-old persons most commonly affected.
- More common after trauma, including repetitive stress injuries.

IMAGING RECOMMENDATIONS

- Radiography:
  - Instability radiographs.
- Dynamic fluoroscopy.
- Arthrography with MRI or CT is the gold standard for demonstration of intrinsic wrist ligaments.
- Conventional MRI is alternative to MR arthrography.

IMAGING FINDINGS

- Volar intercalated segmental instability (VISI) with volar tilt of lunate and decreased scapholunate angle on lateral radiographs.
- LT diastasis or subluxation, which may be apparent only on stress views.
- Abnormal communication through LT joint on arthrography.
- Deficiency of ligament on MRI or MR/CT arthrograms.
- Secondary osteoarthritis (OA) changes.

OTHER RECOMMENDED TESTING

- Laboratory testing to rule out inflammatory arthritis.
- Joint aspiration to rule out crystal arthropathies.
- Joint aspiration to rule out infection if diagnosis is in question.

DIFFERENTIAL DIAGNOSIS

- Ganglion cyst.
- Calcific tendinitis.
- Ulnar styloid fracture.
- Tear of triangular fibrocartilage.
- Distal ulnar fracture.
- Ulnar head chondromalacia.
- Ulnocarpal abutment syndrome.

TREATMENT

- Conservative treatment consisting of local heat, cold, simple analgesics, and nonsteroidal anti-inflammatory agents will improve symptoms in many cases.
- Physical therapy, including gentle stretching, range-of-motion exercises, and deep heat modalities, may be beneficial in selected patients.
- Injection with local anesthetic and steroid will provide symptomatic relief if conservative therapy fails or the pain is limiting activities of daily living.
- Surgery may be required for persistent pain or progressive functional disability.

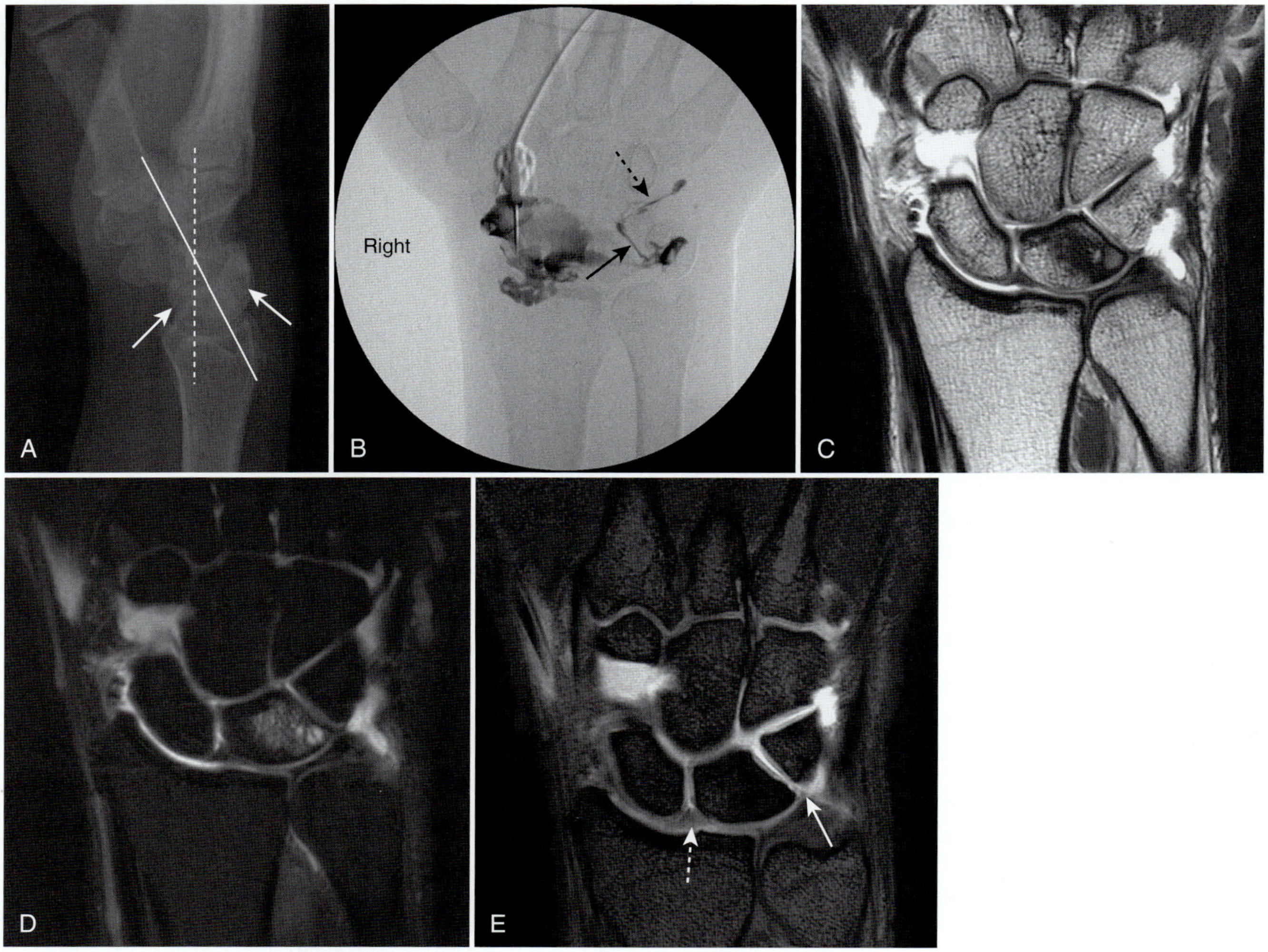

Figure 120.1 (A), Lateral radiograph demonstrating the lunate (*white arrows*) with its axis (*white line*) tilted in a volar direction compared with the axis of capitate and radius (*broken white line*); this tilting is consistent with a VISI deformity. (B), A digital subtraction arthrogram of the same patient after injection of contrast agent into the radiocarpal joint demonstrates contrast agent passing through the LT joint (*black arrow*) and into the midcarpal joint (*broken black arrow*), indicating a tear of the LT ligament. The coronal T1-weighted (T1W) (C) and T2W with fat suppression (FST2W) (D) MR arthrogram images show sclerosis, subchondral cyst formation, and marrow edema within the lunate resulting from secondary OA change in the LT joint. (E), The gradient echo MR image best demonstrates absence of the LT ligament (*white arrow*) and loss of articular cartilage. Compare with the normal appearance of the scapholunate ligament (*broken white arrow*).

CHAPTER 121

Ulnocarpal Abutment Syndrome

DEFINITION

- Degeneration and eccentric sclerosis of the lunate and distal ulna due to excessive loading across the ulnar aspect of the wrist.

SIGNS AND SYMPTOMS

- Gradual onset of dull, ill-defined dorsoulnar wrist pain.
- Swelling over dorsoulnar wrist.
- Crepitus may be present.
- Exacerbation of pain with ulnar deviation and rotation of wrist.
- Tenderness over ulnar head and triquetrum and lunate bones.

DEMOGRAPHICS

- Incidence: Male = Female.
- Forty to 50-year-old persons most commonly affected.
- More common after trauma, including repetitive stress injuries.

IMAGING RECOMMENDATIONS

- Radiography.
- MRI.
- Arthrography with MRI or CT to detect early triangular fibrocartilage (TFC) tears.

IMAGING FINDINGS

- Positive ulnar variance (distal ulna extends beyond distal articular surface of radius).
- Sclerosis and subchondral cyst formation of the lunate.
- Degenerative tear of central portion of TFC.

OTHER RECOMMENDED TESTING

- Laboratory testing to rule out inflammatory arthritis.
- Joint aspiration to rule out crystal arthropathies.
- Joint aspiration to rule out infection if diagnosis is in question.

DIFFERENTIAL DIAGNOSIS

- Ganglion cyst.
- Calcific tendinitis.
- Tear of TFC.
- Distal ulnar fracture.
- Distal radioulnar instability.
- Kienböck disease.

TREATMENT

- Conservative treatment consisting of local heat, cold, simple analgesics, and nonsteroidal anti-inflammatory agents will improve symptoms in many cases.
- Physical therapy, including gentle stretching, range-of-motion exercises, and deep heat modalities, may be beneficial in selected patients.
- Injection with local anesthetic and steroid will provide symptomatic relief if conservative therapy fails or the pain is limiting activities of daily living.
- Surgery may be required for persistent pain or progressive functional disability.

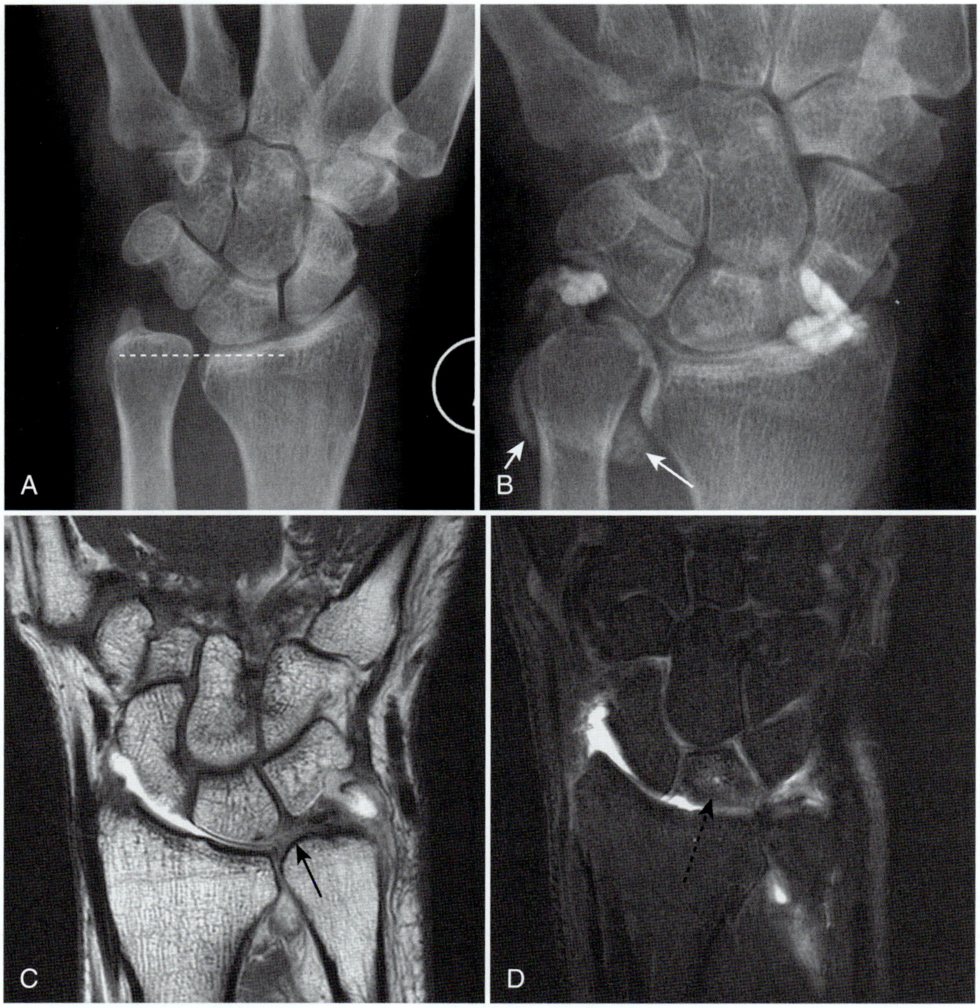

Figure 121.1 (**A**), AP radiograph of a patient with positive ulnar variance. The articular surface of the ulna lies distal to the articular surface of the distal radius (*dotted white line*). (**B**), The MR arthrogram image demonstrates abnormal communication between the radiocarpal joint and the distal radioulnar joint (*white arrows*), which indicates a tear of the TFC. (**C**), The T1-weighted (T1W) MR arthrogram image shows the impaction of the distal ulna on the lunate with a large degenerative-type tear of the TFC (*black arrow*). (**D**), On the T2-weighted with fat suppression (FST2W) MR image, reactive marrow edema can be seen within the scaphoid (*broken black arrow*), due to early secondary osteoarthritis change. There is also early loss of articular cartilage on the lunate and distal radius.

CHAPTER 122

Triangular Fibrocartilage Complex Tear

DEFINITION

- Tear of the triangular fibrocartilage (TFC) complex due to acute trauma or degeneration.

SIGNS AND SYMPTOMS

- Gradual or acute onset of dull, ill-defined ulnar wrist pain.
- Swelling over dorsoulnar wrist.
- Crepitus may be present.
- Catching or clicking with rotation of the wrist.
- Loss of strength.
- Presence of piano key sign.
- Exacerbation of pain with stress loading of the distal radioulnar joint with pronation and supination.
- Tenderness over TFC complex.

DEMOGRAPHICS

- Incidence: Male = Female.
- Twenty to 30-year old persons most commonly affected by traumatic tears.
- Forty to 50-year-old persons most commonly affected by degenerative tears.
- More common after trauma, including repetitive stress injuries.

IMAGING RECOMMENDATIONS

- Arthrography with MRI or CT is the gold standard investigation.
- Conventional MRI is also accurate and is often the primary investigation.

IMAGING FINDINGS

- Degenerative and traumatic patterns:
  - Small central perforations may be asymptomatic.
- May affect central portion, peripheral attachments, or, rarely, the radial attachment.
- Abnormal communication between radiocarpal joint and distal radioulnar joint (DRUJ) on arthrography.
- Tendinopathy of the extensor carpi ulnaris (ECU) tendon may be present.
- Association with ulnar abutment syndrome.

OTHER RECOMMENDED TESTING

- Laboratory testing to rule out inflammatory arthritis.
- Joint aspiration to rule out crystal arthropathies.
- Joint aspiration to rule out infection if diagnosis is in question.

DIFFERENTIAL DIAGNOSIS

- Ganglion cyst.
- Ulnocarpal abutment syndrome.
- Calcific tendinitis of the extensor carpi ulnaris.
- Distal ulnar fracture.
- DRUJ instability.
- Kienböck disease.

TREATMENT

- Conservative treatment consisting of local heat, cold, simple analgesics, and nonsteroidal anti-inflammatory agents will improve symptoms in many cases.
- Physical therapy, including gentle stretching, range-of-motion exercises, and deep heat modalities, may be beneficial in selected patients.
- Injection with local anesthetic and steroid will provide symptomatic relief if conservative therapy fails or the pain is limiting activities of daily living.
- Surgery may be required for persistent pain or progressive functional disability.

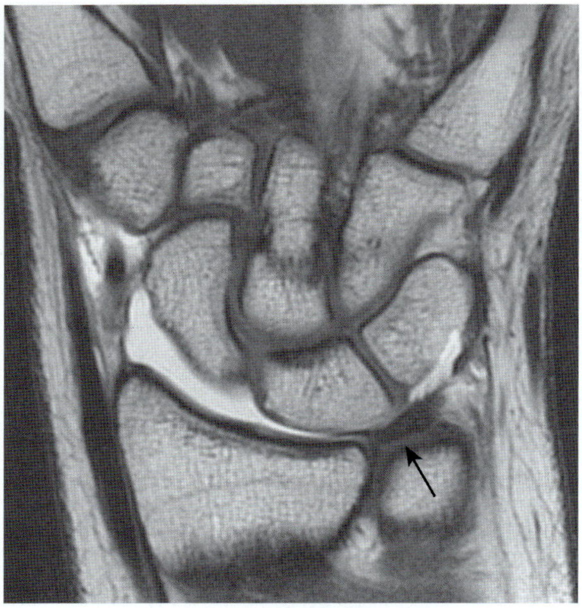

Figure 122.1 Coronal T1-weighted (T1W) MR arthrogram image of a normal TFC, which has low signal intensity (SI) (*black arrow*). There is no contrast agent within the DRUJ.

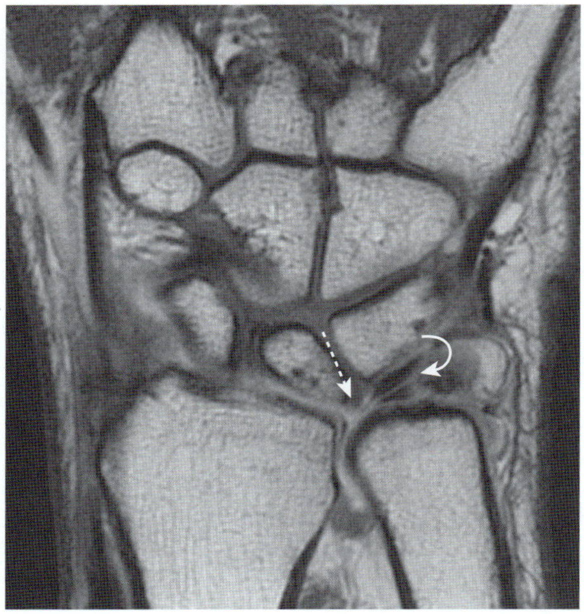

Figure 122.3 Coronal T1W MR image of a complex tear of the TFC. There is a tear of the central portion (*broken white arrow*), and a horizontal component of the tear extends through the periphery of the TFC (*curved white arrow*).

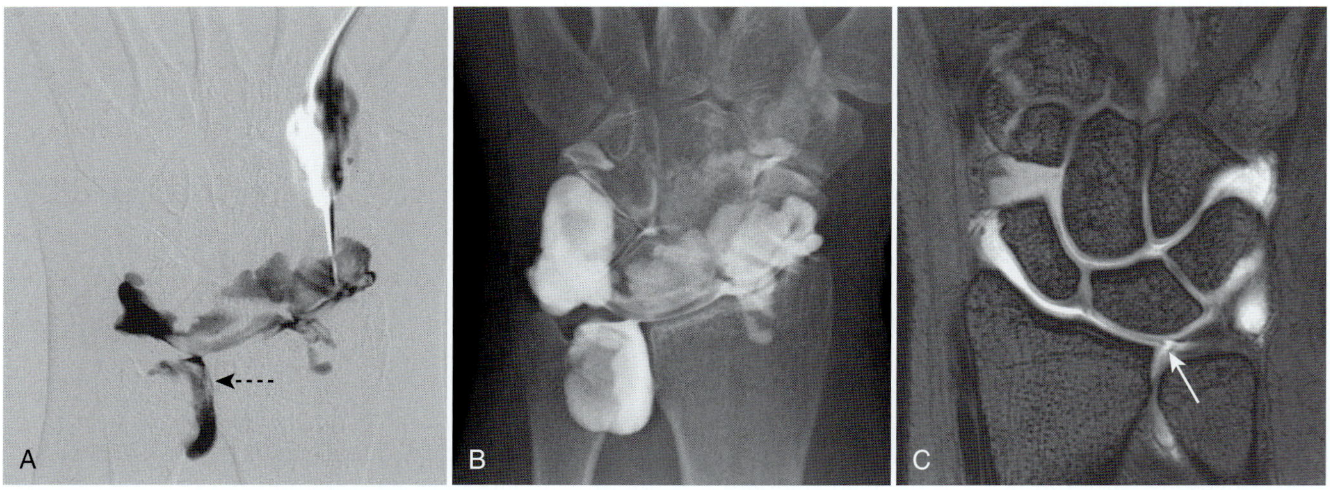

Figure 122.2 (**A**), Digital subtraction MR arthrogram image demonstrating a leak of contrast agent from the radiocarpal joint into the DRUJ (*broken black arrow*) due to a TFC tear. (**B**), The post-injection radiograph also shows contrast agent within the DRUJ. In addition, there is contrast agent in the midcarpal joint because of a leak through an asymptomatic central perforation of the scapholunate ligament. (**C**), The coronal gradient echo MR arthrogram image shows the tear of the TFC (*white arrow*). The articular cartilage of the wrist is well demonstrated and normal.

CHAPTER 123

Non-Union of the Scaphoid

DEFINITION

- Non-union of the scaphoid bone occurring more than 6 months after a fracture.

SIGNS AND SYMPTOMS

- Gradual or acute onset of dull, ill-defined radial wrist pain.
- Swelling over the dorsoulnar wrist.
- Crepitus may be present.
- Catching or clicking with radial and ulnar deviation of wrist.
- Loss of grip strength.
- Loss of dorsiflexion.
- Tenderness over the anatomic snuffbox.

DEMOGRAPHICS

- Incidence: Male > Female.
- 20- to 30-year-old persons most commonly affected.
- More common after severe trauma.

IMAGING RECOMMENDATIONS

- Radiography.
- CT:
  - Fracture non-union.
- Contrast-enhanced MRI
  - Proximal avascular necrosis (AVN).

IMAGING FINDINGS

- Persistent fracture defect with sclerotic and corticated fracture margins.
  - Radiography or CT.
- Proximal AVN:
  - Sclerosis.
  - Subchondral collapse and fragmentation.
  - Low–signal intensity (SI) sclerosis on T1-weighted (T1W) MR images.
  - High-SI edema on T2W with fat suppression (FST2W) MR images.
  - Lack of enhancement on post-contrast (obtained after administration of a contrast agent) MR sequences correlates with loss of perfusion.
- Associated scapholunate diastasis and DISI (dorsal intercalated segmental instability) deformity.

OTHER RECOMMENDED TESTING

- Laboratory testing to rule out inflammatory arthritis.
- Joint aspiration to rule out crystal arthropathies.
- Joint aspiration to rule out infection if diagnosis in question.

DIFFERENTIAL DIAGNOSIS

- Scaphoid fracture.
- Scapholunate ligament tear.
- De Quervain stenosing tenosynovitis.
- Calcific tendinitis.
- Distal radius fracture.
- Distal radioulnar instability.

TREATMENT

- Conservative treatment consisting of local heat, cold, simple analgesics, and nonsteroidal anti-inflammatory agents will improve symptoms in many cases.
- Physical therapy, including gentle stretching, range-of-motion exercises, and deep heat modalities, may be beneficial in selected patients.
- Injection with local anesthetic and steroid will provide symptomatic relief if conservative therapy fails or the pain is limiting activities of daily living.
- Surgery may be required for persistent pain or progressive functional disability.

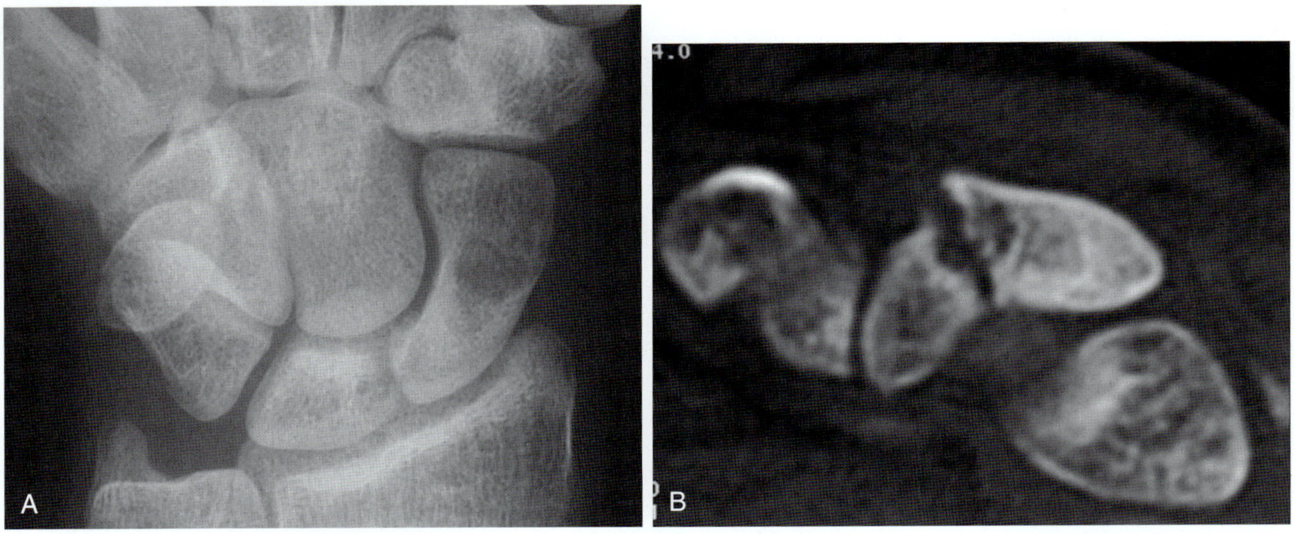

Figure 123.1 (**A**), Radiograph obtained 12 weeks after a scaphoid fracture. There is an apparent cyst in the scaphoid but no fracture line. (**B**), The CT scan, however, confirms fracture non-union.

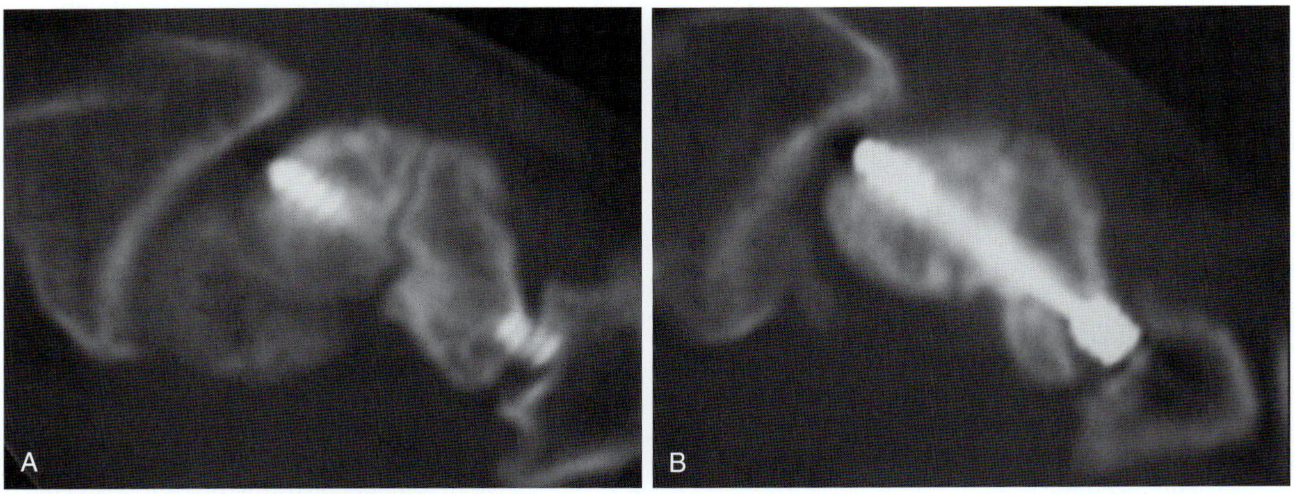

Figure 123.2 (**A** and **B**), CT scans of a patient with previous fixation with a Herbert screw for scaphoid non-union. There is persistent non-union.

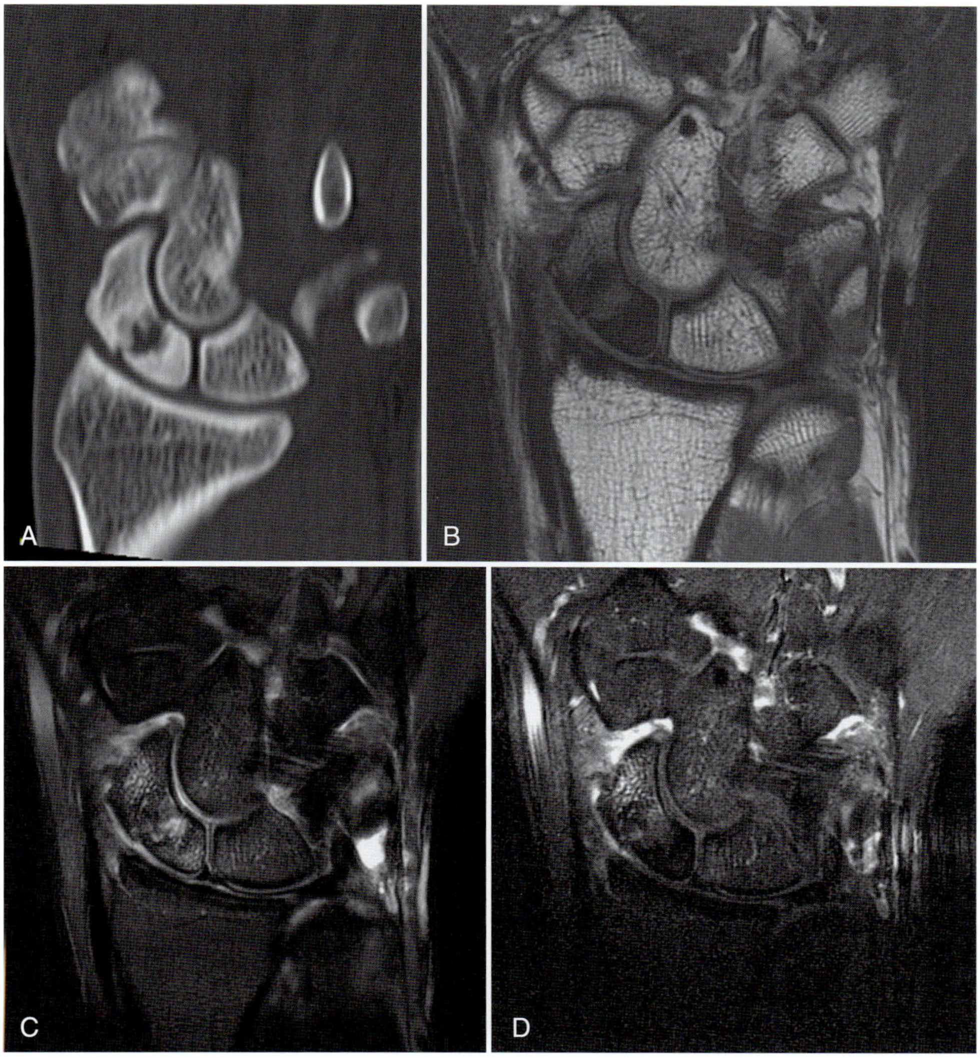

Figure 123.3 (**A**), CT scan of a patient with a scaphoid non-union. The proximal pole is sclerotic, suggesting AVN. (**B**), The T1W MR image shows low SI of the proximal pole. (**C**), The FST2W MR image demonstrates high-SI edema throughout the scaphoid. (**D**), The lack of high-SI enhancement on this post-contrast FST1W MR image confirms AVN in the proximal pole.

CHAPTER 124

Kienböck Disease

DEFINITION

- Avascular necrosis of the lunate bone.

SIGNS AND SYMPTOMS

- Gradual onset of dull, ill-defined wrist pain around the lunate.
- Swelling and synovitis over the lunate.
- Crepitus may be present.
- Catching or clicking with radial and ulnar deviation of the wrist.
- Loss of grip strength.
- Loss of wrist range of motion.

DEMOGRAPHICS

- Incidence: Male > Female.
- Almost always unilateral.
- 20- to 30-year-old persons most commonly affected.
- More common after severe trauma.

IMAGING RECOMMENDATIONS

- Radiography.
- MRI.

IMAGING FINDINGS

- Sclerosis, subchondral collapse, and fragmentation of the lunate.
- MRI:
  - Low signal intensity (SI) on T1-weighted (T1W) MR images.
  - High-SI edema on T2W with fat suppression (FST2W) MR images.
  - Lack of enhancement on post-contrast (obtained after administration of a contrast agent) sequences correlates with loss of perfusion.
- Secondary osteoarthritis change.

OTHER RECOMMENDED TESTING

- Laboratory testing to rule out inflammatory arthritis.
- Joint aspiration to rule out crystal arthropathies.
- Joint aspiration to rule out infection if diagnosis in question.

DIFFERENTIAL DIAGNOSIS

- Scaphoid fracture.
- Lunate fracture.
- Scapholunate ligament tear.
- Ulnocarpal abutment syndrome.
- Calcific tendinitis.
- Carpal instability.

TREATMENT

- Conservative treatment consisting of local heat, cold, simple analgesics, and nonsteroidal anti-inflammatory agents will improve symptoms in many cases.
- Physical therapy, including gentle stretching, range-of-motion exercises, and deep heat modalities, may be beneficial in selected patients.
- Splinting.
- Injection with local anesthetic and steroid will provide symptomatic relief if conservative therapy fails or the pain is limiting activities of daily living.
- Surgery may be required for persistent pain or progressive functional disability.

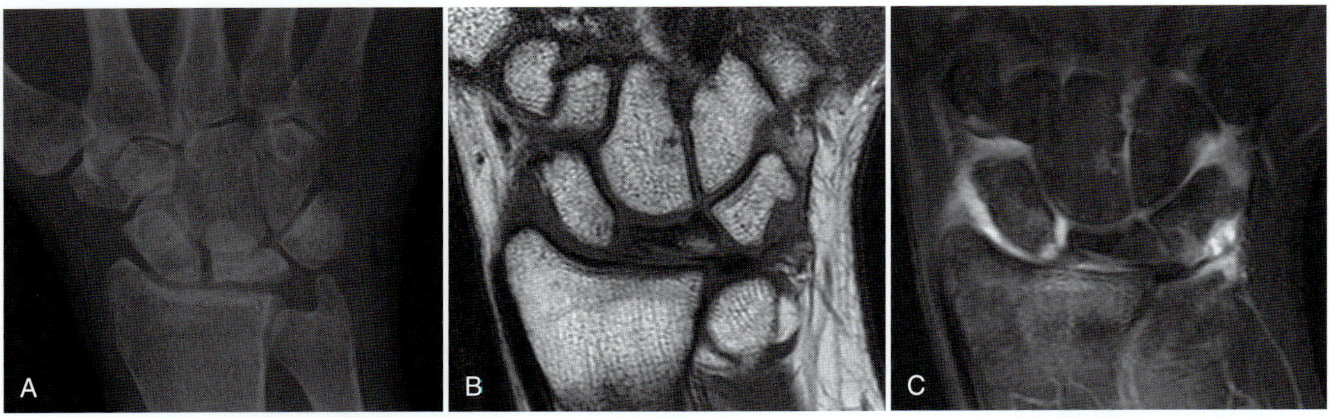

Figure 124.1 (**A**), Radiograph of a patient with established Kienböck disease, showing collapse and sclerosis of the lunate. (**B**), The coronal T1W MR image demonstrates low-SI change throughout most of the lunate that is due to sclerosis, as well as the bony collapse. (**C**), The fat sat T1W MR image acquired after administration of the contrast agent gadolinium shows no enhancement within the lunate, indicating absence of perfusion.

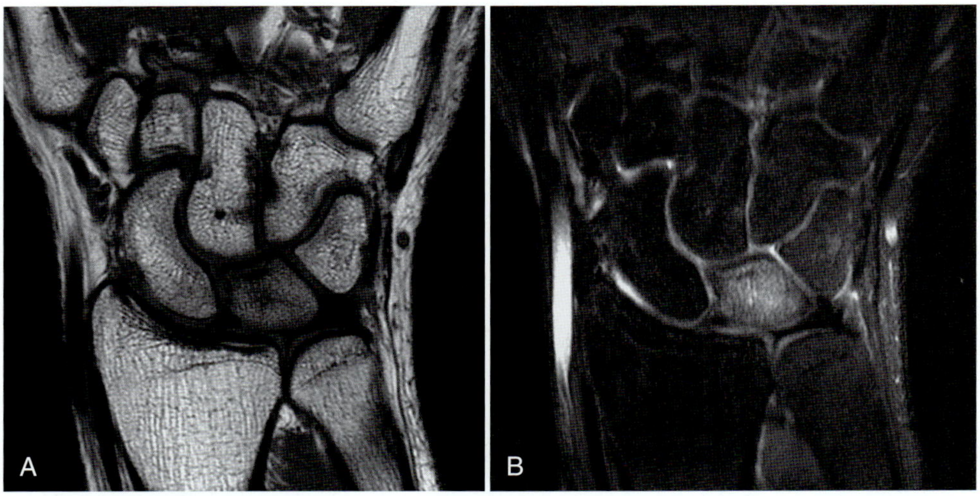

Figure 124.2 Coronal T1W (**A**) and fat sat T2W (**B**) images of early Kienböck disease. There is high-SI marrow edema within the lunate on the fat sat T2W MR image, with only minimal signal change on the T1W MR image, and there is no bony collapse or fragmentation.

CHAPTER 125

Carpal Tunnel Syndrome

DEFINITION

- Entrapment of the median nerve at the wrist as it passes through the carpal tunnel.

SIGNS AND SYMPTOMS

- Pain, numbness, and paresthesias in the hand and wrist that radiate to the thumb, the index finger, the middle finger, and the radial half of the ring finger and are worse at night.
- Associated weakness affecting the thumb, the index finger, the middle finger, and the radial half of the ring finger that is worse at night.
- Symptoms may also radiate proximal to the entrapment, into the forearm.
- Onset of symptoms usually occurs after repetitive wrist motions or as a result of repeated pressure on the wrist, such as from resting the wrist on the edge of a computer keyboard.
- Direct trauma to the median nerve as it enters the carpal tunnel may result in a similar clinical presentation.
- Physical findings include tenderness over the median nerve at the wrist.
- Presence of Tinel sign over the median nerve as it passes beneath the flexor retinaculum is common.
- Positive result of Phalen test is highly suggestive of carpal tunnel syndrome.
- Weakness of thumb opposition and wasting of the thenar eminence are often seen in advanced carpal tunnel syndrome.
- Without treatment, progressive motor deficit and, ultimately, flexion contracture of the affected fingers can result.

DEMOGRAPHICS

- Incidence peaks in the fifth and sixth decades of life.
- Incidence: Female > Male.
- The most common entrapment neuropathy.
- Increased incidence in the last trimester of pregnancy.

IMAGING RECOMMENDATIONS

- Radiography:
  - Identification of associated joint disease.
- MRI or US:
  - Assessment of nerve changes.
  - Identification of synovitis or mass lesion within the carpal tunnel.

IMAGING FINDINGS

- Cross-sectional enlargement at the level of the pisiform:
  - High signal intensity (SI) within the median nerve on T2-weighted with fat suppression (FST2W) or short T1 inversion recovery (STIR) MR images.
  - Loss of fascicular pattern on US.
- Flattening of the median nerve at the level of the hamate.
- Palmar bowing of the transverse carpal ligament at the level of the hamate.
- Pseudoneuroma phenomenon, manifested as swelling of the median nerve proximal to the transverse carpal ligament.
- Other imaging findings:
  - Displaced proximal capitate fracture.
  - Fracture of the radius.
  - Amyloid crystals in the carpal tunnel (low SI on MR images).
  - Ganglion cysts and other masses within the carpal tunnel.
  - Flexor tendon tenosynovitis:
    - Fluid in tendon sheath.
    - Enhancement on post-contrast (obtained after administration of a contrast agent) MR sequences.
- Synovitis associated with rheumatoid arthritis and other arthropathies.

OTHER RECOMMENDED TESTING

- Electromyography and nerve conduction velocity testing are diagnostic except very early in the course of disease.

- Erythrocyte sedimentation rate, rheumatoid factor, and antinuclear antibody determinations if rheumatoid arthritis is suggested.
- Blood glucose determination.

DIFFERENTIAL DIAGNOSIS

- C5-C6 cervical radiculopathy.
- Arthritis of carpometacarpal joints.
- Pronator teres syndrome.
- De Quervain tenosynovitis.
- Thoracic outlet syndrome.
- Carpal instabilities.
- Occult fractures of distal radius.
- Occult fractures of carpal bones.
- Space-occupying lesions involving the carpal tunnel.
- Crystal arthropathies.
- Amyloidosis.

TREATMENT

- Conservative therapy, consisting of simple analgesics, nonsteroidal anti-inflammatory drugs, or cyclooxygenase inhibitors and splinting of the wrist, should be used for mild cases of carpal tunnel syndrome.
- Avoidance of repetitive activities thought to be responsible for the evolution of carpal tunnel syndrome (e.g., typing, hammering) will also help ameliorate the symptoms.
- If there is no response to these conservative measures, injection of the carpal tunnel with local anesthetic and steroid is the next reasonable step.
- Surgical decompression of the compressed median nerve by release of the transverse carpal ligament should be performed for all cases of moderate to severe carpal tunnel syndrome that have not responded to conservative therapy.

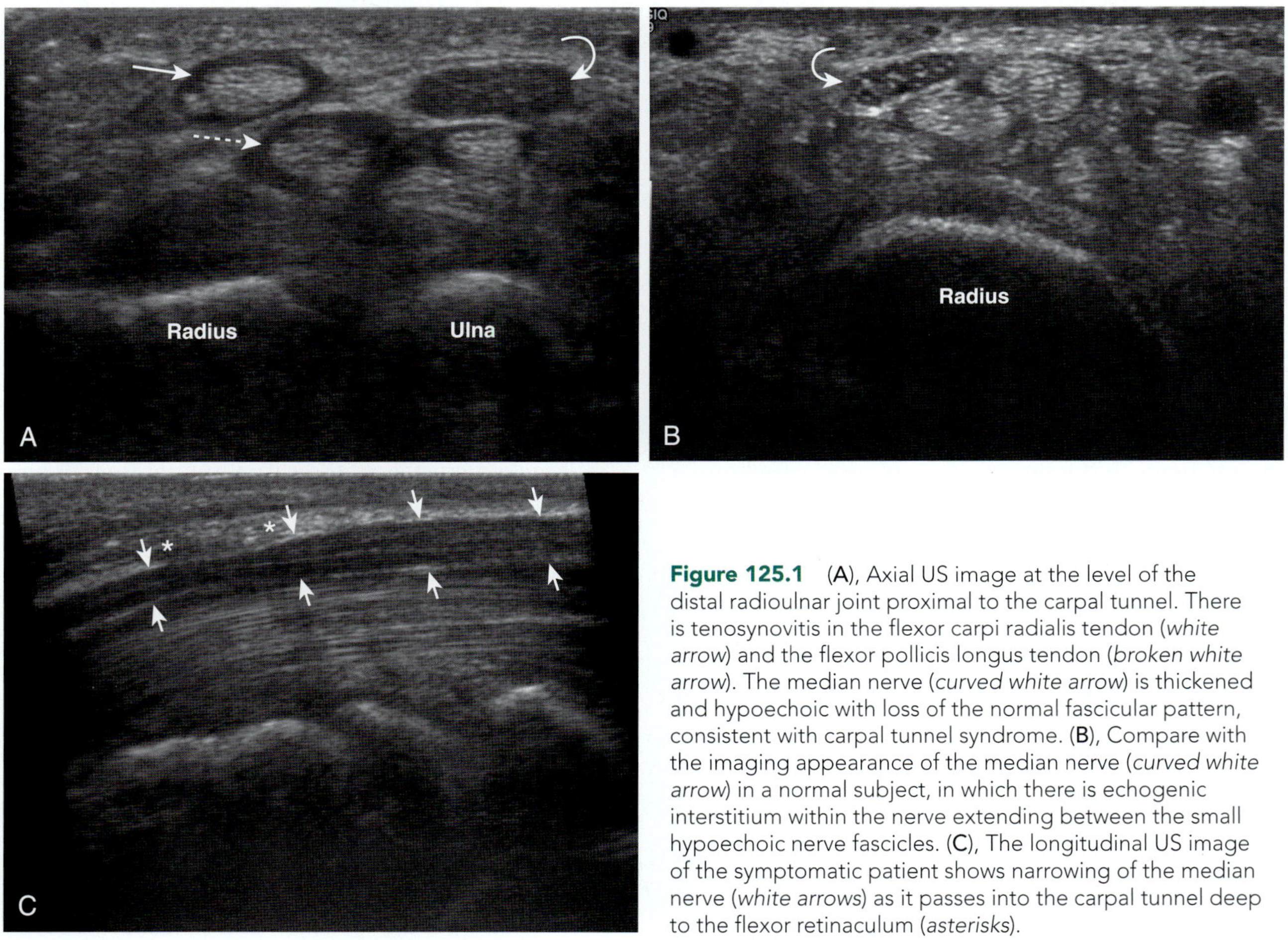

Figure 125.1 (A), Axial US image at the level of the distal radioulnar joint proximal to the carpal tunnel. There is tenosynovitis in the flexor carpi radialis tendon (*white arrow*) and the flexor pollicis longus tendon (*broken white arrow*). The median nerve (*curved white arrow*) is thickened and hypoechoic with loss of the normal fascicular pattern, consistent with carpal tunnel syndrome. (B), Compare with the imaging appearance of the median nerve (*curved white arrow*) in a normal subject, in which there is echogenic interstitium within the nerve extending between the small hypoechoic nerve fascicles. (C), The longitudinal US image of the symptomatic patient shows narrowing of the median nerve (*white arrows*) as it passes into the carpal tunnel deep to the flexor retinaculum (*asterisks*).

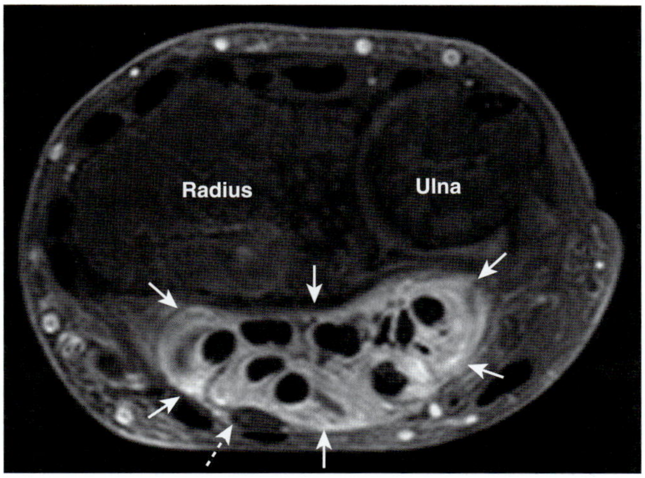

Figure 125.2 Axial FST2W MR image of the wrist in a patient with rheumatoid arthritis and symptoms of carpal tunnel syndrome. Extensive high-SI tenosynovitis surrounds the flexor tendons just proximal to the carpal tunnel (*white arrows*). The median nerve (*broken white arrow*) lies between the inflamed flexor tendons and the normal palmaris longus tendon.

CHAPTER 126

Ulnar Tunnel Syndrome

DEFINITION

- Entrapment of the ulnar nerve at the wrist as it passes through the Guyon canal.

SIGNS AND SYMPTOMS

- Presence of Tinel sign over the entrapped nerve.
- Pain at the wrist that radiates into the little finger and the ulnar side of the ring finger.
- Passive range of motion preserved early on, with clawing of the fingers if left untreated.
- Weakness in ulnar nerve distribution.
- Positive result of little finger abduction test.
- Paresthesias radiating into the ring and little fingers.
- Tenderness to palpation of the ulnar nerve at the point of entrapment.
- Ulnar neurapraxia often present.

DEMOGRAPHICS

- Incidence: Female = Male.
- Can occur acutely following trauma and fracture.
- More common after trauma, including repetitive stress injuries.

IMAGING RECOMMENDATIONS

- MRI or US:
  - Assessment of nerve changes.
  - Identification of mass lesion within the Guyon canal.

IMAGING FINDINGS

- Cross-sectional enlargement of ulnar nerve.
- High signal intensity (SI) within the ulnar nerve on T2-weighted with fat suppression (FST2W) MR images or short T1 inversion recovery (STIR) MR images.
- Loss of fascicular pattern on US.
- Ganglion or other soft tissue mass within the Guyon canal.
- Pseudoaneurysm of ulnar artery.

OTHER RECOMMENDED TESTING

- Electromyography and nerve conduction velocity testing of the cervical nerve roots, brachial plexus, and ulnar, radial, and median nerves.

DIFFERENTIAL DIAGNOSIS

- Parsonage-Turner syndrome.
- Carpal tunnel syndrome.
- Cervical radiculopathy.
- Cubital tunnel syndrome.
- Hamate fracture.
- Hematoma.
- Benign neoplasm.
- Malignant neoplasm.
- Wrist fracture.
- Hansen disease.

TREATMENT

- Conservative treatment consisting of local heat, cold, simple analgesics, and nonsteroidal anti-inflammatory agents will improve symptoms in mild, self-limited cases.
- Physical therapy to maintain function, including gentle stretching, range-of-motion exercises, and local heat modalities, may be beneficial in selected patients.
- Splinting to preserve normal range of motion.
- Injection with local anesthetic and steroid of the ulnar nerve may provide symptomatic relief if conservative therapy fails or the pain is limiting activities of daily living.
- Surgery may be required to relieve entrapment of the ulnar nerve.

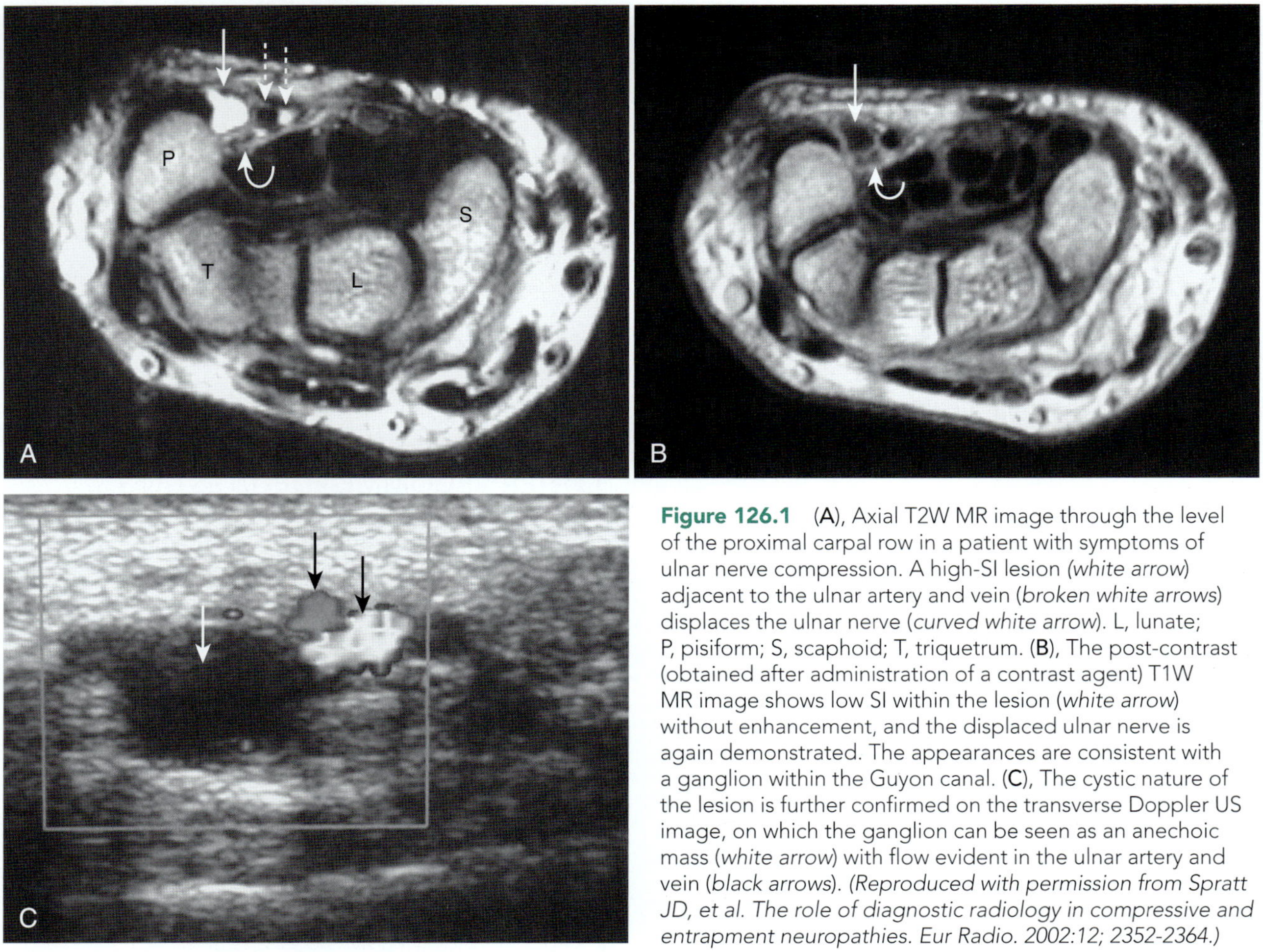

Figure 126.1 (**A**), Axial T2W MR image through the level of the proximal carpal row in a patient with symptoms of ulnar nerve compression. A high-SI lesion *(white arrow)* adjacent to the ulnar artery and vein (*broken white arrows*) displaces the ulnar nerve (*curved white arrow*). L, lunate; P, pisiform; S, scaphoid; T, triquetrum. (**B**), The post-contrast (obtained after administration of a contrast agent) T1W MR image shows low SI within the lesion (*white arrow*) without enhancement, and the displaced ulnar nerve is again demonstrated. The appearances are consistent with a ganglion within the Guyon canal. (**C**), The cystic nature of the lesion is further confirmed on the transverse Doppler US image, on which the ganglion can be seen as an anechoic mass (*white arrow*) with flow evident in the ulnar artery and vein (*black arrows*). *(Reproduced with permission from Spratt JD, et al. The role of diagnostic radiology in compressive and entrapment neuropathies. Eur Radio. 2002:12; 2352-2364.)*

CHAPTER 127

Reflex Sympathetic Dystrophy

DEFINITION

- Complex regional pain syndrome, characterized by allodynia as well as sudomotor, temperature, and trophic skin changes with associated swelling and loss of function, most often occurring after trauma.

SIGNS AND SYMPTOMS

- Gradual onset of pain following seemingly minor trauma.
- Allodynia.
- Sudomotor changes.
- Temperature changes.
- Trophic skin changes.
- Swelling may be present.
- Gradual decrease in range of motion and loss of functional ability.

DEMOGRAPHICS

- Incidence: Female > Male.
- Most common following wrist joint and/or soft tissue trauma.
- Surgery and/or infection may serve as inciting factor.
- All ages affected.
- Hands and feet are most commonly affected.

IMAGING RECOMMENDATIONS

- Radiography
- MRI.
- Triple-phase isotope bone scanning:
  - Alternative to MRI.

IMAGING FINDINGS

- Diffuse or patchy osteopenia.
- Soft tissue swelling.
- MRI:
  - Diffuse subcutaneous edema.
  - Diffuse or patchy marrow edema, which has high signal intensity (SI) on T2-weighted with fat suppression (FST2W) MR images or short T1 inversion recovery (STIR) MR images.
- Bone scanning:
  - Diffuse soft tissue uptake on perfusion and blood pool images.
  - Diffuse skeletal uptake on delayed images.

OTHER RECOMMENDED TESTING

- Laboratory testing to rule out inflammatory arthritis.
- Electromyography and nerve conduction velocity testing to rule out occult plexopathy, radiculopathy, and/or entrapment neuropathy that may be serving as a nidus for the reflex sympathetic dystrophy (RSD).
- Joint aspiration to rule out crystal arthropathies.
- Joint aspiration to rule out infection.

DIFFERENTIAL DIAGNOSIS

- Inflammatory arthritides, especially rheumatoid arthritis.
- Septic wrist joint.
- Osteomyelitis.
- Soft tissue infections.
- Occult foreign bodies.
- Healing wrist joint fractures.
- Metastatic disease.
- Bone infarcts.
- Crystal arthropathy of wrist.
- Avascular osteonecrosis.

TREATMENT

- Conservative treatment consisting of local heat, cold, simple analgesics, and nonsteroidal anti-inflammatory agents will improve symptoms in many cases.
- Physical therapy, including gentle stretching, range-of-motion exercises, tactile desensitization, and contrast baths, may be beneficial in selected patients.
- Stellate ganglion blocks with local anesthetic and steroid will provide symptomatic relief if conservative therapy fails or the pain is limiting activities of daily living.
- Release of coexistent entrapment neuropathies.

- Spinal cord stimulation is a good option for patients who do not experience long-lasting relief from stellate ganglion blocks.
- Surgical sympathectomy or radiofrequency destruction of the stellate ganglion may be required for persistent pain or progressive functional disability.

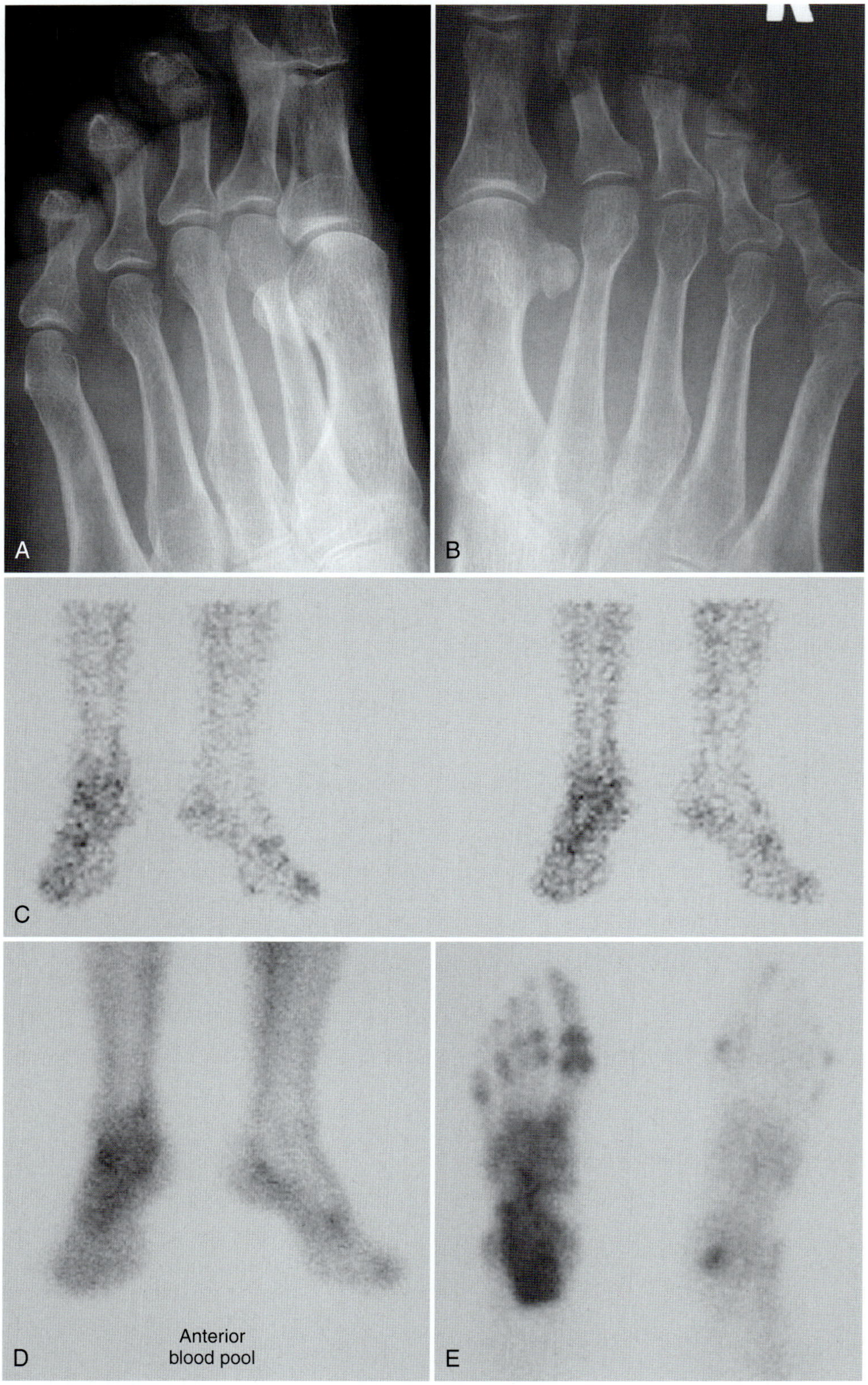

Figure 127.1 Images of a patient with symptoms of RSD affecting the right foot only. (**A**), An oblique radiograph of the left foot demonstrates normal bony density. (**B**), The radiograph of the right foot, however, shows subtle generalized osteopenia. The vascular (**C**) and blood pool (**D**) phases of the isotope bone scan show diffuse soft tissue uptake in the right foot and ankle. (**E**), There is also diffuse skeletal uptake in the right foot on the delayed phase scan.

CHAPTER 128

Ganglion Cyst of the Wrist

DEFINITION

- Cystic mucinous mass occurring most commonly on the dorsal surface of the wrist and less commonly on the volar surface of the wrist.

SIGNS AND SYMPTOMS

- Gradual onset of a soft tissue mass on the dorsal or volar surface of the wrist that is not adhered to the underlying tendon.
- Pain on dorsiflexion and plantarflexion.
- May cause tendinitis and synovitis of adjacent structures.
- No associated neurologic findings unless ganglion cyst impinges on nerve.
- Catching or clicking with radial and ulnar deviation of wrist.
- Loss of grip strength.
- Loss of wrist range of motion.

DEMOGRAPHICS

- Incidence: Female > Male.
- Almost always unilateral.
- Twenty to 40-year-old persons most commonly affected by dorsal ganglion cysts.
- Fifty to 70-year-old persons most commonly affected by volar ganglion cysts.

IMAGING RECOMMENDATIONS

- Imaging not routinely required.
- MRI or US for:
  - Occult ganglia or atypical features.
  - Presurgical planning.
- US for:
  - Guided injections and aspiration.

IMAGING FINDINGS

- Well-demarcated, rounded or ovoid structure.
- Fluid-filled cystic appearance:
  - High signal intensity (SI) on T2-weighted (T2W) MR images or T2W with fat suppression (FST2W) MR images.
  - Low SI on T1W MR images.
  - Anechoic on US (occasionally echogenic).
- Most commonly arises from dorsal component of a degenerated scpholunate ligament.
- May dissect through the soft tissues to become clinically apparent at a site remote from the point of origin.

OTHER RECOMMENDED TESTING

- Laboratory testing to rule out inflammatory arthritis.
- Joint aspiration to rule out crystal arthropathies.
- Joint aspiration to rule out infection if diagnosis is in question.

DIFFERENTIAL DIAGNOSIS

- Abscesses, including fungal and tubercular.
- Tenosynovitis.
- Rheumatoid nodule.
- Foreign body synovitis.
- Gouty tophi.
- Tendon sheath tumors.
- Benign tumors, including lipomas.
- Malignant tumors, including synovial sarcomas.
- Aneurysm.

TREATMENT

- Conservative treatment consisting of local heat, cold, simple analgesics, and nonsteroidal anti-inflammatory agents will improve symptoms in many cases.
- Physical therapy, including gentle stretching, range-of-motion exercises, and deep heat modalities, may be beneficial in selected patients.
- Splinting.
- Injection of ganglion cyst with local anesthetic and steroid will provide symptomatic relief if conservative therapy fails or the pain is limiting activities of daily living.
- Surgery may be required for persistent pain or progressive functional disability or to confirm the diagnosis.

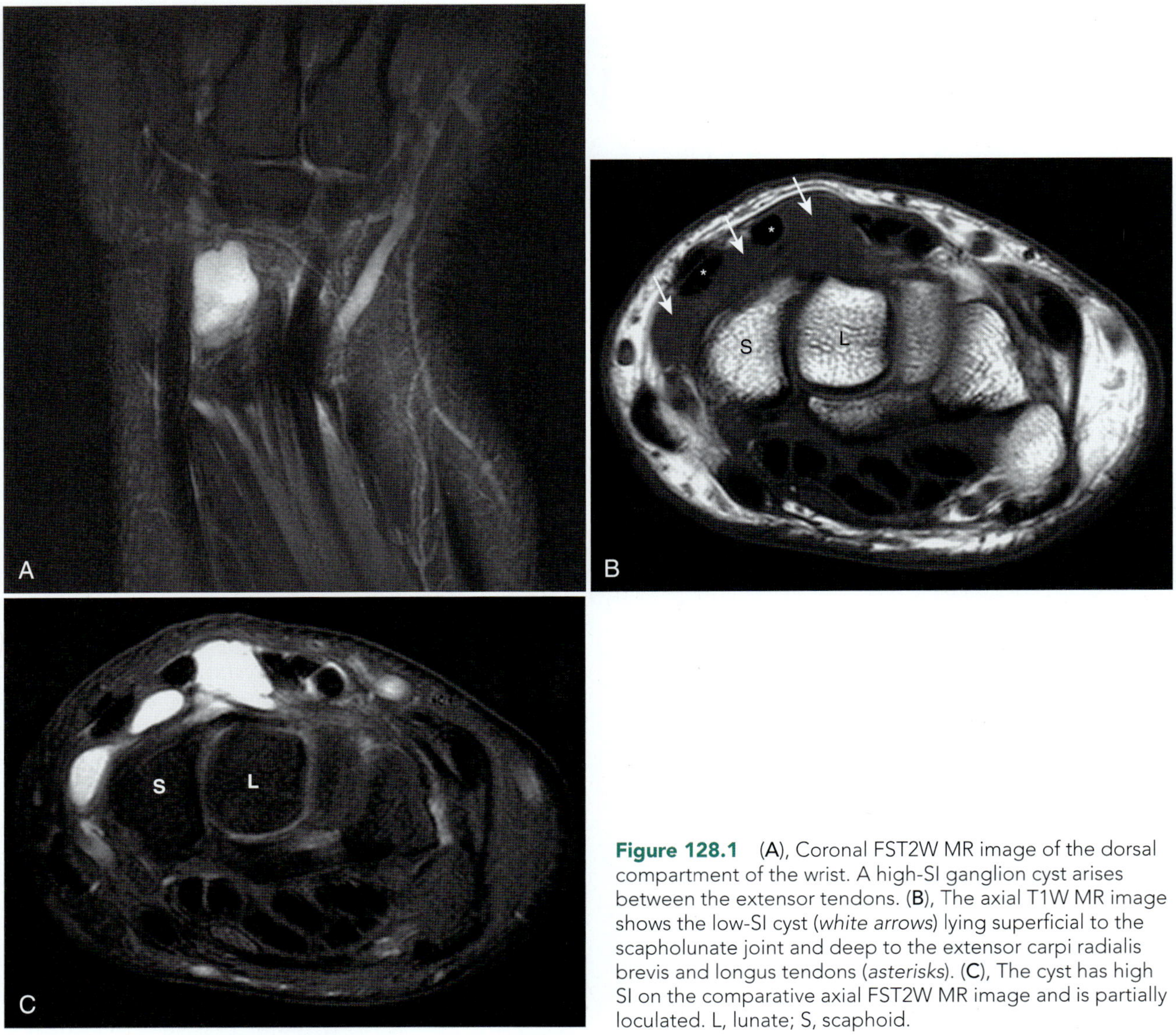

Figure 128.1 (**A**), Coronal FST2W MR image of the dorsal compartment of the wrist. A high-SI ganglion cyst arises between the extensor tendons. (**B**), The axial T1W MR image shows the low-SI cyst (*white arrows*) lying superficial to the scapholunate joint and deep to the extensor carpi radialis brevis and longus tendons (*asterisks*). (**C**), The cyst has high SI on the comparative axial FST2W MR image and is partially loculated. L, lunate; S, scaphoid.

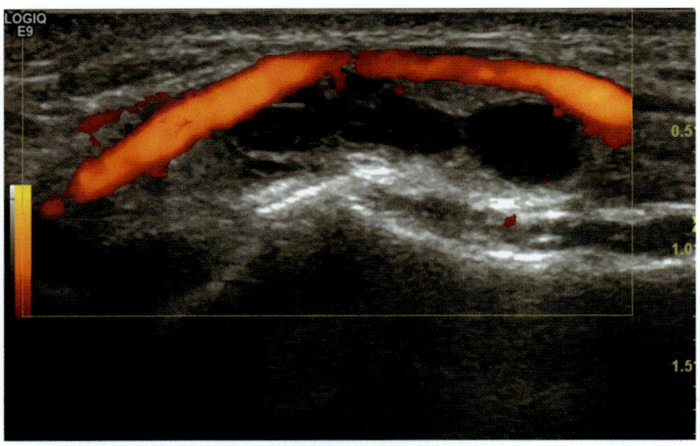

Figure 128.2 Longitudinal power Doppler US image of the volar aspect of the wrist. There is an anechoic and partially loculated ganglion cyst lying deep to the radial artery. This location for a ganglion cyst can be mistaken clinically for an aneurysm of the radial artery.

CHAPTER 129

Extensor Carpi Ulnaris Tendinitis

DEFINITION

- Inflammation of the extensor tendons due to repetitive microtrauma.

SIGNS AND SYMPTOMS

- Acute or gradual onset of pain at the dorsoulnar aspect of the wrist.
- Worse with activity.
- Pain often radiates into forearm.
- Crepitus often present.
- Pain worse with activities such as holding a coffee cup and using a hammer.
- Tenderness and swelling over the tendon.
- Tuck sign often present.
- Pain worse with resisted wrist movement.
- Patient may experience sleep disturbance.

DEMOGRAPHICS

- Incidence: Male = Female.
- Associated with activities that require repeated gripping and stabilizing of the wrist during active range of motion.
- Common in tennis, golf, and raquetball players.
- Common in patients with rheumatoid arthritis.
- More common after trauma, including repetitive stress injuries.

IMAGING RECOMMENDATIONS

- MRI or US.
- US to guide injection therapy.

IMAGING FINDINGS

- Tendinopathy:
  - Tendon thickening.
  - Increased signal intensity (SI) on T1-weighted (T1W) and T2W MR images.
  - Loss of reflectivity on US.
- Tenosynovitis:
  - High SI within tendon sheath on T2W and T2W with fat suppression (FST2W) MR images.
  - Enhancement of inflammatory synovitis on post-contrast (obtained after administration of a contrast agent) images.
  - Anechoic fluid in the tendon sheath on US or hypervascular echogenic synovitis.
- Tendinopathy and tenosynovitis may occur in isolation or in combination.

OTHER RECOMMENDED TESTING

- Electromyography and nerve conduction velocity testing to rule out ulnar tunnel syndrome.
- Laboratory testing to rule out inflammatory arthritis.
- Joint aspiration to rule out crystal arthropathies.
- Joint aspiration to rule out infection if diagnosis in question.

DIFFERENTIAL DIAGNOSIS

- Calcific tendinitis.
- Ulnar tunnel syndrome.
- Kienböck disease.
- Lunotriquetral instability.
- Triangular fibrocartilage disorders.
- Gout.
- Occult distal ulnar fractures.
- Ulnocarpal abutment syndrome.

TREATMENT

- Conservative treatment consisting of local heat, cold, simple analgesics, and nonsteroidal anti-inflammatory agents will improve symptoms in many cases.
- Physical therapy, including gentle stretching, range-of-motion exercises, and deep heat modalities, may be beneficial in selected patients.
- Injection with local anesthetic and steroid will provide symptomatic relief if conservative therapy fails or the pain is limiting activities of daily living.
- Surgery may be required for persistent pain or progressive functional disability.

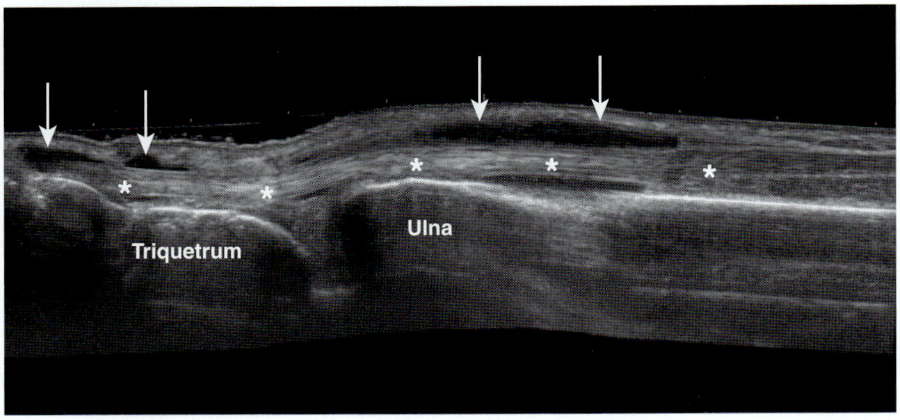

Figure 129.1 Longitudinal US image of a patient with simple tenosynovitis of the extensor carpi ulnaris (ECU) tendon. There is anechoic fluid (*white arrows*) within the ECU tendon sheath. The ECU tendon (*asterisks*) is not thickened.

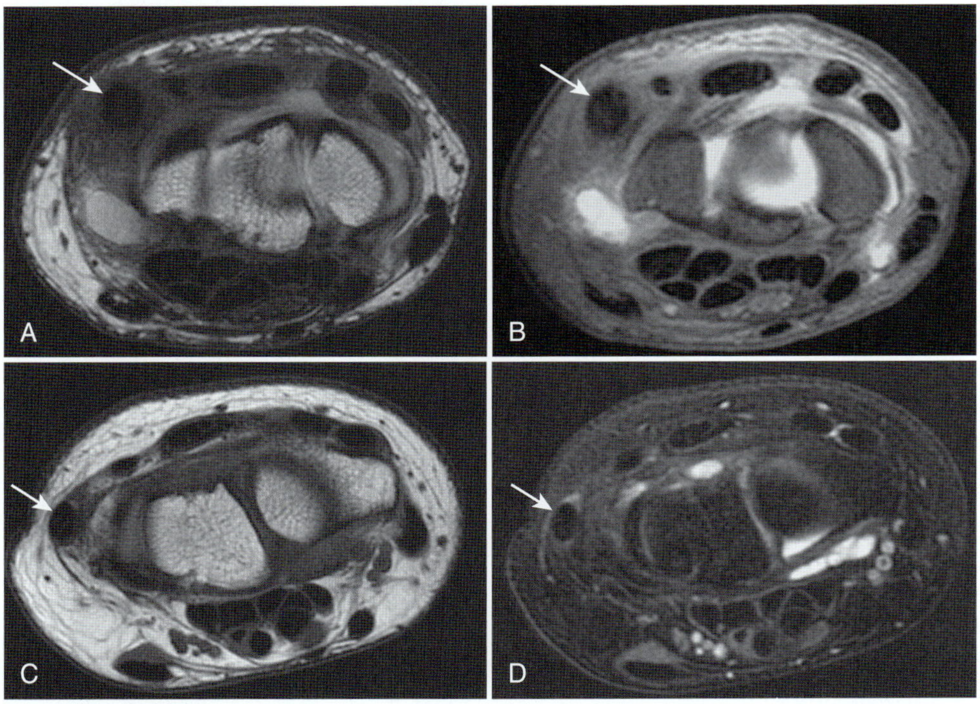

Figure 129.2 Axial T1W (**A**) and FST2W (**B**) MR arthrogram images of a patient being investigated for ulnar-sided wrist pain and exclusion of a triangular fibrocartilage tear. The ECU tendon (*white arrows*) is thickened and rounded with increased SI consistent with tendinopathy. There is also thickening of the tendon sheath. Compare with the normal ECU tendon on T1W (**C**) and FST2W (**D**) MR images (*white arrows*) in another subject, in whom the tendon is more ovoid and smaller with uniformly low SI. The small amount of high-SI fluid within the tendon sheath on the second FST2W MR image is within normal limits and is visible in other tendon groups.

CHAPTER 130

De Quervain Tenosynovitis

DEFINITION

- Inflammation of the extensor tendons of the first dorsal extensor compartment due to repetitive microtrauma.

SIGNS AND SYMPTOMS

- Acute or gradual onset of pain at the radial aspect of the wrist at the radial styloid.
- Worse with thumb and wrist activity.
- Pain often radiates into the forearm.
- Crepitus often present.
- Triggering may occur.
- Positive result of Finkelstein test.
- Pain worse with activity such as pinching or grasping items with the thumb.
- Associated with hyperabduction during golf swing.
- Tenderness and swelling over the first dorsal extensor compartment.
- Pain worse with resisted ulnar deviation of the wrist.
- Patient may experience sleep disturbance.

DEMOGRAPHICS

- Incidence: Male = Female.
- Associated with activities that require repeated gripping and stabilizing of the wrist during active range of motion.
- Common in javelin throwers, fly fisherman, and people who play racquet sports.
- Associated with hyperabduction during golf swing.
- Associated with falls onto the thumb.
- More common after trauma, including repetitive stress injuries.

IMAGING RECOMMENDATIONS

- MRI or US.
- US:
  - To guide injection therapy.

IMAGING FINDINGS

- Tendinopathy:
  - Tendon thickening.
  - Increased signal intensity (SI) on T1-weighted (T1W) and T2W MR images.
  - Loss of reflectivity on US.
- Stenosing tenosynovitis:
  - Low or intermediate SI within tendon sheath on T2W and T2W with fat suppression (FST2W) MR images.
  - Enhancement of inflammatory synovitis on post-contrast (obtained after administration of a contrast agent) MR images.
  - Echogenic thickening of the tendon sheath on US.

OTHER RECOMMENDED TESTING

- Electromyography and nerve conduction velocity testing to rule out radial tunnel syndrome.
- Laboratory testing to rule out inflammatory arthritis.
- Joint aspiration to rule out crystal arthropathies.
- Joint aspiration to rule out infection if diagnosis in question.

DIFFERENTIAL DIAGNOSIS

- Arthritis of first carpometacarpal joint.
- Ganglion cyst.
- Wartenberg syndrome.
- Intersection syndrome.
- Inflammatory arthropathies.
- Calcific tendinitis.
- Scaphoid fracture.
- Radial tunnel syndrome.
- Carpal tunnel syndrome.
- Gout.
- Occult distal radial fractures.

TREATMENT

- Conservative treatment consisting of local heat, cold, simple analgesics, and nonsteroidal anti-inflammatory agents will improve symptoms in many cases.
- Physical therapy, including gentle stretching, range-of-motion exercises, and deep heat modalities, may be beneficial in selected patients.
- Injection with local anesthetic and steroid will provide symptomatic relief if conservative therapy fails or the pain is limiting activities of daily living.
- Surgery may be required for persistent pain or progressive functional disability.

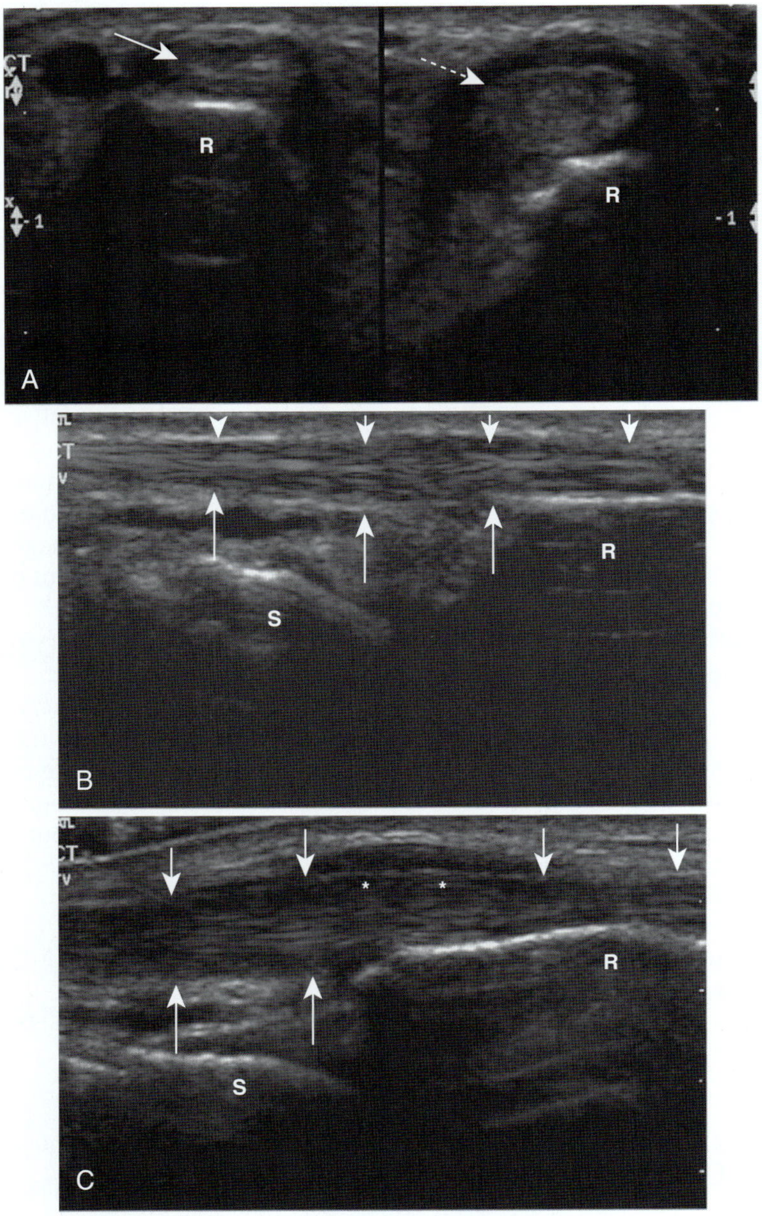

Figure 130.1 (A), Transverse US images of the right (RT) and left (LT) extensor group I tendons acquired at the level of the distal radius (R) in a patient with de Quervain tenosynovitis. The involved tendon and tendon sheath on the left side are thickened (*broken white arrow*) in comparison with the normal tendon on the right side (*white arrow*). Comparison of the longitudinal US images of the normal side (B) and the affected side (C) shows the thickened tendon (*white arrows*) on the affected side as well as echogenic thickening of the tendon sheath (*asterisks*). R, distal radius; S, scaphoid bone.

CHAPTER 131

Giant Cell Tumor of the Tendon Sheath

DEFINITION

- Slow-growing, nonmalignant, multilobulated, extra-articular tumor of the tendon sheath.

SIGNS AND SYMPTOMS

- Gradual onset of a mass, most commonly on the volar surface of the hand.
- Gradual onset of pain in proximity of the mass.
- Mass is well circumscribed.
- Mass does not transilluminate.
- Pain worse with use of affected digit.
- Crepitus often present.
- Triggering may occur.
- Pain worse with activity such as grasping items with affected digit.

DEMOGRAPHICS

- Incidence: Female > Male.
- Most common in third to fifth decade of life.
- Rare in children and the elderly.
- Second most common hand and wrist mass after a ganglion cyst.

IMAGING RECOMMENDATIONS

- Radiography.
- MRI or US.

IMAGING FINDINGS

- Ovoid soft tissue mass arising from tendon sheath.
- Pressure erosion of bone.
- Intermediate signal intensity (SI) on T1-weighted (T1W) and T2W MR images.
- High SI on short T1 inversion recovery (STIR) or T2W with fat suppression (FST2W) MR images.
- Enhancement on post-contrast (obtained after administration of a contrast agent) MR images.
- Hemosiderin may be evident as areas of low SI on T1W and T2W MR images.
- Heterogeneous echo pattern on US with variable internal vascularity on Doppler imaging.
- Less common pattern:
  - Diffuse giant cell tumor of the tendon sheath (GCTTS), usually referred to as extra-articular pigmented villonodular synovitis (PVNS).

OTHER RECOMMENDED TESTING

- Electromyography and nerve conduction velocity testing to rule out associated entrapment neuropathy.
- Laboratory testing to rule out inflammatory arthritis.
- Joint aspiration to rule out crystal arthropathies.
- Joint aspiration to rule out infection if diagnosis is in question.

DIFFERENTIAL DIAGNOSIS

- Tenosynovitis.
- Ganglion cyst.
- Foreign body synovitis.
- Synovial sarcoma.
- Vascular tumors, including hemangiomas.
- Post-traumatic aneurysm.
- Calcific tendonitis.
- Gout.

TREATMENT

- Conservative treatment consisting of local heat, cold, simple analgesics, and nonsteroidal anti-inflammatory agents will improve symptoms in many cases.
- Physical therapy two preserve function, including gentle stretching and range-of-motion exercises, may be beneficial in selected patients.
- Injection should generally be avoided because of the potential of giant cell tumor seeding by the needle.
- Surgery often required for persistent pain or progressive functional disability.

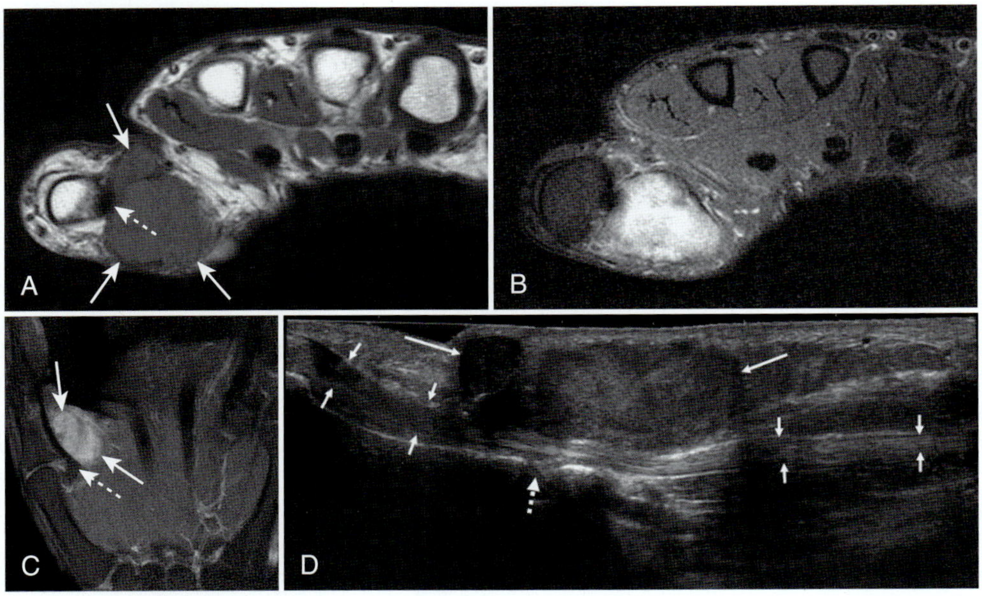

Figure 131.1 (**A**), Axial T1W MR image of a patient with a GCTTS in the thumb. An intermediate-SI mass (*white arrows*) lies superficial to the flexor pollicis longus (FPL) tendon (*broken white arrow*). (**B**), The axial FST2W MR image shows the same mass with high SI. (**C**), The coronal post-contrast FST1W MR image demonstrates diffuse enhancement of the mass (*white arrows*) and its close relationship to the FPL tendon (*broken white arrow*). (**D**), A longitudinal US image acquired at the time of soft tissue biopsy demonstrates the echogenic mass (*long white arrows*) arising from the FPL tendon (*short white arrows*), at the level of the metacarpophalangeal joint (*broken white arrow*).

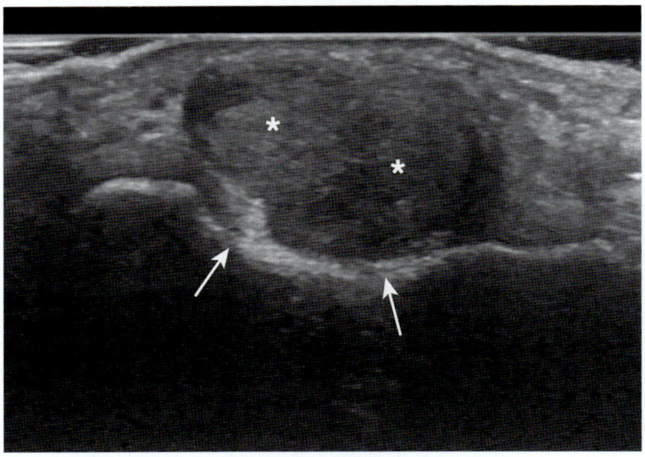

Figure 131.2 Longitudinal US image of a GCTTS (*asterisks*) of the FPL tendon in a different patient. Bony scalloping of the cortex of the underlying metacarpal is due to pressure erosion (*white arrows*).

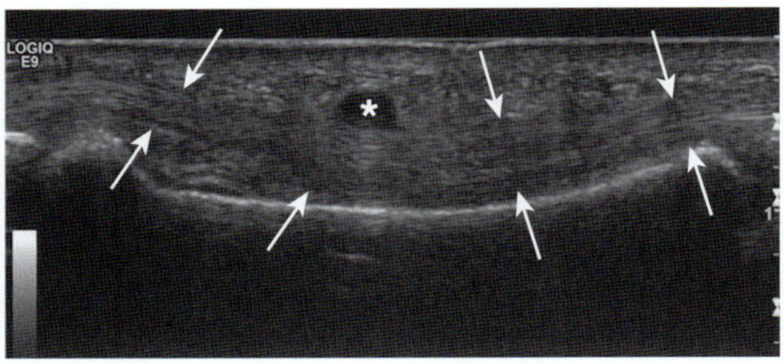

Figure 131.3 Longitudinal US image of the index finger of a patient with a small palpable mass of the flexor tendon. There is a small anechoic mass (*asterisk*) lying on the superficial surface of the flexor tendon (*white arrows*), which is typical of a tendon sheath ganglion.

CHAPTER 132

Anatomy: Special Imaging Considerations of the Pelvis, Hip, and Lower Extremity Pain Syndromes

OSSEOUS STRUCTURES

Femoral Head. An incomplete sphere covered with articular cartilage, with the exception of the fovea on its posteroinferior aspect. The head faces anterosuperiorly and medially to articulate with the acetabulum.

Femoral Neck. Connects the femoral head to the shaft at an angle of 125 degrees and has an anteverted orientation. The femoral neck is roughly cylindrical and flares out as it joins the shaft to produce the intertrochanteric line.

Greater Trochanter. A large quadrangular structure projecting superiorly from the femoral neck–shaft junction. It bears the insertions of the hip abductors and rotators.

Lesser Trochanter. A posteromedial projection on the femoral shaft at the inferior end of the intertrochanteric crest. It bears the attachment of the iliopsoas tendon, which is a powerful hip flexor.

Acetabulum. A deep, slightly ovoid fossa formed by the ischium, ilium, and pubis. The acetabulum has anterior and posterior walls, which merge medially to form the anterior and posterior columns. The columns are continuous medially to form the medial wall and superiorly to form the roof (tectum).

JOINTS

Hip Joint. A multiaxial ball-and-socket type joint formed by articulation of the femoral head with the acetabulum. The acetabular articular cartilage forms an incomplete ring, which is deficient inferiorly.

Acetabular Labrum. A triangular incomplete ring of fibrocartilage that attaches to the acetabular rim and contributes to joint stability by increasing the surface area.

Hip Joint Capsule. A strong fibrous capsule that extends from the acetabular rim medial to the labrum and covers the anterior femoral neck, inserting at the intertrochanteric line with a more medial posterior insertion on the femoral neck.

Pubic Symphysis. A flat vertical synchondrosis formed between the bodies of the pubic bones. It is stabilized inferiorly and superiorly by arcuate ligaments. The symphysis resists rotational stress produced by the medial muscle group (adductors and gracilis), which arises from the pubic bone.

EXTRA-ARTICULAR SOFT TISSUES

Major Muscle Groups

Four major muscle groups surround and act upon the hip:

Lateral Muscle Group. Made up of the tensor fascia lata; gluteus maximus, medius, and minmus; obturator internus and externus; superior and inferior gemelli; and quadratus femoris. The gluteus minimus and medius are hip abductors that insert on the anterior and posterior facets of the greater trochanter, respectively. The obturator and gemelli muscle groups also insert on the greater trochanter and act as hip lateral rotators.

Medial Muscle Group. These consist of the adductors (longus, brevis, magnus), gracilis, and pectineus. The adductors have a common tendon origin at the adductor tubercle on the inferior pubic ramus. They act to perform hip adduction and some hip flexion.

Posterior Muscle Group. The hamstring muscles consist of the semimembranosus, semitendinosus, and biceps femoris. All three have a common origin on the ischial tuberosity and act to perform hip extension. The gluteus maximus is also a powerful hip extensor.

Anterior Muscle Group. This group consists of the rectus femoris, sartorius, and iliopsoas, all of which contribute to hip flexion. The rectus femoris has a direct head that inserts on the anterior-inferior iliac spine and an indirect or reflected head that inserts on the anterior acetabular rim.

Other Soft Tissues

Iliotibial Tract. A dense iliotibial band (ITB) of deep fascia of the lateral thigh into which the tensor fascia lata muscle inserts. The ITB inserts distally onto Gerdy's tubercle on the anteromedial aspect of the proximal tibia.

Bursae. There are three gluteal bursae: the laterally located sub–gluteus maximus or trochanteric bursa, the deeper and more medial sub–gluteus medius bursa, and the anteriorly located sub–gluteus minimus bursa. The iliopsoas bursa lies anterior to the hip, between the capsule and the iliopsoas tendon, and may normally communicate with the hip joint.

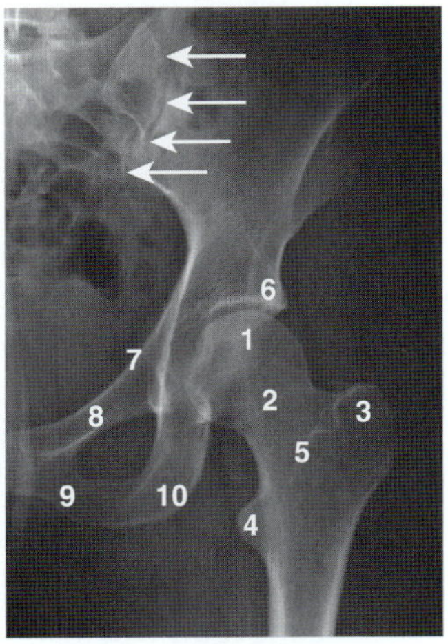

Figure 132.1 AP radiograph of the hip: 1, femoral head; 2, femoral neck; 3, greater trochanter; 4, lesser trochanter; 5, intertrochanteric line; 6, acetabular rim; 7, iliopectineal line; 8, superior pubic ramus; 9, inferior pubic ramus; 10, ischial tuberosity; *white arrows,* sacroiliac joint.

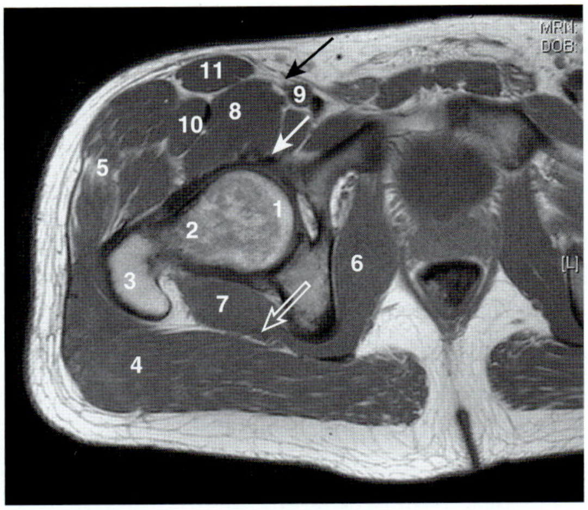

Figure 132.3 Axial T1W MR image of the hip: 1, femoral head; 2, femoral neck; 3, greater trochanter; 4, gluteus maximus; 5, tensor fascia lata; 6, obturator internus; 7, quadratus femoris; 8, iliopsoas muscle; 9, femoral artery; *solid white arrow,* iliopsoas tendon; *black arrow,* femoral nerve; *open white arrow,* sciatic nerve; 10, rectus femoris; 11, sartoris.

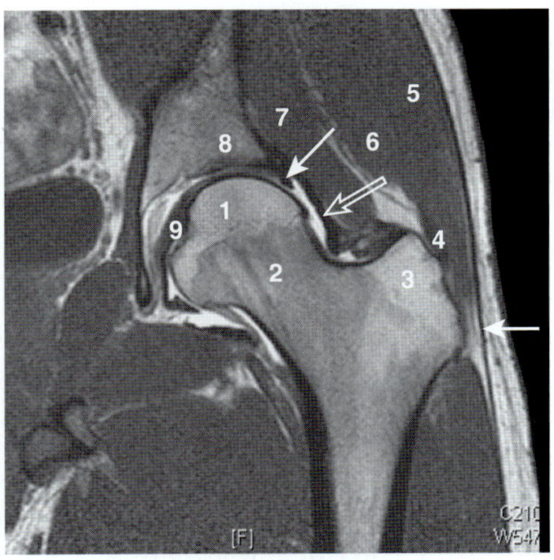

Figure 132.2 Coronal T1-weighted (T1W) MR arthrogram image of the hip: 1, femoral epiphysis; 2, femoral neck; 3, greater trochanter; 4, gluteus medius tendon; 5, tensor fascia lata; 6, gluteus medius muscle; 7, gluteus minimus muscle; 8, acetabular roof; 9, ligamentum teres; *white arrow,* acetabular labrum; *white open arrow,* joint capsule; *black arrow,* iliotibial band.

CHAPTER 133

Meralgia Paresthetica

DEFINITION

- Entrapment of the lateral femoral cutaneous nerve as it passes beneath the inguinal ligament.

SIGNS AND SYMPTOMS

- Paresthesias radiating into the lateral thigh.
- Presence of Tinel sign at the point of nerve entrapment.
- No motor deficit.
- Sensory deficit in the distribution of the lateral femoral cutaneous nerve.
- No symptoms below the knee.
- Passive range of motion preserved.
- Exacerbation of symptoms with sitting or squatting for long periods.
- Exacerbation of symptoms with the wearing of wide belts or tight waistbands.

DEMOGRAPHICS

- Incidence: Male = Female.
- Usually unilateral.
- All ages affected.
- Can occur acutely following trauma to the lateral femoral cutaneous nerve.
- Associated with the wearing of wide belts and tight waistbands.

IMAGING RECOMMENDATIONS

- Imaging not routinely required.
- MRI or US:
  - US may be used to guide injection.

IMAGING FINDINGS

- Nerve not consistently visualized.
- Imaging findings may be normal.
- Inflammatory change or soft tissue mass in region of nerve as it exits into thigh.
- US may show the affected nerve to be low-echo and thickened in comparison with the other nerve.

OTHER RECOMMENDED TESTING

- Electromyography and nerve conduction velocity testing of the lumbar nerve roots, lumbar plexus, and lateral femoral cutaneous nerve.

DIFFERENTIAL DIAGNOSIS

- Lumbar radiculopathy.
- Lumbar plexopathy.
- Benign neoplasm.
- Malignant neoplasm.
- Peripheral neuropathies.

TREATMENT

- Conservative treatment consisting of local heat, cold, simple analgesics, and nonsteroidal anti-inflammatory agents will improve symptoms in mild, self-limited cases.
- Physical therapy to maintain function, including gentle stretching, range-of-motion exercises, and local heat modalities, may be beneficial in selected patients.
- Injection with local anesthetic and steroid of the lateral femoral cutaneous nerve may provide symptomatic relief if conservative therapy fails or the pain is limiting activities of daily living.
- Surgery may be required to relieve entrapment of the lateral femoral cutaneous nerve.

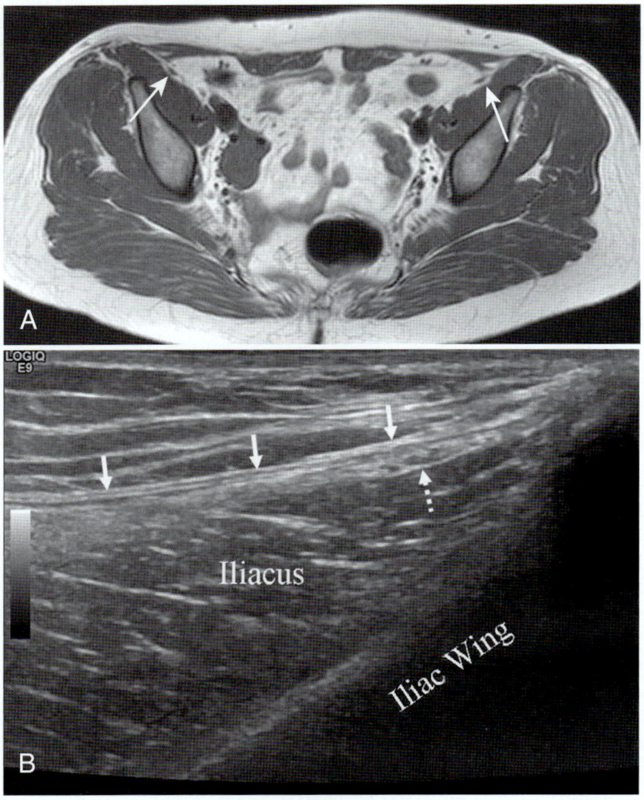

Figure 133.1 (A), Axial T1-weighted MR image demonstrating the lateral cutaneous nerve of the thigh on both sides (*white arrows*), lying on the surface of the iliacus muscle just proximal to the level of the inguinal ligament. (B), An oblique US image in a different subject shows the round nerve (*broken white arrow*) lying on the surface of the iliacus muscle immediately deep to the echo-bright inguinal ligament (*white arrows*).

CHAPTER 134

Osteonecrosis of the Hip

DEFINITION

- The death of cellular components of bone due to interruption of the blood supply with resultant pain, collapse and destruction of bone, and loss of function.

SIGNS AND SYMPTOMS

- Gradual onset of pain with decreasing range of motion of the hip joint.
- Crepitus may be present.
- Functional disability may be severe.

DEMOGRAPHICS

- Incidence: Male > Female.
- Age at onset related to date of trauma or onset of underlying disease, with sickle cell disease being the most common inciting factor in younger patients.
- Most common following hip joint trauma that disrupts vascular supply.
- More common in patients with sickle cell disease, Gaucher disease, Fabry disease, systemic lupus erythematosus (SLE), and gout.
- Often associated with exogenous steroid administration.
- Often associated with heavy alcohol intake.

IMAGING RECOMMENDATIONS

- Radiography.
- MRI:
  - For normal or equivocal radiographic findings: Detects stage I and stage II disease.
  - For preoperative planning:
    To assess extent of femoral head involvement in stage III and stage IV disease.

IMAGING FINDINGS

- Radiography:
  - Sclerosis in the subarticular femoral head.
  - In later stages, subchondral lucency and collapse eventually leading to fragmentation and destruction of the articular surface.
  - Serpiginous lines of sclerosis in intramedullary infarcts.
- MRI:
  - High-signal intensity (SI) edema in femoral head and neck on short T1 inversion recovery (STIR) MR images.
  - Low-SI subchondral sclerosis on T1-weighted (T1W) and T2W MR images.
  - Subchondral crescent sign.
  - Eventual subchondral collapse and fragmentation.
  - Double-line sign of intramedullary infarcts on T2W MR images.
- Ficat staging system:
  - Stage I:
    Contralateral asymptomatic hip.
    MRI: Findings positive.
    Radiography: Findings normal.
  - Stage II:
    Symptomatic hip.
    MRI: Findings positive.
    Radiography: Findings normal or show porosis.
  - Stage III:
    Radiography shows crescentic subchondral sclerosis and early femoral flattening.
  - Stage IV:
    Radiography shows progressive sclerosis and subchondral collapse.

OTHER RECOMMENDED TESTING

- Laboratory testing to rule out SLE.
- Laboratory testing to rule out gout.
- Joint aspiration to rule out crystal arthropathies.
- Joint aspiration to rule out infection.

DIFFERENTIAL DIAGNOSIS

- Inflammatory arthritides, especially SLE.
- Osteoarthritis.
- Bone marrow tumor.
- Primary bone tumor.
- Metastatic tumor.
- Osteochondral injury.

TREATMENT

- Conservative treatment consisting of local heat, cold, simple analgesics, and nonsteroidal anti-inflammatory agents will improve symptoms in many cases.
- Physical therapy, including gentle stretching, range-of-motion exercises, and deep heat modalities, may be beneficial in selected patients.
- Intra-articular injection with local anesthetic and steroid will provide symptomatic relief if conservative therapy fails or the pain is limiting activities of daily living.
- Surgery may ultimately be required for persistent pain or progressive functional disability.

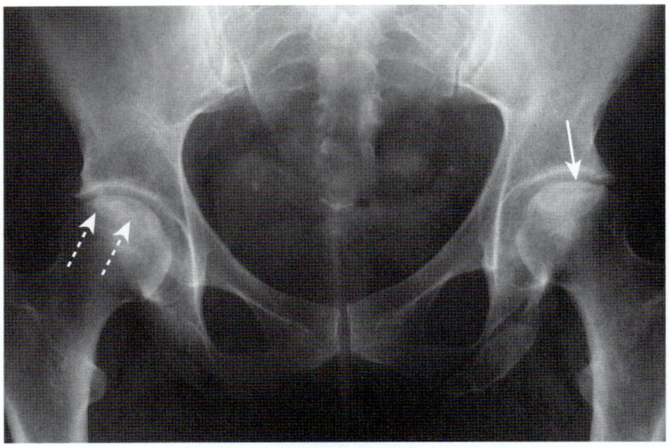

Figure 134.1 AP radiograph of the pelvis demonstrating bilateral avascular necrosis (AVN) of the femoral heads. On the left side there is stage IV disease, with a subchondral sclerotic crescent and subchondral collapse (*white arrow*). On the right side there is stage III AVN with crescentic sclerosis but without subchondral collapse (*broken white arrows*).

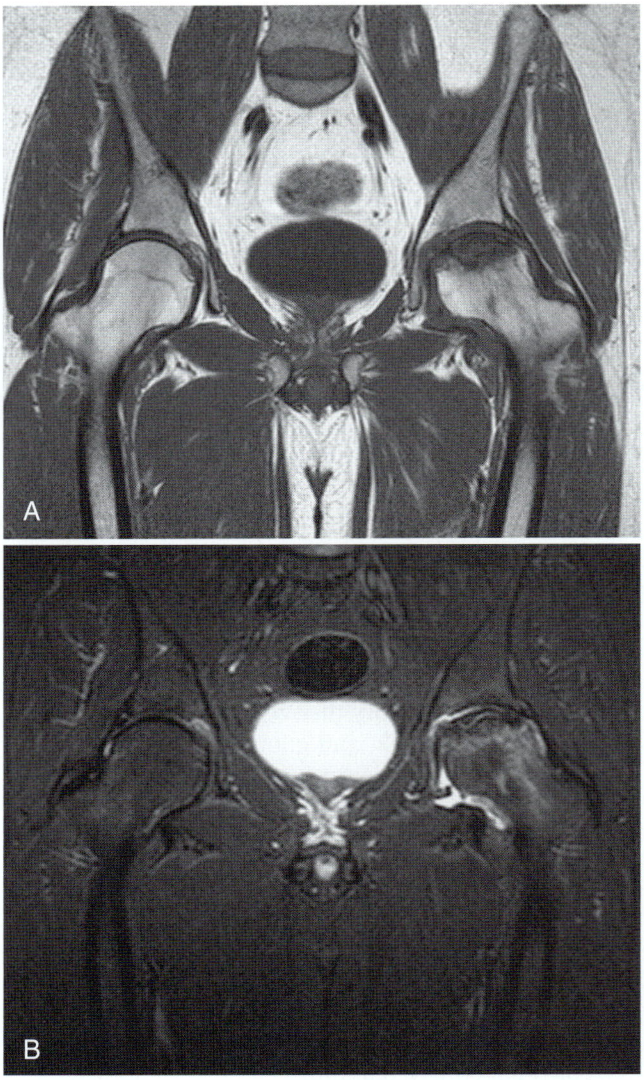

Figure 134.2 (**A**), Coronal T1W MR image of left-sided stage III AVN. There is a crescent of low-SI change in the subchondral bone of the weight-bearing surface of the femoral head. (**B**), The corresponding T2W with fat suppression (FST2W) MR image shows a high-SI linear crescent with more extensive high-SI marrow edema throughout the femoral neck. Early subchondral collapse is present. There is also a joint effusion.

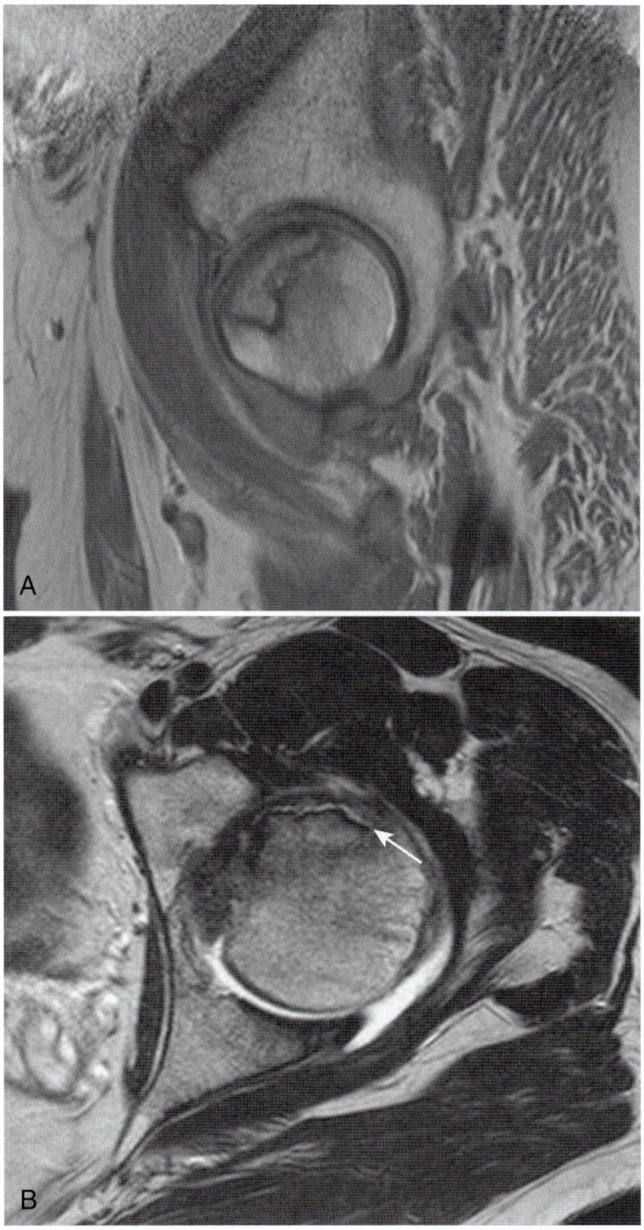

Figure 134.3 Sagittal proton density (**A**) and T2W (**B**) MR images of a different patient with stage II AVN. There is a serpiginous line running through the femoral head, with a double-line sign on the T2W MR image (*white arrow*), which represents a band of sclerosis (low-SI) lined by reactive granulation tissue (high-SI).

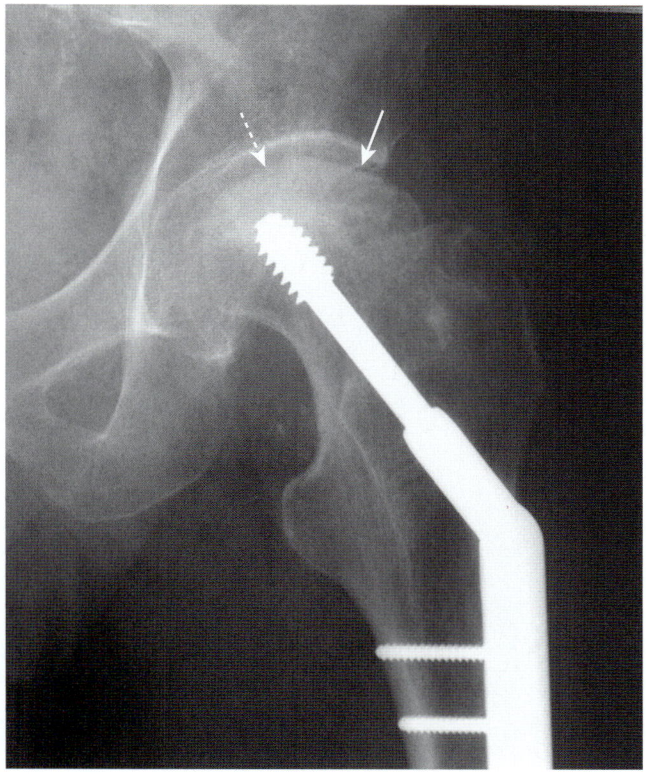

Figure 134.4 AP radiograph of a patient with previous fixation of a femoral neck fracture. There is flattening and sclerosis of the femoral head (*white arrow*), and probable early fragmentation more medially (*broken white arrow*). These findings are due to AVN, which has occurred as a complication of the original fracture.

CHAPTER 135

Ankylosing Spondylitis

DEFINITION

- Chronic, systemic inflammatory arthritis and enthesopathy that cause destruction and ankylosis of the spine and sacroiliac joints.

SIGNS AND SYMPTOMS

- Classic morning back, pelvis, and hip stiffness.
- Pain worse in the morning.
- Radiculopathy common as disease progresses in the cervical spine.
- High incidence of coexistent pathologic fracture.
- Systemic symptoms, including low-grade fever and fatigue.
- Exacerbation and remission of symptoms not uncommon.

DEMOGRAPHICS

- Peak onset in second and third decades of life.
- Incidence: Male > Female.

IMAGING RECOMMENDATIONS

- Radiography of sacroiliac joints (SIJs).
- MRI of SIJs for early disease if radiographic findings are normal.
- CT:
  - Alternative to MRI for assessment of SIJs.
  - Does not, however, show inflammatory changes.

IMAGING FINDINGS

- SIJs:
  - New York diagnostic criteria for ankylosing spondylitis (grades 0–4).
  - Joint widening, later with joint narrowing.
  - Subchondral erosion and sclerosis.
  - Eventual ankylosis.
  - Bilateral and symmetrical: ankylosing spondylitis and enteropathic spondyloarthropathy.
  - Bilateral and asymmetrical: psoriasis and Reiter syndrome.
  - Unilateral: infection.
- Hips:
  - Inflammatory arthropathy.
  - Global joint space narrowing.
  - Enthesopathy with proliferative bone formation.
  - Eventual ankylosis.
- Symphysis pubis:
  - Inflammatory changes and ankylosis.
- Peripheral joint disease:
  - Inflammatory joint disease with proliferative bony changes and enthesitis.

OTHER RECOMMENDED TESTING

- Electromyography and nerve conduction velocity testing to identify radiculopathy and entrapment neuropathy.

DIFFERENTIAL DIAGNOSIS

- Infectious spondyloarthropathies.
- Psoriatic arthritis.
- Reiter syndrome.
- Degenerative disc disease.
- Juvenile chronic arthritis.
- Infection.
- Hemodialysis arthropathy.

TREATMENT

- Cytotoxic drugs, including methotrexate.
- Salicylates, nonsteroidal anti-inflammatory agents, and corticosteroids.
- Physical and occupational therapies.
- Epidural blocks for symptomatic relief of radiculopathy.
- Early surgical treatment of entrapment neuropathies.
- Vertebroplasty and sacroplasty for associated insufficiency fractures.

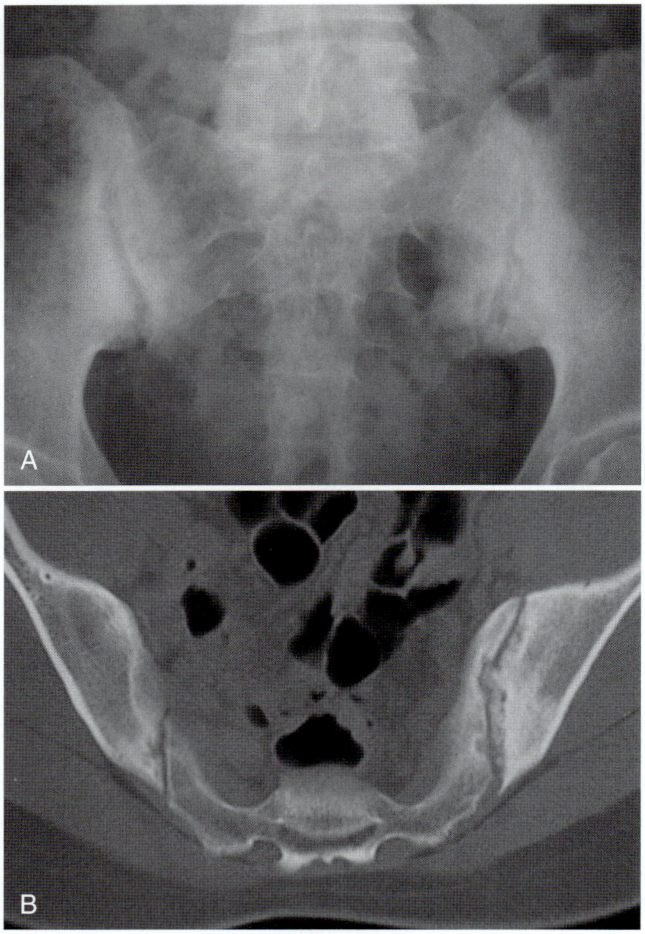

Figure 135.1 (A), Radiograph of bilateral sacroiliitis with subchondral sclerosis, loss of definition of the subchondral bone plate, but no definite erosions. (B), CT scan in the same patient clearly identifies both subchondral sclerosis and erosions.

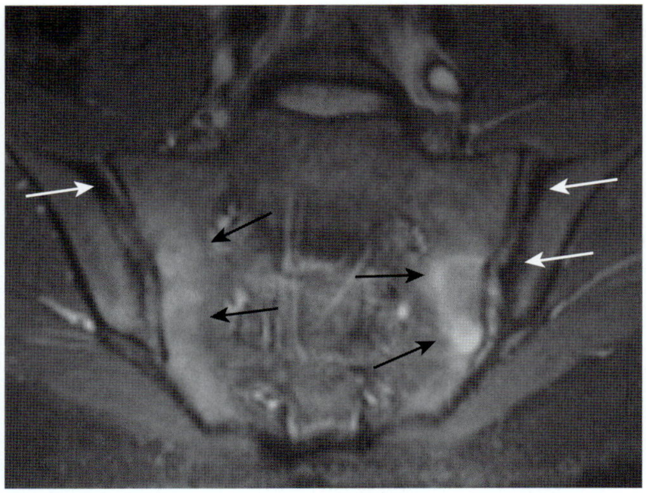

Figure 135.2 Coronal short T1 inversion recovery (STIR) MR image of early sacroiliitis. The presence of high–signal intensity (SI) subchondral marrow edema reflects the inflammatory changes (*black arrows*), and there is high SI within the joint line. Low-SI subchondral sclerosis is also present (*white arrows*).

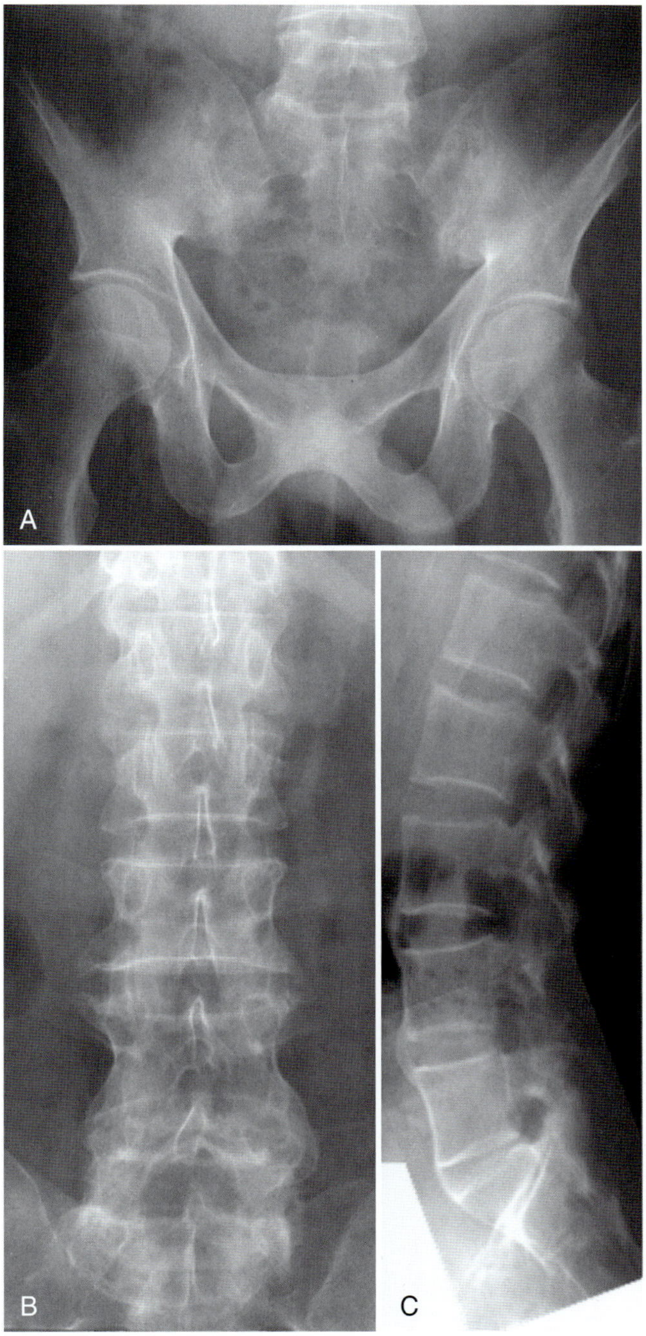

Figure 135.3 (**A**), AP radiograph of a patient with Reiter syndrome and bilateral sacroiliitis. The changes in the SIJs are more typical of ankylosing spondylitis, with symmetrical distribution. However, the AP (**B**) and lateral (**C**) radiographs show a mixed picture of syndesmophytes and osteophytes, which is atypical for classic ankylosing spondylitis. Note also the ankylosis of the symphysis pubis.

CHAPTER 136

Iliopsoas Bursitis

DEFINITION

- Inflammation of the iliopsoas bursa, which lies anterior to the hip joint capsule and medial to the iliopsoas muscle.

SIGNS AND SYMPTOMS

- Pain localized in the anterior that is made worse with any hip movement.
- Pain may radiate to the proximal femur.
- Tenderness to palpation of the iliopsoas bursa.
- Warmth may be present.
- Anterior groin may feel boggy or edematous.
- Crepitus or catching sensation may be present.
- Exacerbation of pain with resisted flexion, abduction, and external rotation of the hip.
- Pain often worse at night.
- Patient unable to sleep on the affected hip.
- Gradual decrease in range of motion.
- May progress to frozen hip if left untreated.

DEMOGRAPHICS

- Incidence: Male = Female.
- Young athletes often affected.
- More common after trauma, including repetitive stress injuries.
- Increased incidence with jobs requiring repeated hip flexion.

IMAGING RECOMMENDATIONS

- MRI or US.

IMAGING FINDINGS

- Fluid within the bursa medial to the iliopsoas tendon and muscle at the level of the groin:
  - High signal intensity (SI) on T2-weighted with fat suppression (FST2W) or short T1 inversion recovery (STIR) MR images.
  - Anechoic fluid on US.
- May extend proximally in the pelvis.
- Tendon may appear normal.

OTHER RECOMMENDED TESTING

- Laboratory testing to rule out inflammatory arthritis.
- Bursa aspiration with Gram staining and culture and sensitivity testing if infection is in question.
- Joint aspiration to rule out crystal arthropathies.
- Joint aspiration to rule out infection if diagnosis is in question.

DIFFERENTIAL DIAGNOSIS

- Calcific tendinitis.
- Avulsion fractures.
- Insufficiency fractures.
- Osteoarthritis of the hip.
- Inflammatory arthritis of the hip.
- Neoplasm.
- Labral tears of the hip with paralabral cyst formation.
- Snapping hip syndrome.
- Septic arthritis of the hip.

TREATMENT

- Conservative treatment consisting of local heat, cold, simple analgesics, and nonsteroidal anti-inflammatory agents will improve symptoms in mild cases.
- Physical therapy, including gentle stretching, range-of-motion exercises, and deep heat modalities, may be beneficial in selected patients.
- Injection with local anesthetic and steroid will provide symptomatic relief if conservative therapy fails or the pain is limiting activities of daily living.
- Surgery may be required for persistent pain or progressive functional disability.

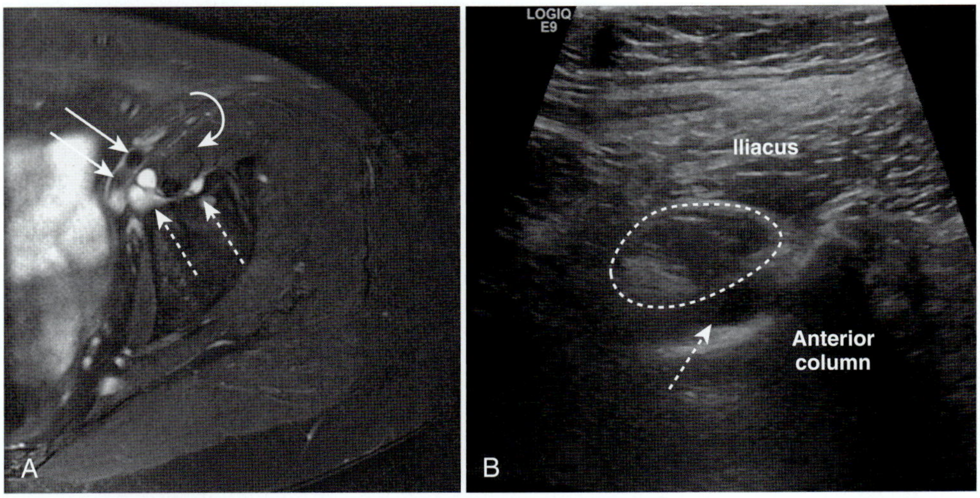

Figure 136.1 (**A**), Axial FST2W MR image demonstrating high-SI fluid (*broken arrows*) medial, deep, and lateral to the psoas tendon (*curved arrow*), due to psoas bursitis. The external iliac vessels lie medially (*white arrows*). (**B**), The corresponding axial US image acquired at time of US-guided injection shoes the low-echo fluid collection (*broken white arrow*) superficial to the anterior column of the acetabulum and inner wall of the pelvis and deep to the psoas tendon (*broken white line*) and iliacus muscle.

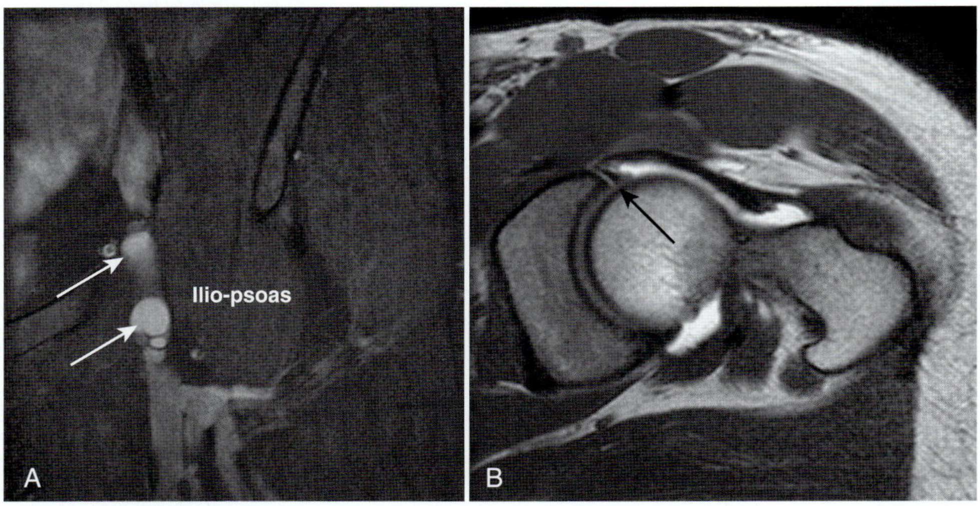

Figure 136.2 (**A**), Coronal FST2W MR image from an MR arthrogram study of the hip, demonstrating a small loculated, high-SI fluid collection (*white arrows*) medial to the iliopsoas muscle and tendon. (**B**), The corresponding axial T1W MR image shows the presence of an acetabular labral tear (*black arrow*) that communicated with the loculated fluid collection, confirming the diagnosis of a paralabral cyst.

CHAPTER 137

Ischiogluteal Bursitis

DEFINITION

- Inflammation of the gluteal bursa, which lies between the gluteus maximus and the ischium.

SIGNS AND SYMPTOMS

- Pain localized in the upper outer quadrant of the buttocks that is made worse with any hip movement.
- Pain may radiate to the proximal femur.
- Tenderness to palpation of the gluteal bursa.
- Warmth may be present.
- Upper outer quadrant of the buttocks may feel boggy or edematous.
- Crepitus or catching sensation may be present.
- Exacerbation of pain with resisted extension, abduction, and external rotation of the hip.
- Pain often worse at night.
- Patient unable to sleep on the affected hip.
- Gradual decrease in range of motion.

DEMOGRAPHICS

- Incidence: Male = Female.
- Young athletes often affected.
- More common after trauma, including repetitive stress injuries.
- Increased incidence with jobs requiring repeated flexion of the trunk or sitting on hard surfaces.

IMAGING RECOMMENDATIONS

- Radiography.
- MRI or US.

IMAGING FINDINGS

- High-signal intensity (SI) fluid interposed between the ischium and gluteus maximus on T2-weighted with fat suppression (FST2W) or T2W MR images.
- Associated findings:
  - Hamstring tendinopathy.
  - Enthesitis of the ischium secondary to inflammatory spondyloarthropathy.
  - Bony avulsions of the ischium.

OTHER RECOMMENDED TESTING

- Laboratory testing to rule out inflammatory arthritis.
- Bursa aspiration with Gram staining and culture and sensitivity testing if infection in question.
- Joint aspiration to rule out crystal arthropathies.
- Joint aspiration to rule out infection if diagnosis in question.

DIFFERENTIAL DIAGNOSIS

- Calcific tendinitis.
- Avulsion fracture.
- Osteoarthritis of the hip.
- Inflammatory arthritis of the hip.
- Neoplasm.
- Labral tears of the hip.
- Piriformis syndrome.
- Sacral insufficiency fracture.
- Septic arthritis of the hip.

TREATMENT

- Conservative treatment consisting of local heat, cold, simple analgesics, and nonsteroidal anti-inflammatory agents will improve symptoms in mild cases.
- Physical therapy, including gentle stretching, range-of-motion exercises, and deep heat modalities, may be beneficial in selected patients.
- Injection with local anesthetic and steroid will provide symptomatic relief if conservative therapy fails or the pain is limiting activities of daily living.
- Surgery may be required for persistent pain or progressive functional disability.

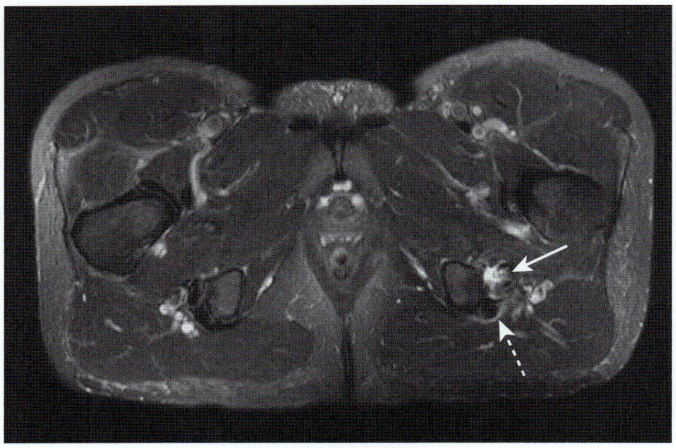

Figure 137.1 Axial FST2W MR image of a patient with tendinopathy of the semimembranosus tendon origin, showing a thickened tendon and high-SI edema (*white arrow*). There is also a thin rim of peritendinous high-SI edema posteriorly between the hamstring origin and the gluteus maximus (*broken white arrow*).

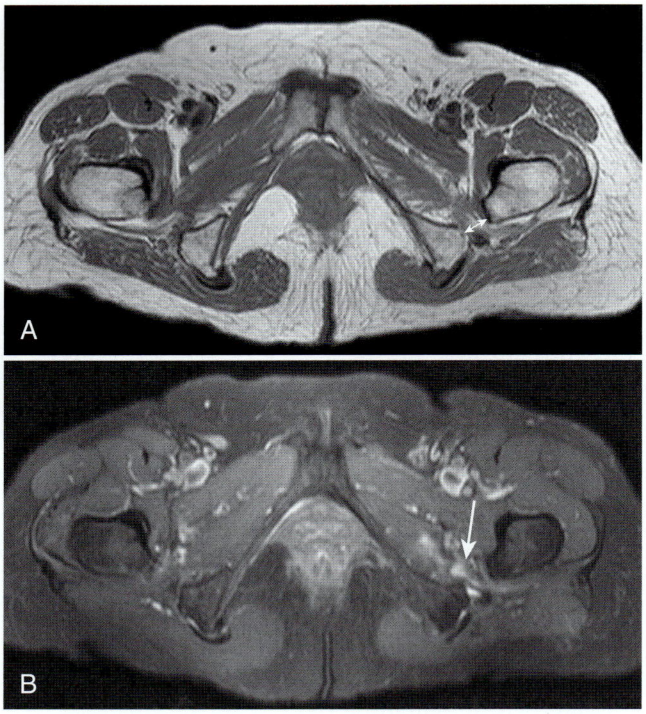

Figure 137.3 (**A**), Axial T1W MR image of a middle-aged woman with poorly localized hip pain demonstrates reduced space between the lesser trochanter and the ischium on the left side (*double-headed white arrow*) due to ischiofemoral impingement. (**B**), The axial FST2W MR image shows high-SI edema within the quadratus femoris muscle and adjacent ischiogluteal bursa (*white arrow*).

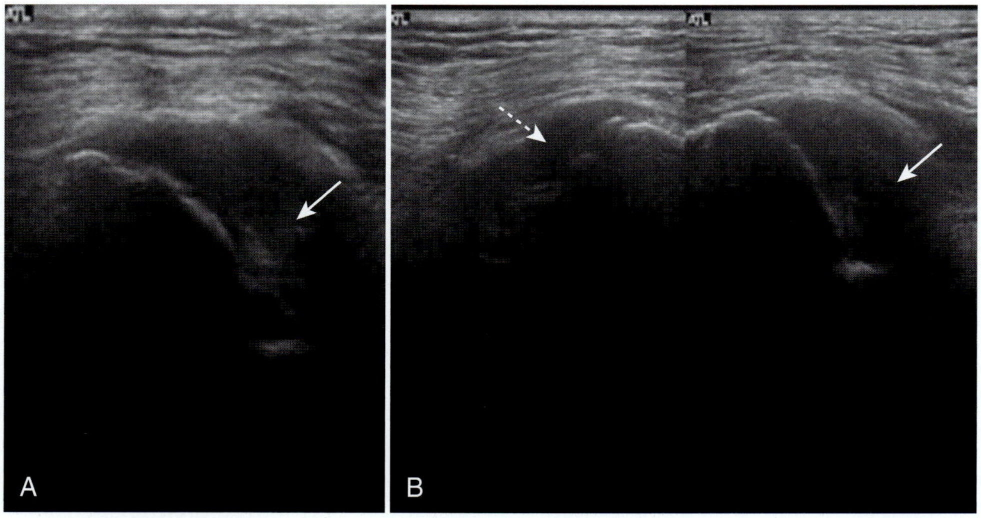

Figure 137.2 (**A**), Transverse US image of a young athlete with buttock pain and thickening of the hamstring tendon (*white arrow*) and some surrounding low-echo fluid within the ischiogluteal bursa. (**B**), A comparative image shows the symptomatic side (*white arrow*) and the asymptomatic side (*broken white arrow*). *(Image courtesy of Dr. M. Reijnierse, Leiden, The Netherlands.)*

CHAPTER 138

Osteoarthritis of the Hip

DEFINITION

- Degenerative arthritis characterized by destruction of the chondral surfaces, subchondral cysts, synovitis, and osteophyte formation.

SIGNS AND SYMPTOMS

- Gradual onset of pain with range of motion of the hip joint.
- Effusion may be present.
- Crepitus may be present.
- Gradual decrease in range of motion.

DEMOGRAPHICS

- Incidence: Male > Female.
- Most common in elderly patients; also seen in younger patients following hip joint trauma and/or surgery.
- Universal finding after the fifth decade of life.
- History of joint trauma common.
- Genetic predisposition possible.

IMAGING RECOMMENDATIONS

- Radiography is the first-line investigation of arthropathy.
- MRI:
  - Assess intra-articular structures.
  - Assess cartilage loss.
- MR/CT arthrography:
  - Specialist investigation for associated abnormalities, such as femoroacetabular impingement and articular cartilage.
- US:
  - To identify effusions and synovitis.
  - To guide joint aspiration and injection.

IMAGING FINDINGS

- Joint space narrowing, subchondral sclerosis, subchondral cysts, and osteophyte formation.
- Joint space narrowing is typically asymmetrical, involving the superior aspect of the joint.
- Supralateral migration of the femoral head.
- Buttressing of the medial aspect of the femoral neck.

OTHER RECOMMENDED TESTING

- Intra-articular injection of contrast agent if labral tear suspected.
- Laboratory testing to rule out inflammatory arthritis.
- Joint aspiration to rule out crystal arthropathies.
- Joint aspiration to rule out infection.

DIFFERENTIAL DIAGNOSIS

- Inflammatory arthritides, especially rheumatoid arthritis.
- Septic hip joint.
- Healing hip joint fracture, especially of the glenoid rim.
- Rotator cuff tear.
- Crystal arthropathy of the hip.
- Avascular osteonecrosis.

TREATMENT

- Conservative treatment consisting of local heat, cold, simple analgesics, and nonsteroidal anti-inflammatory agents will improve symptoms in many cases.
- Physical therapy, including gentle stretching, range-of-motion exercises, and deep heat modalities, may be beneficial in selected patients.
- Intra-articular injection with local anesthetic and steroid will provide symptomatic relief if conservative therapy fails or the pain is limiting activities of daily living.
- Surgery may be required for persistent pain or progressive functional disability.

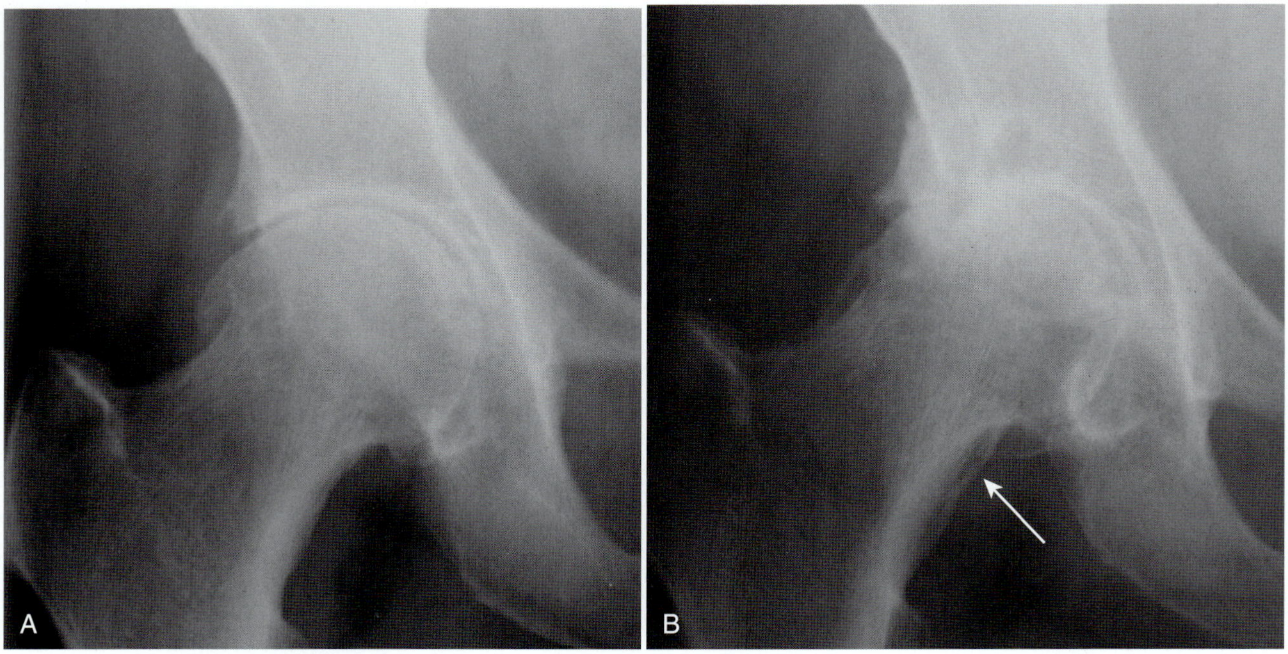

Figure 138.1 (**A**), AP radiograph of a patient with typical osteoarthritis (OA) of the hip with joint space narrowing and osteophyte formation. (**B**), A radiograph of the same patient acquired 18 months later shows rapid progression of the OA changes, with more marked superior joint space narrowing, supralateral migration of the femoral head, prominent subchondral cyst formation, and buttressing of the medial aspect of the femoral neck (*white arrow*).

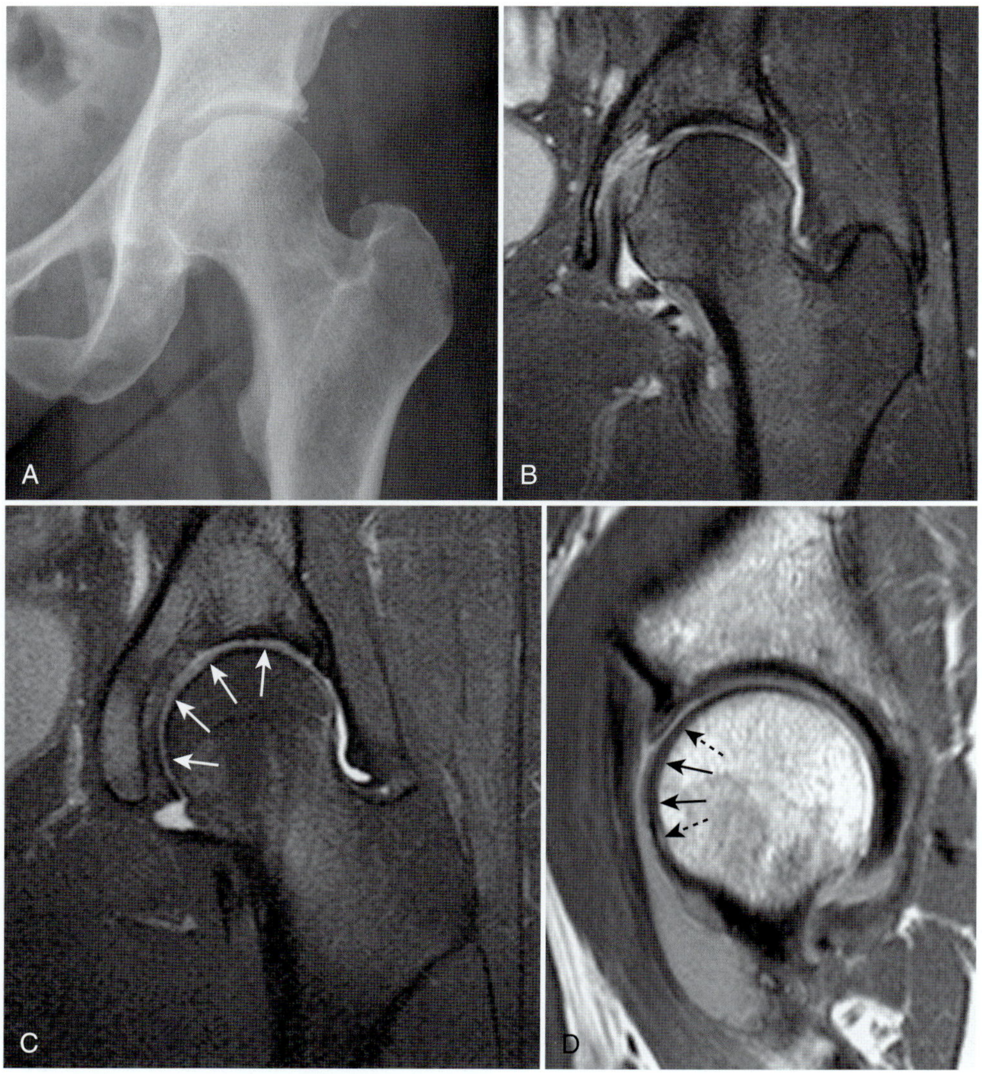

Figure 138.2 (**A**), AP radiograph of a 60-year-old patient with hip pain, which shows no significant OA changes. (**B**), However, the coronal T2-weighted with fat suppression (FST2W) MR image clearly demonstrates a high–signal intensity (SI) hip joint effusion with diffuse areas of cartilage loss across the femoral head, due to early OA. (**C**), Compare with the FST2W MR image of a normal hip with intermediate-SI cartilage overlying the low-SI subchondral bone plate (*white arrows*). (**D**), The cartilage loss is also seen on the sagittal proton density image (*broken black arrows*), but with some areas of cartilage preservation (*black arrows*).

CHAPTER 139

Rheumatoid Arthritis of the Hip Joint

DEFINITION

- Symmetrical inflammatory arthritis characterized by synovitis, joint space narrowing, effusions and erosions, and elevation of serum rheumatoid factor combined with a constellation of other clinical signs and symptoms.

SIGNS AND SYMPTOMS

- Pain with range of motion of the hip joint.
- Synovitis.
- Effusion often present.
- Warmth often present.
- Crepitus may be present.
- Morning stiffness.
- Gelling phenomenon.
- Gradual decrease in range of motion.
- Fatigue, lassitude, and mild fever.
- Symmetrical polyarthritis involving three or more joints invariably present upon careful inspection.

DEMOGRAPHICS

- Incidence: Female > Male.
- Adult form more common, although juvenile form should be considered in any child with polyarthritis.
- Peak onset in the fourth to sixth decade of life.

IMAGING RECOMMENDATIONS

- Radiography is the primary investigation for arthropathy.
- MRI:
  - Assess synovitis, early erosions.
  - Assess cartilage loss.
- US:
  - Identify synovitis, effusions, and early erosions.
  - Guide joint aspiration and injection.

IMAGING FINDINGS

- Joint space narrowing, erosions, osteopenia.
- Joint space narrowing is usually global.
- Reactive bone formation with osteophytes and sclerosis occurs only with secondary osteoarthritis (OA).
- Protrusio acetabuli.
- Secondary avascular necrosis (AVN) may occur with steroid therapy.

OTHER RECOMMENDED TESTING

- Laboratory testing, including complete blood count, blood chemistry profile, and erythrocyte sedimentation rate determination, to rule out extra-articular manifestations of the disease.
- Antinuclear antibody and systemic lupus erythematosus (SLE) testing if diagnosis in doubt.
- Joint aspiration to rule out crystal arthropathies.
- Joint aspiration to rule out infection.

DIFFERENTIAL DIAGNOSIS

- Other inflammatory arthritides, especially SLE arthritis.
- Charcot hip joint.
- Osteoarthritis.
- Psoriatic arthritis.
- Crystal arthropathy of hip.
- Avascular osteonecrosis.

TREATMENT

- Disease-modifying agents, including gold salts, penicillamine, azathioprine, and cyclosporine A, can dramatically slow the progression of the disease, albeit not without side effects.
- Cytotoxic drugs, including methotrexate.
- Biologic agents, including interleukin and tumor necrosis factor-α.
- Salicylates, nonsteroidal anti-inflammatory agents, and corticosteroids.
- Physical and occupational therapy.
- Intra-articular injection of local anesthetic and corticosteroid for symptomatic relief and to aid in physical therapy.
- Surgery may be required for persistent pain or progressive functional disability.

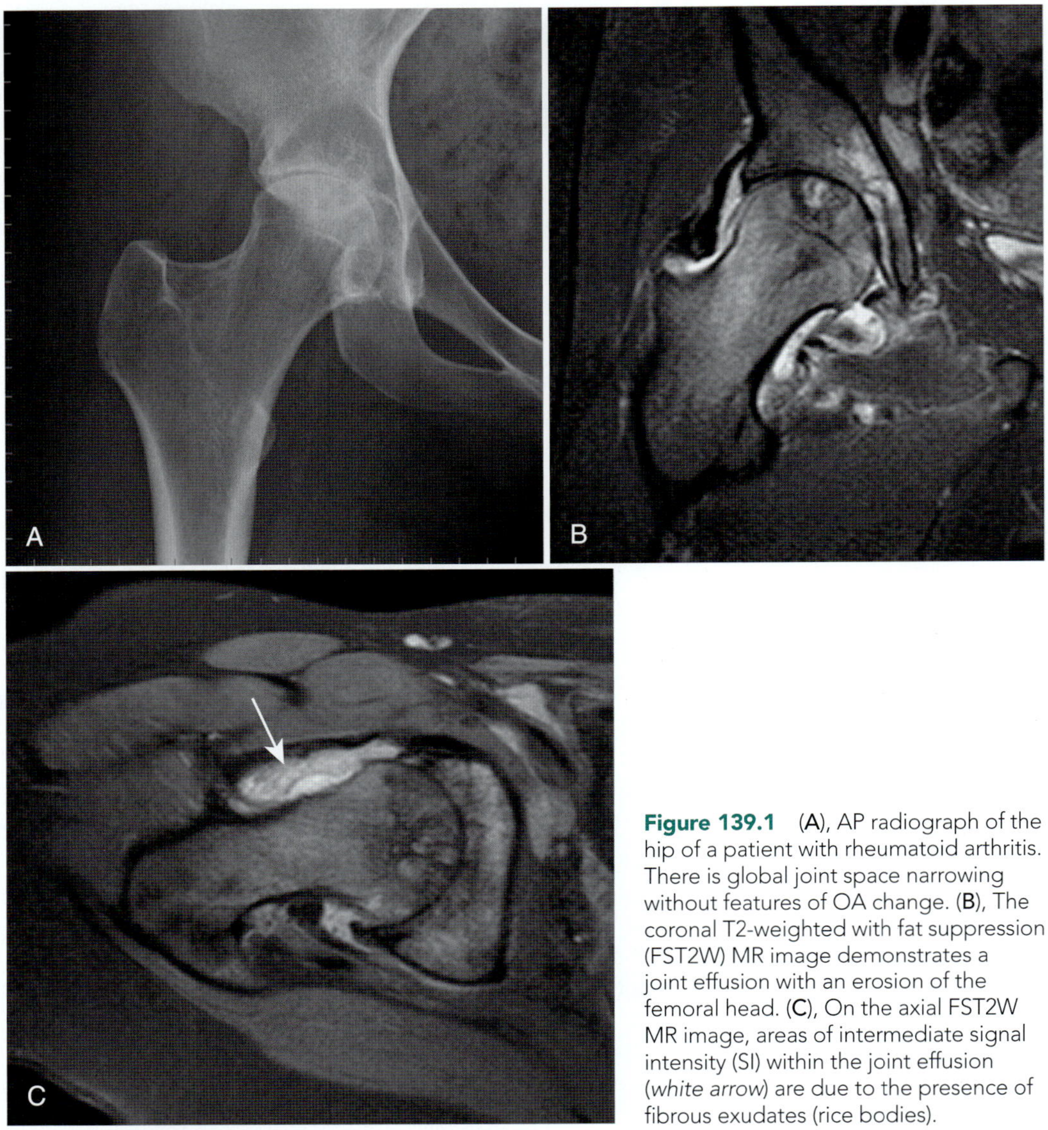

Figure 139.1 (**A**), AP radiograph of the hip of a patient with rheumatoid arthritis. There is global joint space narrowing without features of OA change. (**B**), The coronal T2-weighted with fat suppression (FST2W) MR image demonstrates a joint effusion with an erosion of the femoral head. (**C**), On the axial FST2W MR image, areas of intermediate signal intensity (SI) within the joint effusion (*white arrow*) are due to the presence of fibrous exudates (rice bodies).

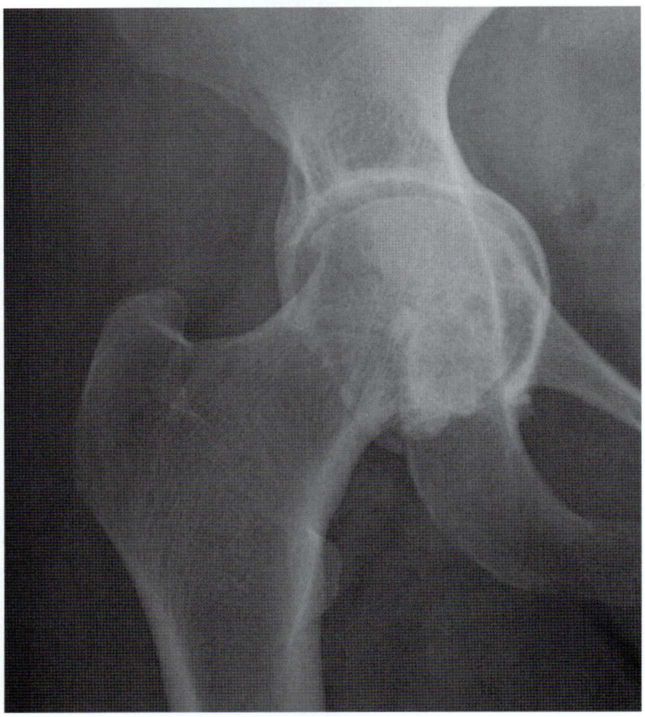

Figure 139.2 Radiograph of a patient with long-standing rheumatoid disease that shows prominent central protrusio deformity of the hip.

CHAPTER 140

Adductor Tendinitis

DEFINITION

- Tendinitis of the gracilis, adductor longus, adductor brevis, and adductor magnus muscles due to repetitive microtrauma to the musculotendinous unit.

SIGNS AND SYMPTOMS

- Gradual onset of sharp, constant, and severe groin and inner thigh pain.
- Pain often radiates into the proximal inner thigh.
- Positive result of Waldman knee squeeze test.
- Adductor lurch type gait often present.
- Patient may walk with the trunk shifted over the affected extremity.
- Catching and creaking may be present.
- Exacerbation of pain with resisted hip and passive abduction.
- Patient unable to sleep on the affected side.

DEMOGRAPHICS

- Incidence: Male = Female.
- Young athletes who use exercise equipments are often affected.
- Bursitis is often present.
- More common after trauma, including repetitive stress injuries.

IMAGING RECOMMENDATIONS

- Radiography:
  - To exclude hip osteoarthritis (OA) in older patients.
- MRI:
  - To assess soft tissue and bony structures.
  - To exclude other causes of groin pain.
- US:
  - Acute muscle tears.
  - To exclude hernias as the cause of groin pain.

IMAGING FINDINGS

- Increased signal intensity (SI) within the common adductor origin on T1-weighted (T1W) and T2W MR images.
- Enhancement within and around the adductor origin on post-contrast (obtained after administration of a contrast agent) T1W with fat suppression (FST1W) MR images.
- High-SI "cleft sign" at the junction between adductor tendon and symphyseal origin on T2W MR images.
- Larger defects indicate a tear or avulsion of the adductor origin.
- Coexistent stress-related osteitis pubis:
  - High-SI marrow edema.
  - Erosion of the bony margins.

OTHER RECOMMENDED TESTING

- Laboratory testing to rule out inflammatory arthritis.
- Joint aspiration to rule out crystal arthropathies.
- Joint aspiration to rule out infection if diagnosis is in question.

DIFFERENTIAL DIAGNOSIS

- Calcific tendinitis.
- Pelvic insufficiency fracture.
- Ilioinguinal neuralgia.
- Genitofemoral neuralgia.
- Hypogastric neuralgia.
- Internal derangement of the hip.
- Labral tear of the hip.
- Neoplasm.

TREATMENT

- Conservative treatment consisting of local heat, cold, simple analgesics, and nonsteroidal anti-inflammatory agents will improve symptoms in many cases.
- Physical therapy, including gentle stretching, range-of-motion exercises, and deep heat modalities, may be beneficial in selected patients.
- Injection with local anesthetic and steroid will provide symptomatic relief if conservative therapy fails or the pain is limiting activities of daily living.
- Surgery may be required for persistent pain or progressive functional disability.

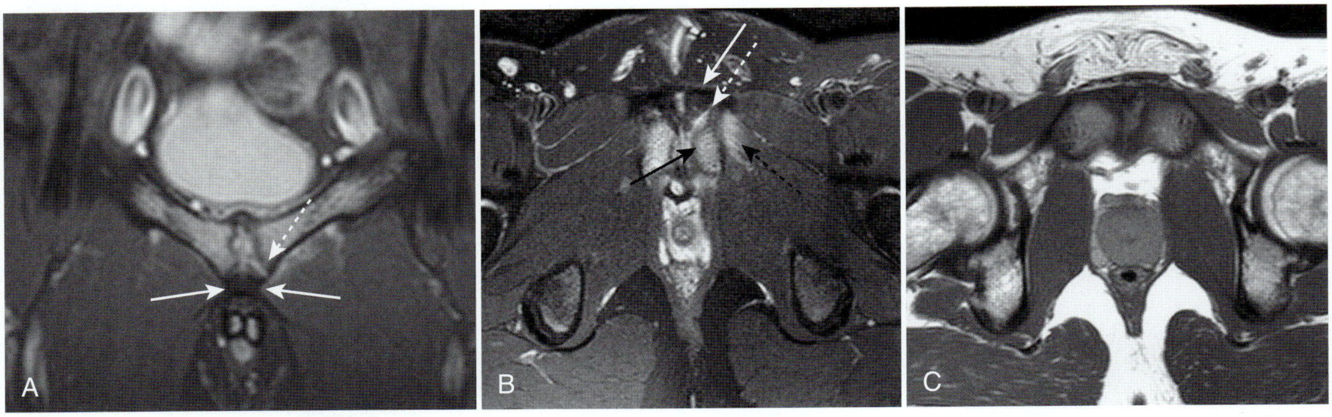

Figure 140.1 (**A**), Coronal FST2W MR image of a young patient with left-sided groin pain. There are stress-related features of osteitis pubis with high-SI marrow edema in both pubic bones. In addition, a high-SI cleft (*broken white arrow*) can be seen between the pubis and the adductor tendon origin (*white arrows*), which is due to chronic adductor tendinopathy. (**B**), The axial FST2W MR image shows the same high-SI cleft (*broken white arrow*) between the adductor tendon (*white arrow*) and the pubis (*black arrow*). There is also high SI within the adjacent adductor muscle because of repetitive strain injury (*broken black arrow*). (**C**), The axial T1W MR image shows the chronic bony erosive changes within the pubic symphysis.

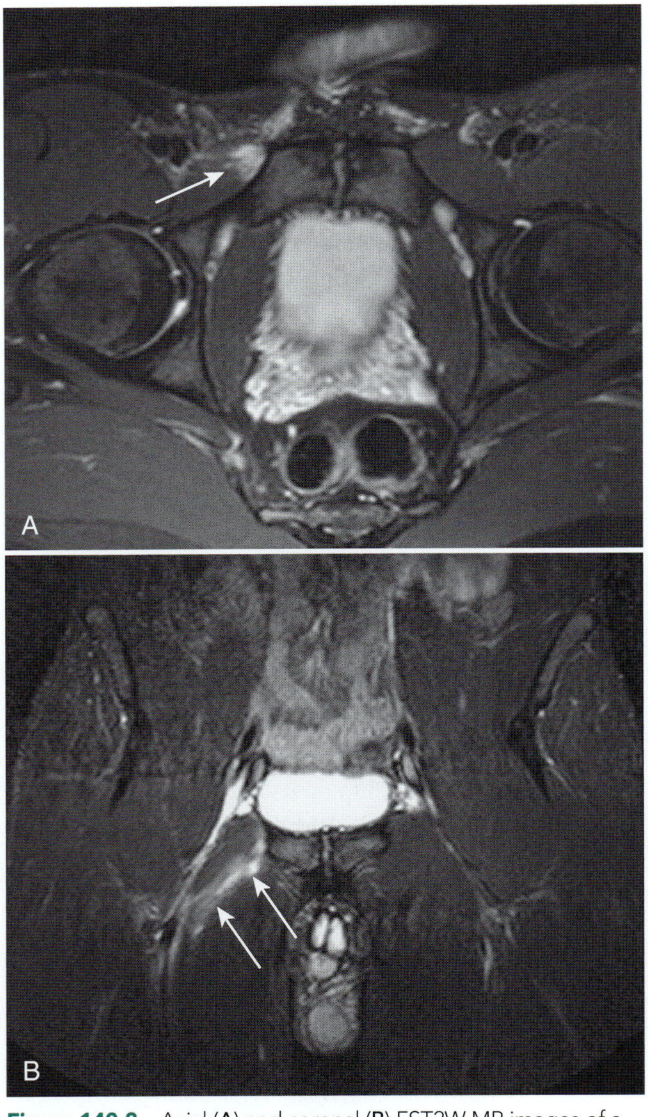

Figure 140.2 Axial (**A**) and coronal (**B**) FST2W MR images of a rugby player with an acute groin injury. There is a high-SI partial tear of the proximal pectineus muscle (*white arrows*) with a normal symphysis and no features of chronic adductor tendonopathy.

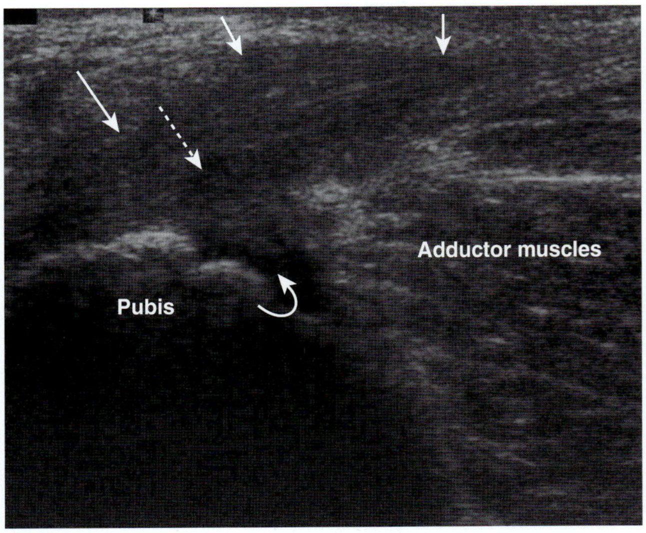

Figure 140.3 US image acquired along the longitudinal plane of the adductor longus tendon. The tendon is thickened (*white arrows*), and there are areas of low-echo change within the tendon substance (*broken white arrow*), consistent with adductor tendinopathy. There is also a low-echo cleft at the adductor origin on the pubis (*curved white arrow*).

CHAPTER 141

Piriformis Syndrome

DEFINITION

- Entrapment of the sciatic nerve as it passes beneath the piriformis muscle.

SIGNS AND SYMPTOMS

- Pain, numbness, and paresthesias in the gluteal region radiating into the L5-S1 derivative.
- Pain often worse at night.
- Pain increased with hip adduction and internal rotation.
- Tenderness on rectal palpation of the piriformis muscle.
- Associated weakness in the distribution of the sciatic nerve.
- Symptoms may also radiate proximal to the entrapment into the buttocks.
- Onset of symptoms usually occurs after repetitive hip motions or as a result of repeated pressure on the sciatic nerve from prolonged sitting.
- Usually unilateral.
- If left untreated, progressive motor deficit and, ultimately, loss of function can result.

DEMOGRAPHICS

- Incidence between the second and fifth decade of life.
- Incidence: Female > Male.
- Increased incidence following direct trauma to gluteal region.

IMAGING RECOMMENDATIONS

- Radiography:
  - To exclude underlying bony abnormality.
- MRI.

IMAGING FINDINGS

- Unilateral hypertrophy of piriformis muscle on the affected side:
  - Normal signal intensity (SI) on MRI.
  - Effacement of adjacent fat planes.
- Anomalous muscle slips.
- Muscle edema pattern:
  - High SI on T2-weighted with fat suppression (FST2W) or short T1 inversion recovery (STIR) MR images.
  - Muscle injury, infection, or tumor.

OTHER RECOMMENDED TESTING

- Electromyography and nerve conduction velocity testing is diagnostic except very early in the course of the disease.
- Erythrocyte sedimentation rate, rheumatoid factor, and antinuclear antibody determinations if rheumatoid arthritis suggested.
- Blood glucose determination.

DIFFERENTIAL DIAGNOSIS

- L5-S1 radiculopathy.
- Arthritis of the hip.
- Adductor tendinitis.
- Gluteal bursitis.
- Neoplasm.
- Pelvic insufficiency fracture.
- Trochanteric bursitis.
- Internal derangement of the hip.
- Internal derangement of the sacroiliac joint.
- Space-occupying lesions involving the sciatic nerve, including aneurysms of the inferior gluteal artery.

TREATMENT

- Conservative therapy, consisting of simple analgesics, nonsteroidal anti-inflammatory drugs, or cyclooxygenase inhibitors and splinting of the wrist, should be used for mild cases of piriformis syndrome.
- Avoidance of repetitive activities thought to be responsible for the evolution of piriformis syndrome will also help ameliorate the symptoms.
- If there is no response to these conservative measures, injection of the carpal tunnel with local anesthetic and steroid is the next reasonable step.
- Surgical decompression of the compressed sciatic nerve by release of the piriformis muscle should be performed in all cases of moderate to severe piriformis syndrome for which conservative therapy has failed.

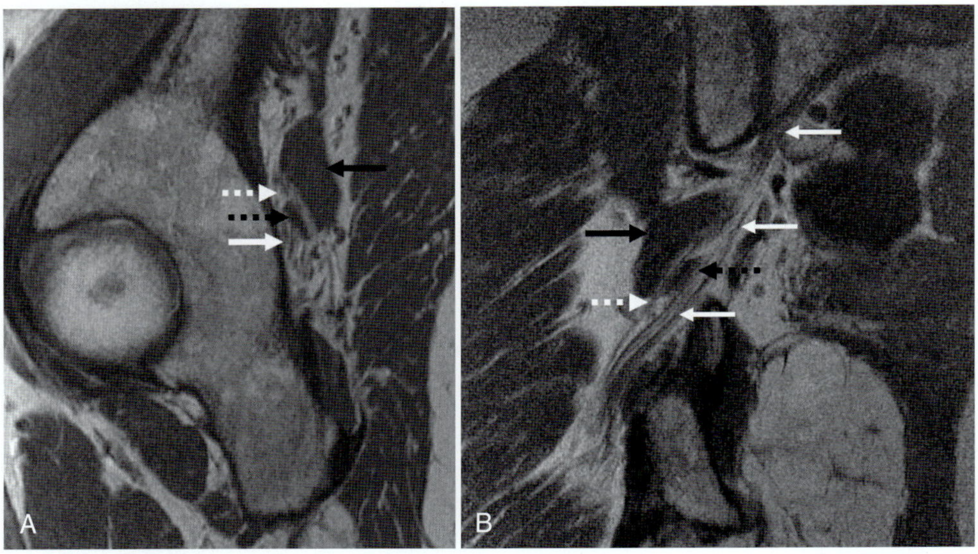

Figure 141.1 Sagittal (**A**) and coronal (**B**) T1W MR images in a patient with sciatic nerve compression symptoms. The piriformis muscle (*black arrow*) and sciatic nerve (*white arrow*) are demonstrated. A separate fascicle of the sciatic nerve (*broken white arrow*) passes between an anomalous slip of the piriformis (*broken black arrow*) and the main muscle belly.

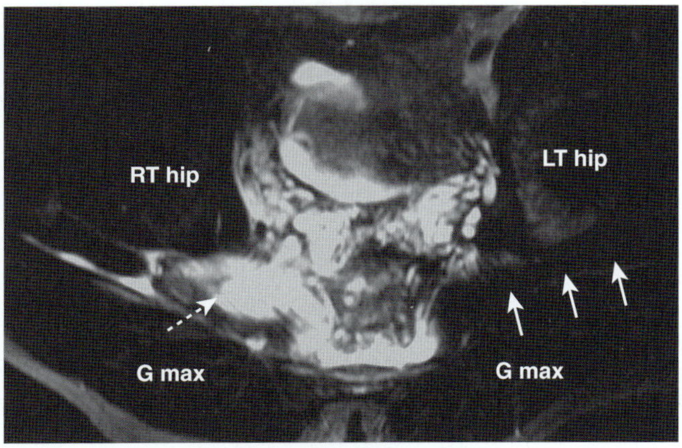

Figure 141.2 Axial T2W MR image of the pelvis in an athlete with an acute injury and tension signs of the sciatic nerve. The right piriformis is enlarged because of a high-SI hematoma (*broken white arrow*) resulting from an acute muscle injury. Compare with the normal left piriformis (*white arrows*). G max, gluteus maximus muscle; LT, left; RT, right. *(Image courtesy of Dr. Phil O'Connor, Leeds, United Kingdom)*

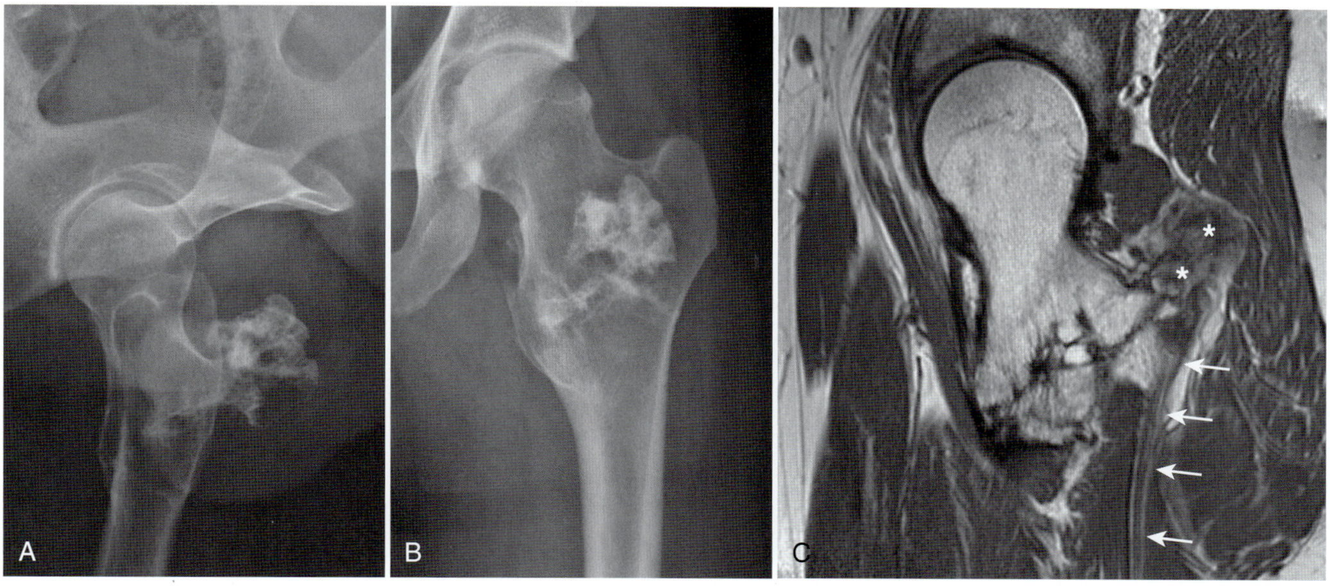

Figure 141.3 AP (**A**) and lateral (**B**) radiographs of a young man with a large osteochondroma arising from the posterior aspect of the proximal femur. (**C**), The sagittal T1W MR image demonstrates the close relationship of the osteochondroma (*asterisks*) to the sciatic nerve (*white arrows*).

CHAPTER 142

Trochanteric Bursitis

DEFINITION

- Inflammation of the trochanteric bursa, which lies between the greater trochanter and the tendon of the gluteus medius muscle and the iliotibial tract.
- Part of trochanteric pain syndrome, which includes bursitis, gluteal tendinopathy, and tendon tears.

SIGNS AND SYMPTOMS

- Pain localized in the outer thigh that is made worse with any hip movement.
- Pain may radiate to proximal femur.
- Tenderness to palpation of the trochanteric bursa.
- Warmth may be present.
- Area over the trochanteric bursa may feel boggy or edematous.
- Crepitus or catching sensation may be present.
- Exacerbation of pain with resisted extension, abduction, and rotation of the hip.
- Pain often worse at night.
- Patient unable to sleep on the affected hip.
- Gradual decrease in range of motion.

DEMOGRAPHICS

- Incidence: Male = Female.
- Young athletes often affected.
- More common after trauma, including repetitive stress injuries.
- Increased incidence with jogging on uneven or soft surfaces.

IMAGING RECOMMENDATIONS

- Radiography to detect underlying bone or joint disease.
- US or MRI to assess the soft tissue structures.
- US to guide injection therapy.

IMAGING FINDINGS

- Radiographic findings are often normal:
  - Insertional bone formation may occur around the greater trochanter as a result of chronic insertional tendinopathy.
- Bursitis is identified as low-echo fluid on US or high–signal intensity (SI) fluid on T2-weighted with fat suppression (FST2W) MR images in the locations of known bursae.
  - Small amounts of fluid may be a normal finding in some individuals.
- Peritendinous inflammatory change or tendon degeneration and tendon tears may be present when bursitis is associated with gluteal tendinopathy:
  - Tendon thickening.
  - Low-echo change on US.
  - Increased SI on FST2W MR images.

OTHER RECOMMENDED TESTING

- Laboratory testing to rule out inflammatory arthritis.
- Bursa aspiration with Gram staining and culture and sensitivity testing if infection in question.
- Joint aspiration to rule out crystal arthropathies.
- Joint aspiration to rule out infection if diagnosis in question.

DIFFERENTIAL DIAGNOSIS

- Calcific tendinitis.
- Avulsion fractures.
- Osteoarthritis of the hip.
- Inflammatory arthritis of the hip.
- Neoplasm.
- Labral tears of the hip.
- Piriformis syndrome.
- Sacral insufficiency fractures.
- Septic arthritis of the hip.

TREATMENT

- Conservative treatment consisting of local heat, cold, simple analgesics, and nonsteroidal anti-inflammatory agents will improve symptoms in mild cases.
- Physical therapy, including gentle stretching, range-of-motion exercises, and deep heat modalities, may be beneficial in selected patients.
- Injection with local anesthetic and steroid will provide symptomatic relief if conservative therapy fails or the pain is limiting activities of daily living.
- Surgery may be required for persistent pain or progressive functional disability.

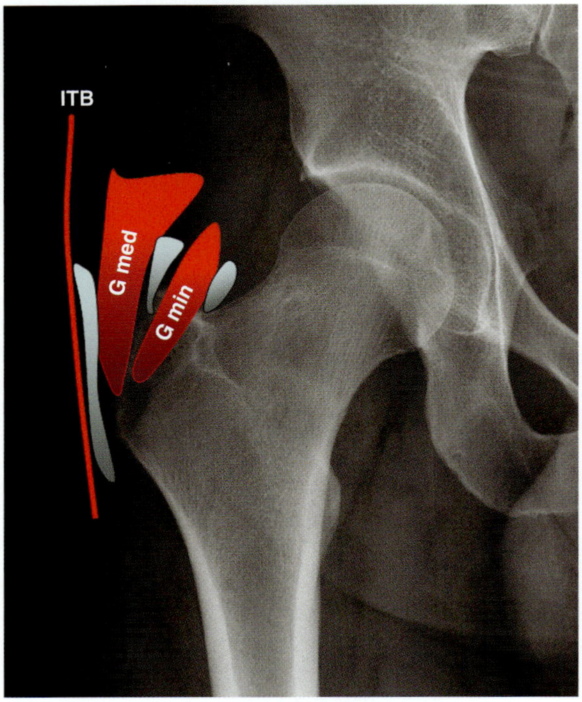

Figure 142.1 Diagrammatic representation of the various bursae (*blue*) around the greater trochanter. The trochanteric bursa lies deep to the iliotibial band (ITB) and superficial to the gluteus medius (G med) and gluteus minimus (G min) tendons. There is also a sub–gluteus medius bursa and a sub–gluteus minimus bursa. The minimus tendon inserts anteriorly, and the medius tendon more posteriorly, on the trochanter.

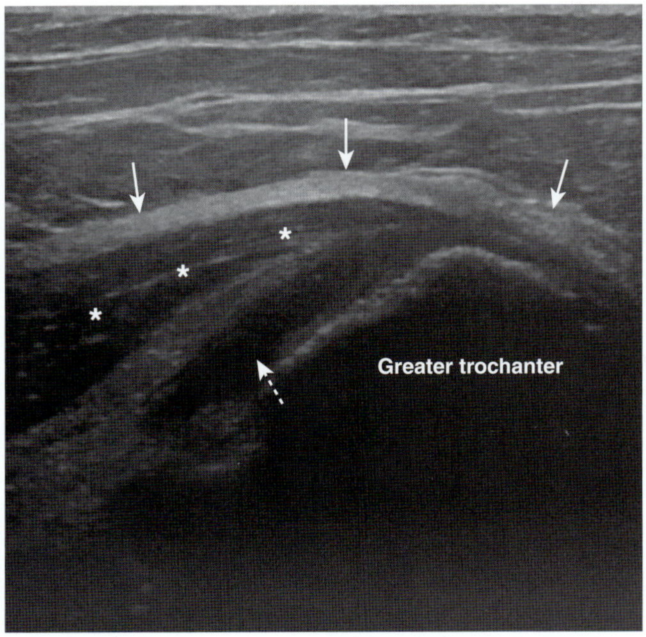

Figure 142.3 Axial US image of the hip in a patient with lateral hip pain. There is low-echo fluid within the sub–gluteus medius bursa (*broken white arrow*), which lies between the gluteus medius muscle and tendon (*asterisks*) and the posterolateral facet of the greater trochanter. The iliotibial band is superficial to the gluteus medius (*white arrows*).

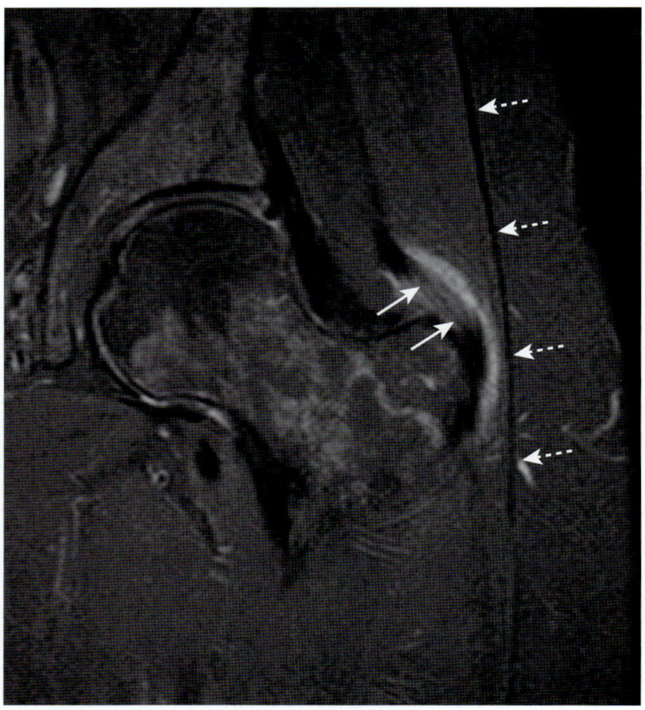

Figure 142.2 Coronal FST2W MR image of a patient with lateral hip pain and trochanteric bursitis with high-SI fluid lying between the iliotibial tract (*broken white arrows*) and the gluteus minimus tendon (*white arrows*).

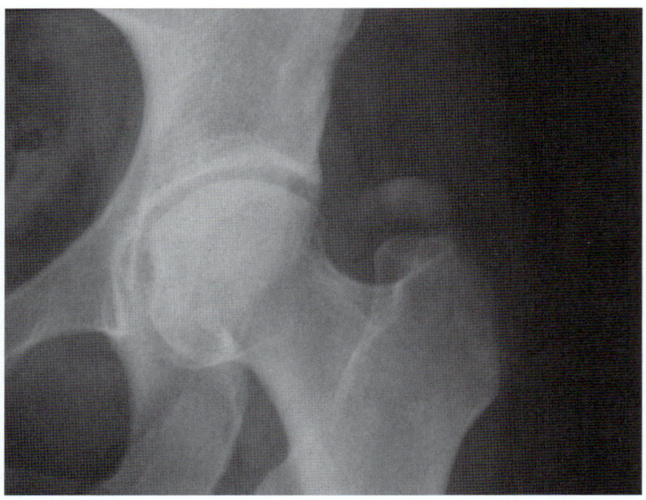

Figure 142.4 Radiograph of the hip of a patient with calcific tendinitis due to hydroxyapatite crystal deposition; it can be identified as a focal area of calcification in the gluteal tendon superior to the greater trochanter. Radiographs obtained 6 months later showed that the calcification had spontaneously resolved.

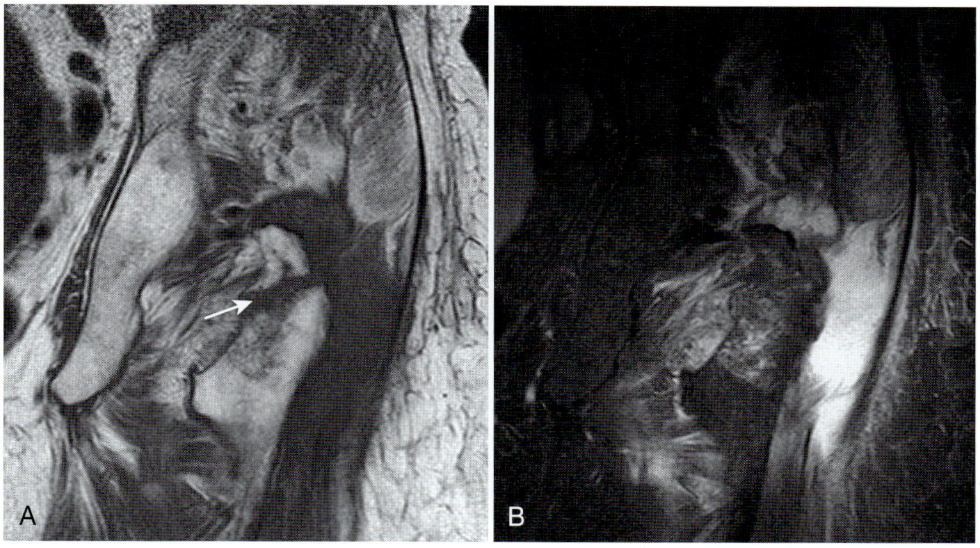

Figure 142.5 (**A**), Coronal T1W MR image of an elderly woman with osteoporosis and lateral hip pain but no history of trauma. Previous radiographic findings had been normal. There is an insufficiency fracture through the base of the greater trochanter (*white arrow*). (**B**), The coronal FST2W MR image shows the extensive high-SI hematoma within the adjacent trochanteric bursa, with more generalized soft tissue edema. The fracture line is not well shown, but there is marrow edema in the proximal femur.

CHAPTER 143

Snapping Hip Syndrome

DEFINITION

- Snapping sensation with movement of the hip:
  - *External*: Iliotibial band snapping over the greater trochanter.
  - *Internal:* Iliopsoas tendon snapping over the iliopectineal eminence, joint capsule, or femoral head.
  - *Intra-articular*: Labral tears or loose bodies.

SIGNS AND SYMPTOMS

- Pain with hip flexion and extension.
- Audible snap with hip flexion and extension.
- Audible snap is eliminated with firm manual pressure over the greater trochanter during hip flexion and extension.
- Tenderness over the greater trochanter.
- Trochanteric bursitis often coexists.
- Patient unable to sleep on the affected hip.
- Gradual decrease in range of motion as patient guards the hip.

DEMOGRAPHICS

- Incidence: Female > Male.
- Most common between the second and fourth decades of life.
- Young athletes often affected.
- More common after trauma, including repetitive stress injuries.
- Increased incidence in ballet dancers.

IMAGING RECOMMENDATIONS

- US for dynamic assessment of snapping tendons.
- MRI to exclude intra-articular disorders of the hip.

IMAGING FINDINGS

- Abnormal motion of tendon on US during range of motion that produces snapping symptoms.
- May be associated with features of iliopsoas or trochanteric bursitis.
- MRI may show thickening and increased signal intensity (SI) within the affected iliopsoas tendon or iliotibial band on T2-weighted with fat suppression (FST2W) MR images.
- Loose bodies or labral tears on MRI or MR arthrography.

OTHER RECOMMENDED TESTING

- Laboratory testing to rule out inflammatory arthritis.
- Bursa aspiration with Gram staining and culture and sensitivity testing if infection in question.
- Joint aspiration to rule out crystal arthropathies.
- Joint aspiration to rule out infection if diagnosis in question.

DIFFERENTIAL DIAGNOSIS

- Calcific tendinitis.
- Avulsion fracture.
- Osteoarthritis of the hip.
- Inflammatory arthritis of the hip.
- Neoplasm.
- Muscle strains and tears.
- Trochanteric bursitis.
- Pelvic insufficiency fracture.
- Septic arthritis of the hip.

TREATMENT

- Conservative treatment consisting of local heat, cold, simple analgesics, and nonsteroidal anti-inflammatory agents will improve symptoms in mild cases.
- Physical therapy, including gentle stretching, range-of-motion exercises, and deep heat modalities, may be beneficial in selected patients.
- Injection with local anesthetic and steroid will provide symptomatic relief if conservative therapy fails or the pain is limiting activities of daily living.
- Surgery may be required for persistent pain or progressive functional disability.

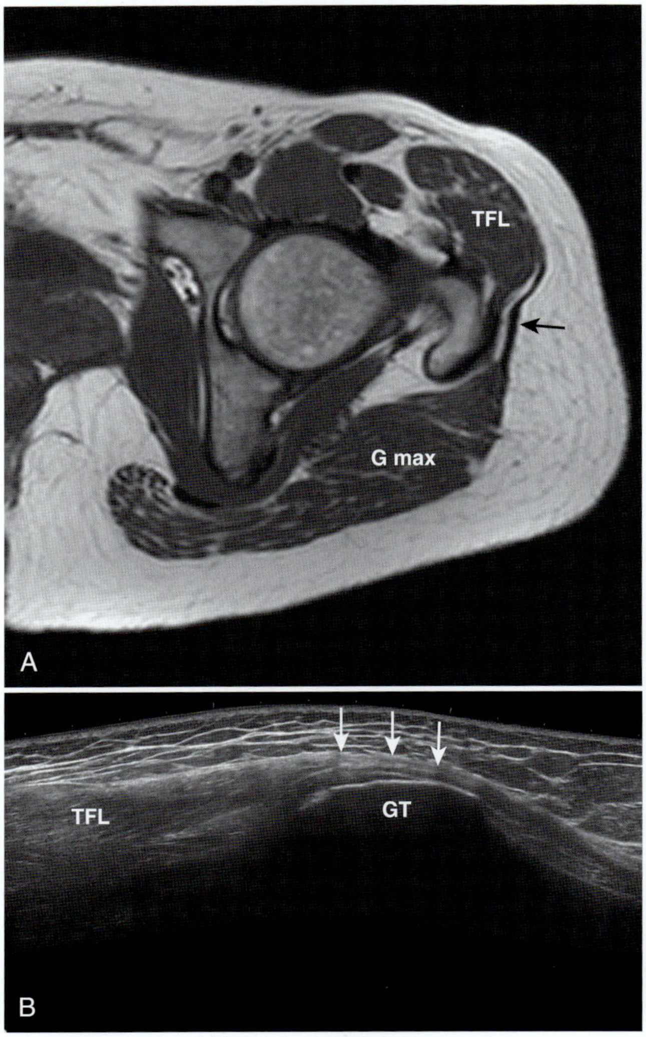

Figure 143.1 (A), Normal axial T1W MR image showing the relationships of the low-SI, thin iliotibial band (ITB) (*black arrow*) which is continuous with the tensor fascia lata (TFL) anteriorly and the gluteus maximus (G max) posteriorly. (B), A longitudinal US image shows the echo-bright ITB lying immediately superficial to the greater trochanter (GT) and its relationship with the TFL muscle proximally.

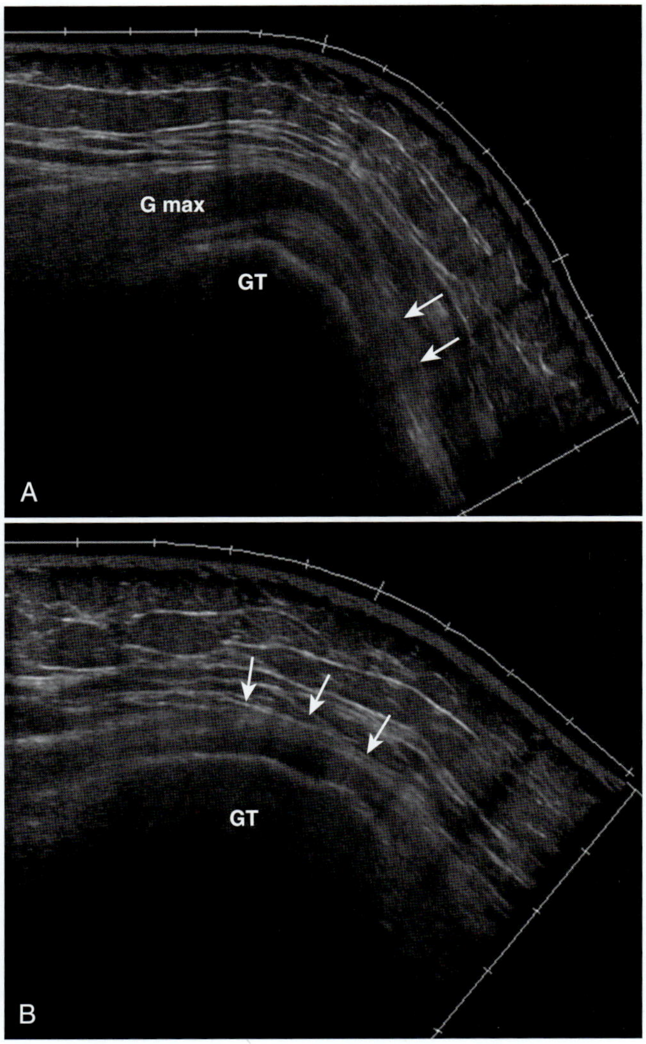

Figure 143.2 Transverse US images of a patient with symptoms of a snapping hip. MRI findings were unremarkable. (A), In flexion, the anterior leading edge of the gluteus maximus (G max), extends around the lateral margin of the greater trochanter (GT), with the echo-bright ITB anteriorly (*white arrows*). (B), In extension, the gluteus maximus moves posteriorly and the ITB (*white arrows*) lies against the lateral margin of the GT. Dynamic US showed that this action did not occur smoothly, but the ITB snapped back suddenly into position as the leg neared full extension. *(Image courtesy of Dr. M. Reijnierse, Leiden, The Netherlands.)*

CHAPTER 144

Anatomy: Special Imaging Considerations of the Knee

The knee, a highly mobile, complex diarthrodial hinge joint, is the largest synovial joint in the body. Knee stability is maintained by a complex ligament structure that is prone to injury. Knowledge of knee anatomy is an essential requirement for performing knee examination and understanding the biomechanics of knee injury.

OSSEOUS STRUCTURES

Femoral Condyles. The medial femoral condyle (MFC) is wider and has a larger articulating surface area than the lateral condyle (LFC), although the LFC is larger anteroposteriorly. The anterior articular surfaces of the condyles become less convex and form a V-shaped groove, known as the trochlear *sulcus,* that articulates with the patella. Posteriorly, the condyles are separated by the intercondylar fossa, which becomes the intercondylar notch anteriorly, through which run the cruciate ligaments.

Tibial Plateau. The proximal articulating surfaces of the tibia form medial and lateral concave plateaus, the medial having a larger surface area. The plateaus are separated by the medial and lateral intercondylar eminences, or tibial spines, which bear the attachments of the meniscal root ligaments.

Patella. The largest sesamoid bone that lies within the quadriceps tendon. It is flat distally and triangular proximally with a convex anterior surface. The posterior articular surface is angled, forming a medial articular facet and a broader lateral facet. The facets articulate with the medial and lateral trochlear surfaces, respectively.

JOINTS

Patellofemoral Joint (PTFJ). A synovial joint formed by the articulation of the patellar facets with the V-shaped trochlear groove of the femoral condyles. There is normal variation in the depth of the trochlear groove and patellar morphology that may contribute to PTFJ instability. Lateral patellar stability is maintained by the medial and lateral patellar retinacula, which are condensations of the fibrous joint capsule. The quadriceps and patellar tendons maintain craniocaudal alignment.

Tibiofemoral Joints. Formed by articulation of the femoral condyles with the tibial plateaus. The concavity of the plateaus is deepened by the menisci, which lie peripherally in each tibiofemoral compartment, thus enhancing joint stability. Posteriorly, the tibiofemoral compartments blend to form the intercondylar fossa. Anteriorly, each tibiofemoral compartment is continuous with the PTFJ compartment.

Menisci. Crescentic fibrocartilaginous structures that are triangular in cross section with an avascular internal apex and a vascularized periphery. Each meniscus can be divided into anterior and posterior horns and a central body. Meniscal stability is provided by the root ligaments that insert centrally on the tibial eminences and by peripheral meniscocapsular attachments. The medial meniscus is C-shaped with a broader posterior horn. The lateral meniscus is four-fifths of a circle and has a uniform breadth covering a larger area than the medial meniscus. The lateral meniscal capsular attachments are deficient posterolaterally, where stability is provided by ligamentous attachment to the popliteus tendon, fibula, and tibia.

LIGAMENTS

Medial Collateral Ligament (MCL). A narrow band-like ligament attaching on the anteromedial aspect of the MFC and inserting distally on the medial surface of the tibia. Its role is to resist valgus stress on the knee.

Lateral Collateral Ligament (LCL). Also referred to as the *fibula collateral ligament,* the LCL attaches on the lateral aspect of the LFC and inserts onto the tip of the proximal tibia. Its role is to resist varus stress. Stability of the posterolateral corner of the knee is also provided by the biceps femoris and popliteus tendons.

TENDONS

Quadriceps Tendon. A thick, broad tendon formed by combination of the rectus femoris and vastus medialis, lateralis, and intermedius tendons that inserts on the superior pole of the patella.

Patella Tendon. A broad tendon arising from the inferior pole of the patella and inserting onto the tibial tuberosity.

BURSAE

Prepatellar Bursa. Potential bursal space within the subcutaneous tissues anterior to the patella and proximal insertion of the patellar tendon.

Semimembranosus Bursa. Potential bursal space located between the medial head of gastrocnemius and the distal semimembranosus tendon. When filled with fluid, the bursa is also referred to as a *popliteal cyst* or *Baker's cyst*.

Pes Anserine Bursa. Potential bursal space located in the anteromedial aspect of the knee overlying the insertion of the pes anserine tendons (sartorius, gracilis, and semimembranosus).

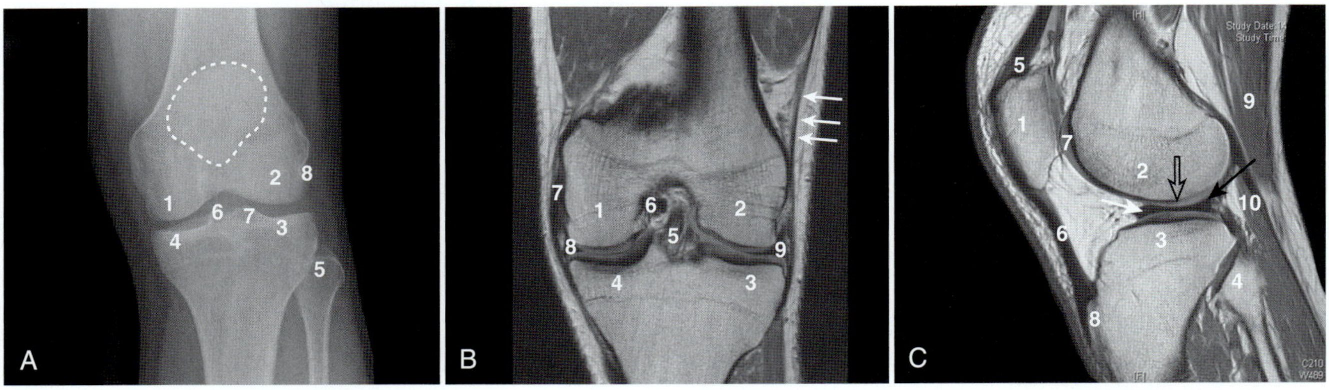

Figure 144.1 (A), Anteroposterior radiograph of the knee: 1, medial femoral condyle; 2, lateral femoral condyle; 3, medial tibial plateau; 4, lateral tibial plateau; 5, fibula head; 6, medial tibial eminence; 7, lateral tibial eminence; 8, popliteal groove; *dashed line,* outline of patella. (B), Coronal proton density MR image of the knee: 1, medial femoral condyle; 2, lateral femoral condyle; 3, medial tibial plateau; 4, lateral tibial plateau; 5, anterior cruciate ligament; 6, posterior cruciate ligament; 7, medial collateral ligament; 8, medial meniscus (body); 9, lateral meniscus (body); *white arrows,* iliotibial band. (C), Sagittal proton density MR image of the knee: 1, patella; 2, lateral femoral condyle; 3, lateral tibial plateau; 4, fibula head; 5, quadriceps tendon; 6, patellar tendon; 7, articular cartilage; 8, tibial tuberosity; 9, biceps femoris muscle; 10, lateral head of gastrocnemius; *black arrow,* anterior horn of lateral meniscus; *open black arrow,* body of lateral meniscus; *white arrow,* posterior horn of lateral meniscus.

CHAPTER 145

Meniscal Degeneration of the Knee

DEFINITION

- Degeneration of the fibrocollagenous elements of the meniscus due to repetitive stress injuries of the meniscus.

SIGNS AND SYMPTOMS

- Gradual onset of knee pain with decreased range of motion of the knee joint as symptoms persist.
- Weakness.
- Clicking usually not present.
- Exacerbation of pain with activity.

DEMOGRAPHICS

- Incidence: Male = Female.
- All ages affected.
- More common after trauma, including repetitive stress injuries.
- May be asymptomatic in many patients until the lesion progresses.

IMAGING RECOMMENDATIONS

- Radiography to exclude osteoarthritis changes in older patients.
- MRI.

IMAGING FINDINGS

- Normal fibrocartilage has low signal intensity (SI) on all MRI pulse sequences.
- Mucoid degeneration:
  - Areas of increased SI within the meniscus on T1-weighted (T1W), proton density, or T2W gradient echo MR images.
  - Does not extend to the surface of the meniscus.
  - Often globular in appearance.
  - Not considered significant in the majority of patients.
- Increased SI within the meniscus may also be due to residual vascularity within the red/red zone in younger individuals.
- Linear areas of high SI that extend to the surface of the meniscus are consistent with degenerative tears:
  - Not all are symptomatic.
- Linear areas of high SI that do not extend to the surface of the meniscus may be a sign of an intrasubstance tear:
  - Significance is uncertain.
  - Difficult to prove.
  - Prominent changes may warrant arthroscopic evaluation.

OTHER RECOMMENDED TESTING

- Laboratory testing to rule out inflammatory arthritis.
- Joint aspiration to rule out crystal arthropathies.
- Joint aspiration to rule out infection if diagnosis in question.

DIFFERENTIAL DIAGNOSIS

- Tendinitis.
- Bursitis.
- Intrasubstance meniscal tear not involving the articular surface.
- Complete meniscal tear.
- Meniscal ossicle containing fat.

TREATMENT

- Conservative treatment consisting of local heat, cold, simple analgesics, and nonsteroidal anti-inflammatory agents will improve symptoms in many cases.
- Physical therapy, including gentle stretching, range-of-motion exercises, and deep heat modalities, may be beneficial in selected patients.
- Injection with local anesthetic and steroid will provide symptomatic relief if conservative therapy fails or the pain is limiting activities of daily living.
- Surgery may be required for persistent pain or worsening functional disability as the lesion progresses.

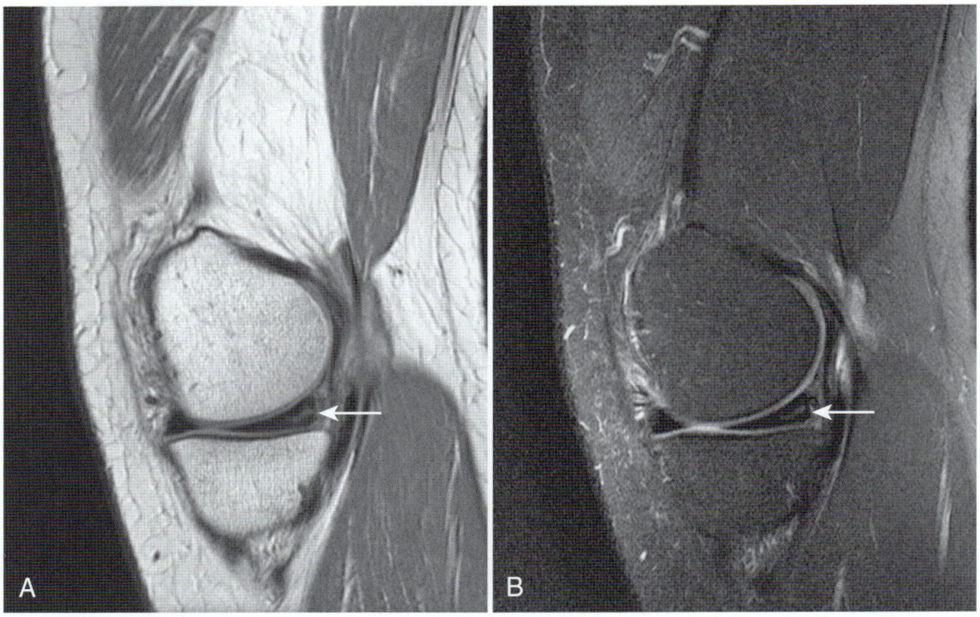

Figure 145.1 Sagittal proton density (**A**) and T2W with fat suppression (FST2W) (**B**) MR images of the medial meniscus. There is linear increased SI within the posterior horn of the meniscus (*white arrows*) that does not extend to the meniscal surface and is not representative of a meniscal tear.

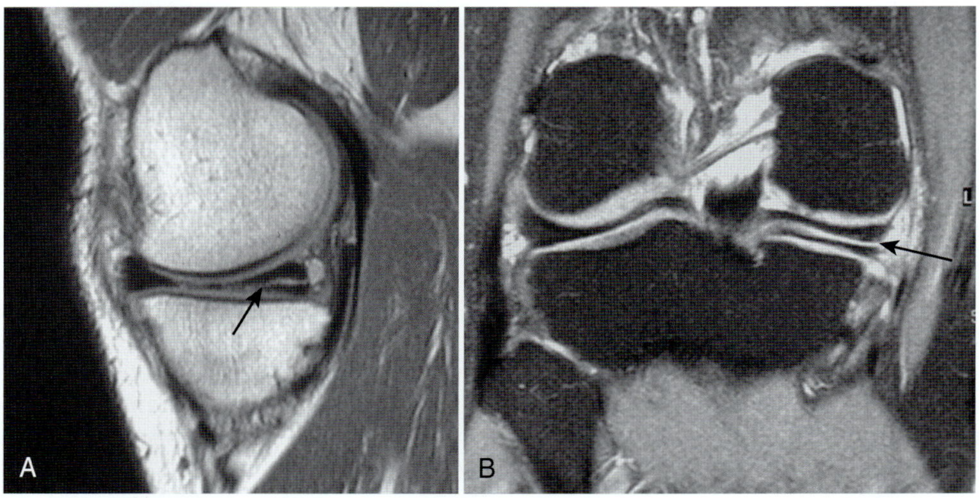

Figure 145.2 Horizontal cleavage tear of the medial meniscus. (**A**), The sagittal proton density MR image demonstrates a linear area of increased SI that extends to the undersurface of the meniscus (*black arrow*). (**B**), The coronal FST2W MR image also shows the horizontal tear as an area of linear high SI within the posterior horn of the meniscus (*black arrow*). Compare with the normal low SI of the lateral meniscus on the coronal image.

CHAPTER 146

Bucket Handle Tear of the Meniscus of the Knee

DEFINITION

- Vertical tear of the meniscus with medial displacement into the intracondylar notch.

SIGNS AND SYMPTOMS

- Acute onset of knee pain after acute trauma.
- Locking of the knee common.
- Decreased full extension of the knee joint.
- Difficulty ambulating on affected knee.
- Feeling of weakness or giving way.
- Clicking often present.
- McMurray test result often positive.
- Apley grinding test result often positive.
- Exacerbation of pain with activity.

DEMOGRAPHICS

- Incidence: Male > Female.
- All ages affected but most commonly younger patients after acute trauma.
- May occur secondary to repetitive stress injuries.
- Common after football and hockey injuries.

IMAGING RECOMMENDATIONS

- Radiography:
  - To exclude osteoarthritis change in older patients.
- MRI.

IMAGING FINDINGS

- Vertical meniscal tears:
  - High-signal intensity (SI) intensity within meniscus extending from superior to inferior surface.
- Bucket-handle tears:
  - Meniscal fragment lies within the intercondylar notch.
  - Fragment remains attached to both anterior and posterior horns.
  - Double posterior cruciate ligament (PCL) sign.
  - Residual meniscal tissue is small and blunted.
- Other patterns of displaced meniscal tears:
  - Flipped fragment (unattached at one end).
  - Completely detached, remote fragments.
- Radial and parrot-beak tears are also associated with symptoms of internal derangement.

OTHER RECOMMENDED TESTING

- Laboratory testing to rule out inflammatory arthritis.
- Joint aspiration to rule out crystal arthropathies.
- Joint aspiration to rule out infection if diagnosis is in question.

DIFFERENTIAL DIAGNOSIS

- Tendinitis.
- Bursitis.
- Anterior cruciate ligament tear.
- Intrasubstance meniscal tear not involving the articular surface.
- Complete meniscal tear.
- Meniscal flap tear.

TREATMENT

- Conservative treatment consisting of local heat, cold, simple analgesics, and nonsteroidal anti-inflammatory agents will improve symptoms in many cases.
- Physical therapy, including gentle stretching, range-of-motion exercises, and deep heat modalities, may be beneficial in selected patients.
- Injection with local anesthetic and steroid will provide symptomatic relief if conservative therapy fails or if the pain is limiting activities of daily living.
- Surgery usually required for persistent pain or progressive functional disability and locking of knee.

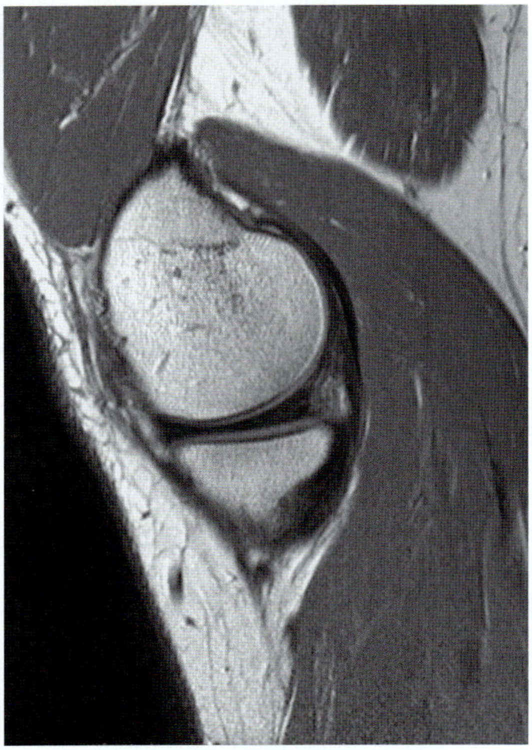

Figure 146.1 Parasagittal proton density MR image of the middle third of the medial meniscus in a normal knee with normal meniscal size and morphology.

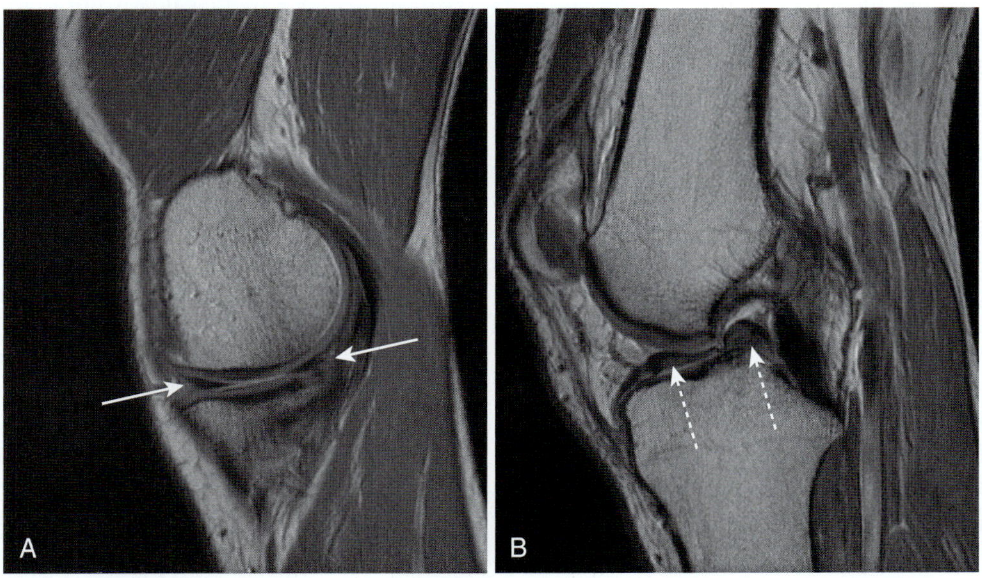

Figure 146.2 Bucket-handle tear of the medial meniscus. **(A)**, The parasagittal proton density MR image shows a much smaller meniscus (*white arrows*) than the normal meniscus shown in Figure 146.1. **(B)**, The sagittal proton density MR image through the level of the intercondylar notch shows the displaced bucket-handle fragment of the medial meniscus (*broken white arrows*) lying inferior and anterior to the PCL.

(Continued)

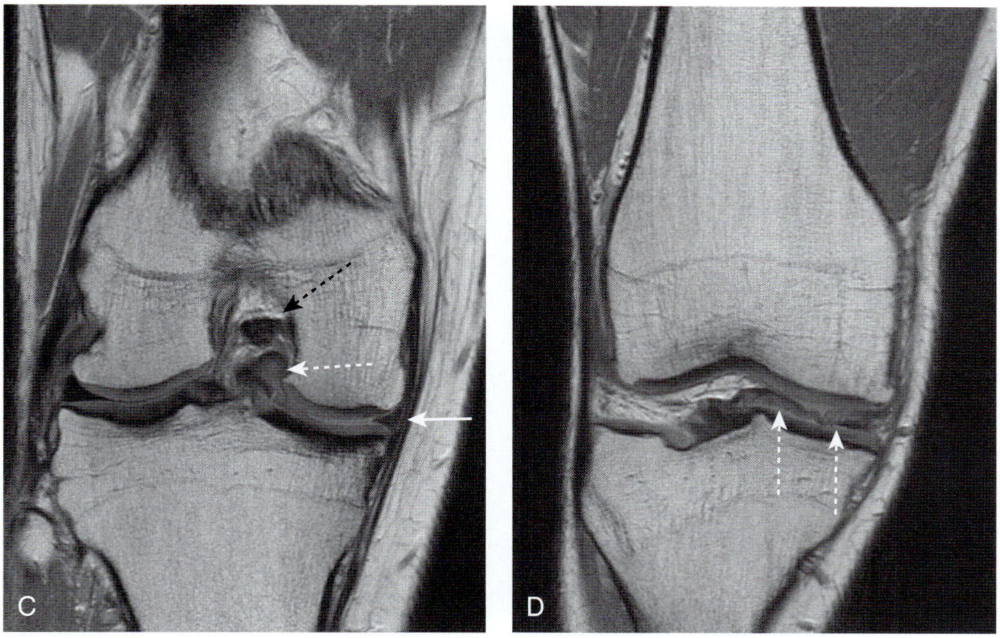

Figure 146.2—Cont'd. (C), The correlative coronal proton density image shows the diminutive meniscal fragment (*white arrow*), with the displaced and degenerated bucket-handle fragment (*broken white arrow*) lying inferior to the PCL (*broken black arrow*). (D), A more anterior coronal proton density MR image shows the intact connection between the meniscal remnant and the bucket handle fragment (*broken white arrows*).

CHAPTER 147

Anterior Cruciate Ligament Tear

DEFINITION

- Tear of the anterior cruciate ligament (ACL) of the knee, most commonly due to trauma involving forward translation of the tibia combined with external rotation of the femur and valgus stress on the joint.

SIGNS AND SYMPTOMS

- Acute onset of knee pain after acute trauma.
- Effusion of the knee common.
- Decreased range of the knee joint due to effusion and pain.
- Difficulty ambulating on affected knee.
- Feeling of weakness or giving way.
- Clicking often present.
- Anterior drawer sign usually present.
- Lachman test result often positive.
- Pivot shift test result often positive.
- Exacerbation of pain with activity.

DEMOGRAPHICS

- Incidence: Female > Male.
- All ages affected but most commonly younger patients after acute trauma.
- May occur secondary to repetitive stress injuries.
- Common after basketball, soccer, football, tennis, snow skiing, and hockey injuries.

IMAGING RECOMMENDATIONS

- Radiography:
  - Acute osteochondral fractures.
- MRI.

IMAGING FINDINGS

- Joint effusion.
- Low-lying ACL within the intercondylar notch:
  - Tears at proximal attachment: "empty notch" sign.
  - Complete absence of the ACL in chronic tears.
- Forward subluxation of tibia and bowing of posterior cruciate ligament (PCL).
- Impaction injuries with contusional bone bruising:
  - Weight-bearing surface of the lateral femoral condyle.
  - Posterior aspect of the lateral tibial plateau.
  - Secondary to pivot-shift injury.
- Associated injuries:
  - Medial collateral ligament (MCL) tear.
  - Meniscal tear.
  - Posterolateral corner of the knee.

OTHER RECOMMENDED TESTING

- Laboratory testing to rule out inflammatory arthritis.
- Joint aspiration to rule out crystal arthropathies.
- Joint aspiration to rule out infection if diagnosis in question.

DIFFERENTIAL DIAGNOSIS

- Tendinitis.
- Bursitis.
- PCL tear.
- Partial-thickness meniscal tear.
- Complete meniscal tear.
- Bucket-handle meniscal tear.
- Mucoid degeneration of the ACL.
- Meniscal flap tear.

TREATMENT

- Conservative treatment consisting of local heat, cold, simple analgesics, and nonsteroidal anti-inflammatory agents will improve symptoms in many cases.
- Physical therapy, including gentle stretching, range-of-motion exercises, and deep heat modalities, may be beneficial in selected patients.
- Injection with local anesthetic and steroid will provide symptomatic relief if conservative therapy fails or the pain is limiting activities of daily living.
- Surgery often required for persistent pain or progressive functional disability of the knee.

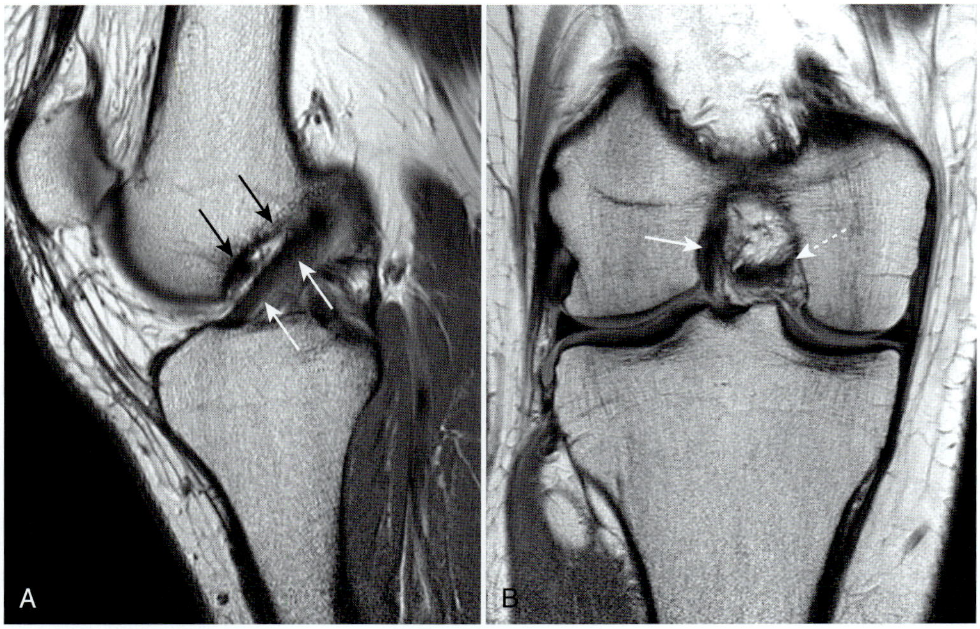

Figure 147.1 Sagittal (**A**) and coronal (**B**) proton density (PD) MR images of a normal ACL. The ligament (*white arrows*) has low signal intensity (SI). It lies parallel to the line of the intercondylar roof (*black arrows*) on the sagittal image, and lateral to the PCL on the coronal image (broken arrow).

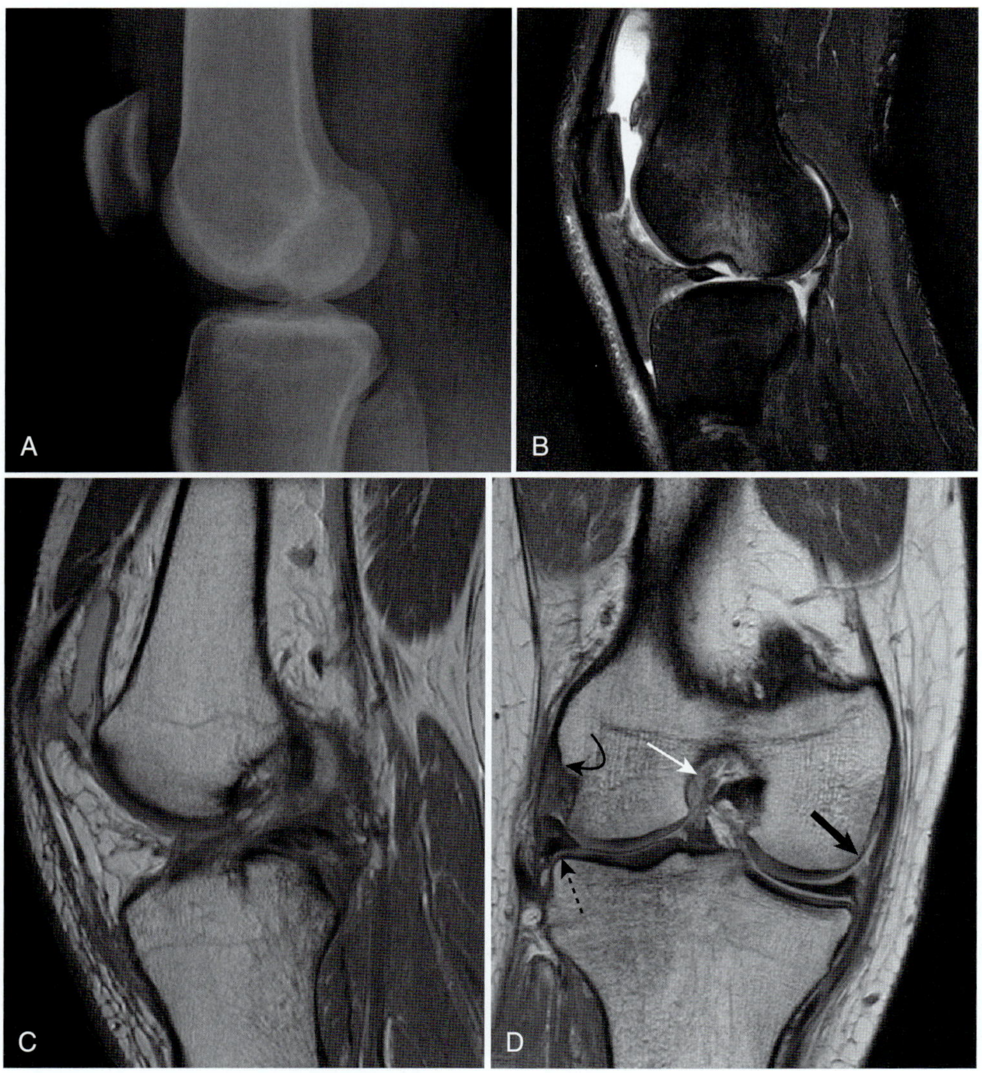

Figure 147.2 Acute complete ACL rupture. (**A**), Lateral radiograph shows an impaction fracture of the lateral femoral condyle. (**B**), The fracture is clearly seen on the sagittal T2-weighted with fat suppression (FST2W) MR image, with associated trabecular bone bruising in the lateral femoral condyle and a large joint effusion. (**C**), On the sagittal PD MR image, there is nonvisualization of the ligament. (**D**), The coronal PD image demonstrates the "empty notch" sign (*white arrow*). There is also a lateral meniscal tear (*broken black arrow*), a partial tear of the lateral collateral ligament (*curved black arrow*), and a grade II tear of the MCL, including disruption of the meniscofemoral component of the deep fibers of the MCL (*black arrow*).

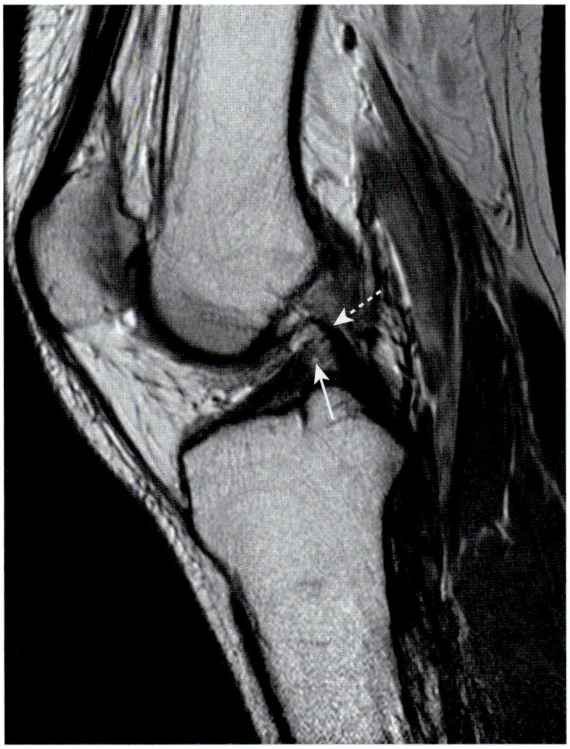

Figure 147.3 Sagittal PD MR image of a chronic ACL tear. The torn end of the ligament lies low within the intercondylar notch (*white arrow*), and the PCL is bowed (*broken white arrow*) because of posterior translation of the tibia on the femur.

CHAPTER 148

Posterior Cruciate Ligament Tear

DEFINITION

- Tear of the posterior cruciate ligament (PCL) of the knee, most commonly due to trauma involving posterior translation of the tibia, often with the knee in flexion.

SIGNS AND SYMPTOMS

- Acute onset of knee pain after acute trauma.
- Effusion of the knee common.
- Decreased range of the knee joint due to effusion and pain.
- Difficulty ambulating on the affected knee.
- Feeling of weakness or giving way.
- Clicking often present.
- Posterior drawer sign usually present.
- Results often positive for:
  - Godfrey sag test.
  - Reverse pivot shift test.
  - Quadriceps active test.
- Exacerbation of pain with activity.

DEMOGRAPHICS

- Incidence: Female = Male.
- All ages affected, but most commonly younger patients after acute trauma.
- May occur secondary to repetitive stress injuries.
- Common after dashboard injuries.
- Common after basketball, soccer, football, tennis, snow skiing, and hockey injuries.

IMAGING RECOMMENDATIONS

- Radiographs
  - Acute osteochondral fractures
- MRI

IMAGING FINDINGS

- Joint effusion
- Partial or interstitial tears are more common than complete ruptures
  - Incomplete: thickened ligament with increased SI on T1W and FST2W MR images
  - Complete: mid-substance disruption or proximal avulsion.
- Impaction injuries with contusional bone bruising
  - Lateral femoral condyle
  - Anterior tibia
- Associated injuries
  - ACL tear
  - Meniscal tears
  - Collateral ligament tears
  - Postero-lateral corner of the knee
  - Bony avulsion of tibial insertion of PCL
  - Anterolateral tibial fractures

OTHER RECOMMENDED TESTING

- Laboratory testing to rule out inflammatory arthritis.
- Joint aspiration to rule out crystal arthropathies.
- Joint aspiration to rule out infection if diagnosis in question.

DIFFERENTIAL DIAGNOSIS

- Tendinitis.
- Bursitis.
- Anterior cruciate ligament tear.
- Partial-thickness meniscal tear.
- Complete meniscal tear.
- Bucket-handle meniscal tear.
- Mucoid degeneration of the PCL.
- Meniscal flap tear.

TREATMENT

- Conservative treatment consisting of local heat, cold, simple analgesics, and nonsteroidal anti-inflammatory agents will improve symptoms in many cases.
- Physical therapy, including gentle stretching, range-of-motion exercises, and deep heat modalities, may be beneficial in selected patients.
- Injection with local anesthetic and steroid will provide symptomatic relief if conservative therapy fails or the pain is limiting activities of daily living.
- Surgery often required for persistent pain or progressive functional disability of the knee.

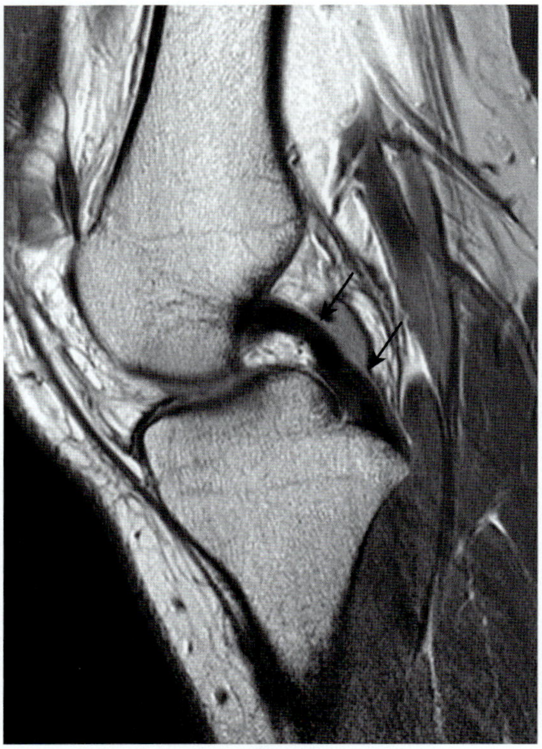

Figure148.1 Sagittal proton density (PD) MR image of a normal PCL (*black arrows*), which is a thick, low–signal intensity (SI) structure.

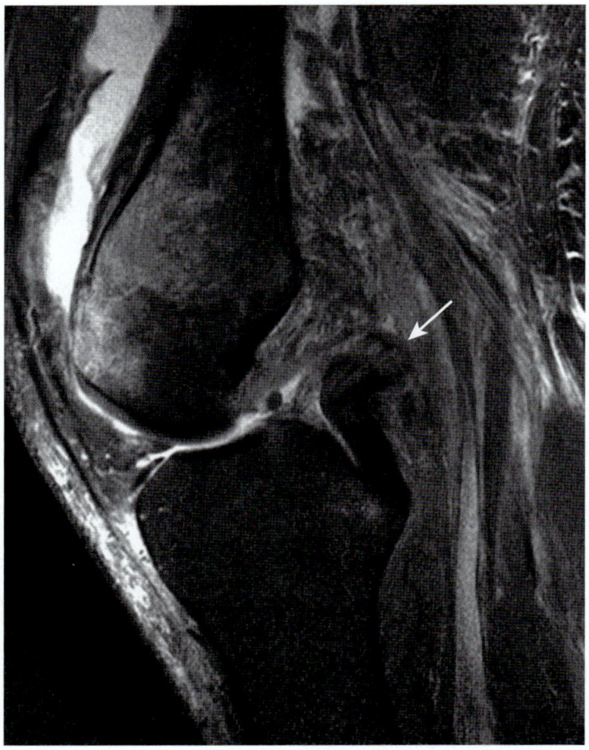

Figure 148.3 Sagittal FST2W MR image of an acute PCL tear. The proximal ligament is completely disrupted from its femoral attachment, and the torn end of the PCL is visualized (*white arrow*). Note also the prominent trabecular bone bruising in the distal femur and the prominent joint effusion.

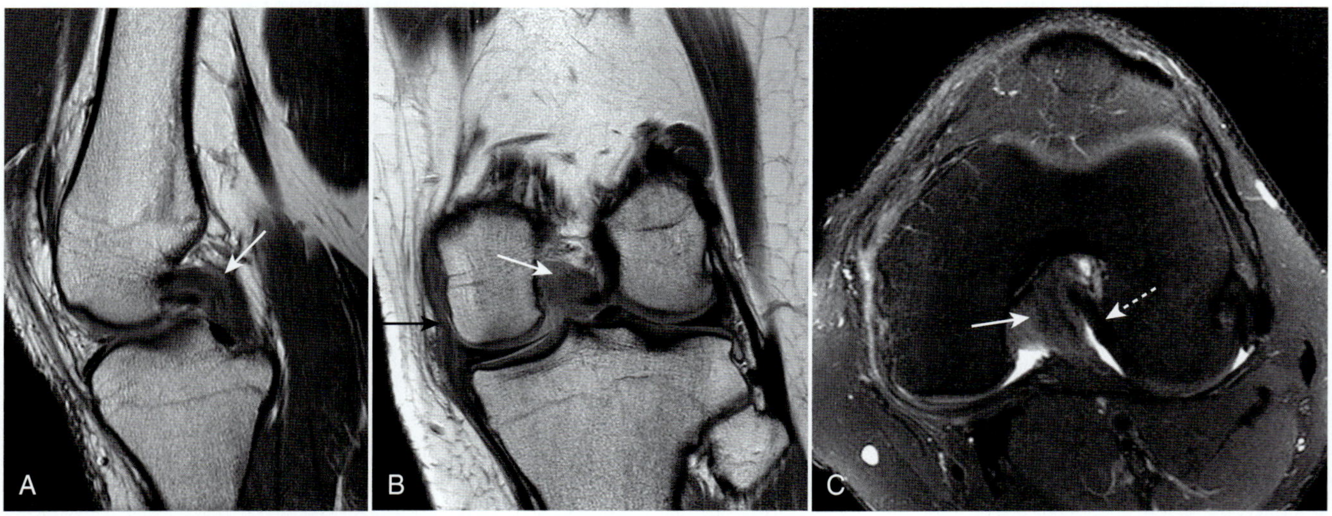

Figure 148.2 (**A**), Subacute PCL tear with diffuse increased SI within the ligament substance (*white arrow*) on the sagittal PD MR image. (**B**), The coronal PD image also shows the abnormal PCL (*white arrow*), and there is an associated grade II tear of the medial collateral ligament (*black arrow*). (**C**), The axial T2-weighted with fat suppression (FST2W) MR image shows the thickened high-SI PCL (*white arrow*) within the intercondylar notch, adjacent to the normal, low-SI anterior cruciate ligament (*broken white arrow*).

CHAPTER 149

Medial Collateral Ligament Tear

DEFINITION

- Tear of the medial collateral ligament (MCL) of the knee, most commonly due to trauma involving valgus injury to the knee.

SIGNS AND SYMPTOMS

- Acute onset of knee pain after acute trauma.
- Effusion of the knee common.
- Decreased range of the knee joint due to effusion and pain.
- Difficulty ambulating on the affected knee.
- Feeling of weakness or giving way.
- Clicking often present.
- Valgus stress test result usually positive.
- Exacerbation of pain with activity.

DEMOGRAPHICS

- Incidence: Male > Female.
- All ages affected, but most commonly younger patients after acute trauma.
- May occur secondary to repetitive stress injuries.
- Common after valgus stress injuries.
- Common after basketball, soccer, football, tennis, snow skiing, and hockey injuries.

IMAGING RECOMMENDATIONS

- Minor isolated injuries may not require imaging.
- MRI.
- US:
  - May be useful in assessing unstable ligaments.

IMAGING FINDINGS

- Usually tear is proximal.
- Three grades:
  - I: Partial tear confined to superficial fibers.
  - II: Higher-grade tear involving deep fibers.
  - III: Complete rupture.
- Increased signal intensity (SI) deep and superficial to the MCL on T2-weighted with fat suppression (FST2W) or short T1 inversion recovery (STIR) MR images.
- Thickening and low SI in chronic tears.
- Cortical bony avulsion of medial femoral epicondyle:
  - Pellegrini-Stieda lesion.
- Associated injuries:
  - Meniscal tear.
  - Anterior cruciate ligament (ACL) injury.
  - Contusional bone injury in lateral joint line.

OTHER RECOMMENDED TESTING

- Laboratory testing to rule out inflammatory arthritis.
- Joint aspiration to rule out crystal arthropathies.
- Joint aspiration to rule out infection if diagnosis in question.

DIFFERENTIAL DIAGNOSIS

- Tendinitis.
- Bursitis, especially involving tibial collateral ligament bursa.
- ACL tear.
- Posterior cruciate ligament (PCL) tear.
- Partial-thickness meniscal tear.
- Complete meniscal tear.
- Bucket-handle meniscal tear.
- Semimembranous tendinitis.
- Partial tear of the MCL.
- Meniscal flap tear.

TREATMENT

- Conservative treatment consisting of local heat, cold, simple analgesics, and nonsteroidal anti-inflammatory agents will improve symptoms in many cases.
- Physical therapy, including gentle stretching, range-of-motion exercises, and deep heat modalities, may be beneficial in selected patients.
- Injection with local anesthetic and steroid will provide symptomatic relief if conservative therapy fails or the pain is limiting activities of daily living.
- Surgery often required for persistent pain or progressive functional disability of the knee.

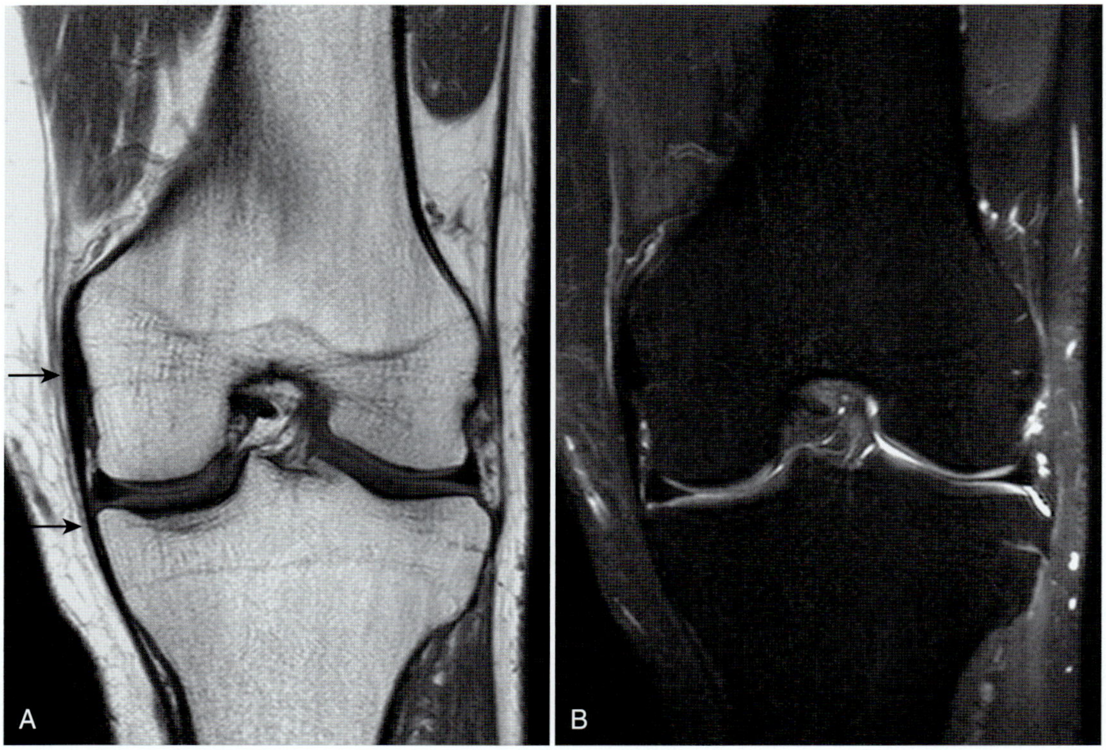

Figure 149.1 (**A**), Coronal proton density (PD) MR image of a normal low-SI MCL (*black arrows*), extending from the medial epicondyle of the femur to the proximal tibial metaphysis. (**B**), The FST2W MR image also shows the low-SI MCL. The adjacent soft tissues are normal, with no soft tissue edema.

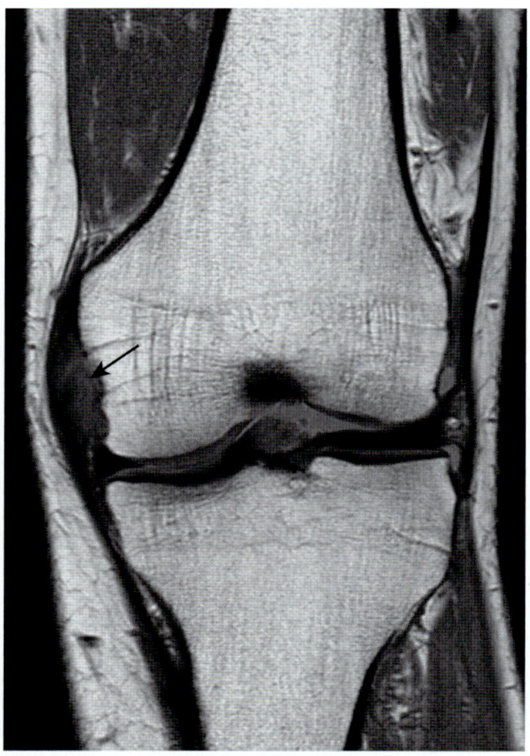

Figure 149.2 Subacute partial tear of the proximal MCL (*broken black arrow*), with thickening and increased SI of the deep fibers of the ligament on a coronal PD MR image.

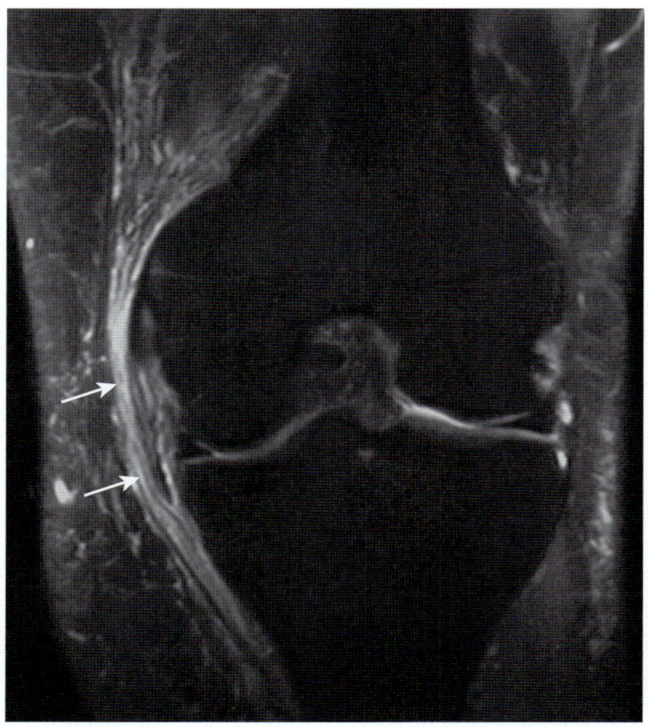

Figure 149.3 Coronal FST2W MR image of an acute grade II tear of the MCL with poorly defined ligament fibers and surrounding soft tissue edema (*white arrows*).

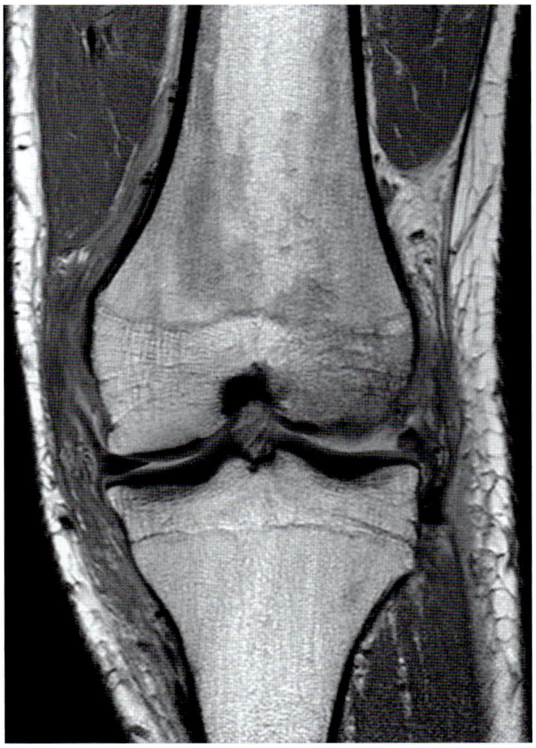

Figure 149.4 Coronal PD MR image of a grade III tear of the MCL with nonvisualization of the ligament. There is also a lateral meniscal tear.

CHAPTER 150

Lateral Collateral Ligament Tear

DEFINITION

- Tear of the lateral collateral ligament (LCL) of the knee, most commonly due to trauma involving varus injury to the knee and often occurring with the knee in external rotation.

SIGNS AND SYMPTOMS

- Acute onset of posterolateral knee pain after acute trauma.
- Effusion of the knee common.
- Decreased range of the knee joint due to effusion and pain.
- Difficulty ambulating on the affected knee.
- Feeling of weakness or giving way.
- Clicking often present.
- Varus stress test result usually positive.
- Exacerbation of pain with activity.

DEMOGRAPHICS

- Incidence: Male = Female.
- All ages affected, but most commonly younger patients after acute trauma.
- May occur secondary to repetitive stress injuries.
- Common after varus stress injuries.
- Common after basketball, soccer, football, tennis, snow skiing, and motorcycle injuries.

IMAGING RECOMMENDATIONS

- MRI.

IMAGING FINDINGS

- Joint effusion.
- Thickening and increased signal intensity (SI) within the LCL.
- Complete disruption of the LCL.
- Surrounding soft tissue edema.
- Associated injury to the popliteus tendon and other structures of the posterolateral corner of the knee.
- Associated anterior cruciate ligament (ACL) or posterior cruciate ligament (PCL) injuries.

OTHER RECOMMENDED TESTING

- Laboratory testing to rule out inflammatory arthritis.
- Joint aspiration to rule out crystal arthropathies.
- Joint aspiration to rule out infection if diagnosis in question.

DIFFERENTIAL DIAGNOSIS

- Tendinitis.
- Bursitis, especially involving the tibial collateral ligament bursa.
- Tibial plateau fracture.
- ACL tear.
- PCL tear.
- Partial-thickness meniscal tear.
- Complete meniscal tear.
- Bucket-handle meniscal tear.
- Lateral gastrocnemius tear.
- Popliteus insertional tear.
- Partial tear of the LCL.
- Meniscal flap tear.

TREATMENT

- Conservative treatment consisting of local heat, cold, simple analgesics, and nonsteroidal anti-inflammatory agents will improve symptoms in many cases.
- Physical therapy, including gentle stretching, range-of-motion exercises, and deep heat modalities, may be beneficial in selected patients.
- Injection with local anesthetic and steroid will provide symptomatic relief if conservative therapy fails or the pain is limiting activities of daily living.
- Surgery often required for persistent pain or progressive functional disability of the knee.

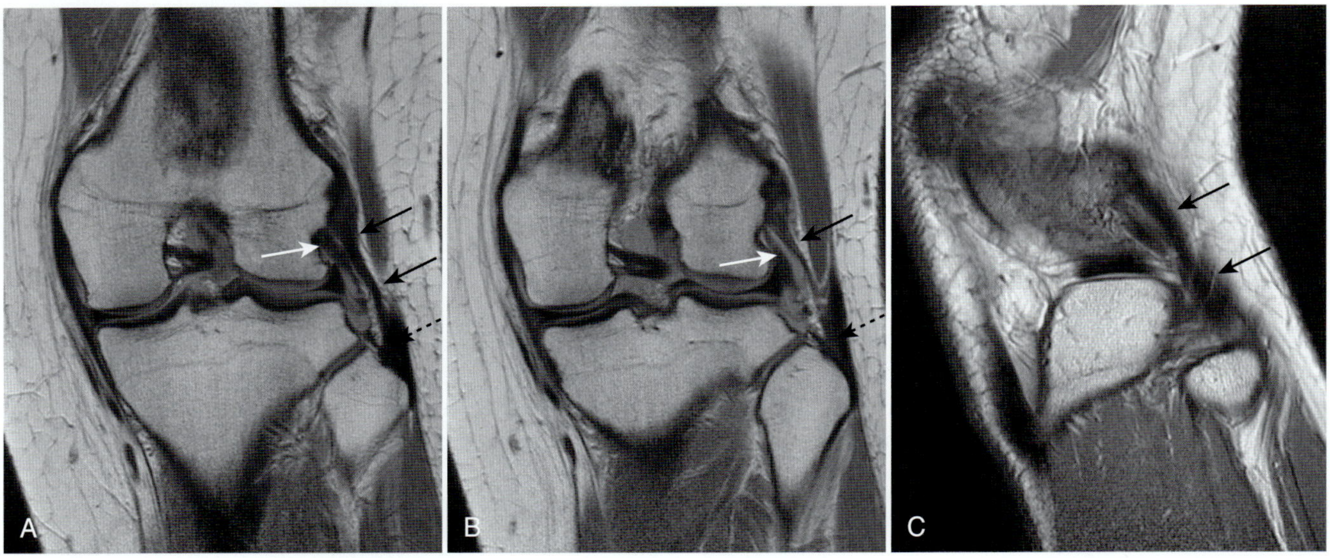

Figure 150.1 Consecutive coronal (**A** and **B**) and sagittal (**C**) proton density (PD) MR images of a normal LCL. The LCL lies in an oblique plane and is identified as a low-SI structure (*black arrows*) lying superficial to the popliteus tendon (*white arrows*). Distally, the ligament fuses with the biceps tendon to form the conjoint tendon (*broken arrows*).

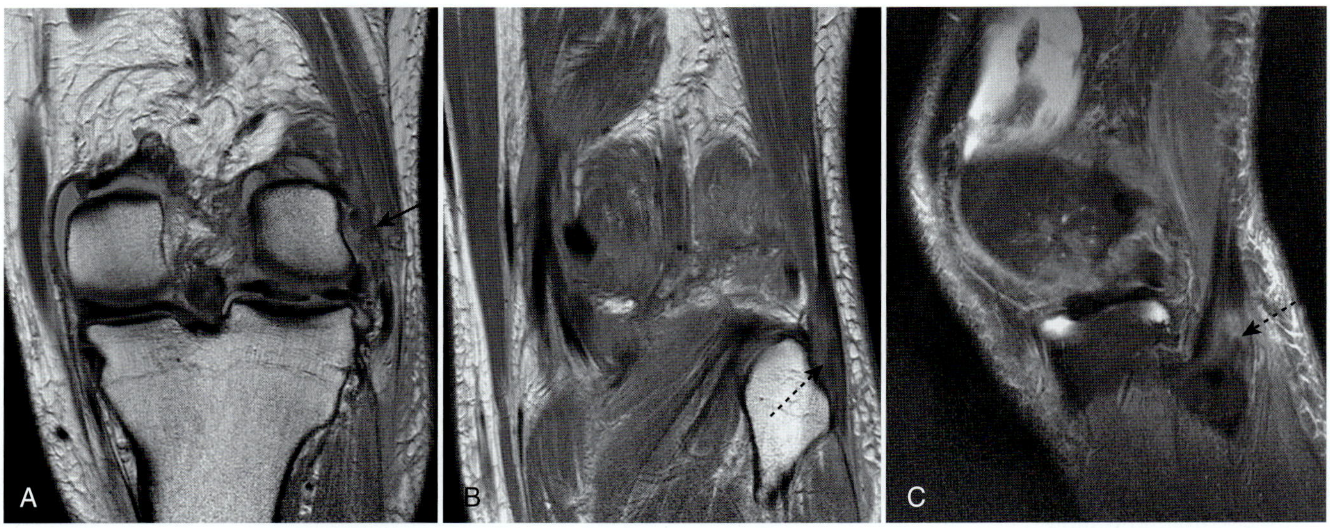

Figure 150.2 MR images of a patient with a combined LCL and PCL injury with lateral meniscal tear. (**A**), The coronal PD MR image demonstrates nonvisualization of the proximal LCL due to complete disruption of the ligament (*black arrow*). There are also thickening and increased SI within the conjoint tendon on the coronal PD MR image (**B**) and the sagittal T2-weighted with fat suppression (FST2W) MR image (**C**), due to associated partial tendon tear (*broken arrows*). Note also the surrounding soft tissue edema and joint effusion.

CHAPTER 151

Iliotibial Band Syndrome

DEFINITION

- Overuse syndrome caused by inflammation of the iliotibial band caused by repetitive frictional trauma as the iliotibial band rubs across the lateral femoral condyle.

SIGNS AND SYMPTOMS

- Pain with flexion and extension of the knee at the point of the lateral condyle of the femur.
- Point tenderness at lateral condyle of the femur.
- Asymptomatic at rest.
- Pain worsens with activity.
- Positive Ober test result.
- Positive Noble test result.
- Bursitis often coexists.
- Patient unable to sleep on the affected knee.

DEMOGRAPHICS

- Incidence: Female = Male.
- Most common between the second and fourth decades of life.
- Young athletes often affected.
- More common after trauma, including repetitive stress injuries.
- Increased incidence in joggers, skiers, weight lifters, and cyclists.

IMAGING RECOMMENDATIONS

- MRI.
- US:
  - Also used to guide therapeutic injection.

IMAGING FINDINGS

- Thickening of iliotibial band at the level of the lateral femoral epicondyle.
- Fluid deep to the iliotibial band.
- Superficial edema.

OTHER RECOMMENDED TESTING

- Laboratory testing to rule out inflammatory arthritis.
- Bursa aspiration with Gram staining and culture and sensitivity testing if infection in question.
- Joint aspiration to rule out crystal arthropathies.
- Joint aspiration to rule out infection if diagnosis in question.

DIFFERENTIAL DIAGNOSIS

- Calcific tendinitis.
- Avulsion fractures.
- Lateral collateral ligament tears.
- Osteoarthritis of the knee.
- Inflammatory arthritis of the knee.
- Neoplasm.
- Muscle strains and tears.
- Infrapatellar bursitis.
- Tibial plateau fractures.
- Septic arthritis of the knee.

TREATMENT

- Conservative treatment consisting of local heat, cold, simple analgesics, and nonsteroidal anti-inflammatory agents will improve symptoms in mild cases.
- Physical therapy, including gentle stretching, range-of-motion exercises, and deep heat modalities, may be beneficial in selected patients.
- Band orthotic devices to prevent friction often helpful.
- Injection with local anesthetic and steroid will provide symptomatic relief if conservative therapy fails or the pain is limiting activities of daily living.
- Surgery may be required for persistent pain or progressive functional disability.

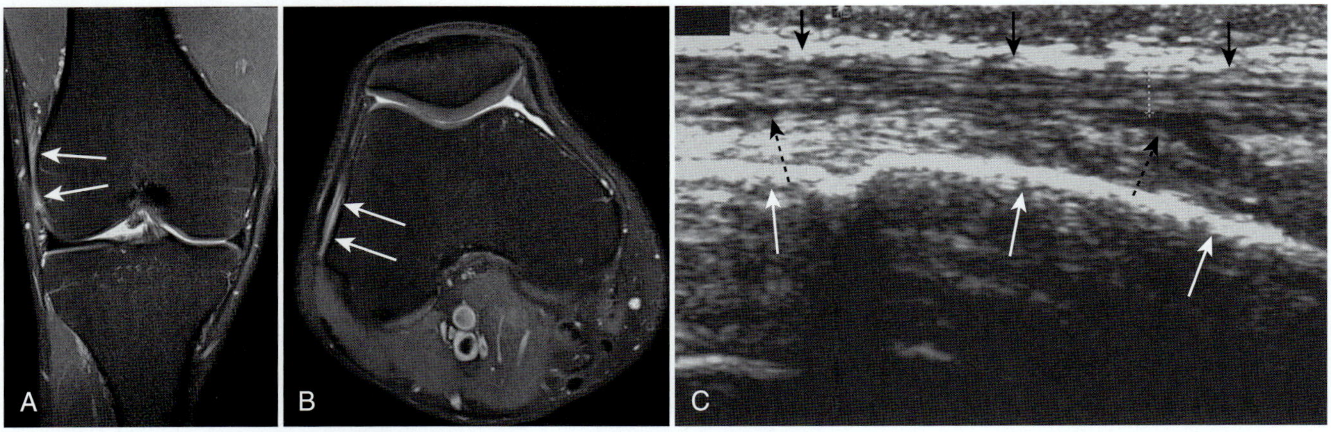

Figure 151.1 Coronal (**A**) and axial (**B**) T2-weighted with fat suppression (FST2W) MR images of a runner with lateral joint pain. There is high–signal intensity (SI) fluid (*white arrows*) lying between the femoral epicondyle and the iliotibial band; it is due to iliotibial band friction syndrome. (*Note:* It is important not to mistake joint fluid in the parapatellar recess for iliotibial bursitis.) (**C**), The correlative transverse US image acquired during imaging-guided injection shows the echo-bright epicondyle (*white arrows*) and the iliotibial band (*black arrows*) with a thin layer of intervening fluid (*broken black arrows*).

CHAPTER 152

Osteochondritis Dissecans of the Knee Joint

DEFINITION

- The death of cellular components of bone due to interruption of the blood supply, with resultant pain and collapse and destruction of bone, followed by reossification and partial healing, with loss of function due to loose intra-articular bone fragments.

SIGNS AND SYMPTOMS

- Gradual onset of pain with decreasing range of motion of the knee joint.
- Crepitus may be present.
- Clicking and catching sensation common.
- Locking common with significant loose fragments.
- Antalgic gait.
- Functional disability may be severe.

DEMOGRAPHICS

- Incidence: Male > Female.
- Most common in 10- to 20-year old patients.
- Age of onset related to date of trauma.
- Most common following knee joint trauma that disrupts vascular supply.
- More common in patients with sickle cell disease.

IMAGING RECOMMENDATIONS

- Radiography.
- MRI.
- MR/CT arthrography:
  - May have a role for differentiating stable from unstable lesions.

IMAGING FINDINGS

- Osteochondral defect on radiographs:
  - Concavity on surface of condyle.
  - Bony fragment with lucency at base.
- Common sites:
  - Lateral aspect of medial femoral condyle: 60%.
  - Weight-bearing medial femoral condyle: 25%.
  - Lateral femoral condyle: 15%.
- Bony fragment may be in situ or remote within the joint.
- Features that favor an unstable in situ fragment:
  - High-signal intensity (SI) rim on T2-weighted (T2W) or short T1 inversion recovery (STIR) MR images at base of lesion.
  - Cyst formation and edema at base of lesion.
  - Breach of articular cartilage.
- CT arthrography may improve accuracy in equivocal cases by better visualizing the breach of the articular cartilage and tracking of contrast agent around the base of the lesion.
- Factors indicating poor prognosis for nonoperative treatment:
  - Adult patient.
  - Lesion > 20 mm.
  - Weight-bearing surface of condyle.
  - Joint effusion.
  - Cartilage breach.

OTHER RECOMMENDED TESTING

- Laboratory testing to rule out juvenile rheumatoid arthritis.
- Laboratory testing to rule out causes of osteoporosis if present.
- Joint aspiration to rule out crystal arthropathies.
- Joint aspiration to rule out infection.

DIFFERENTIAL DIAGNOSIS

- Inflammatory arthritides.
- Osteoarthritis.
- Bone marrow tumors.
- Primary bone tumors.
- Metastatic tumors.
- Osteochondral injuries.
- Stress fractures.
- Insufficiency fractures, especially in older patients.

TREATMENT

- Conservative treatment consisting of local heat, cold, simple analgesics, and nonsteroidal anti-inflammatory agents will improve symptoms in many cases.
- Physical therapy, including gentle stretching, range-of-motion exercises, and deep heat modalities, may be beneficial in selected patients.
- Intra-articular injection with local anesthetic and steroid will provide symptomatic relief if conservative therapy fails or the pain is limiting activities of daily living.
- Surgery may ultimately be required for persistent pain or progressive functional disability, especially in the presence of large joint mice.

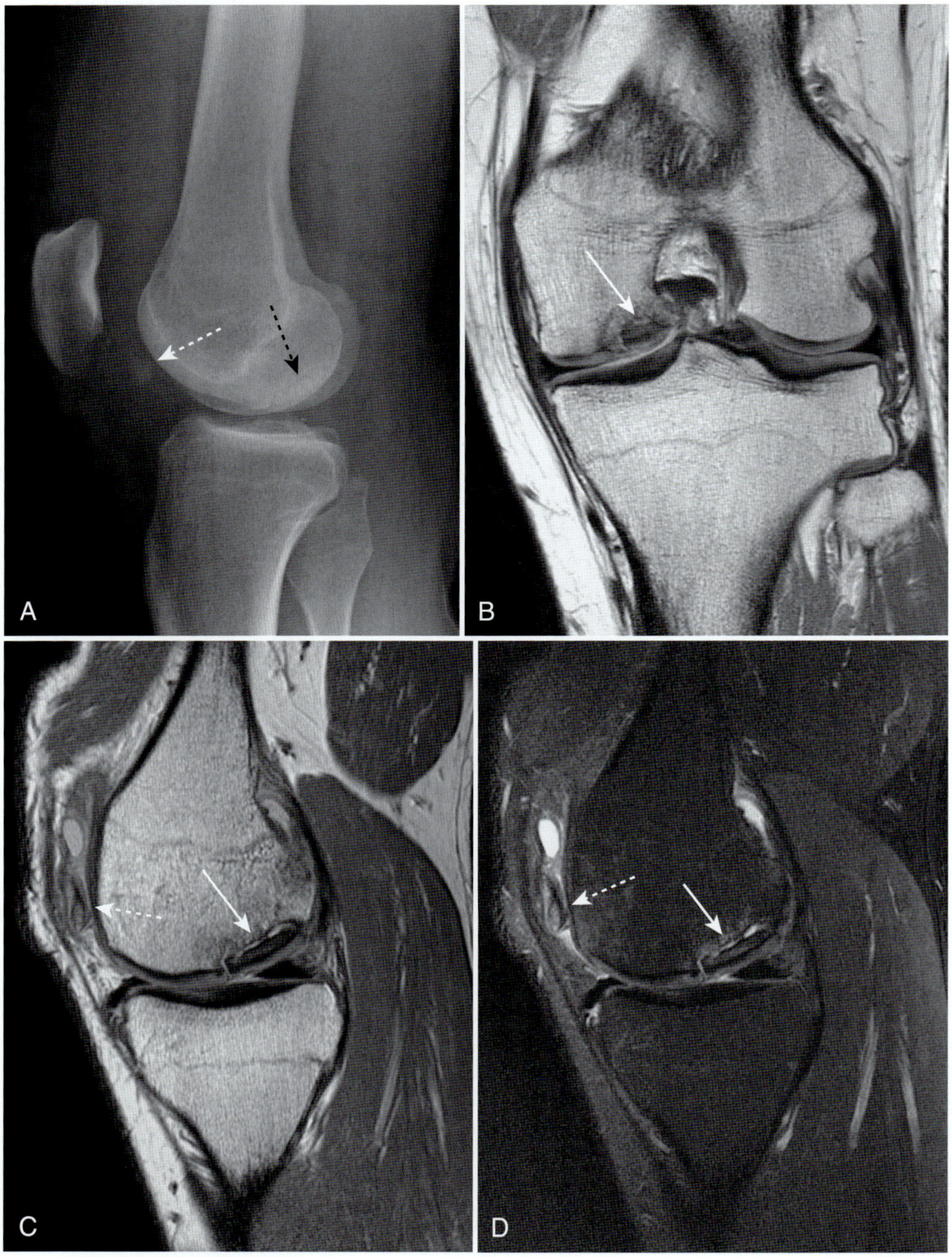

Figure 152.1 (A), Lateral radiograph of the knee demonstrating a focal area of osteochondritis dissecans (OCD) on the medial femoral condyle (*broken black arrow*), with a subchondral lucency. There is also a detached and loose intra-articular body (*broken white arrow*). (B), The corresponding coronal proton density MR image shows the osteochondral fragment (*white arrow*) with high SI at the base of the lesion and a focal breach in the articular cartilage. The high-SI fluid at the rim of the lesion is better appreciated on the sagittal proton density (C) and T2W with fat suppression (FST2W) (D) MR images (*white arrows*). These findings indicate a loose fragment in situ. The detached loose body is also evident (*broken white arrows*).

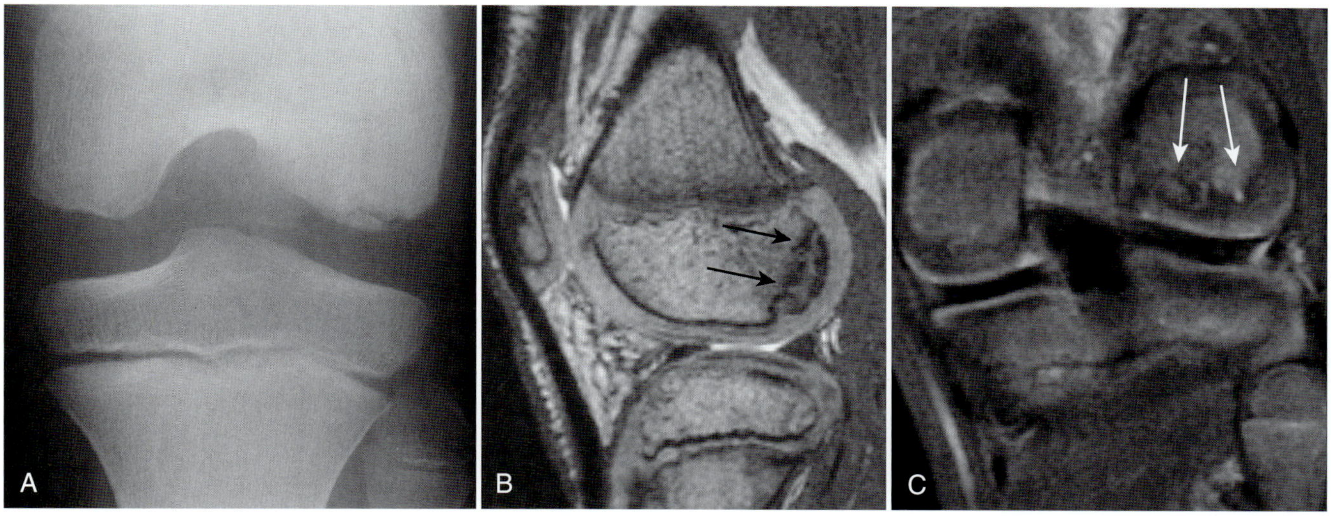

Figure 152.2 (A), AP radiograph of 14-year-old patient with knee pain. There is apparent fragmentation of the lateral femoral condyle. (B), The sagittal gradient echo MR image demonstrates the osseous fragmentation (*black arrows*), but with intact overlying articular cartilage. (C), The coronal STIR image shows relatively normal SI of the adjacent subchondral bone without significant edema or a high-SI rim (*white arrows*). This was considered to be a normal variant of ossification rather than OCD, and follow-up radiographs showed progressive normal bony maturation of the subchondral epiphysis.

CHAPTER 153

Osteonecrosis of the Knee

DEFINITION

- The death of cellular components of bone due to interruption of the blood supply, with resultant pain, collapse and destruction of bone, and loss of function.

SIGNS AND SYMPTOMS

- Gradual onset of pain with decreasing range of motion of the knee joint.
- Crepitus may be present.
- Functional disability may be severe.

DEMOGRAPHICS

- Incidence: Male > Female.
- Age at onset related to date of trauma or onset of underlying disease, with sickle cell disease being the most common inciting factor in younger patients.
- Most common following knee joint trauma that disrupts vascular supply.
- More common in patients with sickle cell disease, Gaucher disease, Fabry disease, systemic lupus erythematosus (SLE), and gout.
- Often associated with administration of exogenous steroids.
- Often associated with heavy alcohol intake.
- Spontaneous osteonecrosis of the knee (SONK) in elderly women is actually usually due to osteochondral insufficiency fractures.

IMAGING RECOMMENDATIONS

- Radiography.
- MRI:
  - Normal or equivocal radiographic findings.
  - Preoperative planning.

IMAGING FINDINGS

- Radiography:
  - Sclerosis in the subarticular femoral condyle: Tibial condyles are less frequently affected.
  - Subchondral lucency and collapse often occur early, leading to fragmentation and destruction of articular surface.
  - Serpiginous lines of sclerosis in intramedullary infarcts.
- MRI:
  - Diffuse high–signal intensity (SI) edema pattern on short T1 inversion recovery (STIR) MR images.
  - Low-SI subchondral sclerosis on T1-weighted (T1W) and T2W MR images.
  - High-SI subchondral rim of fluid on T2W or STIR MR images.
  - Subchondral crescent sign.
  - Eventual subchondral collapse and fragmentation.
  - Double-line sign of intramedullary infarcts on T2W MR images: Granulation tissue lining areas of sclerosis

OTHER RECOMMENDED TESTING

- Laboratory testing to rule out SLE.
- Laboratory testing to rule out gout.
- Joint aspiration to rule out crystal arthropathies.
- Joint aspiration to rule out infection.

DIFFERENTIAL DIAGNOSIS

- Inflammatory arthritides, especially SLE.
- Osteoarthritis.
- Bone marrow tumors.
- Primary bone tumors.
- Metastatic tumors.
- Osteochondral injuries.
- Osteochondrosis dissecans in younger patients.

TREATMENT

- Conservative treatment consisting of local heat, cold, simple analgesics, and nonsteroidal anti-inflammatory agents will improve symptoms in many cases.
- Non–weight-bearing status for osteochondral osteonecrosis or insufficiency fractures.
- Physical therapy, including gentle stretching, range-of-motion exercises, and deep heat modalities, may be beneficial in selected patients.
- Intra-articular injection with local anesthetic and steroid will provide symptomatic relief if conservative therapy fails or the pain is limiting activities of daily living.
- Surgery may ultimately be required for persistent pain or progressive functional disability.

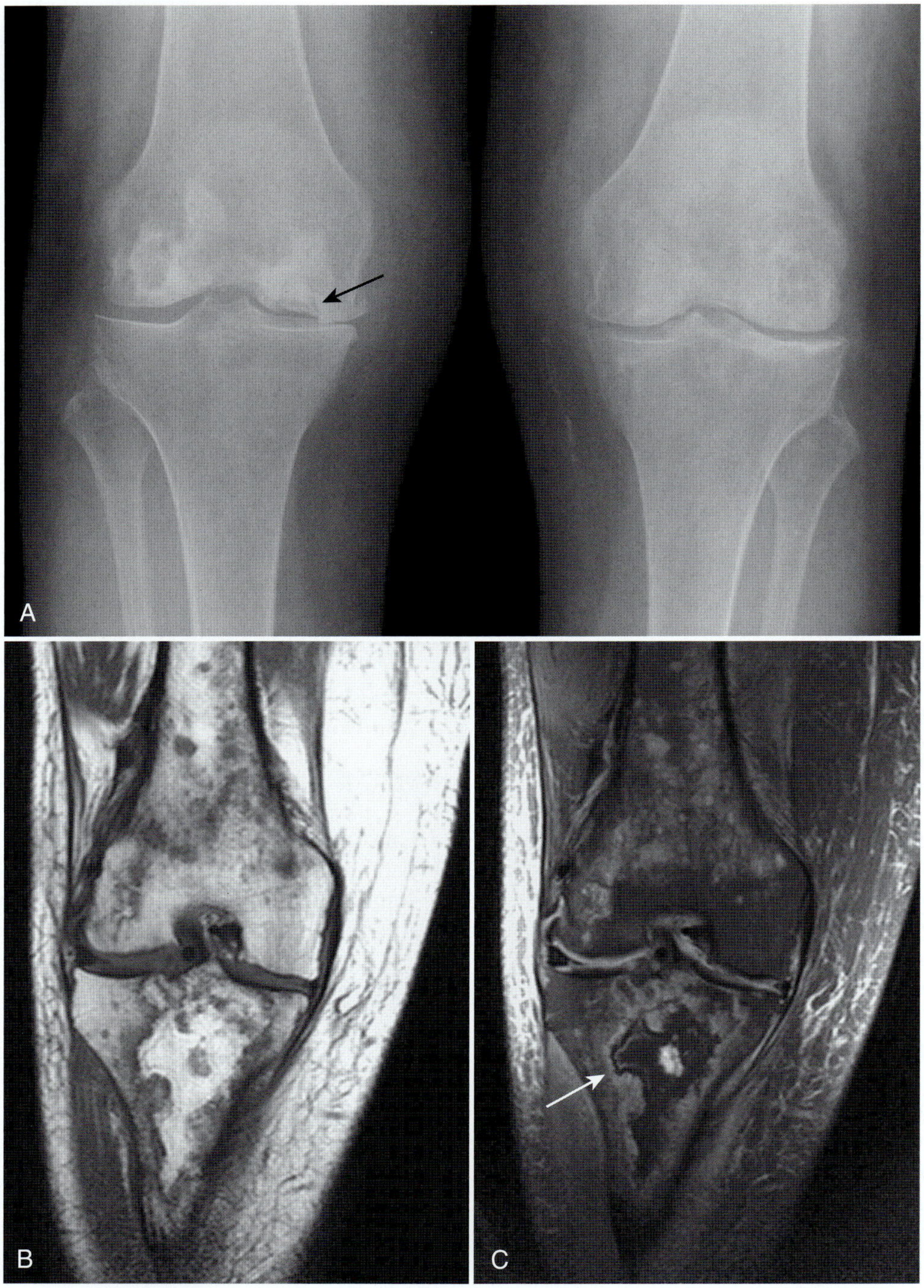

Figure 153.1 (**A**), AP radiographs of both knees in a patient undergoing long-term steroid therapy. There are areas of sclerosis in both distal femoral condyles. This finding is most marked in the right medial femoral condyle, which contains an area of subchondral collapse and fragmentation (*black arrow*). The coronal T1W (**B**) and T2W with fat suppression (FST2W) (**C**) MR images of the right knee also show an intramedullary infarct within the proximal tibia, which was not evident on the radiographs. Note the typical serpiginous lines at the periphery of the infarct (*white arrow*) with a double-line sign.

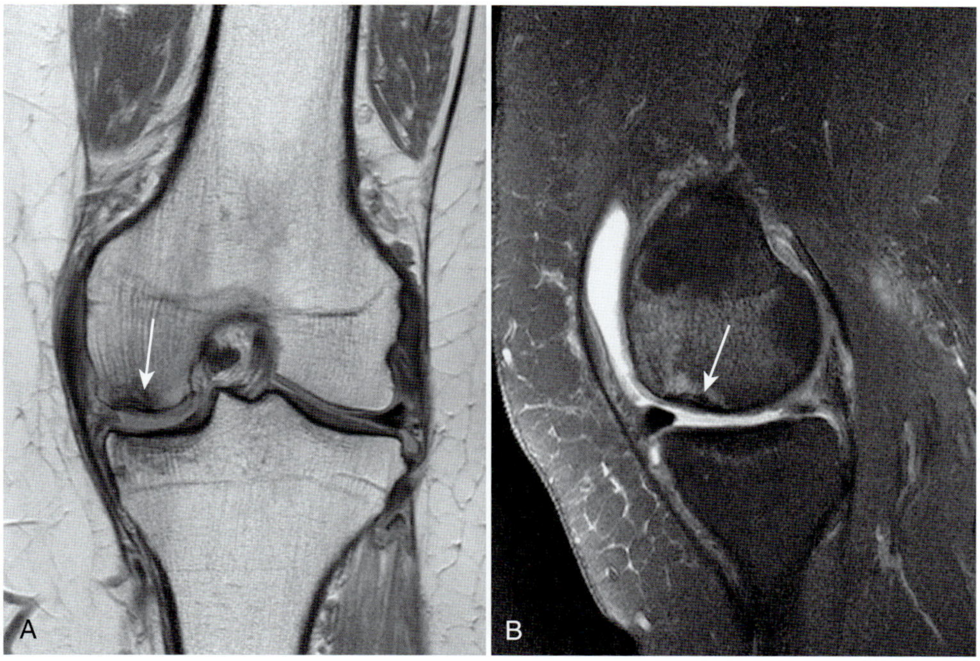

Figure 153.2 Elderly woman with sudden onset of nontraumatic knee pain. The coronal proton density (**A**) and sagittal FST2W (**B**) MR images show a low-SI subchondral crescent with early subchondral collapse (*white arrows*) and a surrounding diffuse edema pattern. The patient had no risk factors for osteonecrosis, and these appearances are consistent with a simple insufficiency fracture rather than avascular necrosis. Note also the presence of a medial meniscal tear.

CHAPTER 154

Patellar Tendinopathy

DEFINITION

- Degeneration of the patellar tendon due to repetitive microtrauma to the musculotendinous unit.

SIGNS AND SYMPTOMS

- Gradual onset of dull, ill-defined anterior knee pain.
- Pain often radiates into the infrapatellar region.
- Tenderness over the infrapatellar tendon.
- Pain with movement of the patella.
- Excessive pronation of the foot often present.
- Crepitus may be present.
- Creaking may be present.
- Exacerbation of pain with resisted extension of the lower leg.
- Patient unable to sleep on the affected knee.

DEMOGRAPHICS

- Incidence: Male = Female.
- Young athletes involved in jumping activities often affected.
- 30- to 50-year-old persons most commonly affected.
- More common after trauma, including repetitive stress injuries.

IMAGING RECOMMENDATIONS

- MRI or US.

IMAGING FINDINGS

- Three patterns of involvement:
  - Proximal tendon (commonest type).
  - Distal tendon.
  - Diffuse tendon involvement.
- Thickening of the affected portion of the tendon.
- Increased signal intensity (SI) on all MR pulse sequences.
- Fluid SI intensity within the tendon substance on T2-weighted (T2W) or T2W with fat suppression (FST2W) MR images is suggestive of partial tendon tear.
- Low reflectivity of tendon on US with neovascularization on Doppler imaging.
- Areas of microcalcification may be seen in chronic tendon degeneration on US.
- Associated prepatellar, superficial, and deep infrapatellar bursitis may be present.

OTHER RECOMMENDED TESTING

- Laboratory testing to rule out inflammatory arthritis.
- Joint aspiration to rule out crystal arthropathies.
- Joint aspiration to rule out infection if diagnosis in question.

DIFFERENTIAL DIAGNOSIS

- Calcific tendinitis.
- Partial-thickness infrapatellar tendon tear.
- Prepatellar bursitis.
- Infrapatellar bursitis.
- Osgood-Schlatter disease.
- Osteoarthritis.
- Inflammatory arthritis.
- Sinding-Larsen-Johansson disease.

TREATMENT

- Conservative treatment consisting of local heat, cold, simple analgesics, and nonsteroidal anti-inflammatory agents will improve symptoms in many cases.
- Physical therapy, including gentle stretching, range-of-motion exercises, and deep heat modalities, may be beneficial in selected patients.
- Injection with local anesthetic and steroid will provide symptomatic relief if conservative therapy fails or the pain is limiting activities of daily living.
- Surgery may be required for persistent pain or progressive functional disability.

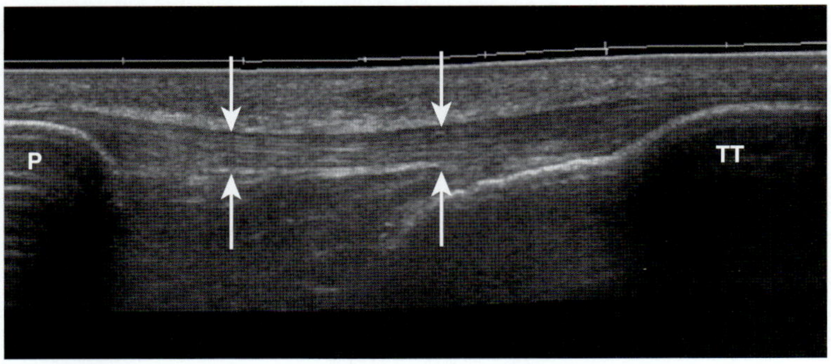

Figure 154.1 Longitudinal US image of a normal patellar tendon. The tendon is demonstrated as an echogenic structure with an echo-bright tendon sheath (*white arrows*) extending from the patella (P) to the tibial tuberosity (TT).

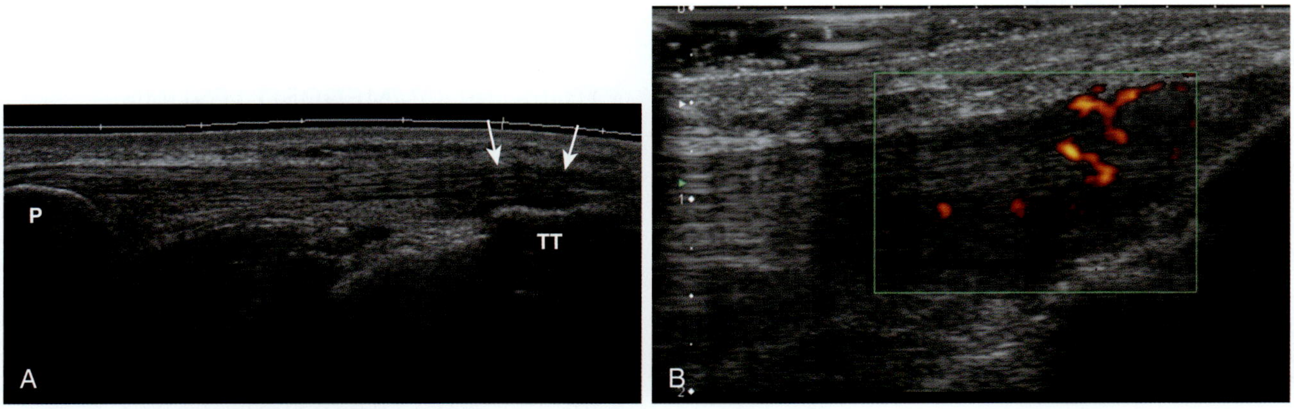

Figure 154.2 (A), Longitudinal US image of a patient with distal patellar tendinopathy. The distal tendon (*white arrows*) is thickened, hyporeflective, and poorly defined. (B), The Doppler US image demonstrates the tendon thickening and neovascularization.

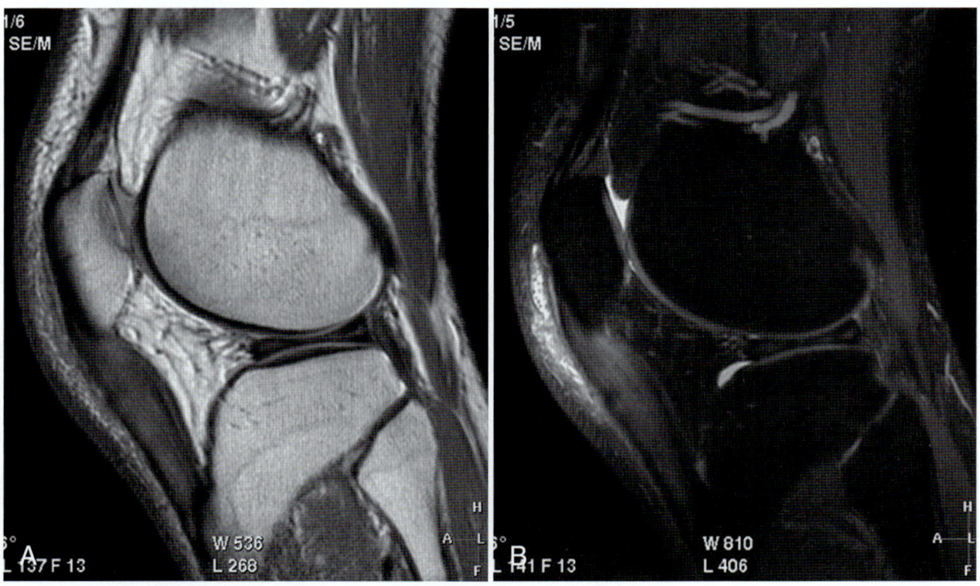

Figure 154.3 Sagittal T1W (A) and FST2W (B) MR images of a patient with diffuse patellar tendinopathy. The tendon is thickened and of increased SI on both pulse sequences, but the SI is not as bright as that of fluid on the FST2W MR image. High-SI prepatellar bursitis is also evident on the FST2W MR image.

CHAPTER 155

Osgood-Schlatter Disease

DEFINITION

- Apophysitis at the site of the patellar ligament insertion on the anterior tibial tubercle due to repetitive microtrauma.

SIGNS AND SYMPTOMS

- Gradual onset of dull, ill-defined anterior knee pain.
- Pain often radiates into the infrapatellar region.
- Tenderness over the anterior tibial tubercle.
- Swelling of the anterior tibial tubercle.
- Pain with resisted knee extension.
- Worse with activity.
- Antalgic gait.
- Patient unable to sleep on the affected knee.

DEMOGRAPHICS

- Incidence: Male > Female.
- Young athletes involved in jumping activities often affected.
- Eight to 15-year old persons most commonly affected.
- More common after trauma, including repetitive stress injuries.
- Bilateral in 20% to 25% of patients.

IMAGING RECOMMENDATIONS

- Imaging not routinely required.
- Radiography.
- MRI or US.

IMAGING FINDINGS

- Bony fragmentation of tibial tuberosity.
- Associated tendinopathy:
  - Distal patellar tendon thickening.
  - Increased signal intensity (SI) in distal tendon on MRI.
- Associated deep and superficial infrapatellar bursitis.

OTHER RECOMMENDED TESTING

- Laboratory testing to rule out inflammatory arthritis.
- Joint aspiration to rule out crystal arthropathies.
- Joint aspiration to rule out infection if diagnosis is in question.

DIFFERENTIAL DIAGNOSIS

- Calcific tendinitis.
- Partial-thickness infrapatellar tendon tear.
- Prepatellar bursitis.
- Infrapatellar bursitis.
- Osteochondritis dissecans.
- Osteoarthritis.
- Inflammatory arthritis.
- Neoplasm.
- Sinding-Larsen-Johansson disease.

TREATMENT

- Conservative treatment consisting of local heat, cold, simple analgesics, and nonsteroidal anti-inflammatory agents will improve symptoms in many cases.
- Physical therapy, including gentle stretching, range-of-motion exercises, and deep heat modalities, may be beneficial in selected patients.
- Injection with local anesthetic and steroid will provide symptomatic relief if conservative therapy fails or the pain is limiting activities of daily living.
- Surgery may be required for persistent pain or progressive functional disability.

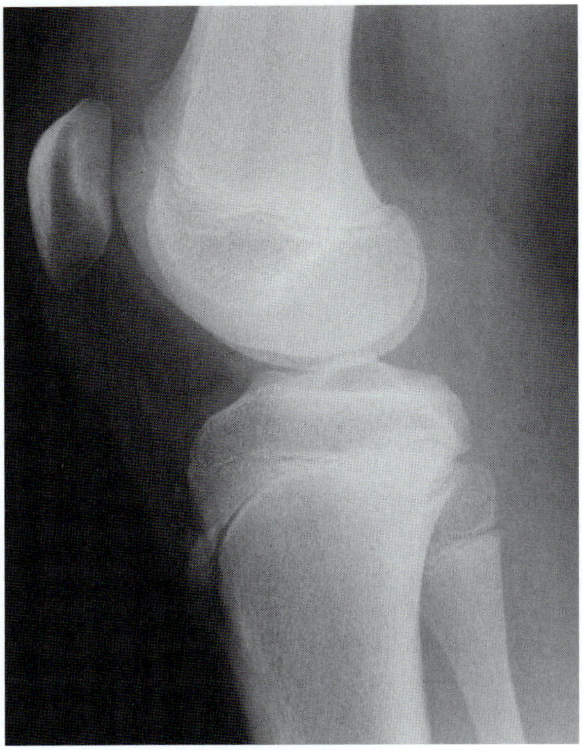

Figure 155.1 Lateral radiograph of an adolescent with anterior knee pain, demonstrating fragmentation of the tibial tuberosity due to Osgood-Schlatter disease.

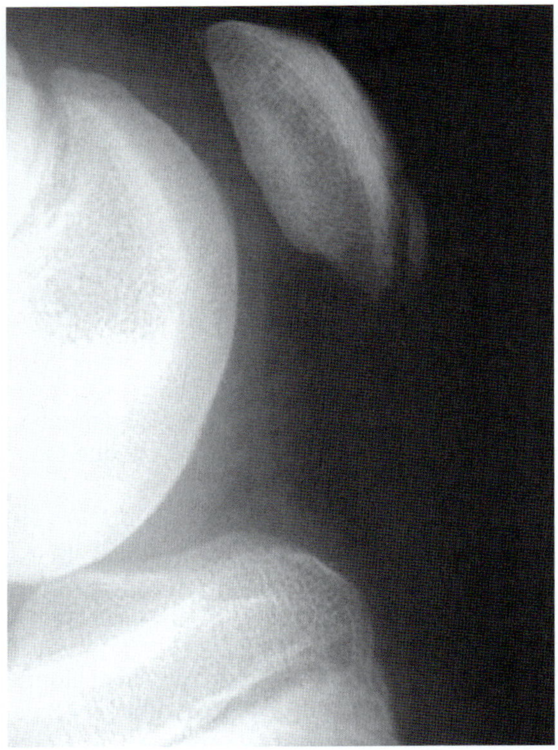

Figure 155.3 Lateral radiograph of a juvenile with pain over the patella. There is fragmentation of the lower pole of the patella due to apophysitis (Sinding-Larsen-Johansson disease), which is the same process as Osgood-Schlatter disease.

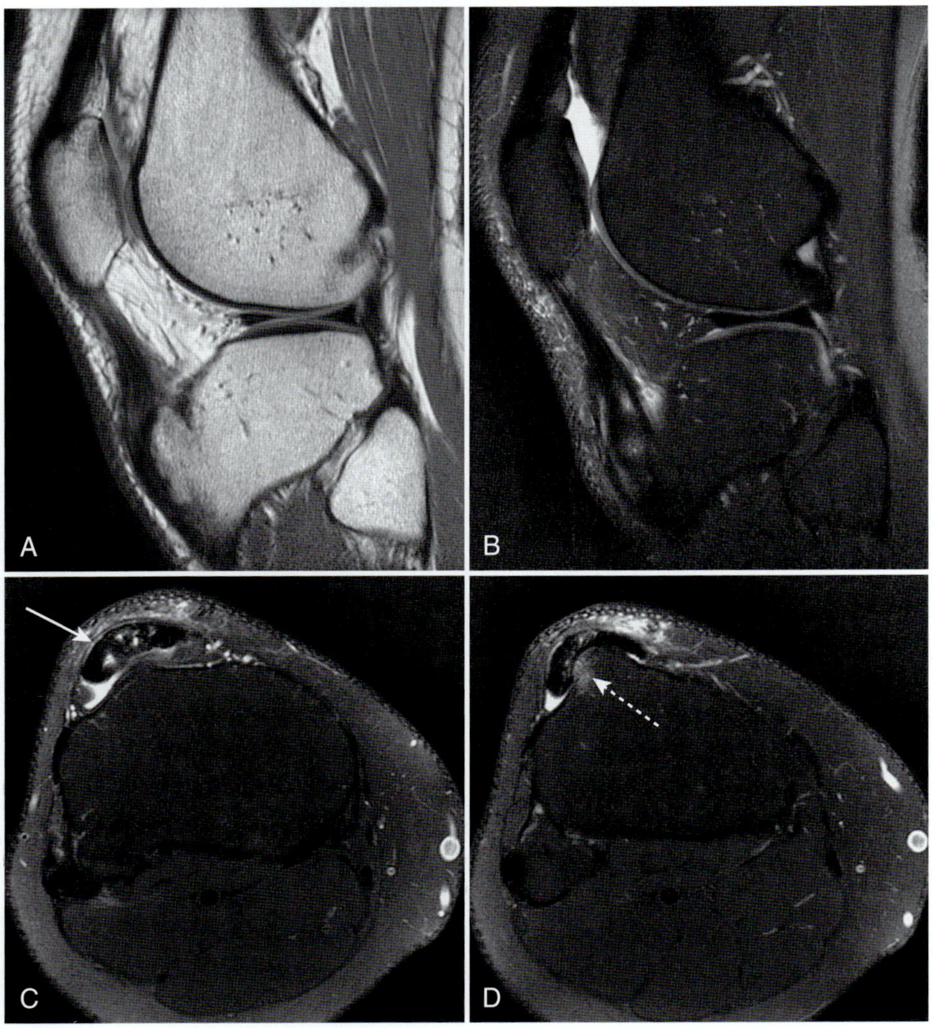

Figure 155.2 (A), Sagittal proton density MR image of a young adult with anterior knee pain. The tibial tuberosity is prominent as a result of adolescent Osgood-Schlatter disease. (B), The sagittal T2-weighted with fat suppression (FST2W) MR image shows associated increased SI within a thickened distal patellar tendon. The axial FST2W MR images (C and D) also show the tendon changes (*white arrow*) and the marrow edema in the tibial tuberosity (*broken white arrow*) due to chronic insertional tendinopathy.

CHAPTER 156

Suprapatellar Bursitis

DEFINITION

- Inflammation of the bursa that lies superior to the patella and deep to the quadriceps femoris muscle.
- The bursa normally communicates with the knee joint and is distended by any cause of joint effusion or synovitis.
- Imperforate superior plica may manifest as a localized suprapatellar bursitis.

SIGNS AND SYMPTOMS

- Pain localized underneath the distal quadriceps femoris muscle that is made worse with any knee movement.
- Pain may radiate to the distal anterior thigh.
- Tenderness to palpation of the suprapatellar bursa.
- Warmth may be present.
- Knee may feel boggy or edematous.
- Crepitus or catching sensation may be present.
- Exacerbation of pain with resisted knee extension.
- Gradual decrease in range of motion.

DEMOGRAPHICS

- Patients with inflammatory synovitis.
- Sporadic cases of imperforate plicae.

IMAGING RECOMMENDATIONS

- MRI:
  - To exclude internal derangement of knee and simple effusion.

IMAGING FINDINGS

- High–signal intensity (SI) fluid in the bursa on T2-weighted (T2W) MR images.
- Synovial thickening and enhancement in inflammatory arthritis.
- Low-SI superior plica.

OTHER RECOMMENDED TESTING

- Laboratory testing to rule out inflammatory arthritis.
- Bursa aspiration with Gram staining and culture and sensitivity testing if infection in question.
- Joint aspiration to rule out crystal arthropathies.
- Joint aspiration to rule out infection if diagnosis in question.

DIFFERENTIAL DIAGNOSIS

- Simple joint effusion.
- Calcific tendinitis.
- Patellar tendon tear.
- Prepatellar bursitis.
- Internal derangement of the knee.
- Hemarthrosis.
- Septic arthritis of the knee.

TREATMENT

- Conservative treatment consisting of local heat, cold, simple analgesics, and nonsteroidal anti-inflammatory agents will improve symptoms in mild cases.
- Physical therapy, including gentle stretching, range-of-motion exercises, and deep heat modalities, may be beneficial in selected patients.
- Injection with local anesthetic and steroid will provide symptomatic relief if conservative therapy fails or the pain is limiting activities of daily living.
- Surgery may be required for persistent pain or progressive functional disability.

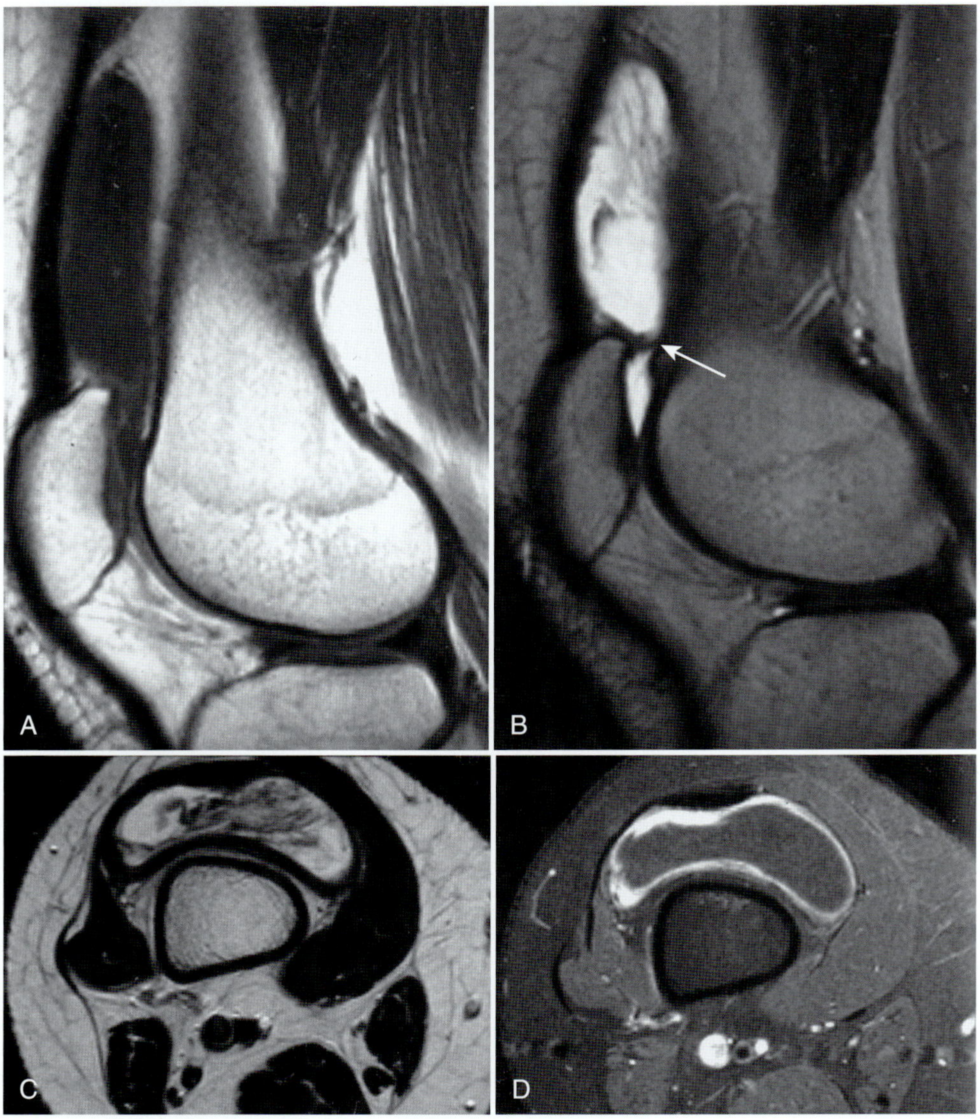

Figure 156.1 Sagittal T1W (**A**) and T2W (**B**) MR images of a patient with an imperforate superior plica (*white arrow*). There is a loculated effusion within the suprapatellar bursa but no significant effusion in the other recesses of the knee joint. A few low-SI fronds of synovium within the bursa can be seen on the sagittal T2W MR image and on an axial T2W MR image (**C**). (**D**), An axial T1W with fat suppression (FST1W) MR image obtained after administration of a contrast agent shows minor enhancement of the synovial lining of the bursa.

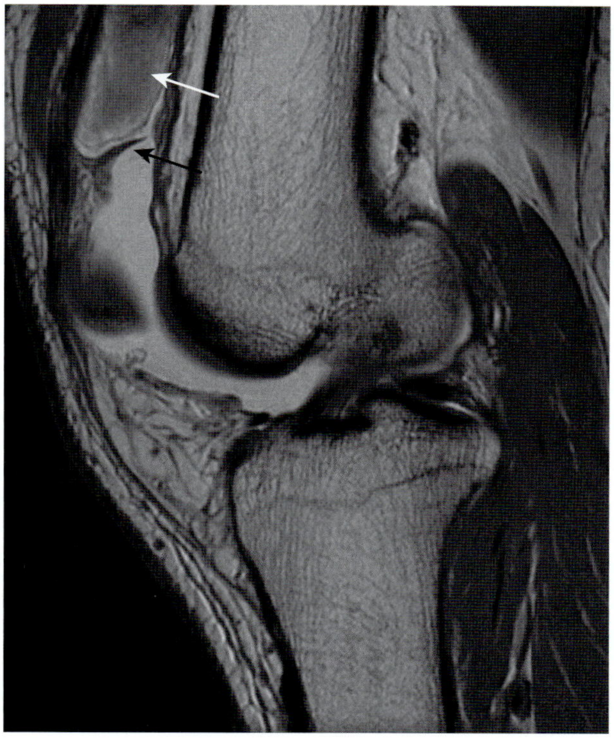

Figure 156.2 Sagittal T2W MR image of an imperforate plica (*black arrow*) in a patient with a loculated hematoma in the suprapatellar bursa (*white arrow*) following an acute injury.

CHAPTER 157

Prepatellar Bursitis

DEFINITION

- Inflammation of the bursa that lies between the subcutaneous tissues and patella.

SIGNS AND SYMPTOMS

- Pain localized to the anterior knee that is worse with any knee movement.
- Pain may radiate to the distal anterior thigh and infrapatellar region.
- Tenderness to palpation of the prepatellar bursa.
- Significant effusions often present.
- Warmth may be present.
- Knee may feel boggy or edematous.
- Crepitus or catching sensation may be present.
- Exacerbation of pain with resisted knee extension.
- Pain often worse at night.
- Patient unable to sleep on the affected knee.
- Gradual decrease in range of motion.
- May progress to frozen knee if left untreated.

DEMOGRAPHICS

- Incidence: Female > Male.
- Young athletes often affected.
- Common:
  - After running on soft or uneven surfaces.
  - In people who scrub floors on their hands and knees; hence the term "housemaid's knee."
  - In jobs that require crawling.
- All adult ages affected.
- More common after direct trauma to the patella, including repetitive stress injuries.

IMAGING RECOMMENDATIONS

- Imaging not routinely required.
- MRI or US.

IMAGING FINDINGS

- Fluid within the subcutaneous soft tissues anterior to the patella.
- May overlap with superficial infrapatellar bursitis.
- Infected bursitis and bursitis associated with crystal and inflammatory arthropathy may demonstrate:
  - Echogenic effusions on US.
  - Increased vascularity on power Doppler imaging.
  - Enhancement on post-contrast (obtained after administration of a contrast agent) T1-weighted (T1W) MR images.
  - Surrounding soft tissue edema.

OTHER RECOMMENDED TESTING

- Laboratory testing to rule out inflammatory arthritis.
- Bursa aspiration with Gram staining and culture and sensitivity testing if infection in question.
- Joint aspiration to rule out crystal arthropathies.
- Joint aspiration to rule out infection if diagnosis in question.

DIFFERENTIAL DIAGNOSIS

- Calcific tendinitis.
- Partial-thickness patellar tear.
- Complete patellar tendon tear.
- Reflex sympathetic dystrophy of the knee.
- Joint effusion.
- Internal derangement of the knee.
- Hemarthrosis.
- Septic arthritis of the knee.

TREATMENT

- Conservative treatment consisting of local heat, cold, simple analgesics, and nonsteroidal anti-inflammatory agents will improve symptoms in mild cases.
- Physical therapy, including gentle stretching, range-of-motion exercises, and deep heat modalities, may be beneficial in selected patients.
- Injection with local anesthetic and steroid will provide symptomatic relief if conservative therapy fails or the pain is limiting activities of daily living.
- Surgery may be required for persistent pain or progressive functional disability.

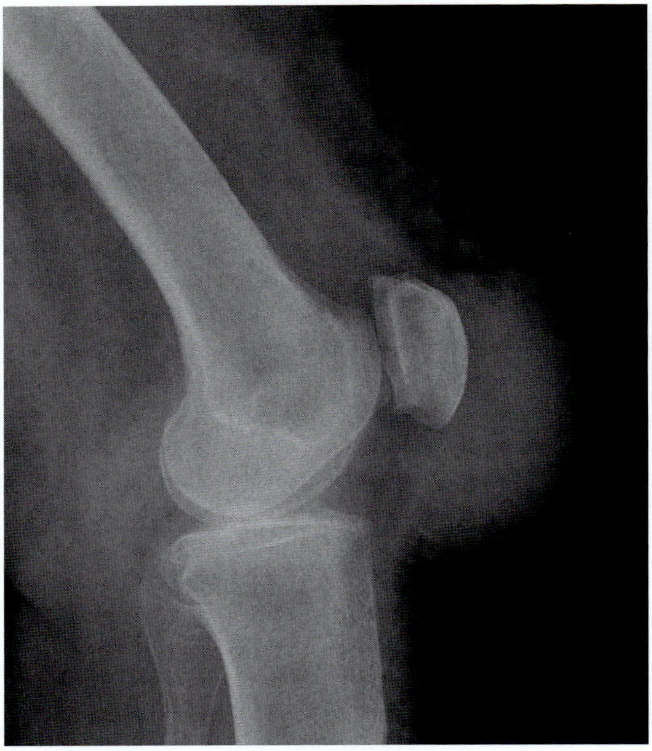

Figure 157.1 Lateral radiograph of the knee in a patient with an acute attack of gout. There is prominent prepatellar soft tissue swelling due to gouty bursitis.

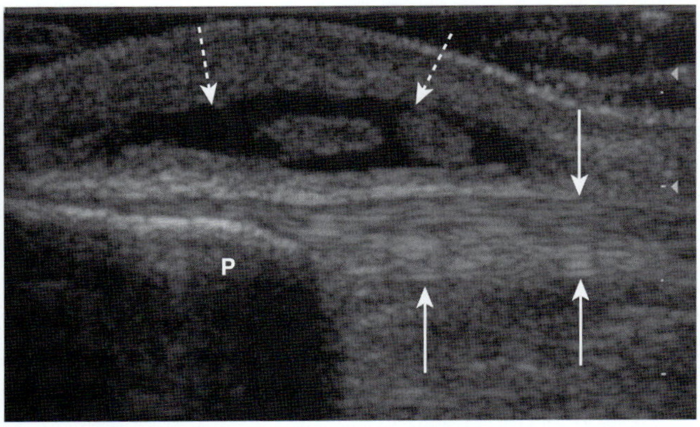

Figure 157.2 US image of a patient with simple prepatellar bursitis. The patella (P) and patellar tendon (*white arrows*) are normal. There is an anechoic fluid collection within the prepatellar soft tissues (*broken white arrows*), partly surrounding small echogenic fat lobules.

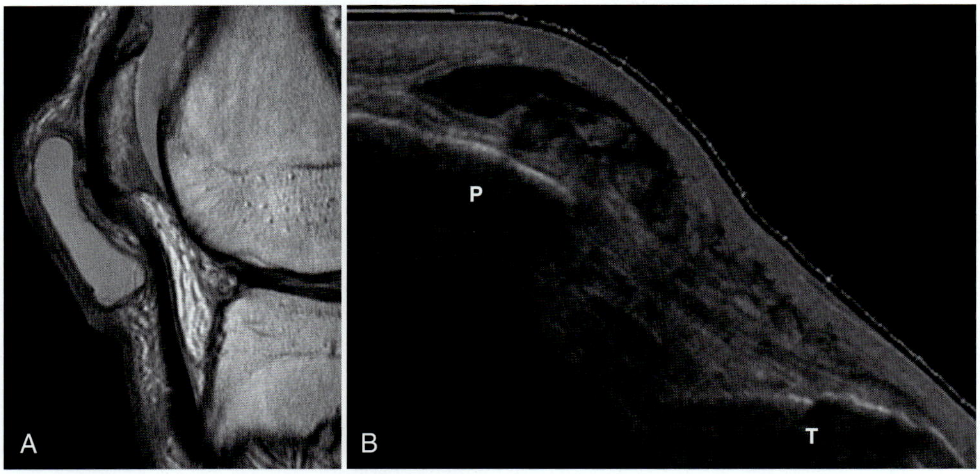

Figure 157.3 (**A**), Sagittal T2W MR image showing prominent high–signal intensity (SI) fluid within the prepatellar bursa. There is also an advance osteoarthritic change in the patellofemoral joint. (**B**), The corresponding longitudinal US image shows the extensive low-echo fluid collection. P, patella; T, tibia.

CHAPTER 158

Superficial Infrapatellar Bursitis

DEFINITION

- Inflammation of the bursa that lies between the subcutaneous tissues and the upper part of the ligamentum patellae.

SIGNS AND SYMPTOMS

- Pain localized to the inferoanterior knee that is worse with any knee movement.
- Pain may radiate to the infrapatellar region.
- Tenderness to palpation of the superficial infrapatellar bursa.
- Significant effusions often present.
- Warmth may be present.
- Knee may feel boggy or edematous.
- Crepitus or catching sensation may be present.
- Exacerbation of pain with resisted knee extension.
- Patient often unable to walk stairs.
- Patient often unable to kneel.
- Pain often worse at night.
- Patient unable to sleep on the affected knee.
- Gradual decrease in range of motion.
- May progress to frozen knee if left untreated.

DEMOGRAPHICS

- Incidence: Male > Female.
- Young athletes often affected.
- Common after running on soft or uneven surfaces.
- Common in jobs that require crawling.
- All adult ages affected.
- More common after direct trauma to patella, including repetitive stress injuries.

IMAGING RECOMMENDATIONS

- Imaging not routinely required.
- MRI or US.

IMAGING FINDINGS

- Fluid within the subcutaneous soft tissues inferior to the patella.
- May overlap with prepatellar bursitis.
- Prominent surrounding soft tissue edema is present with infected bursitis.
- Echogenic effusions on US or enhancement on post-contrast (obtained after administration of a contrast agent) MR images suggests possible crystal or inflammatory arthropathy.
- Associated patellar tendinopathy may be present.

OTHER RECOMMENDED TESTING

- Laboratory testing to rule out inflammatory arthritis.
- Bursa aspiration with gram staining and culture and sensitivity testing if infection in question.
- Joint aspiration to rule out crystal arthropathies.
- Joint aspiration to rule out infection if diagnosis in question.

DIFFERENTIAL DIAGNOSIS

- Calcific tendinitis.
- Partial-thickness patellar tear
- Complete patellar tendon tear.
- Reflex sympathetic dystrophy of the knee.
- Prepatellar bursitis.
- Internal derangement of the knee.
- Hemarthrosis.
- Septic arthritis of the knee.

TREATMENT

- Conservative treatment consisting of local heat, cold, simple analgesics, and nonsteroidal anti-inflammatory agents will improve symptoms in mild cases.
- Physical therapy, including gentle stretching, range-of-motion exercises, and deep heat modalities, may be beneficial in selected patients.
- Injection with local anesthetic and steroid will provide symptomatic relief if conservative therapy fails or the pain is limiting activities of daily living.
- Surgery may be required for persistent pain or progressive functional disability.

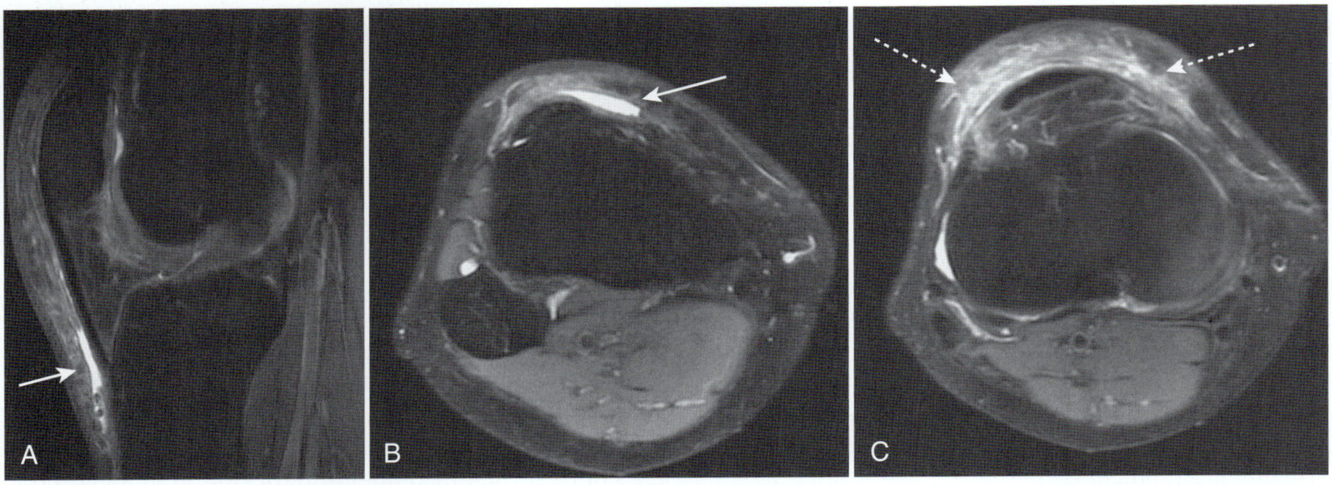

Figure 158.1 (**A**), Sagittal T2-weighted with fat suppression (FST2W) MR image demonstrating a small area of high–signal intensity (SI) fluid superficial to the distal patellar tendon and tibial tuberosity (*white arrow*). (**B**), This area of fluid is also evident on the axial FST2W MR image. A small amount of fluid may be a normal finding. (**C**), In this case, however, more extensive diffuse high-SI edema *(broken white arrows)* is demonstrated in the adjacent soft tissues on the proximal axial FST2W MR image, representing a diffuse adventitial bursitis.

CHAPTER 159

Deep Infrapatellar Bursitis

DEFINITION

- Inflammation of the bursa that lies between the patellar ligament and the tibia.

SIGNS AND SYMPTOMS

- Pain localized to the inferoanterior knee that is worse with any knee movement.
- Pain may radiate to infrapatellar region.
- Tenderness to palpation of the deep infrapatellar bursa.
- Significant effusions often present.
- Warmth may be present.
- Knee may feel boggy or edematous.
- Crepitus or catching sensation may be present.
- Exacerbation of pain with resisted knee extension.
- Patient often unable to walk stairs.
- Patient often unable to kneel.
- Pain often worse at night.
- Patient unable to sleep on the affected knee.
- Gradual decrease in range of motion.
- May progress to frozen knee if left untreated.

DEMOGRAPHICS

- Incidence: Male > Female.
- Young athletes often affected.
- Common after running on soft or uneven surfaces.
- Common in jobs that require crawling or kneeling.
- All adult ages affected.
- More common after direct trauma to the patella, including repetitive stress injuries.

IMAGING RECOMMENDATIONS

- MRI or US.

IMAGING FINDINGS

- Fluid within soft tissues deep to the distal patellar tendon:
  - Small amounts of fluid are a normal finding.
- Often associated with insertional tendinopathy and Osgood-Schlatter disease.
- Prominent surrounding soft tissue edema is present with infected bursitis.

OTHER RECOMMENDED TESTING

- Laboratory testing to rule out inflammatory arthritis.
- Bursa aspiration with Gram staining and culture and sensitivity testing if infection in question.
- Joint aspiration to rule out crystal arthropathies.
- Joint aspiration to rule out infection if diagnosis in question.

DIFFERENTIAL DIAGNOSIS

- Calcific tendinitis.
- Partial-thickness patellar tear.
- Complete patellar tendon tear.
- Reflex sympathetic dystrophy of the knee.
- Prepatellar bursitis.
- Superficial infrapatellar bursitis.
- Internal derangement of the knee.
- Hemarthrosis.
- Septic arthritis of the knee.

TREATMENT

- Conservative treatment consisting of local heat, cold, simple analgesics, and nonsteroidal anti-inflammatory agents will improve symptoms in mild cases.
- Physical therapy, including gentle stretching, range-of-motion exercises, and deep heat modalities, may be beneficial in selected patients.
- Injection with local anesthetic and steroid will provide symptomatic relief if conservative therapy fails or the pain is limiting activities of daily living.
- Surgery may be required for persistent pain or progressive functional disability.

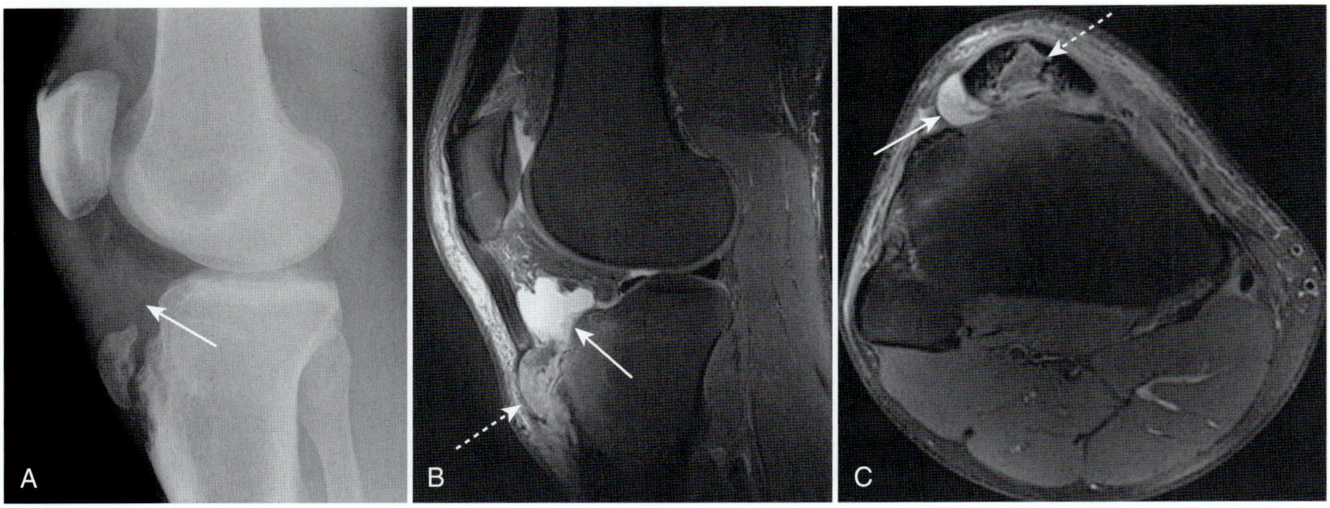

Figure 159.1 (**A**), Lateral radiograph of a patient with chronic insertional tendinopathy of the patellar tendon with nonfused tibial apophysis. There is soft tissue shadowing deep to the distal patellar tendon (*white arrow*) that partly obliterates the Hoffa fat pad. The sagittal (**B**) and axial (**C**) T2-weighted with fat suppression (FST2W) MR images clearly show the high–signal intensity (SI) fluid within the deep infrapatellar bursa (*white arrows*). There is also high-SI marrow edema within the unfused apophysis and adjacent tibia (*broken white arrows*).

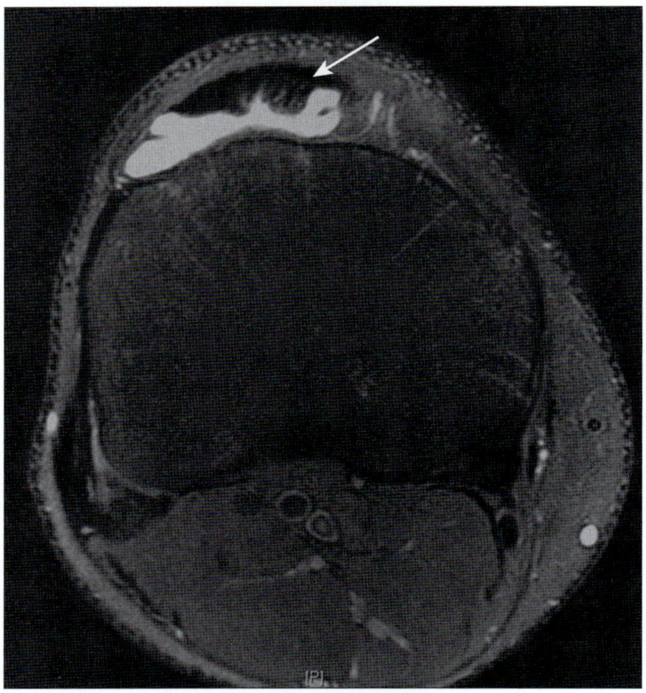

Figure 159.2 Axial FST2W MR image of a patient with minor patellar tendinopathy but prominent infrapatellar bursitis. The distal tendon is thickened and irregular in contour, with areas of increased SI (*white arrow*), and there is high-SI fluid within the bursa deep to the tendon.

CHAPTER 160

Medial Plica Syndrome

DEFINITION

- Chronic inflammation and microhemorrhage of the synovial plica, leading to proliferation and thickening, which results in joint pain, clicking, and pseudo-locking of the knee.

SIGNS AND SYMPTOMS

- Gradual onset of medial knee pain most often after trauma.
- Pain is dull and aching.
- Pain often worse after sitting for prolonged periods.
- Locking of the knee common.
- Decrease in full extension of the knee joint.
- Difficulty ambulating on the affected knee.
- Feeling of weakness or giving way.
- Clicking or popping sensation often present at 60 to 50 degrees of joint flexion.
- Exacerbation of pain with activity.

DEMOGRAPHICS

- Incidence: Male = Female.
- All ages affected, but most commonly younger patients after acute trauma.
- May occur secondary to repetitive stress injuries.
- Common after rowing, cycling, and swimming injuries.

IMAGING RECOMMENDATIONS

- MRI.
- Radiography:
  - In older patients to exclude osteoarthritis.

IMAGING FINDINGS

- Fold of synovium in medial parapatellar recess.
- Best demonstrated on axial T2-weighted (T2W) or T2W with fat suppression (FST2W) MR images.
  - Joint effusion improves visualization.
- Small plicae are often asymptomatic.
- Factors suggestive of symptomatic plica:
  - Plica extends into patellofemoral joint.
  - Thickened synovial fold > 2 mm.
- Plicae may occur at other sites.
  - Imperforate suprapatellar plica may manifest as a mass in the distal thigh because of a loculated effusion.

OTHER RECOMMENDED TESTING

- Laboratory testing to rule out inflammatory arthritis.
- Joint aspiration to rule out crystal arthropathies.
- Joint aspiration to rule out infection if diagnosis in question.

DIFFERENTIAL DIAGNOSIS

- Tendinitis.
- Bursitis.
- Anterior cruciate ligament tear.
- Hoffa impingement.
- Partial-thickness meniscal tear not involving the articular surface.
- Complete medial meniscal tear.
- Medial meniscal flap tear.
- Patellar chondromalacia.
- Bursitis.

TREATMENT

- Conservative treatment consisting of local heat, cold, simple analgesics, and nonsteroidal anti-inflammatory agents will improve symptoms in many cases.
- Physical therapy, including gentle stretching, range-of-motion exercises, and deep heat modalities, may be beneficial in selected patients.
- Injection with local anesthetic and steroid will provide symptomatic relief if conservative therapy fails or the pain is limiting activities of daily living.
- Surgery usually required for persistent pain or progressive functional disability and locking of the knee.

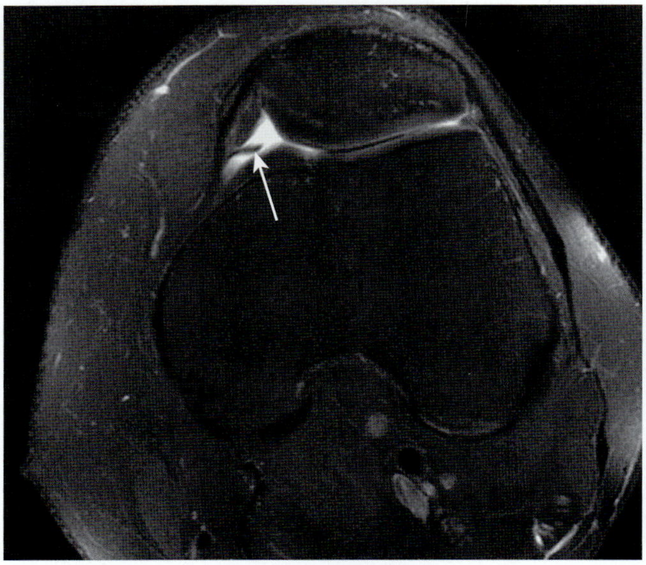

Figure 160.1 Axial FST2W MR image demonstrating a small medial plica (*white arrow*), which is not thickened and does not impinge within the patellofemoral joint.

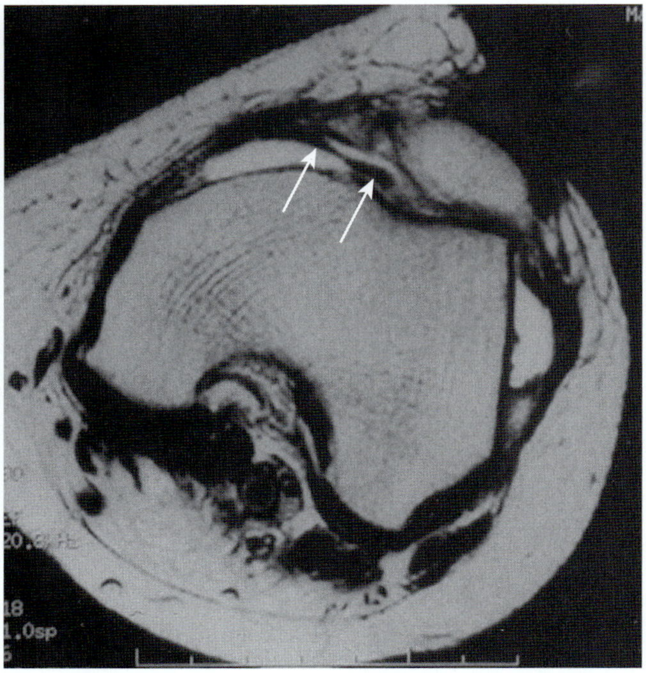

Figure 160.2 Axial T2W MR image of a patient with impingement symptoms of the extensor mechanism. There is a medial plica (*black arrows*), which is thickened as it extends into the patellofemoral joint.

CHAPTER 161

Baker Cyst

DEFINITION

- Cyst of the popliteal space, usually involving the gastrocnemius-semimembranosus bursa, which communicates with the intra-articular space.

SIGNS AND SYMPTOMS

- Popliteal swelling or mass.
- Pain localized to the posterior knee that is made worse with any knee movement.
- Tenderness to palpation of the popliteal fossa.
- Significant swelling may be present.
- Warmth may be present.
- Posterior knee may feel boggy or edematous.
- Crepitus or catching sensation may be present.
- Exacerbation of pain with resisted knee flexion.
- Patient is often unable to walk stairs.
- Patient is often unable to kneel.
- Pain often worse at night.
- Patient is unable to sleep on the affected knee.
- Gradual decrease in range of motion.
- May become infected.

DEMOGRAPHICS

- Incidence: Male > Female.
- Common after posterior knee trauma.
- All adult ages affected.
- Cyst may regress or spontaneously rupture.

IMAGING RECOMMENDATIONS

- Radiography:
  - To assess for knee joint arthropathy.
  - To exclude loose bodies.
- MRI or US.

IMAGING FINDINGS

- Fluid-filled cyst extending out between the medial head of the gastrocnemius muscle and the semimembranosus tendon.
  - "Speech bubble" sign.
- Synovial thickening may be present, especially in association with inflammatory arthropathies.
- Loose bodies may be present within the cyst.
- Cyst rupture:
  - Superficial edema extending distally within the calf.
  - Fluid collections in calf, both superficial and deep to the gastrocnemius muscle.

OTHER RECOMMENDED TESTING

- Laboratory testing to rule out inflammatory arthritis.
- Bursa aspiration with Gram staining and culture and sensitivity testing if infection in question.
- Joint aspiration to rule out crystal arthropathies.
- Joint aspiration to rule out infection if diagnosis in question.

DIFFERENTIAL DIAGNOSIS

- Calcific tendinitis.
- Popliteal artery aneurysm.
- Ganglion cyst.
- Deep vein thrombosis.
- Complete patellar tendon tear.
- Reflex sympathetic dystrophy of the knee.
- Bursitis.
- Internal derangement of the knee.
- Hemarthrosis.
- Septic arthritis of the knee.

TREATMENT

- Conservative treatment consisting of local heat, cold, simple analgesics, and nonsteroidal anti-inflammatory agents will improve symptoms in mild cases.
- Physical therapy, including gentle stretching, range-of-motion exercises, and deep heat modalities, may be beneficial in selected patients.
- Injection with local anesthetic and steroid will provide symptomatic relief if conservative therapy fails or the pain is limiting activities of daily living.
- Surgery may be required for persistent pain or progressive functional disability.

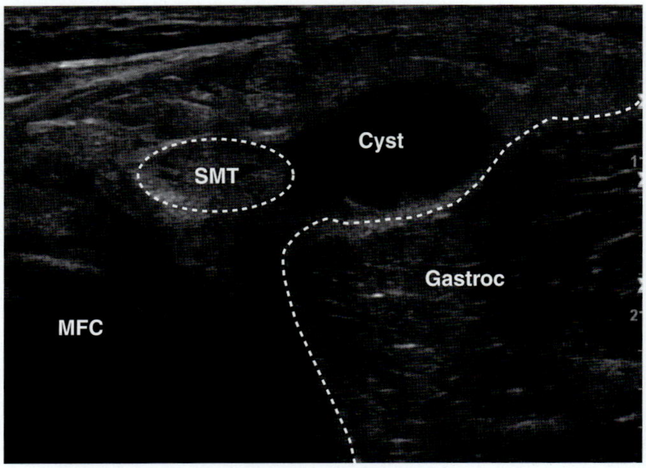

Figure 161.1 US image of a Baker cyst arising out of the knee joint between the medial head of the gastrocnemius muscle (Gastroc) and the semimembranosus tendon (SMT). The cyst is anechoic, consistent with simple fluid. The back of the medial femoral condyle is also visible (MFC).

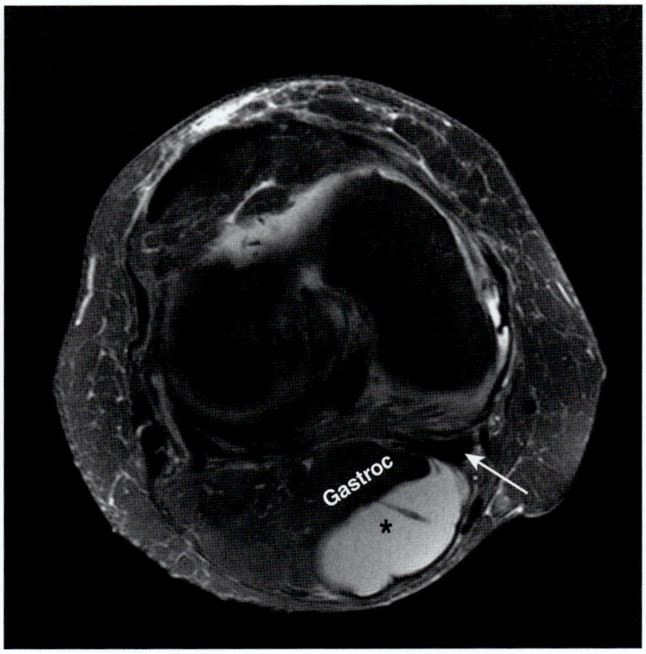

Figure 161.2 A T2-weighted with fat suppression (FST2W) MR image of a Baker cyst in a different patient. The features are identical, with the high–signal intensity (SI), fluid-filled cyst (*asterisk*) arising between the gastrocnemius muscle (Gastroc) and the semimembranosus tendon (*white arrow*).

CHAPTER 162

Reflex Sympathetic Dystrophy and Regional Migratory Osteoporosis

DEFINITION

- Migrating arthralgia of the weight-bearing joints with localized areas of osteoporosis.

SIGNS AND SYMPTOMS

- Rapid onset of pain and swelling.
- Spontaneous resolution.
- Recurrence at other sites.
- Occasional history of minor trauma.

DEMOGRAPHICS

- Mainly affects middle-aged men.
- Limited to weight-bearing joints, but knees are often affected.
- Associated with generalized osteoporosis.
- Possible overlap with reflex sympathetic dystrophy and transient osteoporosis of the hip.

IMAGING RECOMMENDATIONS

- Radiography.
- MRI.
- Isotope bone scanning is an alternative to MRI.

IMAGING FINDINGS

- Localized areas of periarticular osteopenia:
  - Not all of the joint may be involved.
- Preservation of joint space.
- Bone marrow edema on MRI corresponding to areas of osteoporosis.
- Other features of avascular necrosis are absent.

OTHER RECOMMENDED TESTING

- Laboratory testing to rule out inflammatory arthritis.
- Electromyography and nerve conduction velocity testing to rule out occult plexopathy, radiculopathy, and/or entrapment neuropathy that may be serving as a nidus for the reflex sympathetic dystrophy.
- Joint aspiration to rule out crystal arthropathies.
- Joint aspiration to rule out infection.

DIFFERENTIAL DIAGNOSIS

- Inflammatory arthritides, especially rheumatoid arthritis.
- Septic knee joint.
- Osteomyelitis.
- Soft tissue infections.
- Occult foreign bodies.
- Healing fractures.
- Metastatic disease.
- Bone infarcts.
- Crystal arthropathy of the knee.
- Avascular osteonecrosis.

TREATMENT

- Conservative treatment consisting of local heat, cold, simple analgesics, and nonsteroidal anti-inflammatory agents will improve symptoms in many cases.
- Intravenous pamidronate may be effective.
- Physical therapy, including gentle stretching, range-of-motion exercises, tactile desensitization, and contrast baths, may be beneficial in selected patients.
- Lumbar sympathetic blocks with local anesthetic and steroid will provide symptomatic relief if conservative therapy fails or the pain is limiting activities of daily living.
- Release of coexistent entrapment neuropathies.
- Spinal cord stimulation a good option for patients who do not experience long-lasting relief from lumbar sympathetic blocks.
- Surgical sympathectomy or radiofrequency destruction of the lumbar sympathetic ganglion may be required for persistent pain or progressive functional disability.

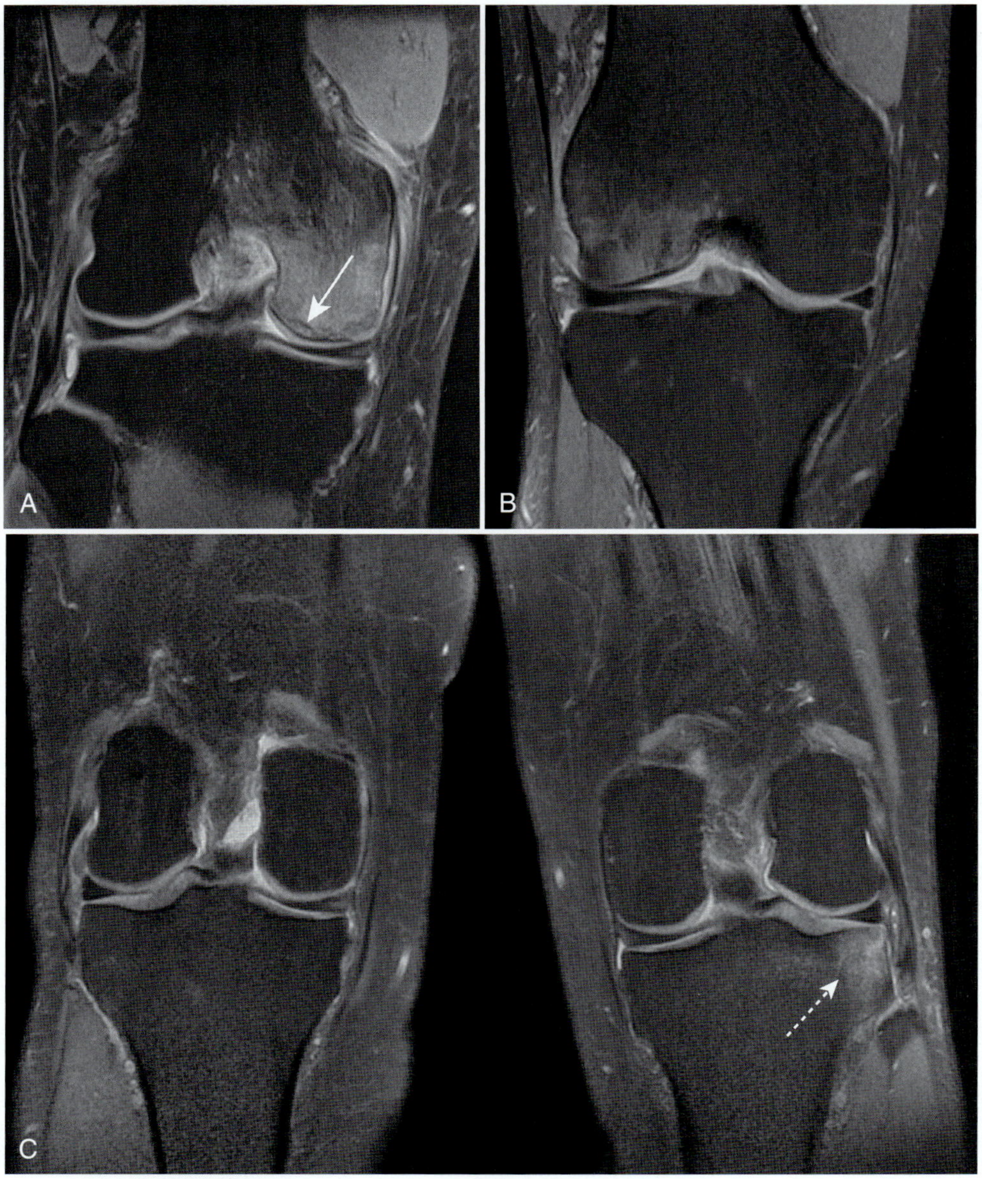

Figure 162.1 (A), Coronal T2-weighted with fat suppression (FST2W) MR image of a patient with right-sided medial knee pain but no history of trauma. Radiographs showed a joint effusion but findings were otherwise normal. There is diffuse high–signal intensity (SI) marrow edema in the medial femoral condyle. A low-SI subchondral line (*white arrow*) could indicate early avascular necrosis or an insufficiency fracture, although there is no subchondral collapse. Symptoms resolved with non–weight-bearing treatment, but new-onset right lateral knee pain developed a few months later. (B), A second MR image shows recovery of the edema in the medial condyle, but new edema in the lateral condyle. Symptoms again responded to conservative treatment, but the patient presented once more with left knee pain. (C), A repeat MR image shows normal appearances in the right knee, but with marrow edema in the lateral tibial condyle (*broken white arrow*). This pattern of flitting marrow edema is typical of regional migratory osteoporosis. *(Images courtesy of Dr Abdul Gafoor, Derriford Hospital, Plymouth, United Kingdom.)*

CHAPTER 163

Anatomy: Special Imaging Considerations of the Ankle and Foot

OSSEOUS STRUCTURES

Tibia

The distal tibia bears medial and posterior prominences known as the medial malleolus and posterior tibial process, respectively. The medial malleolus is longer than the lateral tibial surface and articulates with the medial surface of the talus to form the medial gutter of the ankle joint. The lateral tibial surface is concave, forming a groove for the distal fibula. The tibial articular surface, known as the plafond, forms a sagittal concavity covered with articular cartilage.

Fibula

The fibular diaphysis is thin and gracile; it is slightly triangular in cross section, with a bulbous and pointed distal end known as the lateral malleolus. The anterior surface of the lateral malleolus lies partly within the ankle joint. The fibula is longer than the tibia, and the medial surface of the lateral malleolus articulates with the lateral border of the talus to form the lateral gutter of the ankle joint.

Talus

The talus possesses a sagittally convex superior articular surface known as the dome, which articulates with the tibial plafond to form the ankle joint. Anterior to the dome is the talar neck, through which most of the talar blood supply is derived. The talar neck has a bulbous distal head that articulates with the navicular to form the talonavicular joint. The inferior talar surface has a large, anteromedially down-sloping articular facet that articulates with the calcaneus to form the posterior subtalar joint (PSTJ). There are smaller medial and anterior facets that form the anterior and medial subtalar joints.

Calcaneus

The largest of the tarsal bones, the calcaneus is cuboidal with an anteriorly directed long axis. The bulbous posterior process bears the attachment of the Achilles tendon. The superior surface of the calcaneal body has an articular facet that forms the PSTJ with the talus. Anterior to the PSTJ lies a notch on the superior surface that forms the floor of a space known as the sinus tarsi. The calcaneus has an anterior process as well as a superomedially directed process called the sustentaculum, which articulates with the talus to form the middle subtalar joint.

Navicular

A broad, but narrow and slightly curved bone that articulates with the talar head proximally and the three cuneiforms distally.

Cuboid

A pyramidal bone on the lateral side of the foot. The cuboid articulates proximally with the calcaneum and distally with the fourth and fifth metatarsals.

Cuneiforms

Three wedge shaped bones comprising the first (medial), second (middle) and third (lateral) cuneiforms. All three articulate with the navicular proximally. The first cuneiform articulates distally with the first and second metatarsals. The second and third cuneiforms articulate with the corresponding metatarsals.

Metatarsals

A typical metatarsal has a base that is broad superiorly and narrow inferiorly with facets for articulation with the cuneiforms. Each shaft tapers distally, with a bulbous and rounded head that is covered with articular cartilage to form the metatarsal phalangeal (MTP) joint with the corresponding proximal phalanx. The first metatarsal is much broader and stouter than the second to fifth metatarsals.

Phalanges

These correspond in number and arrangement to those in the hand. They are broader at their bases with concave proximal articular surfaces and rounded distal articular surfaces. As in the thumb, the hallux possesses only two phalanges and one interphalangeal joint.

Tibiofibular Syndesmosis

The distal fibula forms a relatively rigid fibrous and ligamentous attachment to the groove on the lateral tibial surface known as the tibiofibular syndesmosis. The syndesmosis is stabilized by the inferior tibiofibular ligaments both anteriorly and posteriorly.

TENDONS

Peroneal Tendons

The peroneus brevis and peroneus longus tendons are located on the lateral aspect of the ankle, posterior to the distal fibula. The peroneus brevis lies adjacent to the fibula, within the fibular groove, and passes distal to the tip of the lateral malleolus to insert on the base of the fifth metatarsal. The peroneus longus covers the brevis as it also passes over the fibula tip to course over the lateral and plantar border of the foot to insert on the first metatarsal and first cuneiform. Each tendon has its own sheath distal to the malleolus. The peroneal tendons are stabilized within the fibular groove by the superior peroneal retinaculum.

Medial Flexor Tendons

These are located posterior to the medial malleolus. From medial to lateral they are: tibialis posterior (TP), flexor digitorum longus (FDL), and flexor hallucis longus (FHL). The TP tendon, an important plantarflexor and inverter of the foot, inserts on a tubercle on the medial navicular surface with additional slips that insert on the plantar surfaces of the cuneiforms, cuboid, and metatarsal bases. The FDL tendon is a singular structure as it passes round the medial malleolus and under the foot, where it divides into four slips that insert on the second to fifth distal phalanges. The FHL tendon carries its muscle quite distally, almost to the level of the ankle joint. It passes over a groove in the posterior surface of the tibia before passing distally under the sustentaculum of the calcaneus to insert on the distal phalanx of the hallux, where it acts as a powerful plantar-flexor.

Anterior Extensor Tendons

At the level of the ankle joint, the anterior extensor tendons lie beneath the extensor retinaculum. From medial to lateral they are the tendons of tibialis anterior, extensor hallucis longus (EHL), extensor digitorum longus (EDL), and peroneus tertius muscles. The last may be absent. The tibialis anterior inserts on the plantar aspect of the first cuneiform and the base of the first metatarsal to act as a foot inverter and dorsiflexor. The EHL tendon inserts on the first distal phalanx to act as a powerful dorsiflexor. The EDL tendon divides into four slips just distal to the ankle joint, which insert on the second to fifth distal phalanges and act to produce toe extension. The peroneus tertius is an extension of the EDL tendon that inserts on the dorsal surface of the base of the fifth metatarsal.

Achilles Tendon

The strongest tendon in the body, the Achilles is the common tendon of the gastrocnemius and soleus muscles. The medial and lateral muscle bellies of the gastrocnemius muscle join at a central fibrous septum before blending to contribute fibers to the Achilles tendon, which are joined more distally by the soleus contribution to the tendon. The gastrocnemius and soleus muscles are separated by an aponeurosis. The Achilles tendon broadens at its insertion on the posterior surface of the calcaneal posterior process. The tendon is accompanied by the thin plantaris tendon, the muscle of which lies between the gastrocnemius and soleus muscles in the proximal calf.

Plantar Fascia

A structure composed of medial, central, and lateral bundles of dense fascia that arise from the plantar surface of the posterior calcaneal process and extend distally, fanning out to blend with the flexor tendon sheaths of the toes.

NERVES

Tibial Nerve and Branches

The largest branch of the sciatic nerve descends with the posterior tibial vessels between the gastrocnemius and soleus muscles proximally, giving off muscular branches. Distally, it courses medially to lie between the medial ankle flexor tendons and the heel. The tibial nerve extends under the flexor retinaculum in a region known as the tarsal tunnel, where it may undergo entrapment, before dividing into the medial and lateral plantar nerves. The medial and lateral plantar nerves course distally in the foot deep to the plantar fascia, giving off muscular and articular branches and finally dividing into the paired common digital nerves that supply each toe.

Sural Nerve

A branch of the tibial nerve that descends between the heads of gastrocnemius to course laterally to lie between the lateral malleolus and the Achilles tendon at the level of the ankle. It then extends distally to the lateral malleolus to supply the skin on the lateral border of the foot.

Common Peroneal Nerve

This nerve divides into superficial and deep branches after wrapping around the fibular head and passing through the fibular tunnel located behind the peroneus longus muscle. The superficial peroneal nerve gives off motor branches to the peroneal muscles and sensory branches to supply the anterolateral leg and the dorsum of the foot. The deep peroneal nerve gives off motor branches to the EHL, EDL, peroneus tertius, and extensor digitorum brevis muscles, with sensory branches supplying the dorsa of the first and second toes.

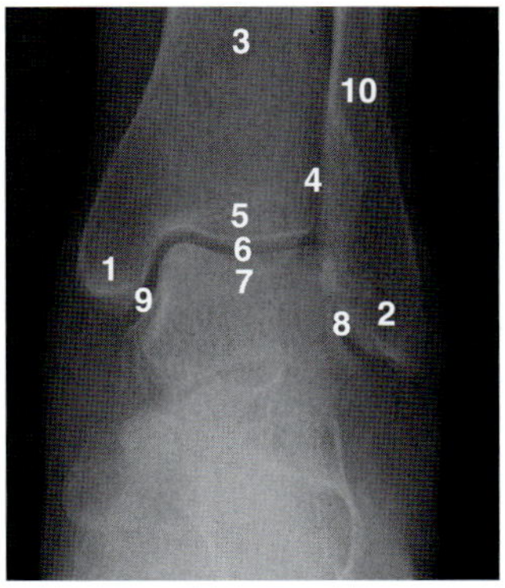

Figure 163.1 Anteroposterior radiograph of the ankle: 1, medial malleolus; 2, lateral malleolus; 3, tibial diaphysis; 4, tibiofibular syndesmosis; 5, anterior tibial plafond; 6, ankle joint space; 7, talar dome; 8, lateral gutter; 9, medial gutter; 10, fibular diaphysis.

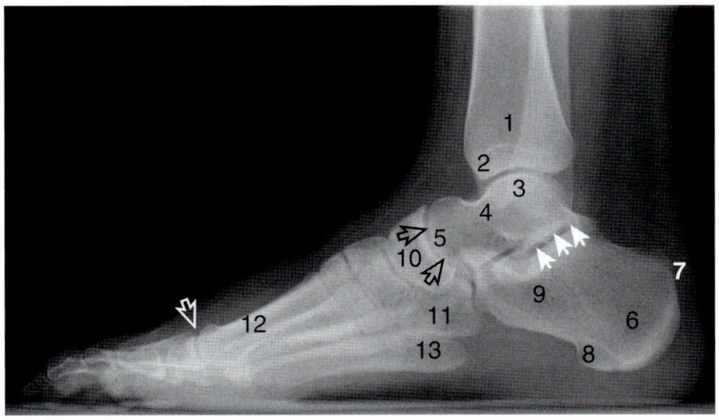

Figure 163.2 Lateral radiograph of the ankle and foot: 1, tibial metaphysis; 2, anterior rim of tibial plafond; 3, talar dome; 4, talar neck; 5, talar head; 6, posterior process of calcaneus; 7, Achilles tendon insertion; 8, origin of plantar fascia; 9, body of calcaneus; 10, navicular; 11, cuboid; 12, first metatarsal; 13, fifth metatarsal; *white arrows,* posterior subtalar joint; *open white arrow,* first metatarsal joint; *open black arrows,* talonavicular joint.

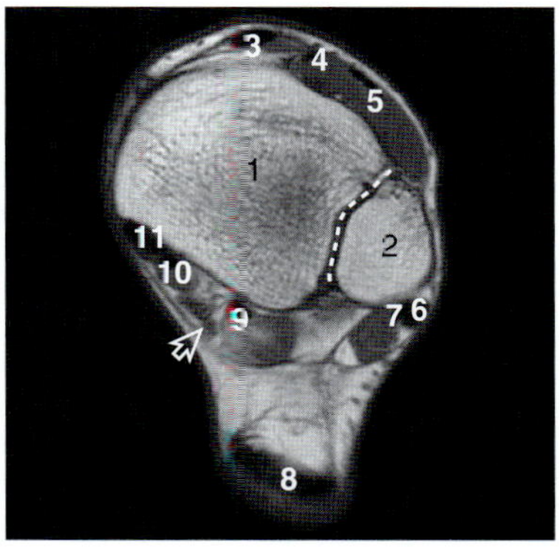

Figure 163.3 Axial T1-weighted MR image above the level of the ankle joint: 1, tibia; 2, fibula; 3, tibialis anterior tendon; 4, extensor hallucis longus tendon; 5, extensor digitorum longus tendon and muscle; 6, peroneus longus tendon; 7, peroneus brevis tendon; 8, Achilles tendon; 9, flexor hallucis longus tendon and muscle; 10, flexor digitorum longus tendon; 11, tibialis posterior tendon; *dashed white line,* tibiofibular syndesmosis; *open white arrow,* posterior tibial nerve.

CHAPTER 164

Anterior Tarsal Tunnel Syndrome

DEFINITION

- Entrapment of the deep peroneal nerve at the ankle as it passes beneath the superficial fascia of the ankle.

SIGNS AND SYMPTOMS

- Presence of Tinel sign over the entrapped nerve.
- Pain at the ankle radiating into the first dorsal space.
- Paresthesias at the ankle radiating into the first dorsal space.
- Passive range of motion preserved.
- Usually no motor involvement unless the lateral branch of deep peroneal nerve is affected.
- Night-time foot pain common.
- Patient may hold the foot in everted position to relieve symptoms.
- Active plantar-flexion may exacerbate symptoms.
- Weakness of extensor digitorum brevis if the lateral branch of the deep peroneal nerve is involved.

DEMOGRAPHICS

- Incidence: Female > Male.
- Much less common than posterior tarsal tunnel syndrome.
- Can occur acutely following trauma and fracture.
- More common after trauma, including repetitive stress injuries.
- Wearing of too-tight shoes often implicated.

IMAGING RECOMMENDATIONS

- Deep peroneal nerve not consistently visualized on US or MRI.
- Radiography to assess bony compression.
- MRI or US to assess soft tissue compression.

IMAGING FINDINGS

- Bony compression:
  - Osteophytes.
  - Fractures.
- Soft tissue compression:
  - Synovial disease in ankle.
  - Ganglia or other soft tissue masses.
  - Tenosynovitis.
  - Nerve sheath tumors of deep peroneal nerve.

OTHER RECOMMENDED TESTING

- Electromyography and nerve conduction velocity testing of the lumbar nerve roots, lumbar plexus, and associated peripheral nerves.

DIFFERENTIAL DIAGNOSIS

- Lumbar radiculopathy.
- Arthritis.
- Occult fracture.
- Diabetic polyneuropathy.
- Benign neoplasm.
- Malignant neoplasm.
- Ganglion.
- Tendinitis.

TREATMENT

- Conservative treatment consisting of local heat, cold, simple analgesics, and nonsteroidal anti-inflammatory agents will improve symptoms in mild, self-limited cases.
- Physical therapy to maintain function, including gentle stretching, range-of-motion exercises, and local heat modalities, may be beneficial in selected patients.
- Splinting to preserve normal range of motion.
- Avoidance of shoes that are too tight.
- Injection of the deep peroneal nerve with local anesthetic and steroid may provide symptomatic relief if conservative therapy fails or the pain is limiting activities of daily living.
- Surgery may be required to relieve entrapment of the deep peroneal nerve

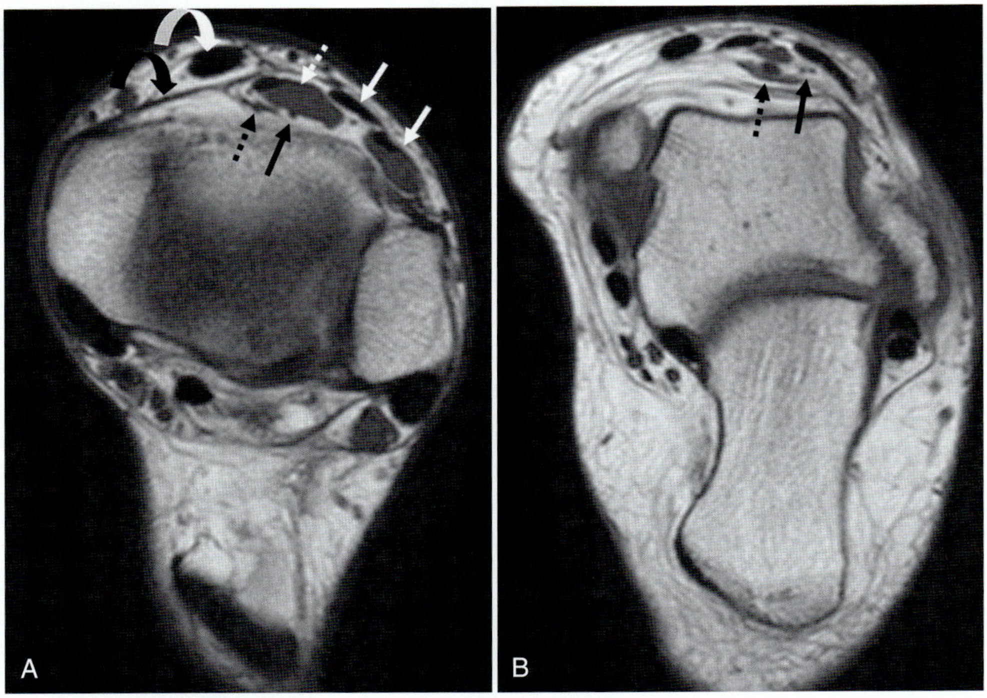

Figure 164.1 (A), Axial T1-weighted (T1W) MR image of the normal anatomy of the anterior tarsal tunnel. The extensor retinaculum (*curved black arrow*) is identified as a linear, low–signal intensity (SI) structure. The extensor tendons—extensor digitorum (*white arrows*), extensor hallucis longus (*broken white arrows*), and tibialis anterior (*curved white arrow*)—are demonstrated. The deep peroneal nerve (*black arrow*) lies lateral to the anterior tibial artery and veins (*broken black arrow*). (B), Distally, the axial T1W MR image shows the division of the deep peroneal nerve into its two terminal branches (*black arrow*), lateral to the tibial artery and vein (*broken black arrow*).

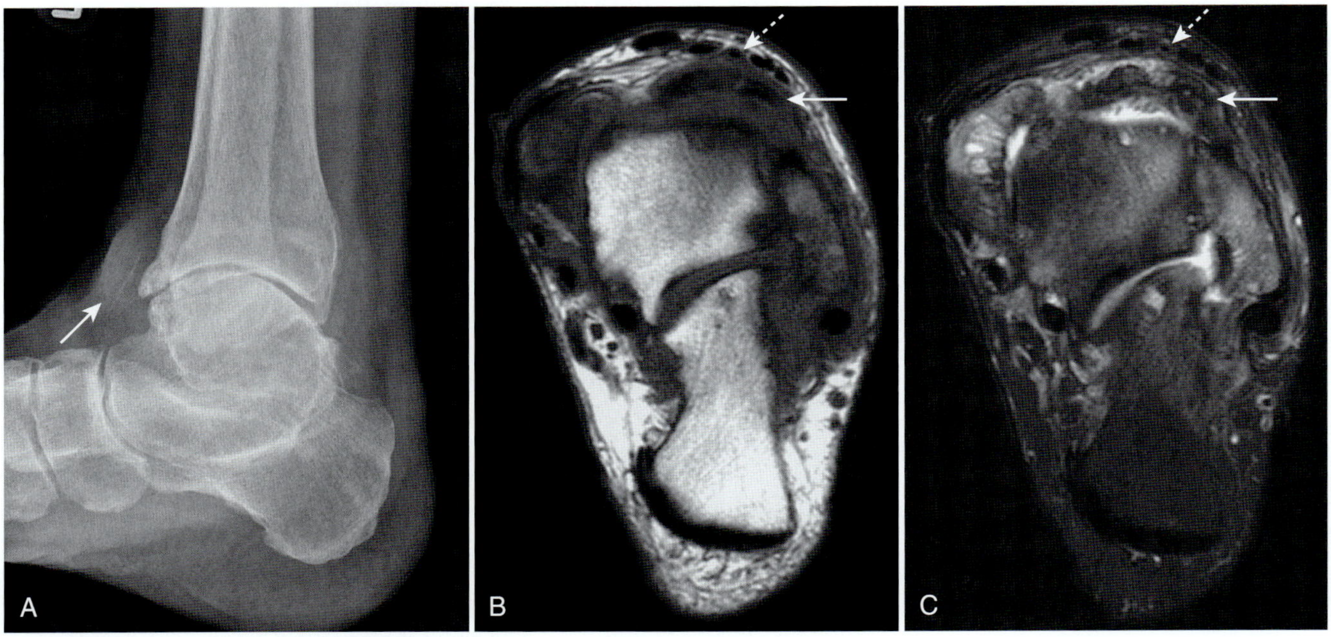

Figure 164.2 (A), Lateral radiograph of a patient with osteoarthritis of the ankle and subtalar joint. There is prominent anterior osteophyte formation at the anterior aspect of the joint with associated soft tissue shadowing (*white arrow*). The axial T1W (B) and T2W with fat suppression (FST2W) (C) MR images show the anterior osteophytosis and associated synovitis (*white arrows*) impinging on the extensor tendons. The anterior tibial artery is displaced anteriorly (*broken white arrows*) between the extensor tendons. The deep peroneal nerve is not visualized.

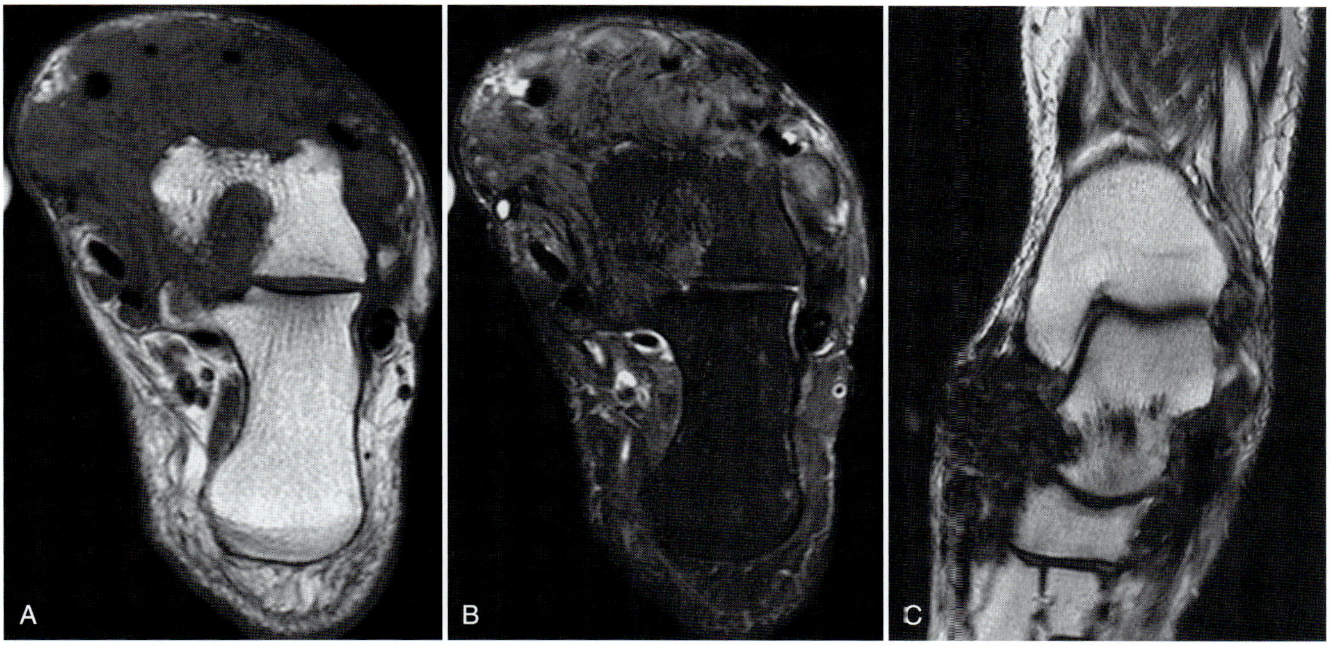

Figure 164.3 Axial T1W (**A**) and FST2W (**B**) MR images of a patient with ankle pain and paresthesia over the dorsal aspect of the foot. A mass of synovitis arising from the ankle joint surrounds the extensor tendons and the anterior neurovascular bundle. The synovium has intermediate SI on both images and also on the coronal T2W MR image (**C**). There is also bony erosion. These appearances are typical of pigmented villonodular synovitis.

CHAPTER 165

Posterior Tarsal Tunnel Syndrome

DEFINITION

- Entrapment of the posterior tibial nerve at the ankle as it passes through the posterior tarsal tunnel.

SIGNS AND SYMPTOMS

- Presence of Tinel sign over the entrapped nerve.
- Pain at the ankle that radiates into the sole of the foot.
- Paresthesias at the ankle that radiate into the sole of the foot.
- Symptoms may radiate proximally from the site of entrapment.
- Passive range of motion preserved.
- Weakness of the flexor digitorum brevis.
- Weakness of the lumbricals, causing a sensation of foot instability.
- Night-time foot pain is common.
- Active inversion of the foot may exacerbate symptoms.

DEMOGRAPHICS

- Incidence: Female > Male.
- Much more common than anterior tarsal tunnel syndrome.
- Can occur acutely following trauma and fracture.
- More common after trauma, including repetitive stress injuries.
- Associated with rheumatoid arthritis.
- Wearing of shoes that are too tight often is implicated.
- Occasionally associated with thrombophlebitis involving the posterior tibial artery.

IMAGING RECOMMENDATIONS

- MRI or US:
  - Identification of mass lesion within tarsal tunnel.
- Radiography:
  - To exclude associated ankle joint arthropathy.

IMAGING FINDINGS

- Common masses within tarsal tunnel:
  - Fluid-filled ganglion cyst.
  - Giant cell tumor of the tendon sheath of the tibialis posterior tendon.
- Inflammatory tenosynovitis of flexor tendons:
  - Enhancement of thickened tendon sheath on post-contrast (obtained after administration of a contrast agent) MR images.
  - Echogenic, thickened tendon sheath on US with hypervascularity.
- Synovitis arising from the ankle joint.
  - Enhancing synovial tissue in ankle joint extending into the tarsal tunnel on post-contrast MR images.
  - Echogenic and hypervascular synovitis on US.

OTHER RECOMMENDED TESTING

- Electromyography and nerve conduction velocity testing of the lumbar nerve roots, lumbar plexus, and associated peripheral nerves.
- Laboratory testing for rheumatoid arthritis if suspected.

DIFFERENTIAL DIAGNOSIS

- Lumbar radiculopathy.
- Arthritis.
- Occult fracture.
- Diabetic polyneuropathy.
- Benign neoplasm.
- Malignant neoplasm.
- Ganglion.
- Tendinitis.

TREATMENT

- Conservative treatment consisting of local heat, cold, simple analgesics, and nonsteroidal anti-inflammatory agents will improve symptoms in mild, self-limited cases.
- Physical therapy to maintain function. including gentle stretching, range-of-motion exercises, and local heat modalities. may be beneficial in selected patients.
- Splinting to preserve normal range of motion.
- Avoidance of shoes that are too tight.
- Injection with local anesthetic and steroid of the posterior tibial nerve may provide symptomatic relief if conservative therapy fails or if the pain is limiting activities of daily living.
- Surgery may be required to relieve entrapment of posterior tibial nerve.

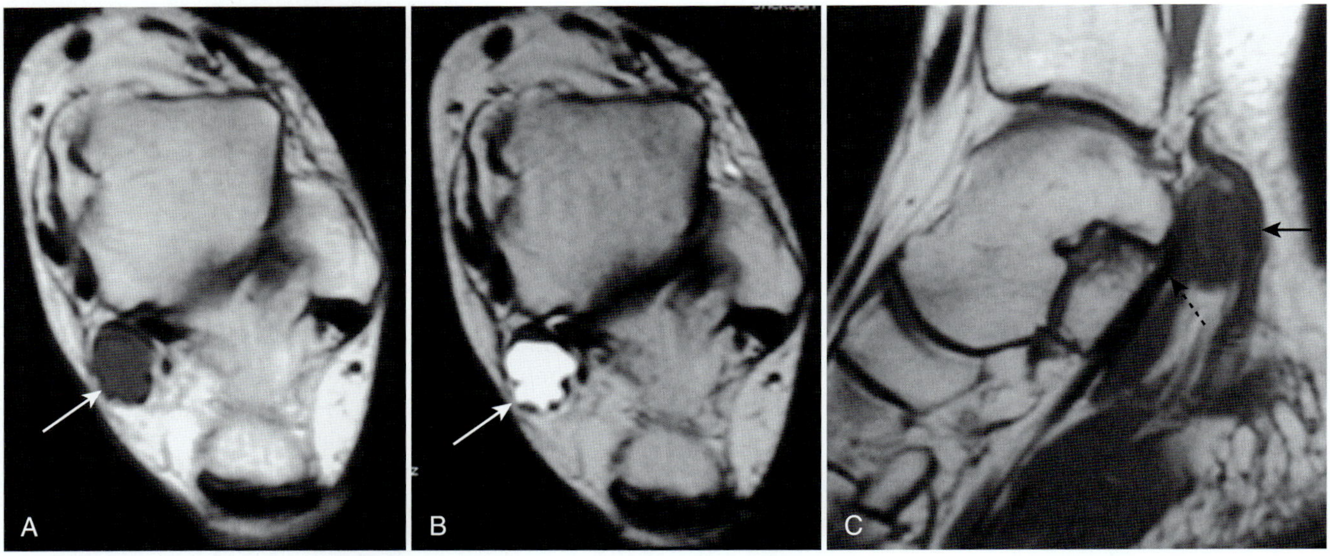

Figure 165.1 Axial proton density (PD) (**A**) and T2-weighted (T2W) (**B**) MR images of the ankle in a patient with medial foot pain. There is a discrete rounded lesion (*white arrow*) within the tarsal tunnel. It has intermediate signal intensity (SI) on the PD MR images and high SI on the T2W MR images consistent with a fluid-filled ganglion cyst. (**C**) The sagittal T1W MR image demonstrates the mass posterior to the talus and the flexor hallucis longus tendon (*broken arrow*), and one of the posterior tibial vessels runs over the superficial surface of the mass (*black arrow*). The cyst is causing mass effect within the tarsal tunnel, compressing the posterior tibial nerve and producing symptoms of posterior tarsal tunnel syndrome. *(Reproduced with permission from Spratt JD et al. The role of diagnostic radiology in compressive and entrapment neuropathies. European Radiology 2002:12; 2352-2364.)*

CHAPTER 166

Achilles Tendinitis

DEFINITION

- Inflammation of the Achilles tendon occurring most commonly at its narrowest part, approximately 5 cm above its insertion or at the calcaneus muscles, due to repetitive microtrauma to the musculotendinous unit.

SIGNS AND SYMPTOMS

- Acute onset of sharp, constant, and severe posterior ankle pain.
- Positive Achilles creak test result.
- Antalgic gait often present.
- Catching and creaking may be present.
- Exacerbation of pain with resisted plantar-flexion.
- Patient often unable to sleep on the affected side.

DEMOGRAPHICS

- Incidence: Male = Female.
- Young athletes who participate in running and in sports that involve sudden stopping and starting often affected.
- Bursitis often present.
- More common after trauma, including repetitive stress injuries.

IMAGING RECOMMENDATIONS

- MRI or US:
  - US may be also be used to guide therapeutic injections.
- Radiography:
  - Not routinely indicated.

IMAGING FINDINGS

- Fusiform thickening of the mid-Achilles tendon:
  - Distal tendon less commonly involved: Insertional tendinopathy (Haglund syndrome).
- MRI:
  - Diffuse increased signal intensity (SI) on all pulse sequences.
  - Focal areas of fluid SI on T2-weighted (T2W) and T2W with fat suppression (FST2W) MR images are suggestive of partial tears or mucoid degeneration.
- US:
  - Ill-defined areas of low-reflective change and loss of fibrillar pattern.
  - Microcalcification.
  - Neovascularization on Doppler imaging.
  - Discrete hyporeflective clefts on US are suggestive of partial tears.
- Reactive paratenonitis of the adventitial tendon sheath, with fluid encompassing the tendon.
- Associated retrocalcaneal bursitis.

OTHER RECOMMENDED TESTING

- Laboratory testing to rule out inflammatory arthritis.
- Joint aspiration to rule out crystal arthropathies.
- Joint aspiration to rule out infection if diagnosis in question.

DIFFERENTIAL DIAGNOSIS

- Calcific tendinitis.
- Occult ankle fractures.
- Posterior tarsal tunnel syndrome.
- Diabetic polyneuropathy.
- Thrombophlebitis of the posterior tibial artery.
- Internal derangement of the ankle.
- Neoplasm.

TREATMENT

- Conservative treatment consisting of local heat, cold, simple analgesics, and nonsteroidal anti-inflammatory agents will improve symptoms in many cases.
- Physical therapy, including gentle stretching, range-of-motion exercises, and deep heat modalities, may be beneficial in selected patients.
- Injection with local anesthetic and steroid will provide symptomatic relief if conservative therapy fails or the pain is limiting activities of daily living.
- Surgery may be required for persistent pain or progressive functional disability.

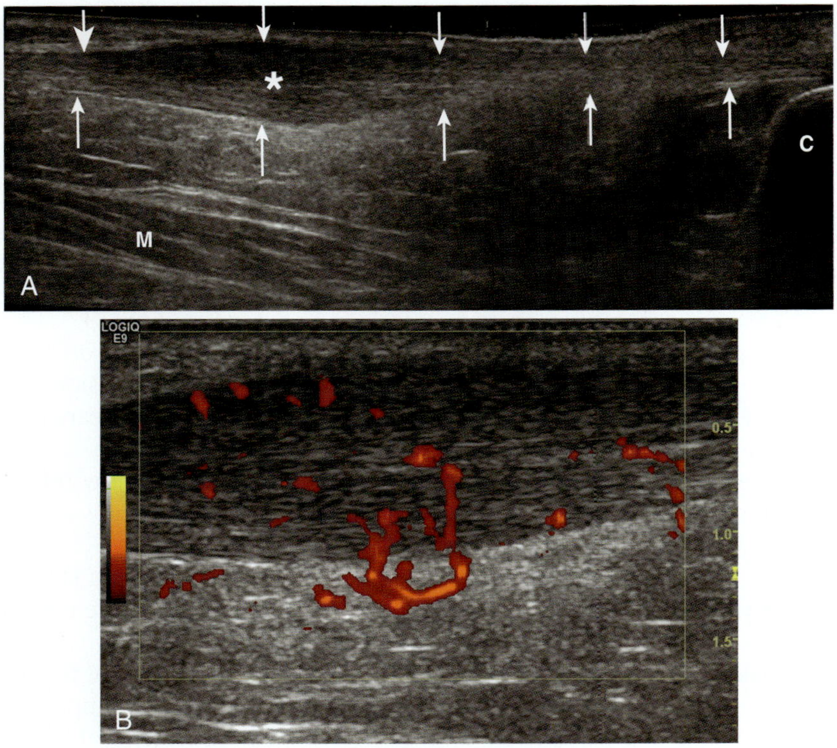

Figure 166.1 (A) Longitudinal US image of a patient with Achilles tendinopathy. The tendon (*white arrows*) inserts on the calcaneus (C), and lies superficial to Kager fat pad and the underlying posterior compartment muscle group (M). The mid-portion of the tendon demonstrates fusiform thickening with low-reflective change (*asterisk*). (B) A localized power Doppler image also shows the tendon thickening as well as prominent areas of neovascularization within the tendon substance.

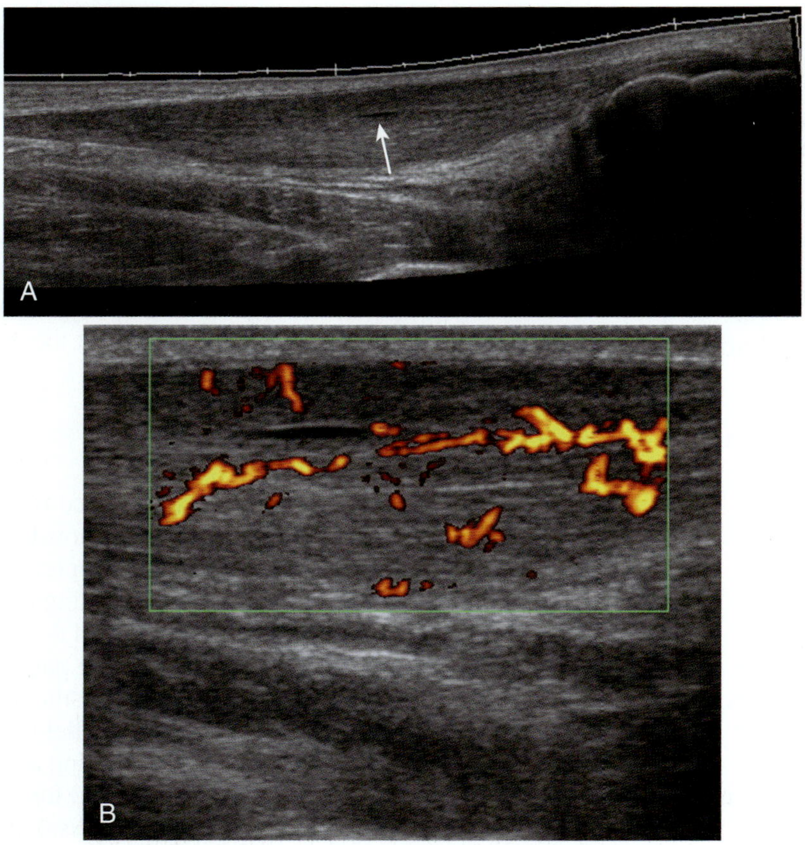

Figure 166.2 (A) Longitudinal US image of a small intrasubstance cleft (*white arrow*) of a thickened and tendinopathic Achilles tendon. (B) The power Doppler image demonstrates prominent neovascularization.

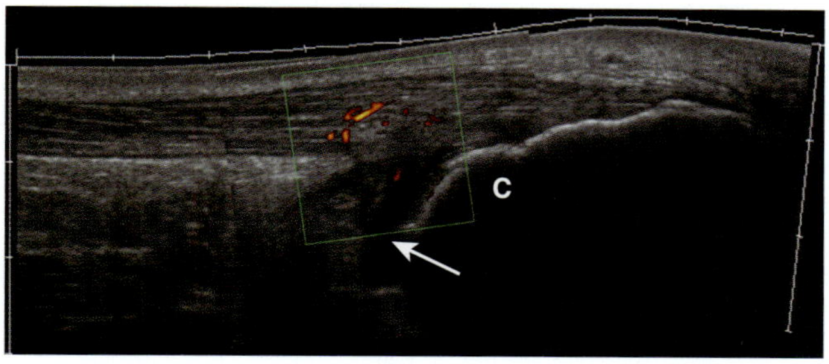

Figure 166.3 Longitudinal US of a patient with insertional tendinopathy of the Achilles tendon. Thickening, low-reflective change, and neovascularization are present close to the insertion on the calcaneus (C). In addition, anechoic fluid can be seen within the retrocalcaneal bursa (*white arrow*) that is due to associated bursitis.

CHAPTER 167

Achilles Tendon Rupture

DEFINITION

- Complete disruption of the Achilles tendon occurring most commonly at its narrowest part, approximately 5 cm above its insertion.

SIGNS AND SYMPTOMS

- Acute onset of sharp, constant, and severe posterior ankle pain.
- Positive Achilles squeeze test result.
- Ecchymosis.
- Swelling over the posterior ankle.
- Obvious tendon defect on palpation.
- Weak plantar-flexion.
- Exacerbation of pain with resisted plantar-flexion.
- Patient often unable to sleep on the affected side.

DEMOGRAPHICS

- Incidence: Male > Female.
- Young athletes who run or who play sports that involve sudden stopping and starting, such as basketball, racquetball, and tennis, often affected.
- Increased incidence in third to fifth decade of life.
- Bursitis often present.
- More common after trauma, including repetitive stress injuries.

IMAGING RECOMMENDATIONS

- US or MRI.
- Radiography not routinely indicated.

IMAGING FINDINGS

- US:
  - Localized defect in the tendon.
  - Hyporeflective hematoma in the tendon gap in early stages.
  - Hematoma becomes hyperreflective as granulation tissue develops.
  - Paradoxic movement of tendon ends on passive plantar-flexion and dorsiflexion of the foot.
- MRI:
  - Focal defect of the tendon.
  - Tendon gap filled with high-signal intensity (SI) fluid hematoma in early stages.
  - In later stages, enhancing granulation tissue seen on post-contrast (obtained after administration of a contrast agent) images.
- Preexisting tendinopathic changes are frequently present in the remaining tendon.
- Imaging can help guide surgical management, depending on the size of the tendon gap.

OTHER RECOMMENDED TESTING

- Laboratory testing to rule out inflammatory arthritis.
- Joint aspiration to rule out crystal arthropathies.
- Joint aspiration to rule out infection if diagnosis in question.

DIFFERENTIAL DIAGNOSIS

- Calcific tendinitis.
- Achilles bursitis.
- Achilles tendinitis.
- Occult ankle fractures.
- Posterior tarsal tunnel syndrome.
- Diabetic polyneuropathy.
- Thrombophlebitis of the posterior tibial artery.
- Internal derangement of the ankle.
- Neoplasm.

TREATMENT

- Conservative treatment consisting of local heat, cold, simple analgesics, and nonsteroidal anti-inflammatory agents will improve symptoms in many cases.
- Physical therapy, including gentle stretching, range-of-motion exercises, and deep heat modalities, may be beneficial in selected patients.
- Surgery usually required for persistent pain or progressive functional disability.

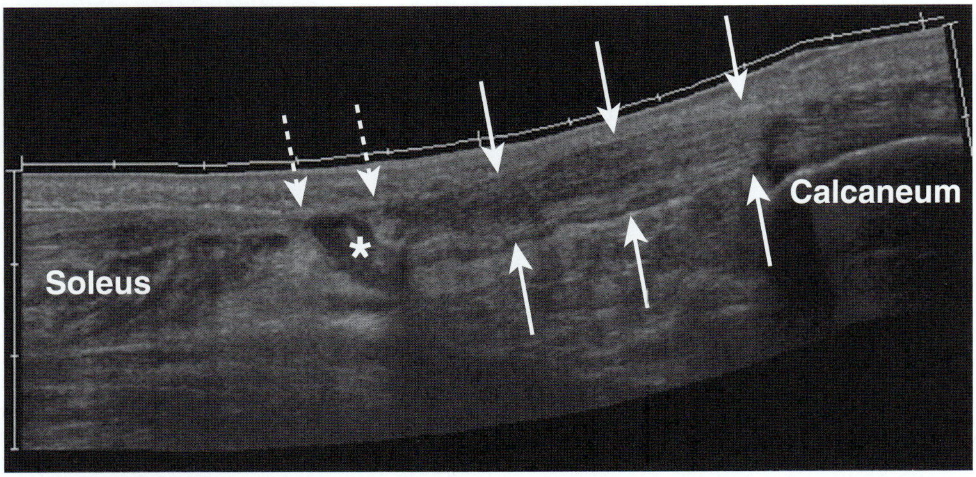

Figure 167.1 Longitudinal US image of an acute mid–Achilles tendon rupture. The distal tendon (*white arrows*) appears relatively normal, although there is some low-reflective fluid within the deep portion of the paratenon. The torn ends of the tendon are visualized (*broken white arrows*), and there is a low-reflective hematoma in the tendon gap (*asterisk*).

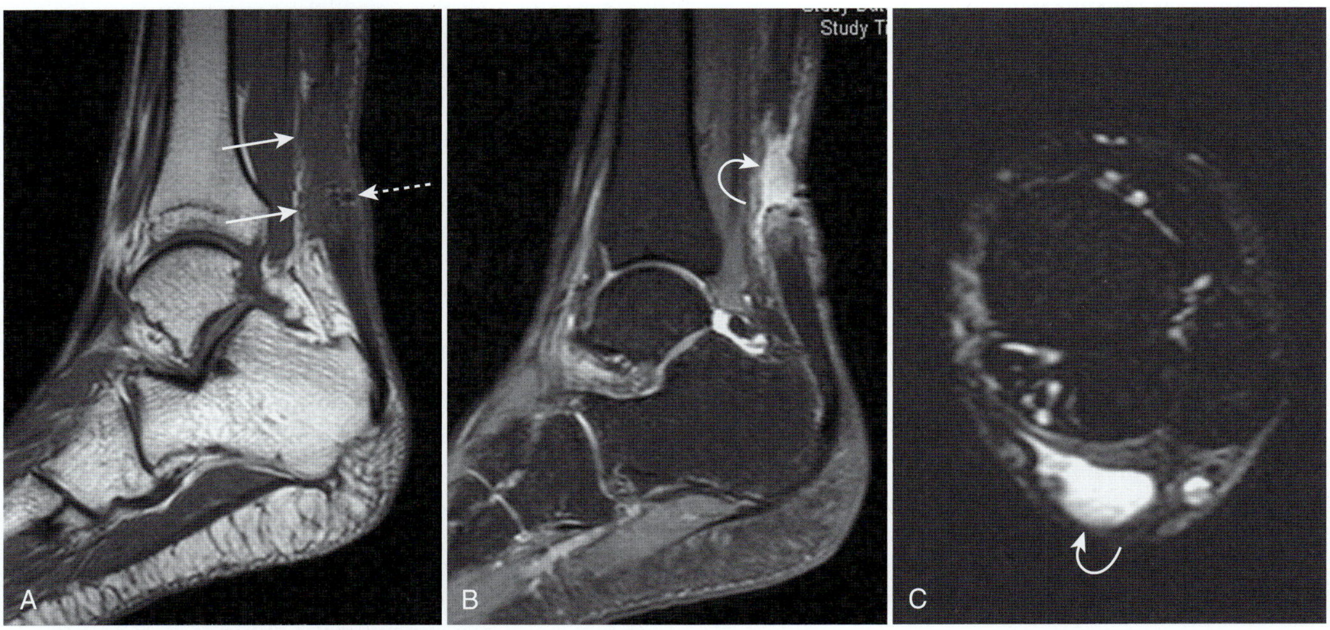

Figure 167.2 (**A**), Sagittal T1-weighted (T1W) MR image of a patient with a failed Achilles tendon repair. The midportion of the tendon is thickened, irregular, and of intermediate SI (*white arrows*). There are some areas of susceptibility artifact due to previous tendon repair (*broken white arrow*). The sagittal (**B**) and axial (**C**) T2W with fat suppression (FST2W) MR images demonstrate the tendon gap filled by high-SI hematoma (*curved white arrows*).

CHAPTER 168

Anterior Tibial Tendon Rupture

DEFINITION

- Complete disruption of the anterior tibial tendon, occurring most commonly between the flexor retinaculum and the insertion of the tendon onto the medial aspect of the first cuneiform and the base of the adjacent first metatarsal.

SIGNS AND SYMPTOMS

- Acute onset of sharp, constant, and severe anteromedial ankle pain.
- Footdrop.
- Ecchymosis.
- Swelling over the anteromedial ankle.
- Defect at the site of tendon rupture often palpable.
- Steppage gait often present.
- Heel walking on the affected side difficult.
- Forefoot eversion with active dorsiflexion.
- Pain with resisted foot dorsiflexion.
- Patient often unable to sleep on the affected side.

DEMOGRAPHICS

- Incidence: Male > Female.
- Often associated with posterior tibial tendon rupture.
- Increased incidence in fifth and sixth decades of life.
- Bursitis often present.
- Common in runners and soccer players.
- More common after trauma, including repetitive stress injuries.

IMAGING RECOMMENDATIONS

- MRI or US.
- Radiography not routinely indicated.

IMAGING FINDINGS

- Focal defect of the distal tendon.
- Proximal tendon end often retracted to the level of the retinaculum.
- Thickening of the proximal tendon.
- Fluid within the proximal tendon sheath.
- Surrounding hemorrhage and edema in acute cases.

OTHER RECOMMENDED TESTING

- Laboratory testing to rule out inflammatory arthritis.
- Joint aspiration to rule out crystal arthropathies.
- Joint aspiration to rule out infection if diagnosis in question.

DIFFERENTIAL DIAGNOSIS

- Calcific tendinitis.
- Occult ankle fractures.
- Deltoid ligament pathology.
- Anterior tarsal tunnel syndrome.
- Peroneal nerve entrapment.
- Diabetic polyneuropathy.
- Thrombophlebitis.
- Tibiotalar synovitis.
- Internal derangement of the ankle.
- Neoplasm.

TREATMENT

- Conservative treatment consisting of local heat, cold, simple analgesics and nonsteroidal anti-inflammatory agents will improve symptoms in many cases.
- Physical therapy, including gentle stretching, range-of-motion exercises and deep heat modalities, may be beneficial in selected patients.
- A weight-bearing cast may be effective in more sedentary individuals.
- Surgery often required for persistent pain or progressive functional disability.

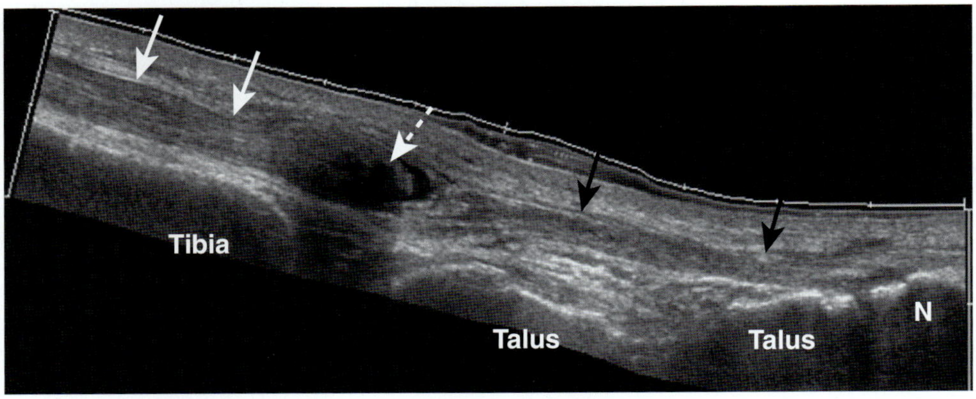

Figure 168.1 Longitudinal US image of rupture of the anterior tibialis tendon. The proximal tendon is visualized at the level of the distal tibia (*white arrows*), and the torn tendon end is retracted, lying at the level of the ankle joint (*broken white arrow*). The distal tendon sheath (*black arrows*) is filled with echogenic granulation tissue and extends down the insertion on the navicular (N).

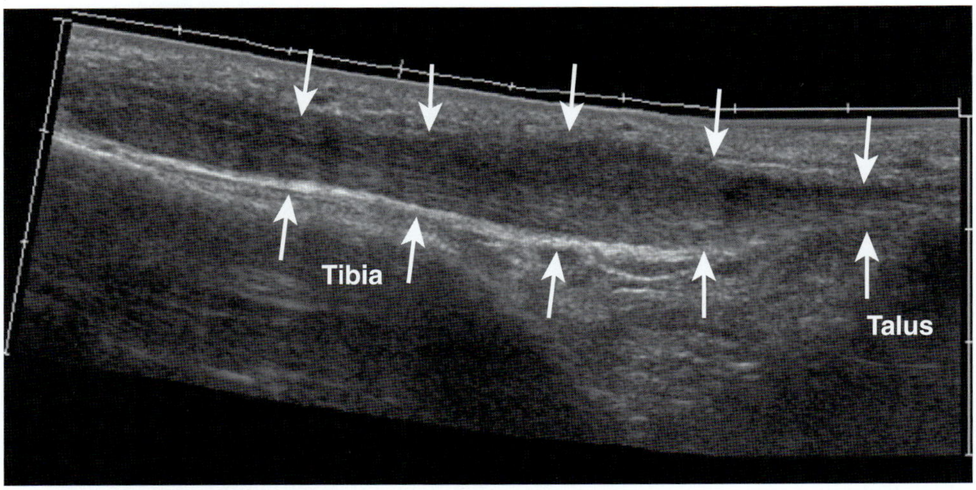

Figure 168.2 Longitudinal image of a thickened and tendinopathic anterior tibialis tendon (*white arrows*), with poorly defined and irregular margins. There is no tendon rupture.

CHAPTER 169

Posterior Tibial Tendon Rupture

DEFINITION

- Complete disruption of the posterior tibial tendon, occurring most commonly at the medial malleolus.

SIGNS AND SYMPTOMS

- Acute onset of sharp, constant, and severe medial ankle pain.
- Flattening of the medial longitudinal arch resulting in pes valgus deformity.
- Ecchymosis.
- Swelling over the medial ankle.
- Heel valgus often present.
- Forefoot abduction often present.
- Pain with resisted foot inversion and plantarflexion.
- Patient often unable to sleep on affected side.

DEMOGRAPHICS

- Incidence: Female > Male.
- Left-sided rupture more common.
- Increased incidence in fifth and sixth decades of life.
- Bursitis often present.
- More common after trauma, including repetitive stress injuries.

IMAGING RECOMMENDATIONS

- MRI or US.
- Radiography not routinely indicated.

IMAGING FINDINGS

- Staging of posterior tibial tendon dysfunction:
  - Grade I: Tendinopathy.
  - Grade II: Partial tear.
  - Grade III: Complete rupture.
- Defect of tendon at the level of the malleolus or distally.
- Fluid within the proximal and distal tendon sheath.
- Thickening and heterogeneity of the remaining tendon due to preexisting tendinopathy.
- Surrounding hemorrhage and edema in acute cases.

OTHER RECOMMENDED TESTING

- Laboratory testing to rule out inflammatory arthritis.
- Joint aspiration to rule out crystal arthropathies.
- Joint aspiration to rule out infection if diagnosis in question.

DIFFERENTIAL DIAGNOSIS

- Calcific tendinitis.
- Achilles bursitis.
- Achilles tendinitis.
- Occult ankle fractures.
- Deltoid ligament pathology.
- Posterior tarsal tunnel syndrome.
- Diabetic polyneuropathy.
- Thrombophlebitis of the posterior tibial artery.
- Internal derangement of the ankle.
- Neoplasm.

TREATMENT

- Conservative treatment consisting of local heat, cold, simple analgesics, and nonsteroidal anti-inflammatory agents will improve symptoms in many cases.
- Physical therapy, including gentle stretching, range-of-motion exercises, and deep heat modalities, may be beneficial in selected patients.
- Surgery often required for persistent pain or progressive functional disability.

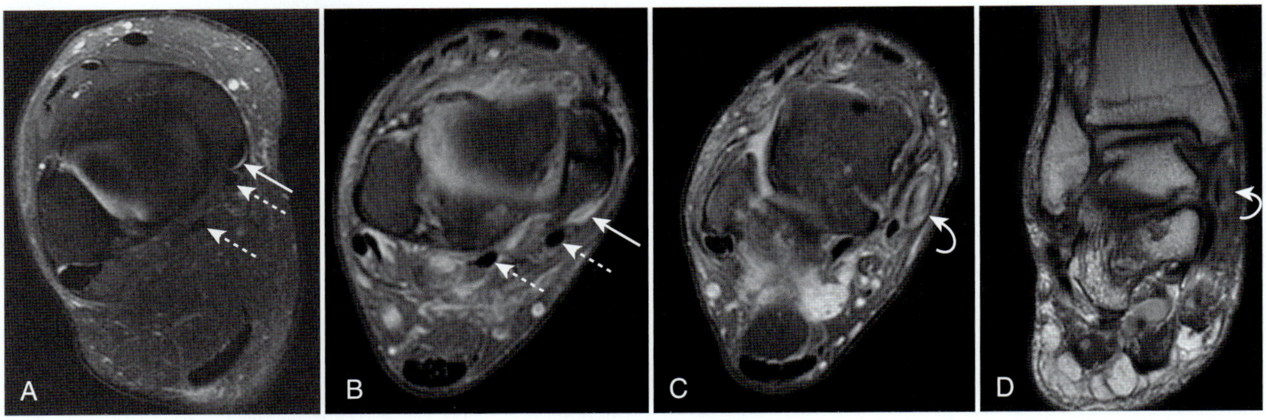

Figure 169.1 (A), Axial T2-weighted with fat suppression (FST2W) MR image of a normal posterior tibial tendon (*white arrow*) within the tarsal tunnel adjacent to the other flexor tendons of the flexor digitalis longus and flexor hallucis longus (*broken arrows*). (B), The axial FST2W MR image in a patient with a posterior tibial tendon rupture shows an empty tendon sheath filled with high-signal intensity (SI) fluid (*solid white arrow*). The inferior axial FST2W MR image (C) and coronal proton density (PD) MR image (D) show the thickened degenerated distal tendon remnant (*curved arrows*).

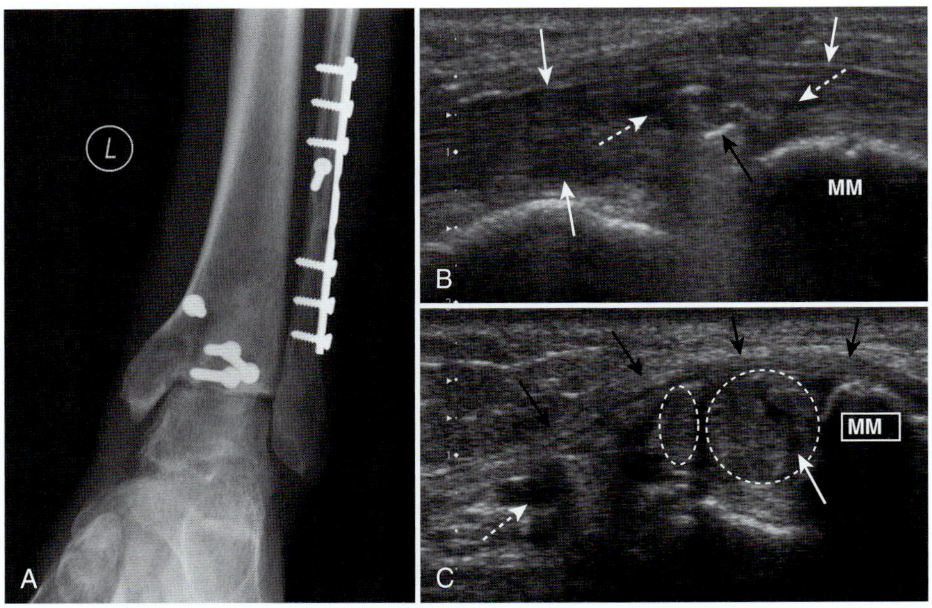

Figure 169.2 (A), Radiograph of a patient with symptoms of posterior tibial tendon dysfunction after a previous instrumented fixation of the distal tibia and fibula. (B), The longitudinal US image shows the tibial tendon (*white arrows*) at the level of the medial malleolus (MM), with the head of one of the orthopedic screws (*black arrow*) impinging on the tendon. There is a low-echo tear within the tendon substance (*broken arrows*). (C), The tranverse US image shows the tendons of the tibialis posterior and flexor digitalis longus (*white circles*) deep to the flexor retinaculum (*black arrows*) and posterior to the medical malleolus (MM). There is a split within the tibial tendon (*white arrow*). The posterior tibial vessels can also be seen (*broken white arrow*).

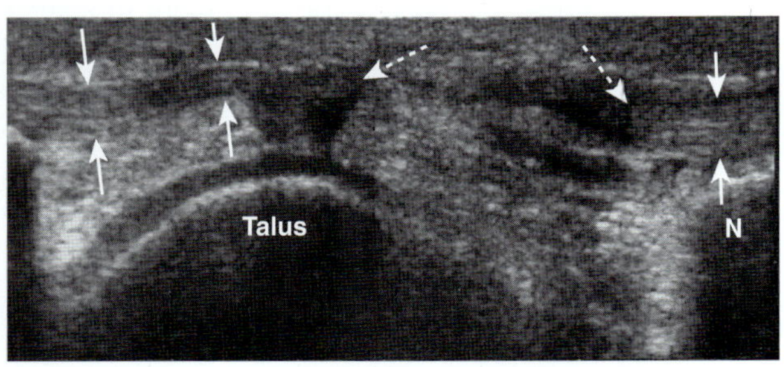

Figure 169.3 Longitudinal US image of a complete rupture of the posterior tibial tendon. The proximal and distal tendon (*white arrows*) is visualized inferior to the level of the medial malleolus, superficial to the talus, and inserting on the navicular (N). The torn ends of the tendon (*broken arrows*) can be seen, with some anechoic fluid within the tendon sheath.

CHAPTER 170

Anterior Talofibular Ligament Tear

DEFINITION

- Disruption of the fibers of the anterior talofibular ligament, occurring most commonly along its course from the anterior lateral malleolus to its insertion just anterior to the lateral articular facet.

SIGNS AND SYMPTOMS

- Acute onset of sharp, constant, and severe lateral ankle pain.
- Patient also describes hearing a pop at the time of injury.
- Ecchymosis.
- Swelling over the lateral ankle.
- Antalgic gait often present.
- Patient unable to stand unassisted on the affected ankle.
- Pain with resisted foot inversion.
- Pain with weight bearing.
- Patient often unable to sleep on the affected side.

DEMOGRAPHICS

- Incidence in Male > Female until fourth decade of life; then female preponderance.
- The most common ankle sprain.
- Often associated with running and jumping.
- Bursitis and tendinitis often present.
- More common after trauma, including repetitive stress injuries.
- Associated with hypoplastic ligament in some cases.

IMAGING RECOMMENDATIONS

- Imaging not routinely required for most simple ankle sprains:
  - May be used for acute injuries in sports injuries.
- Radiography to exclude bony injury.
- MRI or US is the primary modality for investigation of ankle instability.
- Stress radiography in equivocal cases.

IMAGING FINDINGS

- Acute injuries:
  - Localized soft tissue swelling and edema.
  - Focal disruption of the ligament.
- Chronic injuries:
  - Scarring and thickening in the anterolateral gutter: May be associated with reactive synovitis. Part of anterolateral impingement.
  - Irregular thickened ligament.
  - Absence of ligament.

OTHER RECOMMENDED TESTING

- Laboratory testing to rule out inflammatory arthritis.
- Joint aspiration to rule out crystal arthropathies.
- Joint aspiration to rule out infection if diagnosis in question.

DIFFERENTIAL DIAGNOSIS

- Calcific tendinitis.
- Occult ankle fracture, especially of the lateral malleolus.
- Occult tarsal fractures.
- Often associated with deltoid ligament pathology.
- Diabetic polyneuropathy.
- Thrombophlebitis.
- Ankle synovitis.
- Internal derangement of the ankle.
- Neoplasm.

TREATMENT

- Conservative treatment consisting of local heat, cold, simple analgesics, and nonsteroidal anti-inflammatory agents will improve symptoms in many cases.
- Physical therapy, including gentle stretching, range-of-motion exercises, and deep heat modalities, may be beneficial in selected patients.
- Weight-bearing cast or controlled ankle motion (CAM) walker boot may be effective in more sedentary individuals.
- Surgery often required for persistent pain or progressive functional disability.

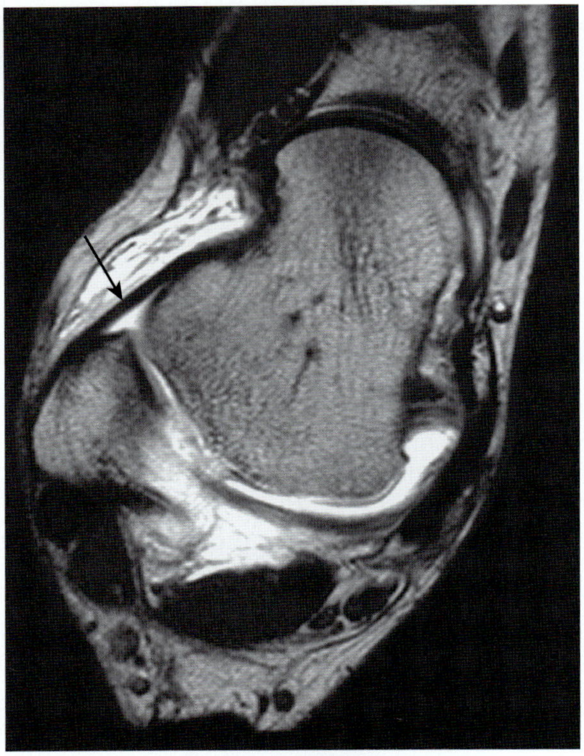

Figure 170.1 Axial T1-weighted (T1W) MR arthrogram image outlining a normal low–signal intensity (SI) anterior talofibular ligament (*arrow*).

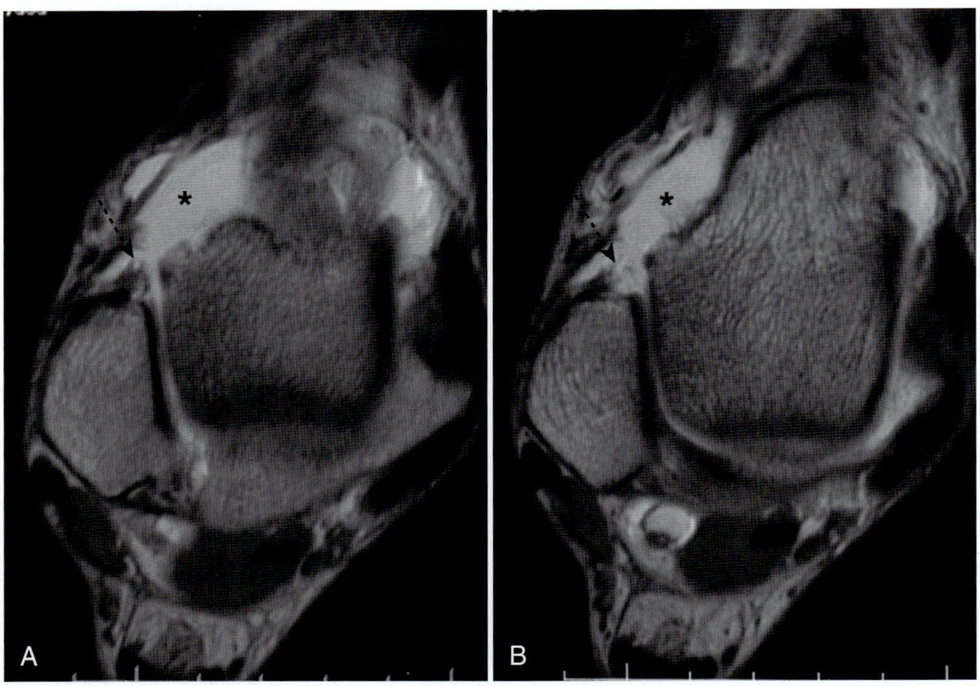

Figure 170.2 (A and B), Consecutive axial T1W MR arthrogram images demonstrating complete rupture of the talofibular ligament with only a small proximal remnant (*broken arrows*). High-SI fluid has extravasated outside the normal joint recesses (*asterisks*).

CHAPTER 171

Deltoid Ligament Tear

DEFINITION

- Disruption of the fibers of the deltoid ligament, occurring most commonly at the medial malleolus:
  - Minor strain injuries are common.
  - Complete rupture is usually associated with major ankle injury.

SIGNS AND SYMPTOMS

- Acute onset of sharp, constant, and severe medial ankle pain.
- Patient also notes a pop heard at time of injury.
- Ecchymosis.
- Swelling over the medial ankle.
- Antalgic gait often present.
- Patient unable to stand unassisted on the affected ankle.
- Pain with resisted foot eversion.
- Pain with weight bearing.
- Patient often unable to sleep on the affected side.

DEMOGRAPHICS

- Incidence in Male > Female until fourth decade of life; then female preponderance.
- Fairly common ankle sprain.
- Often associated with running and jumping.
- Bursitis and tendinitis often present.
- More common after trauma, including repetitive stress injuries.
- Associated with hypoplastic ligament in some cases.

IMAGING RECOMMENDATIONS

- Radiography:
  - Associated bony avulsion injuries.
- MRI or US not routinely indicated for acute injuries.

IMAGING FINDINGS

- Disruption of ankle mortise indicates complete ligament disruption associated with major ankle injuries.
- Small bony avulsions at tip of medial malleolus associated with simple ligament sprains.
- Soft tissue swelling and joint effusion.
- Associated osteochondral injuries of the talus.
- Thickening of ligament in partial tears with high signal intensity (SI) on T2-weighted with fat suppression (FST2W) MR images.
- Chronic tears may lead to fibrosis with anteromedial impingement.

OTHER RECOMMENDED TESTING

- Laboratory testing to rule out inflammatory arthritis.
- Joint aspiration to rule out crystal arthropathies.
- Joint aspiration to rule out infection if diagnosis in question.

DIFFERENTIAL DIAGNOSIS

- Calcific tendinitis.
- Occult ankle fracture, especially of medial malleolus.
- Occult tarsal fractures.
- Often there is associated deltoid ligament pathology.
- Diabetic polyneuropathy.
- Thrombophlebitis.
- Ankle synovitis.
- Internal derangement of the ankle.
- Neoplasm.

TREATMENT

- Conservative treatment consisting of local heat, cold, simple analgesics, and nonsteroidal anti-inflammatory agents will improve symptoms in many cases.
- Physical therapy, including gentle stretching, range-of-motion exercises, and deep heat modalities, may be beneficial in selected patients to preserve range of motion.
- Weight-bearing cast or CAM (controlled ankle motion) walking boot may be effective in more sedentary individuals.
- Surgery often required for persistent pain or progressive functional disability.

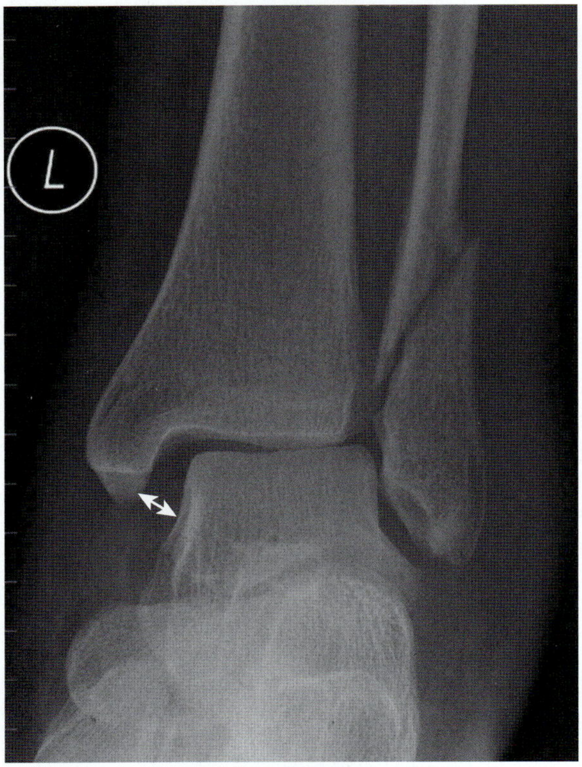

Figure 171.1 AP radiograph of a severe acute eversion ankle injury. There is an oblique fracture of the distal fibula. Disruption of the ankle mortise with widening of the medial joint line (*double-headed arrow*) indicates a tear of the deltoid ligament. This pattern of injury is less common than an avulsion fracture of the entire medial malleolus with an intact ligament.

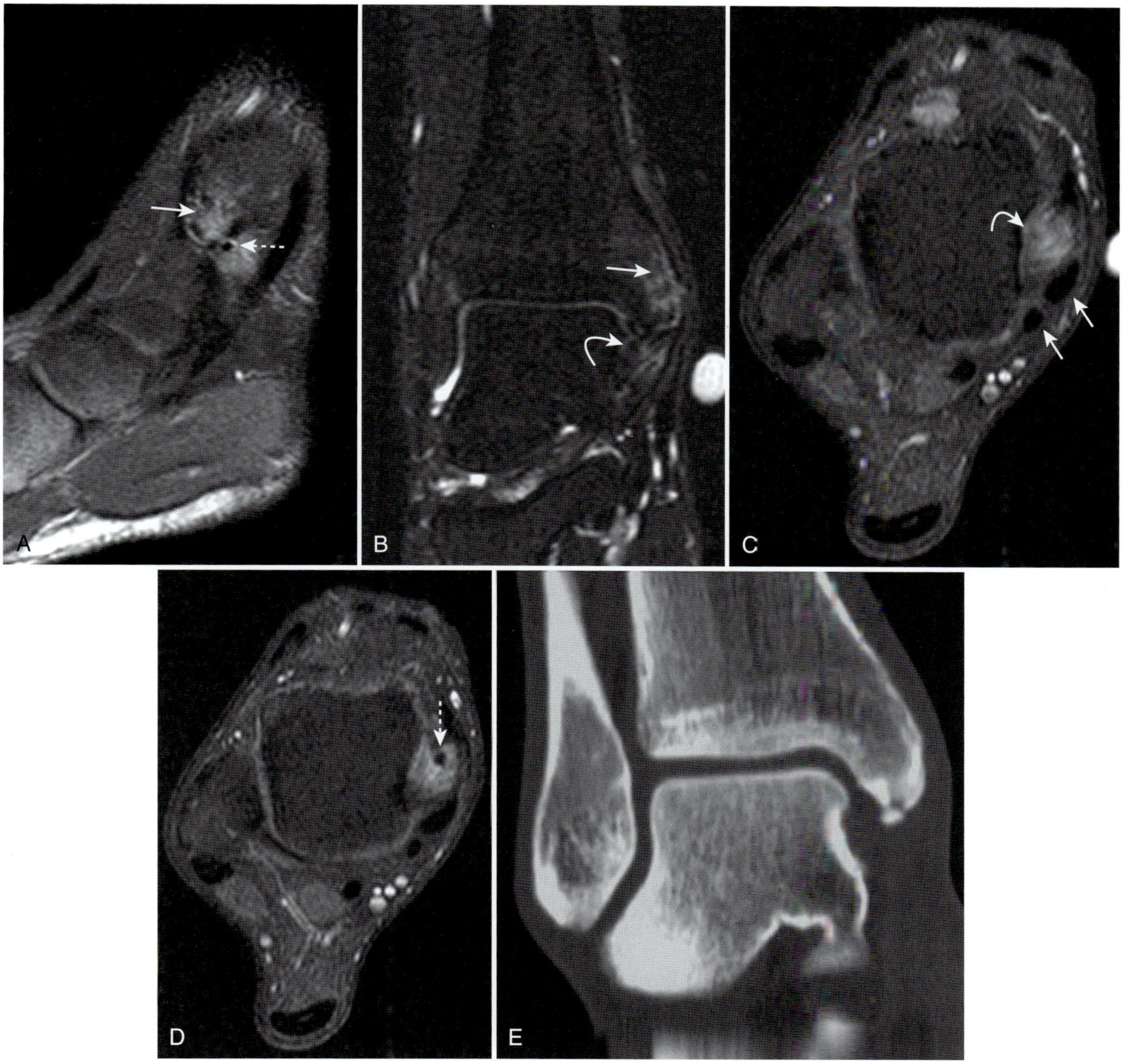

Figure 171.2 (**A**), Sagittal FST2W MR image of an athlete with a subacute eversion ankle sprain. There is marrow edema in the tip of the medial malleolus (*white arrow*) and a possible small bony avulsion injury (*broken white arrow*). (**B**), The coronal FST2W MR image also shows the marrow edema (*white arrow*), and there is high SI within the deltoid ligament (*curved white arrow*) as a result of partial tearing. (**C** and **D**), Consecutive axial FST2W MR images more clearly demonstrate the deltoid ligament edema (*curved white arrow*) anterior to the flexor tendons (*white arrows*). The bony avulsion fragment is demonstrated as a small round area of low SI (*broken white arrow*). (**E**), The coronal CT scan confirms the presence of an avulsion fracture of the tip of the medial malleolus.

CHAPTER 172

Tennis Leg

DEFINITION

- Complete disruption of the plantaris tendon or tear of medial gastrocemenius, occurring most commonly at the myotendinous junction.

SIGNS AND SYMPTOMS

- Acute onset of sharp, constant, and severe posterior calf pain.
- Patient often notes hearing a pop immediately prior to the onset of symptoms.
- Ecchymosis that is often out of proportion to the pain.
- Swelling over posterior calf that is often out of proportion to the pain.
- Pain on weight bearing.
- Pain on ambulation.

DEMOGRAPHICS

- Incidence: Male = Female.
- Middle-aged atheletes who play sports that involve pushing off and sudden stopping and starting, such as basketball, diving, and tennis.
- Increased incidence in fourth to fifth decade of life.
- More common after trauma including repetitive stress injuries.

IMAGING RECOMMENDATIONS

- MRI or US.
- Radiography not routinely indicated.

IMAGING FINDINGS

- Fluid extending between myotendinous junction of soleus and medial gastrocnemius muscles in the mid-calf.
- Superficial edema.
- Associated muscle tear:
  - High-signal intensity (SI) diffuse muscle edema on short T1 inversion recovery (STIR) MR images with focal fluid SI defect.
  - Ill-defined hyper-reflective muscle tear on US, becoming more focal and hyporeflective within the first few days.
- Intact Achilles tendon.
- Occasionally, the plantaris tendon may rupture distally.

OTHER RECOMMENDED TESTING

- Laboratory testing to rule out inflammatory arthritis.
- Joint aspiration to rule out crystal arthropathies.
- Joint aspiration to rule out infection if diagnosis in question.

DIFFERENTIAL DIAGNOSIS

- Calcific tendinitis
- Achilles bursitis.
- Achilles tendinitis.
- Occult ankle fracture.
- Posterior corner sprain.
- Gastrocnemius muscle and tendon pathology.
- Soleus muscle and tendon pathology.
- Thromboplebitis.
- Posterior compartment syndrome.
- Neoplasm.

TREATMENT

- Conservative treatment consisting of local heat, cold, simple analgesics, and nonsteroidal anti-inflammatory agents will improve symptoms in many cases.
- Physical therapy, including gentle stretching, range-of-motion exercises, and deep heat modalities, may be beneficial in selected patients.
- Surgery rarely required unless neurovascular compromise secondary to bleeding occurs.

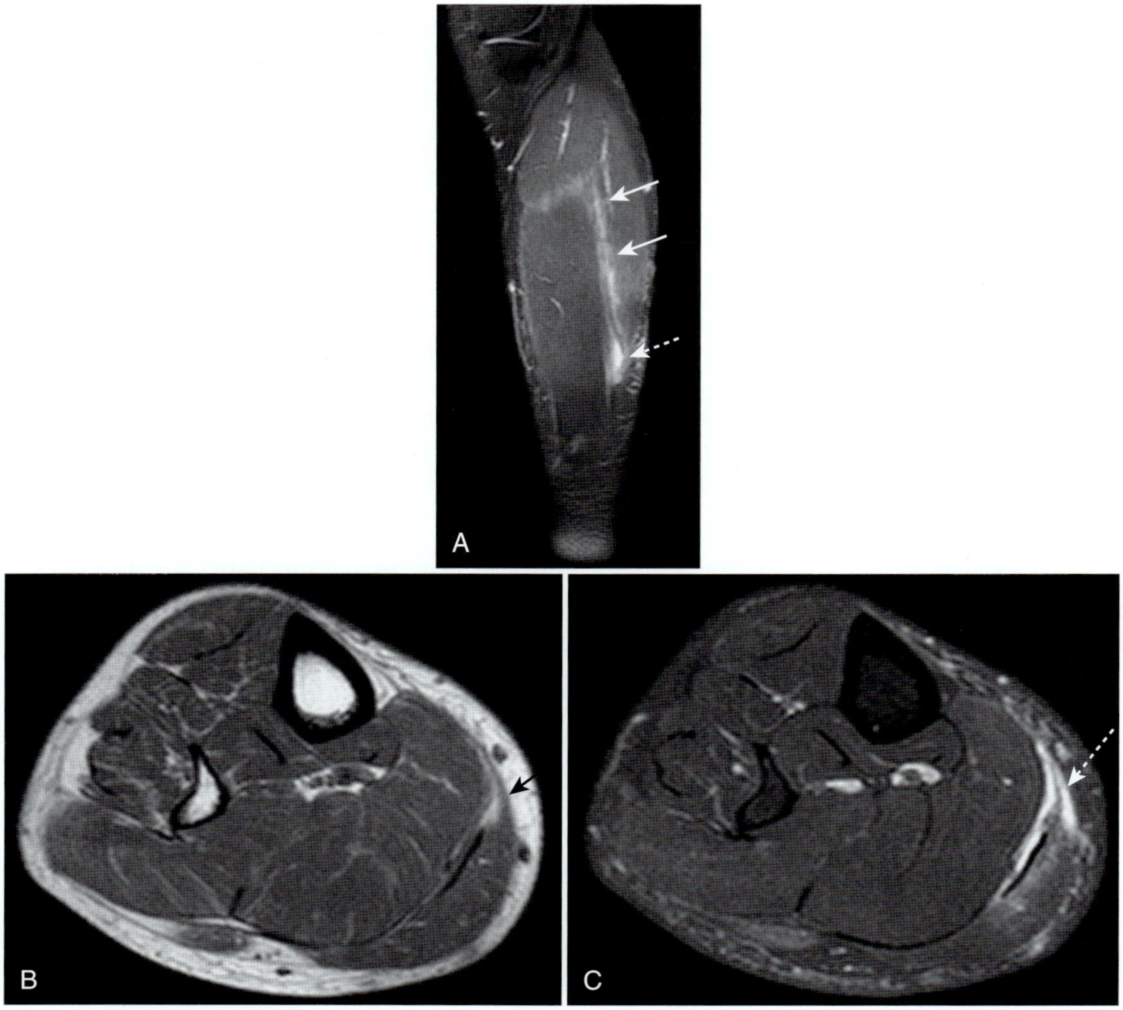

Figure 172.1 (A), Sagittal STIR MR image of a patient with an acute medial gastrocnemius muscle tear. There are high-SI diffuse edema within the muscle belly (*white arrows*) and a focal area of high-SI hematoma (*broken white arrow*). (B), The axial T1W MR image shows the partly retracted muscle belly (*black arrow*). (C), The high-SI hematoma (*white arrow*) can be seen on the axial T2W with fat suppression (FST2W) MR image.

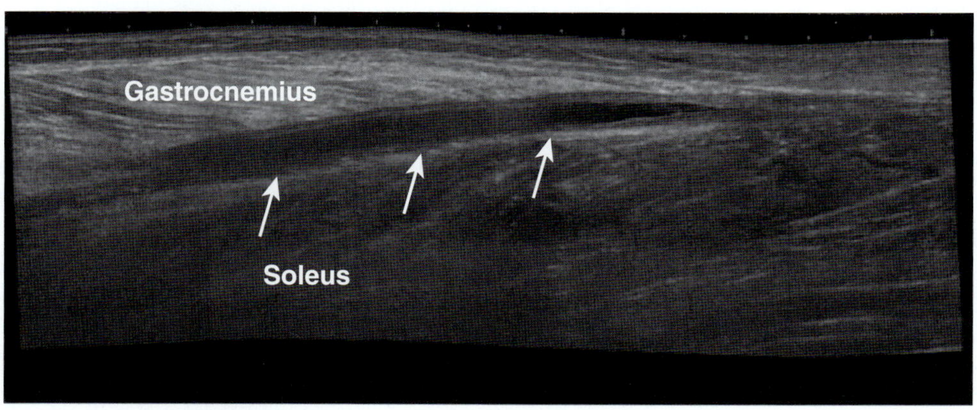

Figure 172.2 Longitudinal US image of a patient with tennis leg, showing a low-echo fluid-density hematoma extending along the myofascial plane between the gastrocnemius and soleus muscles.

CHAPTER 173

Osteonecrosis of the Ankle Joint

DEFINITION

- The death of cellular components of bone due to interruption of the blood supply, with resultant pain, collapse and destruction of bone, and loss of function.

SIGNS AND SYMPTOMS

- Gradual onset of pain with decreasing range of motion of the ankle joint.
- Crepitus may be present.
- Functional disability may be severe.

DEMOGRAPHICS

- Incidence: Male = Female.
- Age at onset related to date of trauma or onset of underlying disease, with sickle cell disease being the most common inciting factor in younger patients.
- Most common following ankle joint trauma that disrupts the vascular supply.
- More common in patients with sickle cell disease, Gaucher disease, Fabry disease, systemic lupus erythematosus (SLE), and gout.
- Often associated with exogenous steroid administration.
- Often associated with heavy alcohol intake.

IMAGING RECOMMENDATIONS

- Radiography.
- MRI:
  - Normal or equivocal radiographic findings.
- CT:
  - Alternative to MRI in patient with previous screw fixation of the talar neck.

IMAGING FINDINGS

- Radiography:
  - Evidence of a previous talar neck fracture or non-union.
  - Sclerosis in the talar dome.
  - In later stages, subchondral lucency and collapse, eventually leading to fragmentation and destruction of the articular surface.
- MRI:
  - High-signal intensity (SI) edema in the talar dome on short T1 inversion recovery (STIR) images.
  - Low-SI subchondral sclerosis on T1-weighted (T1W) and T2W MR images.
  - Eventual subchondral collapse and fragmentation.

OTHER RECOMMENDED TESTING

- Laboratory testing to rule out SLE.
- Laboratory testing to rule out gout.
- Joint aspiration to rule out crystal arthropathies.
- Joint aspiration to rule out infection.

DIFFERENTIAL DIAGNOSIS

- Inflammatory arthritides, especially SLE.
- Osteoarthritis.
- Bone marrow tumors.
- Primary bone tumors.
- Metastatic tumors.
- Osteochondral injuries.
- Osteochondrosis dissecans in younger patients.

TREATMENT

- Conservative treatment consisting of local heat, cold, simple analgesics, and nonsteroidal anti-inflammatory agents will improve symptoms in many cases.
- Physical therapy, including gentle stretching, range-of-motion exercises, and deep heat modalities, may be beneficial in selected patients.
- Intra-articular injection with local anesthetic and steroid will provide symptomatic relief if conservative therapy fails or the pain is limiting activities of daily living.
- Surgery may ultimately be required for persistent pain or progressive functional disability.

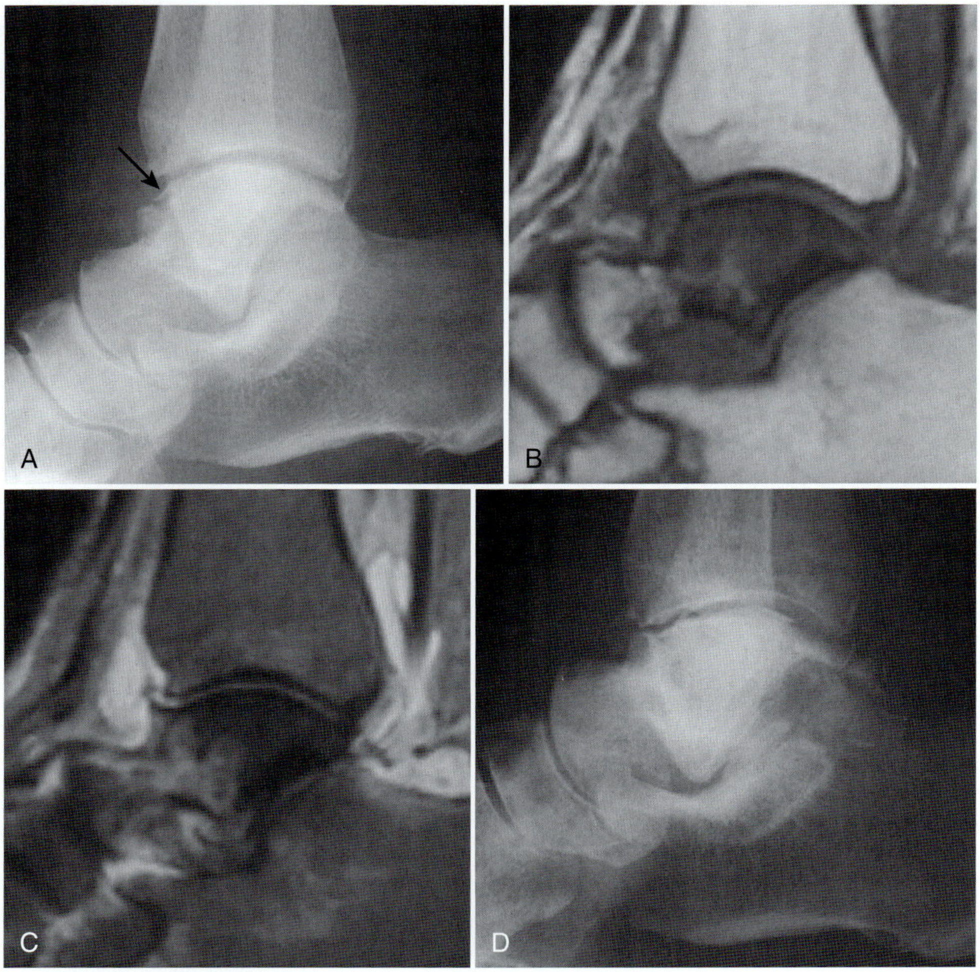

Figure 173.1 (A), Lateral radiograph of the ankle of a patient with ankle pain and a history of previous injury without fracture. There are early flattening and sclerosis of the talar dome, with a small articular fragment (*black arrow*). The sagittal T1W (B) and STIR (C) MR images show low-SI sclerosis in the dome of the talus. There is also high-SI marrow edema in the talar neck and a joint effusion is apparent on the STIR image. The appearances are consistent with avascular necrosis (AVN) of the talus. (D), A follow-up radiograph, taken a few months later, shows progressive collapse of the talus with increased sclerosis.

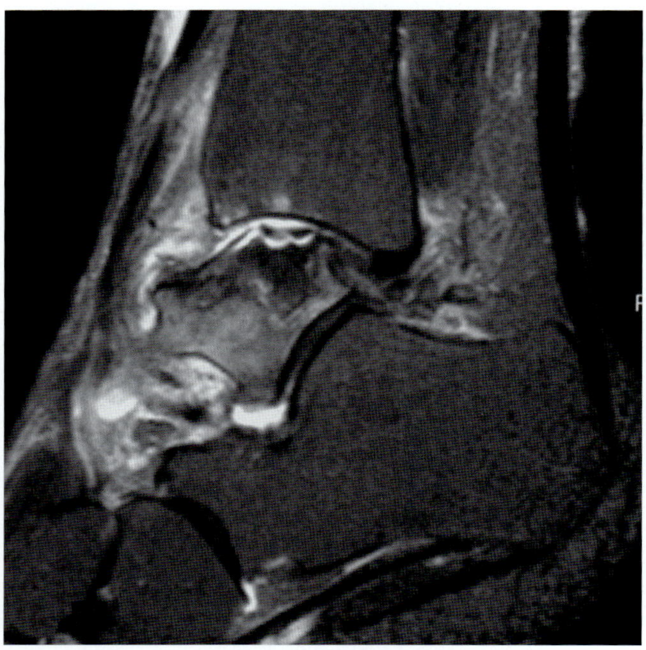

Figure 173.2 Sagittal T2W MR image of established AVN of the talus. There is a joint effusion, along with areas of subchondral collapse and fragmentation as well as reactive low-SI sclerosis and high-SI marrow edema.

CHAPTER 174

Freiberg's Disease

DEFINITION

- Avascular necrosis of the articular surface of the head of the metatarsal bone.

SIGNS AND SYMPTOMS

- Gradual onset of dull, ill-defined foot pain involving the metatarsal head.
- Swelling and synovitis over the affected joint.
- Crepitus may be present.
- Catching or clicking with weight bearing.
- Pain with range of motion.
- Antalgic gait.
- Loss of range of motion of the affected joint.

DEMOGRAPHICS

- Incidence: Male > Female.
- Almost always unilateral.
- 10- to 18-year-old persons most commonly affected.
- More common after severe trauma.

IMAGING RECOMMENDATIONS

- Radiographic findings are usually diagnostic.
- MRI not routinely indicated.

IMAGING FINDINGS

- Second and third metatarsals are most frequently involved.
- Features of avascular necrosis:
  - Sclerosis and subchondral collapse of the metatarsal head.
  - Fragmentation is uncommon.
  - In late stages, simple flattening of articular surface is the only abnormality.
- Secondary osteoarthritis changes are uncommon in young adults.
- Absence of changes on proximal phalanx helps exclude arthropathy.
- Multiple metatarsal involvement suggests a possible systemic cause of avascular necrosis, such as systemic lupus erythematosus (SLE).

OTHER RECOMMENDED TESTING

- Laboratory testing to rule out inflammatory arthritis.
- Joint aspiration to rule out crystal arthropathies.
- Joint aspiration to rule out infection if diagnosis in question.

DIFFERENTIAL DIAGNOSIS

- Metatarsal fracture.
- Forefoot arthritis.
- Crystal arthropathies.
- Charcot arthropathy.
- Rheumatoid arthritis.
- Diabetic polyneuropathy.
- Metatarsalgia.
- Scapulolunate ligament tear.
- Sesamoiditis.

TREATMENT

- Conservative treatment consisting of local heat, cold, simple analgesics, and nonsteroidal anti-inflammatory agents will improve symptoms in many cases.
- Physical therapy, including gentle stretching, range-of-motion exercises, and deep heat modalities, may be beneficial in selected patients.
- Splinting.
- Injection with local anesthetic and steroid will provide symptomatic relief if conservative therapy fails or the pain is limiting activities of daily living.
- Surgery may be required for persistent pain or progressive functional disability.

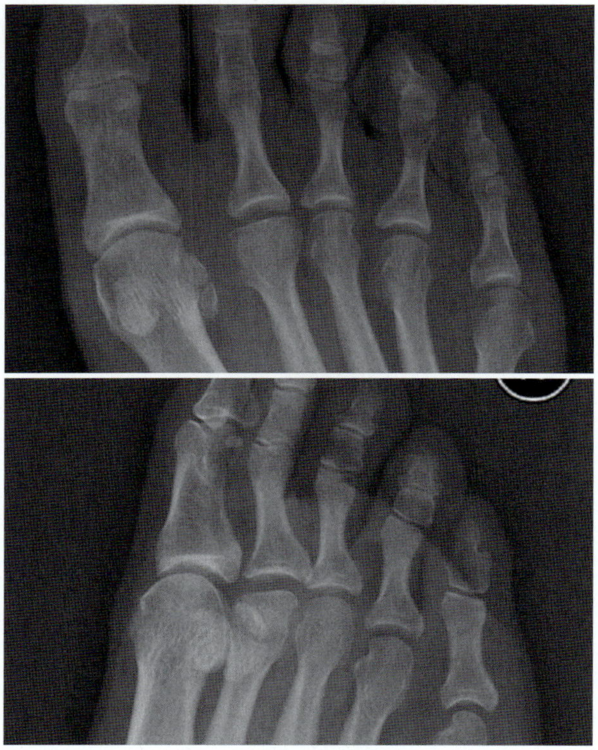

Figure 174.1 AP (*top*) and oblique (*bottom*) radiographs of the forefoot demonstrating flattening of the second metatarsal head in an adult patient secondary osteoarthritis changes in the metatarsophalangeal joint. These features, which are consistent with long-standing Freiberg's disease, are probably incidental findings.

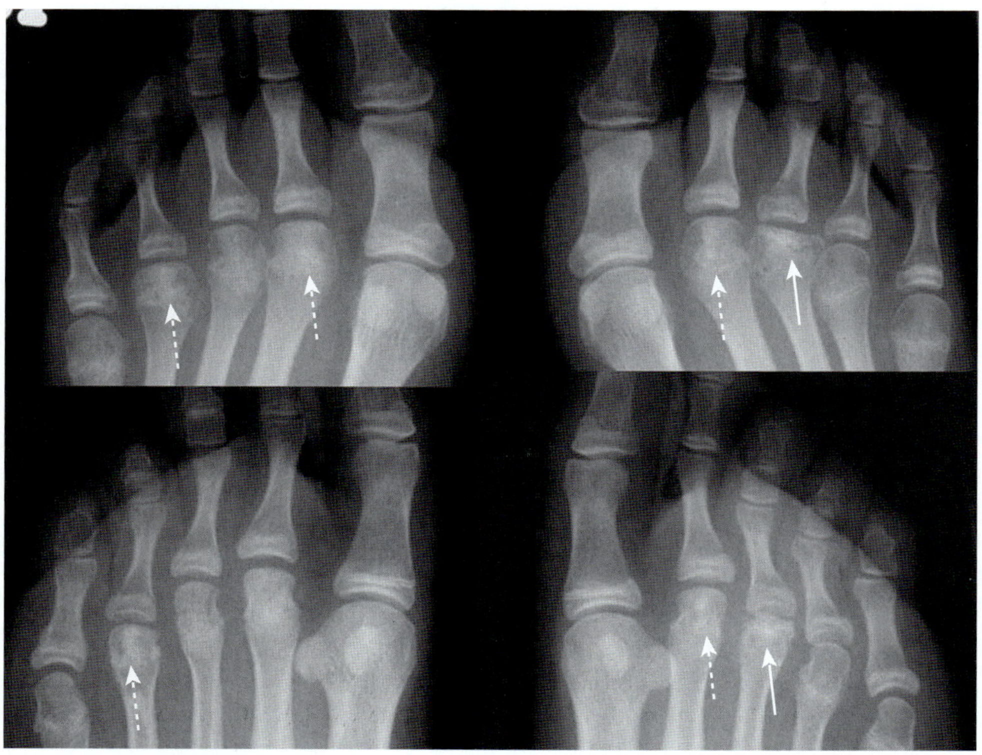

Figure 174.2 AP (*top*) and oblique (*bottom*) radiographs of both forefeet in a female adolescent. There is flattening, sclerosis, and fragmentation of the right third metatarsal head (*white arrows*). The features are the same as those of osteochondritis due to Freiberg's disease. However, there are also areas of sclerosis in several other metatarsal heads bilaterally, with some areas of subtle articular flattening (*broken white arrows*). The widespread changes are atypical for simple Freiberg's disease, and the diagnosis in this case is avascular necrosis secondary to a combination of SLE and steroid therapy.

CHAPTER 175

Os Trigonum

DEFINITION

- Failure of normal fusion of one or more of the ossification centers of the talus, resulting in separate posterior ossicles that may cause posterior impingement.

SIGNS AND SYMPTOMS

- Gradual onset of posterior ankle pain.
- Swelling of the posterior ankle.
- Exacerbation of pain with plantarflexion of ankle.
- Exacerbation of pain with weight bearing.
- Decreased subtalar range of motion.
- Clicking or catching sensation may be present.

DEMOGRAPHICS

- Incidence: Female > Male.
- Most common in the early third decade of life.
- Commonly associated with posterior ankle impingement syndromes.
- Commonly affects ballet dancers.

IMAGING RECOMMENDATIONS

- Radiography.
- MRI:
  - Diagnosis of posterior impingement.

IMAGING FINDINGS

- Bony ossicle at the posterior margin of the talus on lateral radiographs.
- Often a normal asymptomatic finding.
- Features of posterior impingement:
  - Marrow edema in os trigonum and posterior talus.
  - Effusion in ankle joint and posterior subtalar joint.
  - High-signal intensity (SI) fluid around os trigonum on T2-weighted (T2W) or T2W with fat suppression (FST2W) MR images.
  - Minor enhancing reactive synovitis in posterior ankle recess on post-contrast (obtained after administration of a contrast agent) MR images.
- Occasionally an elongated posterior Stieda process of the talus may cause posterior impingement.

OTHER RECOMMENDED TESTING

- Laboratory testing to rule out inflammatory arthritis if diagnosis in question.
- Joint aspiration to rule out crystal arthropathies if diagnosis in question.
- Joint aspiration to rule out infection if diagnosis in question.

DIFFERENTIAL DIAGNOSIS

- Pathology of flexor hallucis longus.
- Internal derangement of the ankle.
- Osteonecrosis of the talus.
- Shepard fracture.
- Post-traumatic arthritides.
- Inflammatory arthritides, especially rheumatoid arthritis.
- Dancer's foot.

TREATMENT

- Conservative treatment consisting of local heat, cold, simple analgesics, and nonsteroidal anti-inflammatory agents will improve symptoms in many cases.
- Physical therapy, including gentle stretching, range-of-motion exercises, and deep heat modalities, may be beneficial in selected patients.
- Intra-articular injection with local anesthetic and steroid will provide symptomatic relief if conservative therapy fails or the pain is limiting activities of daily living.
- Surgery may be required for persistent pain or progressive functional disability.

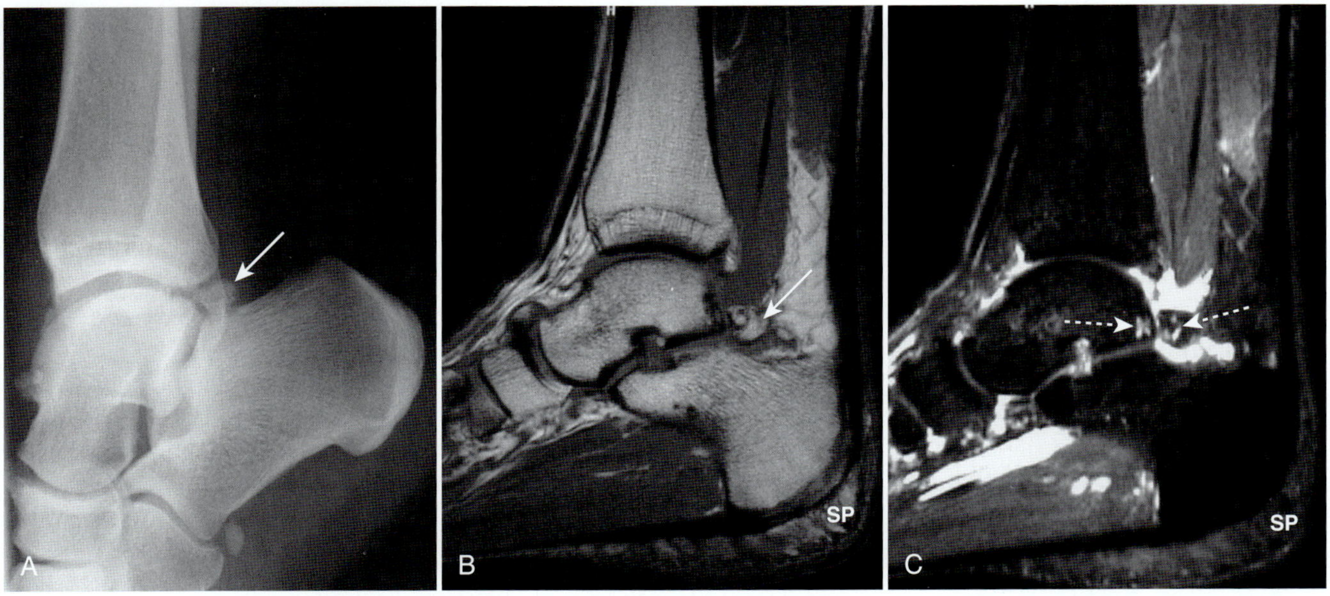

Figure 175.1 (A), Lateral radiograph of the ankle in a patient with posterior impingement. The os trigonum (*white arrow*) is compressed between the posterior tibia and calcaneus. (B), The corresponding sag ttal T1W MR image shows the fatty marrow within the os trigonum (*white arrow*). (C), On the FST2W MR image, there is high-SI fluid around the os trigonum, with reactive high-SI marrow edema in the ossicle and posterior talus (*broken white arrows*).

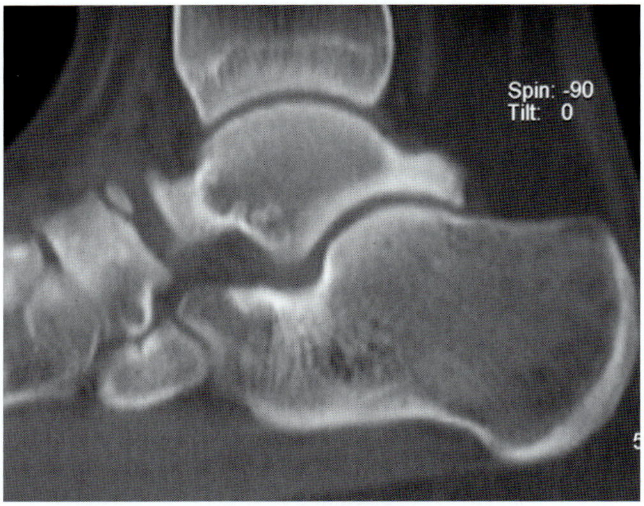

Figure 175.2 Sagittal CT scan of a patient with symptoms of posterior impingement, demonstrating a prominent posterior Stieda process of the talus.

CHAPTER 176

Navicular Secundum Syndrome

DEFINITION

- Failure of normal fusion of one or more of the ossification centers of the navicular bone of the ankle, resulting in separate ossicles attached by a synchondrosis to the main body of the navicular bone.

SIGNS AND SYMPTOMS

- Gradual onset of medial ankle pain.
- Swelling of the medial ankle.
- Common presenting complaint is shoe irritation.
- Exacerbation of pain with range of motion involving the navicular bone of the ankle.
- Exacerbation of pain with weight bearing.
- Clicking or catching sensation may be present.

DEMOGRAPHICS

- Incidence: Female > Male.
- Most common in children and adolescents.
- Commonly associated with trauma and overuse syndromes.
- Commonly associated with ballet dancing.

IMAGING RECOMMENDATIONS

- Radiography.
- MRI or US.
- For assessment of associated soft tissue changes.

IMAGING FINDINGS

- Radiography:
  - Smooth rounded ossicle adjacent to the medial aspect of the navicular.
- MRI or US:
  - Ossicle lies within the fibers of the tibial posterior tendon.
  - Marrow edema in the ossicle and navicular on MRI.
  - Tendinopathy of the distal tibialis tendon in symptomatic cases:
    Tendon thickening.
    High signal intensity (SI) on MRI.
    Low-echo change and neovascularity on US.

OTHER RECOMMENDED TESTING

- Laboratory testing to rule out inflammatory arthritis if diagnosis in question.
- Joint aspiration to rule out crystal arthropathies if diagnosis in question.
- Joint aspiration to rule out infection if diagnosis in question.

DIFFERENTIAL DIAGNOSIS

- Pathology of the posterior tibial tendon.
- Internal derangement of the ankle and forefoot.
- Osteonecrosis of the navicular.
- Occult fracture.
- Osteomyelitis.
- Post-traumatic arthritides.
- Inflammatory arthritides, especially rheumatoid arthritis.
- Kohler disease.

TREATMENT

- Conservative treatment consisting of local heat, cold, simple analgesics, and nonsteroidal anti-inflammatory agents will improve symptoms in many cases.
- Physical therapy, including gentle stretching, range-of-motion exercises, and deep heat modalities, may be beneficial in selected patients.
- Shoe modifications may help.
- Intra-articular injection with local anesthetic and steroid will provide symptomatic relief if conservative therapy fails or the pain is limiting activities of daily living.
- Surgery may be required for persistent pain or progressive functional disability.

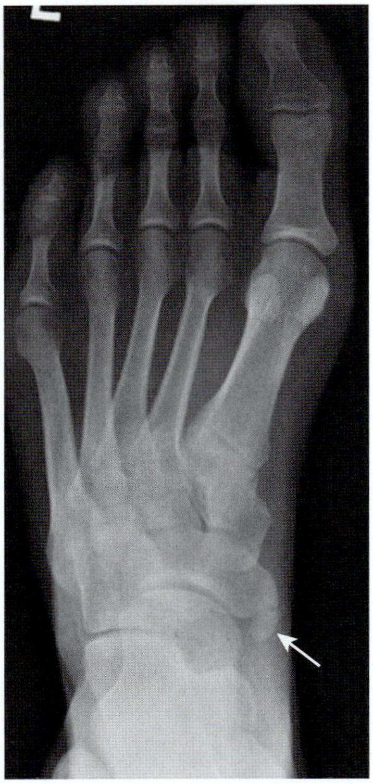

Figure 176.1 AP radiograph demonstrating a smooth rounded and well-defined secondary os naviculare (*arrow*) medial to the navicular.

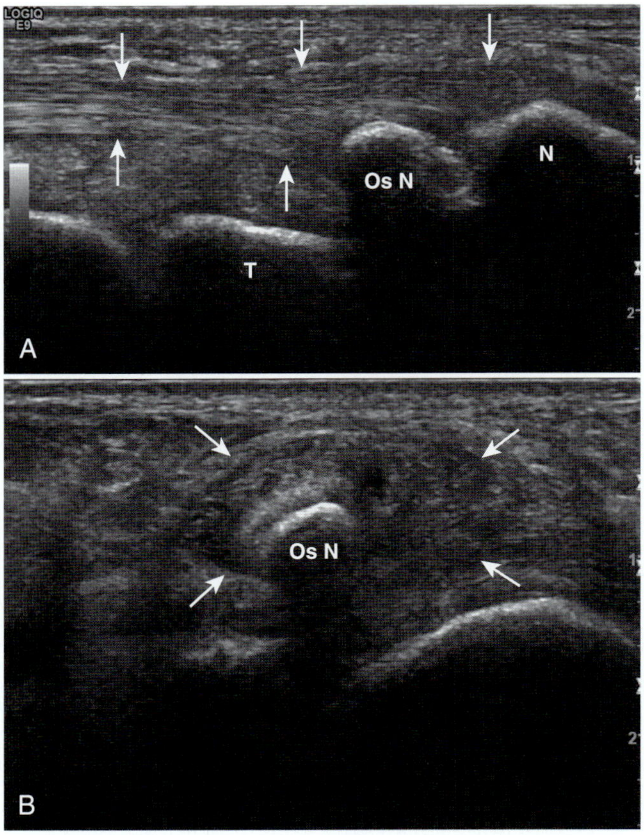

Figure 176.2 Longitudinal (A) and transverse (B) US images of an os naviculare. The ossicle lies within the fibers of the posterior tibial tendon (*arrows*), which demonstrates a normal appearance and echo pattern, widening as it inserts on the navicular. This was an incidental finding. N, navicular; Os N, os naviculare; T, talus.

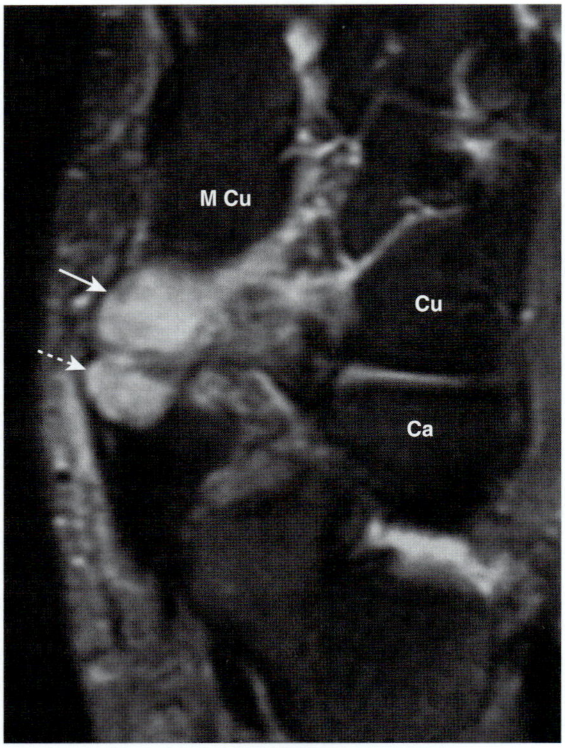

Figure 176.3 Coronal T2-weighted with fat suppression (FST2W) MR image of a patient with medial foot pain. There is prominent marrow edema in the navicular (*solid arrow*) and the accessory os naviculare (*broken arrow*), indicating a symptomatic ossicle. Ca, calcaneum; Cu, cuboid; M Cu, medial cuneiform.

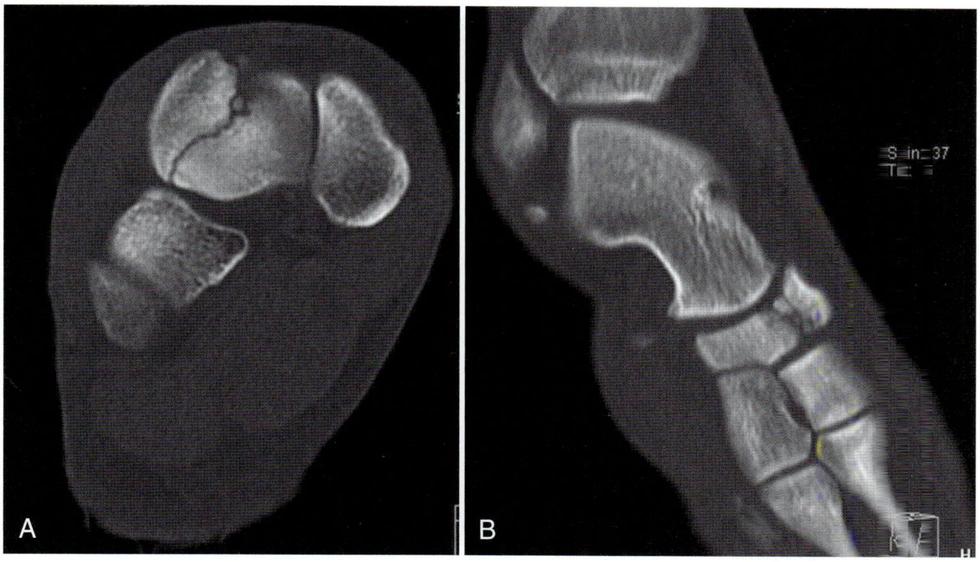

Figure 176.4 Coronal (**A**) and axial (**B**) CT scans demonstrating a stress fracture of the navicular. A sharply demarcated linear lucent line runs through the body of the navicular, which has some fragmentation. This appearance is quite different from that of an accessory ossicle.

CHAPTER 177

Sesamoiditis

DEFINITION

- Inflammation of the sesamoid bones of the flexor tendons of the feet and the surrounding structures, most commonly involving the first metatarsal head.

SIGNS AND SYMPTOMS

- Acute or gradual onset of metatarsal head pain.
- Patient frequently complains of the sensation of walking on a stone.
- Point tenderness over the affected sesamoid bone.
- Exacerbation of pain with standing.
- Exacerbation of pain with walking.
- Antalgic gait.
- Exacerbation of pain with weight bearing on affected foot.

DEMOGRAPHICS

- Incidence: Female = Male.
- Most common in second and third decades of life.
- Commonly associated with trauma and overuse syndromes.
- Commonly associated with jogging and long distance running.

IMAGING RECOMMENDATIONS

- Radiography:
  - Profile views of sesamoids may be helpful to assess articulation.
- MRI.

IMAGING FINDINGS

- Sesamoids may be bipartite or tripartite:
  - Often asymptomatic finding.
  - Obvious bony fragmentation is typical of sesamoiditis.
- High-signal intensity (SI) marrow edema on T2-weighted with fat suppression (FST2W) or short T1 inversion recovery (STIR) MR images within sesamoids.
- Effusion in first metatarsophalangeal joint.
- Superficial soft tissue edema.
- Minor enhancing reactive synovitis on post-contrast (obtained after administration of a contrast agent) FST1W MR images.

OTHER RECOMMENDED TESTING

- Laboratory testing to rule out inflammatory arthritis if diagnosis in question.
- Joint aspiration to rule out crystal arthropathies if diagnosis in question.
- Joint aspiration to rule out infection if diagnosis in question.

DIFFERENTIAL DIAGNOSIS

- Pathology of flexor tendons of the foot.
- Sesamoid fractures.
- Internal derangement of the ankle and forefoot.
- Freiberg disease.
- Occult fracture.
- March fracture.
- Osteomyelitis.
- Post-traumatic arthritides.
- Inflammatory arthritides, especially rheumatoid arthritis.
- Charcot arthropathy.
- Morton neuroma.

TREATMENT

- Conservative treatment consisting of local heat, cold, simple analgesics, and nonsteroidal anti-inflammatory agents will improve symptoms in many cases.
- Physical therapy, including gentle stretching, range-of-motion exercises, and deep heat modalities, may be beneficial in selected patients.
- Shoe modifications may help.
- Local injection with local anesthetic and steroid will provide symptomatic relief if conservative therapy fails or the pain is limiting activities of daily living.
- Surgery may be required for persistent pain or progressive functional disability.

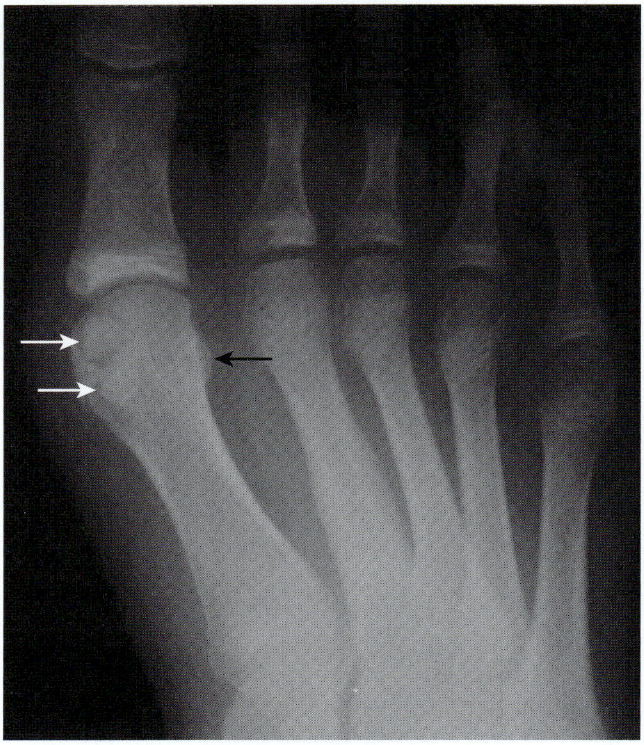

Figure 177.1 Radiograph of a patient with an asymptomatic bipartite medial sesamoid (*white arrows*) and a normal lateral sesamoid (*black arrow*).

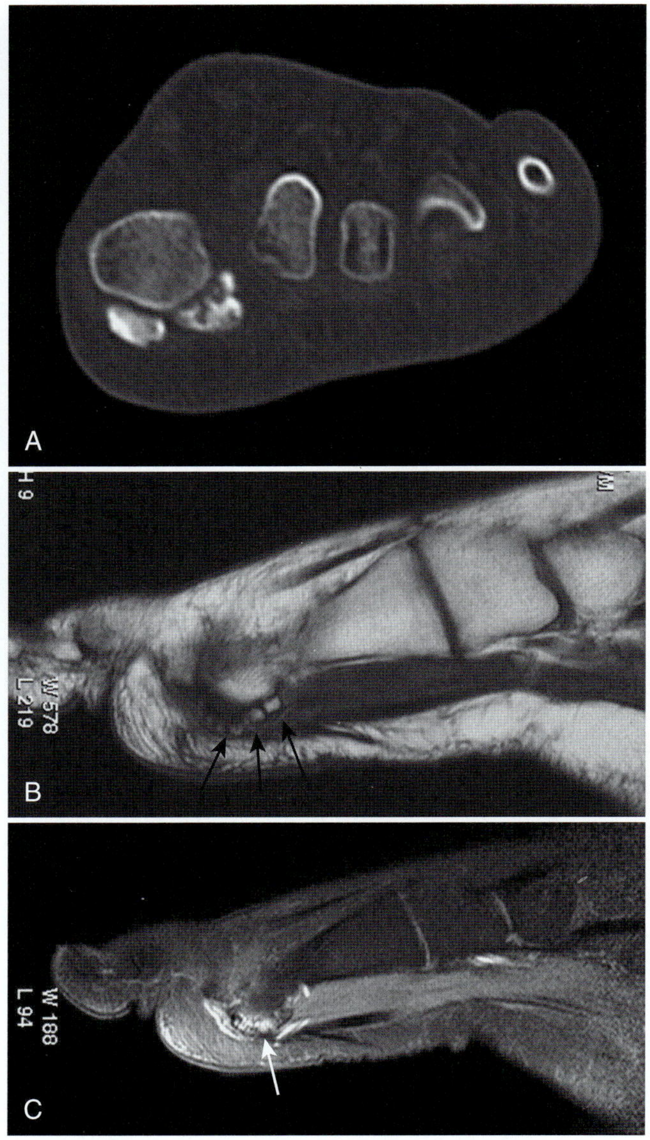

Figure 177.2 (A), Coronal CT scan of a patient with sesamoiditis, demonstrating fragmentation and sclerosis of the lateral sesamoid. (B), The sagittal T1W MR image also demonstrates the bony fragmentation *(black arrows)*. (C), High-SI reactive edema is present on the corresponding FST2W MR image (*white arrow*).

CHAPTER 178

Plantar Fasciitis

DEFINITION

- Inflammation of the plantar aponeurosis at the os calcis attachment and adjacent fascia.

SIGNS AND SYMPTOMS

- Gradual onset of medial calcaneal pain.
- Patient frequently complains of the sensation of walking on a stone.
- Point tenderness over the heel.
- Exacerbation of pain with dorsiflexion of the toes.
- Exacerbation of pain with walking.
- Antalgic gait.
- Exacerbation of pain with weight bearing on the affected heel.
- Pain worse in morning.
- Pain improves during the day.

DEMOGRAPHICS

- Incidence: Female > Male.
- Most common in fourth decade of life.
- Associated with seronegative spondyloarthropathies.
- Commonly associated with trauma and overuse syndromes involving twisting injuries to the foot.
- Commonly associated with jogging and long distance running.

IMAGING RECOMMENDATIONS

- Imaging not routinely indicated.
- Radiography:
  - Demonstrate plantar spurs.
  - To exclude insufficiency fractures of the os calcis.
- MRI or US.
  - US also useful to guide injections.

IMAGING FINDINGS

- Bony enthesophytes/spurs on calcaneal origin of fascia:
  - But do not correlate with symptoms.
- Thickening of the proximal medial head of the plantar fascia.
- Increased signal intensity (SI) in the fascia on T2-weighted with fat suppression (FST2W) or short T1 inversion recovery (STIR) MR images with surrounding soft tissue edema.
- Low reflectivity of fascia on US.
- Associated bony erosion and marrow edema suggest possible enthesopathy related to seronegative spondylarthropathy.
- Fasciitis occasionally manifests as diffuse thickening of the entire plantar fascia.
- Focal areas of thickening of the mid–plantar fascia are more likely to be due to plantar fibromas.

OTHER RECOMMENDED TESTING

- Laboratory testing to rule out inflammatory arthritis if diagnosis in question.
- HLA-B27 antigen testing.
- Joint aspiration to rule out crystal arthropathies if diagnosis in question.
- Joint aspiration to rule out infection if diagnosis in question.

DIFFERENTIAL DIAGNOSIS

- Pathology of the flexor tendons of the foot.
- Sesamoid fractures.
- Posterior tarsal tunnel syndrome.
- Entrapment of the first branch of the plantar nerve.
- Internal derangement of the ankle and hindfoot.
- Plantar fibromatosis.
- Sarcoidosis.
- Occult fracture of the calcaneus.
- March fracture.
- Osteomyelitis.
- Post-traumatic arthritides.
- Inflammatory arthritides, especially rheumatoid arthritis.
- Charcot arthropathy.

TREATMENT

- Conservative treatment consisting of local heat, cold, simple analgesics, and nonsteroidal anti-inflammatory agents will improve symptoms in many cases.

- Physical therapy, including gentle stretching, range-of-motion exercises, and deep heat modalities, may be beneficial in selected patients.
- Shoe modification including a heel cup may help.
- Local injection with local anesthetic and steroid will provide symptomatic relief if conservative therapy fails or the pain is limiting activities of daily living.
- Surgery may be required for persistent pain or progressive functional disability.

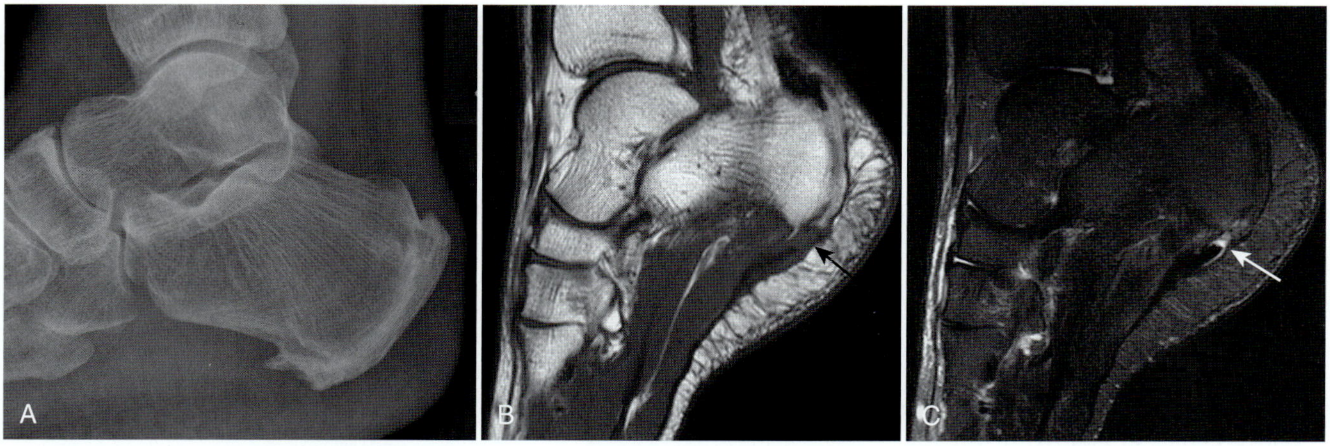

Figure 178.1 (A), Lateral radiograph of a plantar spur on the calcaneus. (B), The sagittal T1W MR image demonstrates thickening and increased SI within the plantar fascia origin (*black arrow*). There is high-SI fatty marrow within the bony spur. (C), High-SI fluid (*white arrow*) is seen within the plantar fascia origin on the sagittal FST2W MR image. The appearances are consistent with plantar fasciitis and partial tearing of the origin of the fascia.

CHAPTER 179

Morton Neuroma

DEFINITION

- Neuromatous enlargement of the interdigital nerve, most commonly occurring between the third and fourth metatarsal heads.

SIGNS AND SYMPTOMS

- Gradual onset of pain in the area between the metatarsal heads.
- Pain may be dull, burning, or neuritic.
- Patient frequently complains of the sensation of walking on a stone.
- Point tenderness over the neuroma.
- Exacerbation of pain with standing.
- Exacerbation of pain with walking.
- Antalgic gait.
- Exacerbation of pain with wearing shoes.
- Presence of Mulder sign.

DEMOGRAPHICS

- Incidence: Female > Male.
- Most common in fourth and fifth decades of life.
- Commonly associated with wearing high-heeled shoes.
- Common associated with shoes with toe boxes that are too tight.
- Commonly associated with jogging and long distance running.

IMAGING RECOMMENDATIONS

- Radiography not routinely indicated.
  - May be useful to exclude osteoarthritis of the MTP (metatarsophalangeal) joints.
- MRI or US.
  - US useful to guide therapeutic injections.

IMAGING FINDINGS

- Focal nodule of soft tissue in an inter-metatarsal web space.
  - Usually affects the second-third or third-fourth space.
- Intermediate signal intensity (SI) on T1-weighted (T1W), T2W, and T2W with fat suppression (FST2W) MR images.
  - High SI on FS T2W MR images suggests bursitis.
- Hyporeflective nodule on US:
  - Compressible areas suggests bursitis:
    Lesion compression can be demonstrated with use of increased probe pressure (sonopalpation).
  - Tissue may prolapse on lateral compression (US equivalent of Mulder click).

OTHER RECOMMENDED TESTING

- Laboratory testing to rule out inflammatory arthritis if diagnosis in question.
- Joint aspiration to rule out crystal arthropathies if diagnosis in question.
- Joint aspiration to rule out infection if diagnosis in question.

DIFFERENTIAL DIAGNOSIS

- Pathology of the flexor tendons of the foot.
- Sesamoid fractures.
- Sesamoiditis.
- Internal derangement of the ankle and forefoot.
- Freiberg disease.
- Occult fracture.
- March fracture.
- Osteomyelitis.
- Post-traumatic arthritides.
- Inflammatory arthritides, especially rheumatoid arthritis.
- Charcot arthropathy.
- Metatarsalgia.

TREATMENT

- Conservative treatment consisting of local heat, cold, simple analgesics, and nonsteroidal anti-inflammatory agents will improve symptoms in many cases.
- Physical therapy, including gentle stretching, range-of-motion exercises, and deep heat modalities, may be beneficial in selected patients.
- Shoe modifications may help.
- Patient should avoid wearing high-heeled shoes.
- Local injection with local anesthetic and steroid will provide symptomatic relief if conservative therapy fails or the pain is limiting activities of daily living.
- Surgery may be required for persistent pain or progressive functional disability.

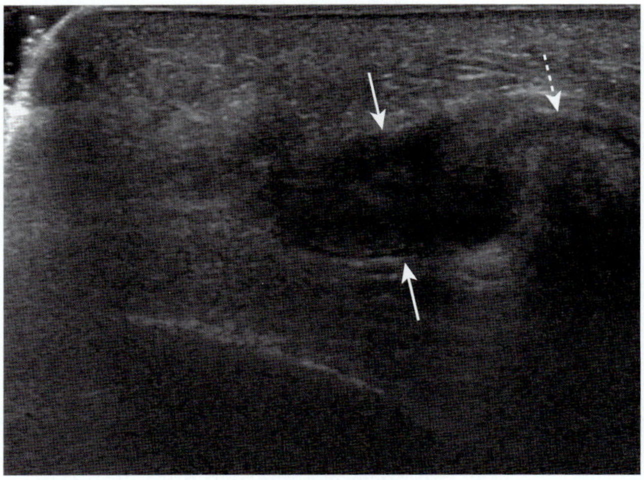

Figure 179.1 Longitudinal US image of an ovoid hyporeflective mass in the inter-metatarsal space (*white arrows*) arising from the digital nerve (*broken white arrow*), which is typical of Morton neuroma.

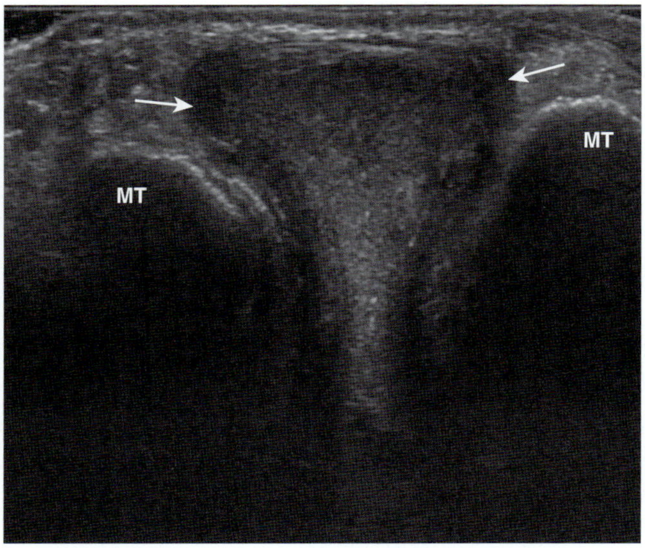

Figure 179.3 Transverse US image of an echogenic inter-metatarsal bursa (*white arrows*) arising between the metatarsal necks (MT). The mass was easily compressible with sonopalpation.

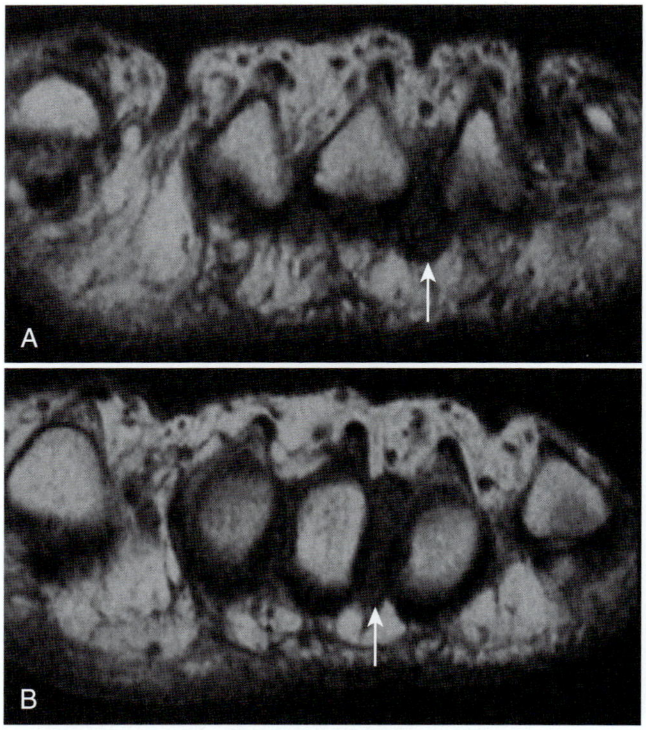

Figure 179.2 (**A** and **B**), Consecutive coronal T1W MR images of a low-SI Morton neuroma (*white arrows*) arising between the third and fourth metatarsal heads.

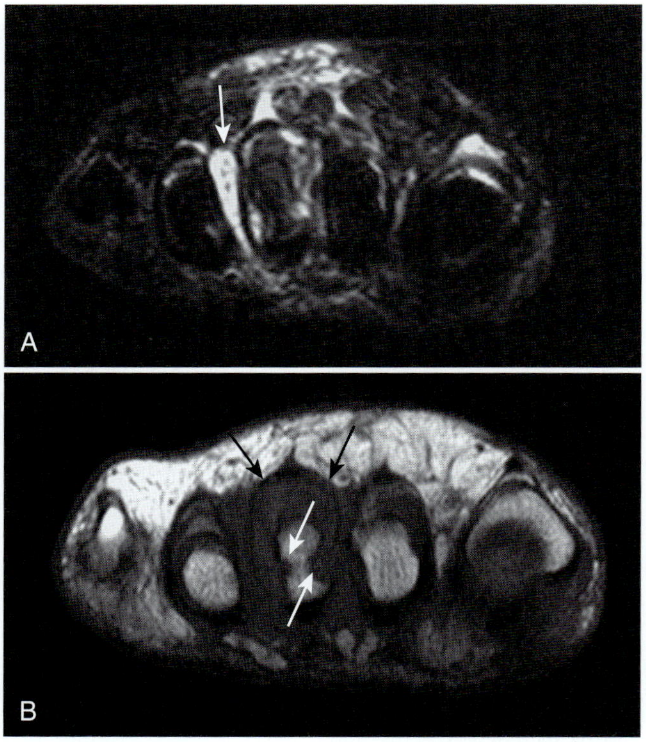

Figure 179.4 (**A**), Coronal T2W MR image of a patient with rheumatoid arthritis demonstrating an inflammatory bursa in the intermetatarsal space (*white arrow*). There is associated synovitis in the third MTP joint. (**B**), The corresponding T1W MR image shows the synovial thickening (*black arrows*), and the associated bony erosions (*white arrows*).

INDEX

Note: Page numbers followed by *f* indicate figures.

B

C

D

E

F

G

H

I

J

O